Best Wishes

Kerlin L. Bird

Disorders of Hemostasis and Thrombosis

Principles of Clinical Practice

Disorders of Hemostasis and Thrombosis

Principles of Clinical Practice

Rodger L. Bick, M.D., F.A.C.P.
Medical Director, San Joaquin Hematology
 Oncology Medical Group
Chief of Medicine and Hematology/Oncology
San Joaquin Community Hospital
Bakersfield, California

Clinical Faculty, Division of Hematology/
 Oncology
Department of Medicine
UCLA Center for the Health Sciences
Los Angeles, California

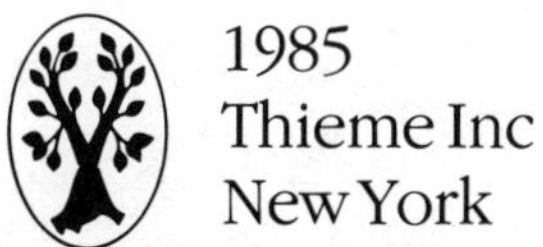
1985
Thieme Inc
New York

Georg Thieme Verlag
Stuttgart • New York

Thieme Inc.
381 Park Avenue South
New York, New York 10016

Library of Congress Cataloging-in-Publication Data

Bick, Rodger L.
  Disorders of hemostasis and thrombosis.

  Includes bibliographies and index.
  1. Blood—Coagulation, Disorders of.
2. Hemostasis. 3. Thrombosis. I. Title.
[DNLM: 1. Blood Coagulation Disorders.
2. Hemostasis. 3. Thrombosis. WH 322 B583da]
RC647.C55B53 1985   616.1'57   85-12567
ISBN 0-86577-196-0

cover design by Patrice Giusto

Printed in the United States of America

DISORDERS OF HEMOSTASIS AND THROMBOSIS:
Principles of Clinical Practice
Rodger L. Bick, M.D.

TI ISBN 0-86577-196-0
GTV ISBN 3-13-680301-9

5 4 3 2 1

Dedicated to

Marcy and Shauna

Without their patience, understanding, and love,
this book could not have been written

Acknowledgments

The author wishes to sincerely thank Ms. Julie De Armon, his administrative assistant. Ms. De Armon typed the entire manuscript, checked all spelling, all tables, figures, and references, and without her tremendous help, persistance, and dedication this work would not have been possible. The author also wishes to thank Ms. Sally Ott and Ms. Linda Garner for library searches. In addition, the impeccable editing provided by Mr. Peter Klamkin of Thieme Inc. is gratefully acknowledged; special thanks is due to Mr. Klamkin for bringing this book to fruition.

Rodger L. Bick, M.D., F.A.C.P.

Contents

Preface

Disorders of hemostasis and thrombosis span all medical specialities, and most clinicians are familiar with the catastrophic consequences of these disorders. Most physicians are frequently faced with the awesome responsibility of diagnosing and treating these thrombotic and hemorrhagic disorders, and the importance of a quick diagnosis and specific efficacious therapy is recognized by all, since these disorders can lead to very rapid irreversible consequences with respect to morbidity and mortality of patients.

In this book I have attempted a logical review of basic mechanisms of hemostasis and thrombosis. Each disease category or chapter, when appropriate, is intended to flow logically with respect to the etiology, pathophysiology, clinical and laboratory diagnosis, and management. With this approach, it is hoped that the clinician or laboratorian can quickly use this book as a reference source with respect to diagnosis and management. In addition, an attempt at completeness with respect to each disease topic is intended to allow the nonhematology specialist to pinpoint key areas of interest as they pertain to a particular speciality.

This book deals with a systematic and practical approach to the diagnosis and therapy of disorders of hemostasis and thrombosis. It is hoped that it will be useful in all areas of clinical and laboratory medicine and to all varieties of medical specialities. I hope all who read it find it useful and enhance the ability of all to ultimately render the utmost in patient care.

I thank my many ASCP workshop students for encouraging the development of a textbook of this nature.

Rodger L. Bick, M.D., F.A.C.P.
Bakersfield, California

1
Basic Physiology of Hemostasis and Thrombosis

Many individuals are hesitant to learn basic physiology of hemostasis and thrombosis; however, it cannot be overemphasized that the clinically related rewards will be highly significant if one is willing to master these basic concepts. An understanding and mastering of basic thrombohemorrhagic physiology is quite important for multiple reasons. Firstly, by such understanding, one can interpret new hemostasis and thrombosis testing modalities now available. Secondly, one can now appreciate and understand what is known of the pathophysiology of most disease processes in hemostasis and thrombosis as well as the intermediary mechanism that the hemostasis system plays in many seemingly unrelated disorders. Thirdly, and perhaps more importantly from the standpoint of clinicians, is that major and specific pharmacologic investigations and advances are now being made with respect to treating disorders of hemostasis and thrombosis. These specific pharmacologic agents and the concepts from which they are being developed come simply from understanding basic physiology of the hemostasis system.

Figure 1–1 depicts the so-called waterfall, or cascade, scheme of hemostasis. This outdated concept did serve a major historical purpose in terms of leading us into new mechanisms of hemostasis and thrombosis and was primarily developed through the concepts and early investigations of Davies and Ratnoff[24,65] However, as we understand hemostasis today, this cascade scheme is incomplete and fails to recognize the important role of inhibitors, the interactions between different blood protein systems, and the important and key interactions between the blood proteins and the platelet and the endothelial-vascular components of hemostasis.[9]

Figure 1–2 serves to exemplify the extremely significant point that there are three equally important and interrelated hemostatic compartments:[9] the platelets, which must be normal in both number and function, the blood proteins, which can no longer be simply thought of as the coagulation proteins but many other blood proteins as well (all of which will be discussed in this chapter), and the vasculature, which probably remains the "last frontier" and most poorly understood with respect to disorders of hemostasis and thrombosis. Normal physiology as well as pathophysiology of the vasculature and its components have only recently been elucidated. Because these three hemostatic compartments are intricately interrelated, disturbances of these interrelationships or defects within any compartment may lead to serious clinical consequences.

Figure 1–3 represents a more realistic, although highly complicated, view of the hemostasis system and is included to exemplify the numerous interrelationships that occur among the platelets, the blood proteins, and the vasculature, and the important roles of the contact activation, the inhibitor, and the fibrinolytic enzyme systems.[9,112]

Vasculature

Normal vascular morphology is comprised of *three* discrete layers; the intima, media, and adventitia.[23,44,63] The intima is comprised of a monolayer of nonthrombogenic endothelial cells and an internal elastic membrane. The media is comprised of smooth muscle cells; the size of the media will vary, depending on the type

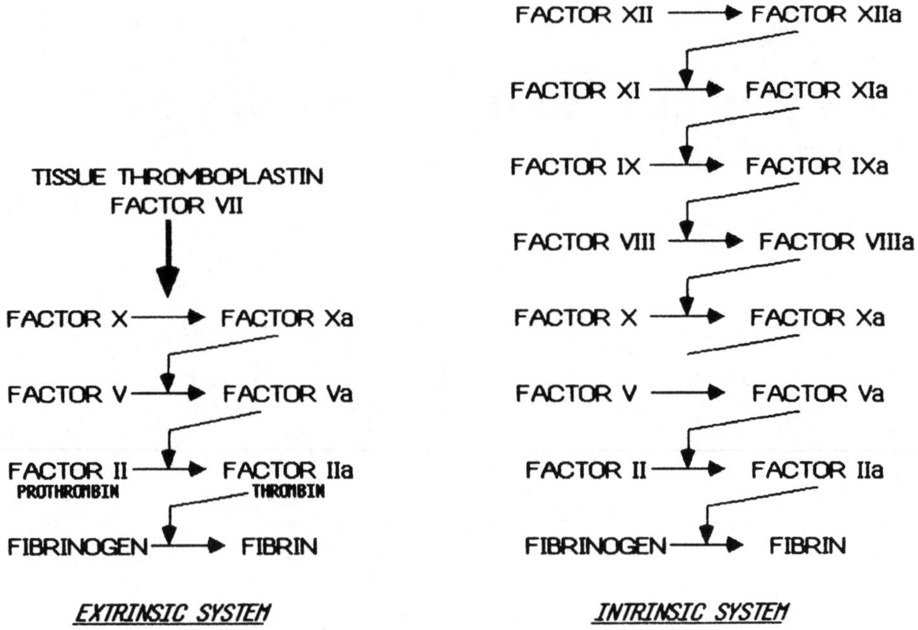

Fig. 1–1. Cascade, or waterfall, scheme of coagulation.

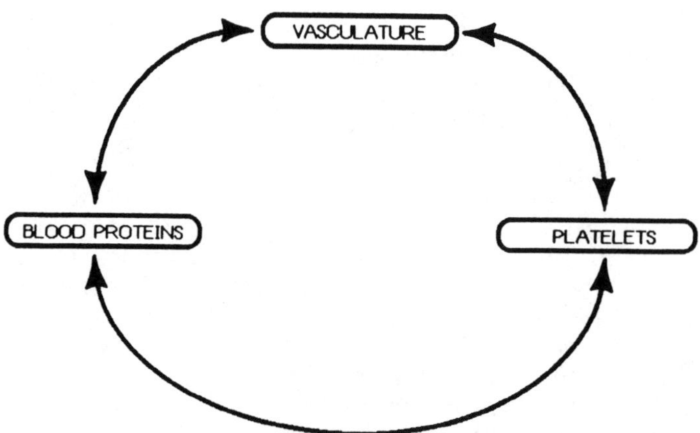

Fig. 1–2. Three hemostatic compartments.

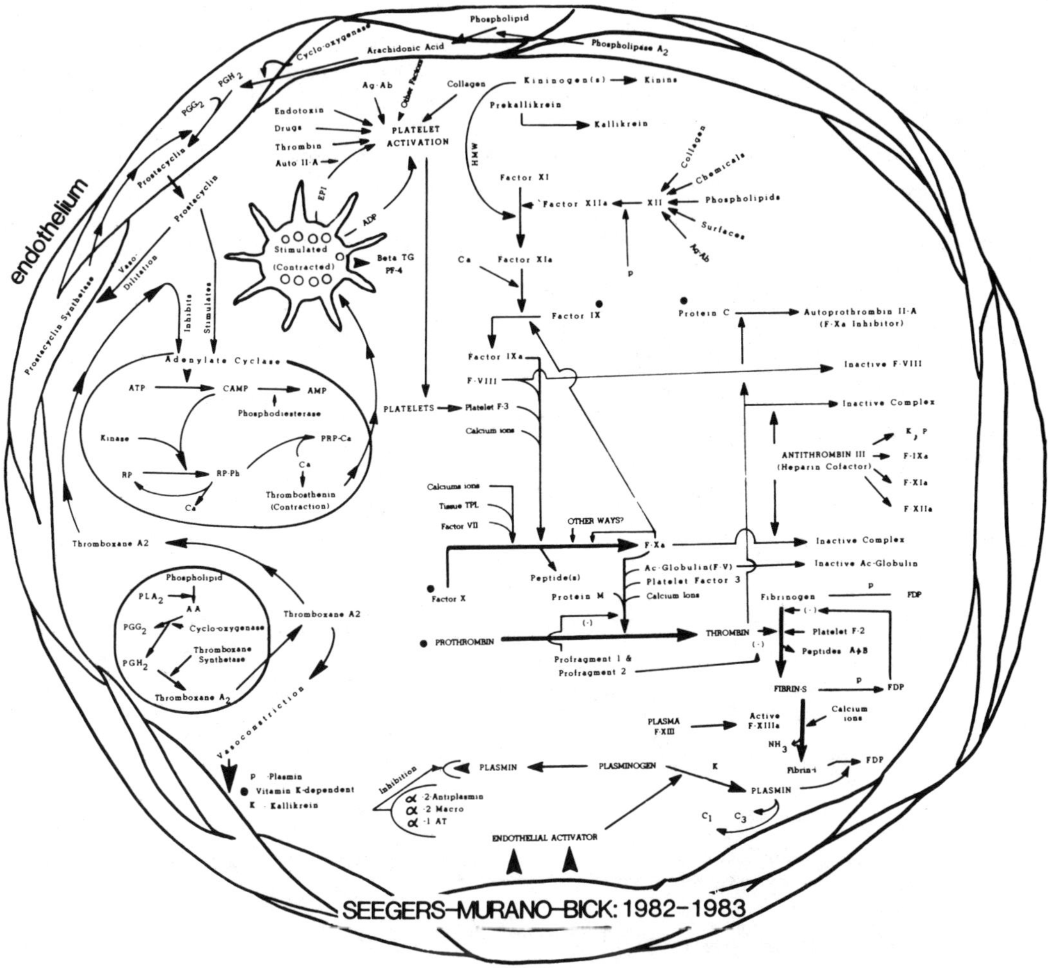

Fig. 1–3. A comprehensive scheme of hemostasis.

(arterial or venous) and size of the vasculature. The adventitia is comprised of an external elastic lamina or membrane and supportive connective tissue.

Figure 1–4 depicts an important pathophysiologic event that commonly occurs in the vasculature, that is, endothelial sloughing.[7,136] Endothelial sloughing may be induced by a wide variety of pathophysiologic events, including acidosis, hypoxia, endotoxin, circulating antigen-antibody complex, and many other insults.[10,81,107]

The first event occurring after endothelial sloughing, with the subsequent exposure of subendothelial collagen and base-ment membrane, is the recruitment of platelets to fill this endothelial gap[89,124] (Fig. 1–5). Both subendothelial collagen and basement membrane recruit platelets and a primary hemostatic plug is formed that stops blood from leaving the vascular compartment. As the primary hemostatic plug is formed, and if a normal reparative process is to occur, the subsequent reparative events are thought to be as follows: smooth muscle or other cells from the media will dedifferentiate, migrate through the internal elastic membrane, and then redifferentiate into new nonthrombogenic endothelial cells. If this is a one time event, then a normal reparative

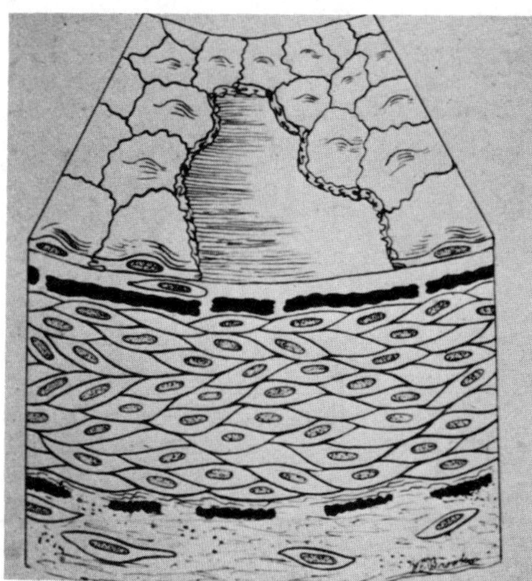

Fig. 1–4. Endothelial sloughing in the vasculature.

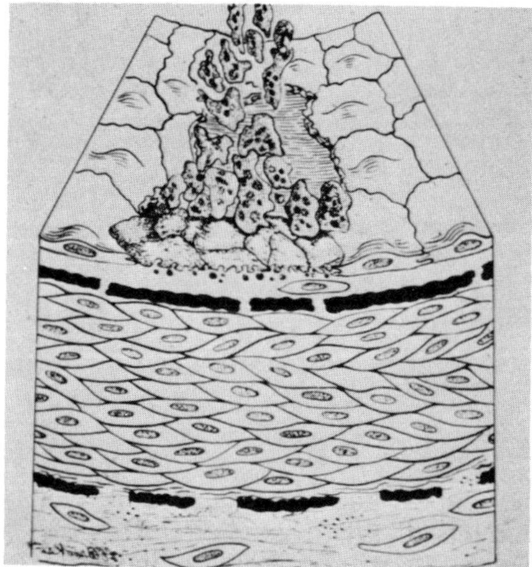

Fig. 1–5. Plate filling of endothelial gap.

process is completed. However, it should be noted that forming the primary hemostatic plug may be an overwhelming event leading to a large platelet and fibrin thrombus, impedence of blood flow, and resultant end organ damage from ischemia. Another event that may occur when endothelial sloughing and damage occurs is the formation of an atherosclero-

tic plaque[34,35,100] (Fig. 1–6). If endothelial sloughing and endothelial damage occur in the same area over a protracted period on numerous occasions, then as smooth muscle or other cells dedifferentiate and migrate into the intima of the vessel, compounds are released that are thought to call forth macrophages that then ingest cholesterol and other materials, eventually resulting in an atherosclerotic plaque. If normal pathophysiologic events and an appropriate reparative process occurs, endothelial sloughing will be followed by platelets filling the endothelial gaps and the formation of an appropriate primary hemostatic plug, the dedifferentiation of muscle cells, redifferentiation into a new nonthrombogenic monolayer of endothelial cells and a normal vascular lining.[72] All of these potential events are summarized in Figure 1–7.

Vascular function is comprised of vascular permeability, vascular integrity, and vasoconstriction (Table 1–1). If vascular permeability is disrupted or increased, blood will leave the vessel, which will be seen clinically as petechiae and purpura or, in some instances, large ecchymoses. If increased vascular fragility occurs, there can be rupture of the vasculature with sub-

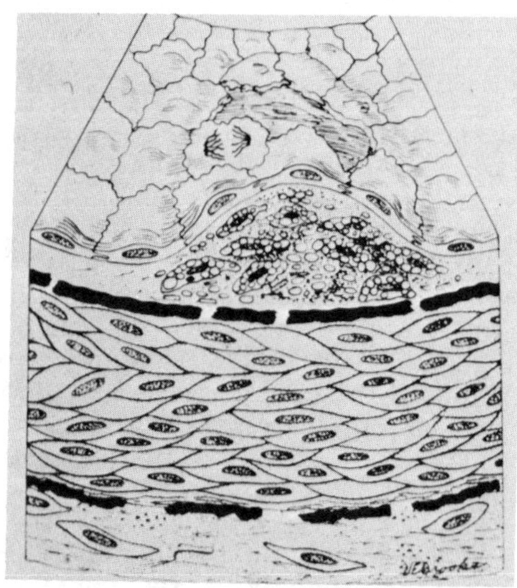

Fig. 1–6. Atherosclerotic plaque formation.

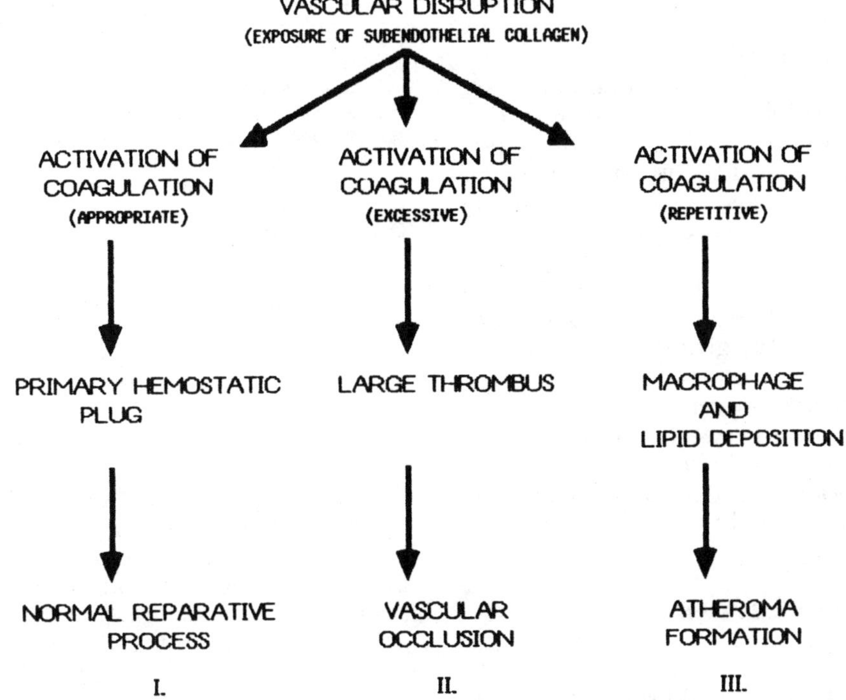

Fig. 1–7. Vascular damage (endothelial sloughing) followed by three alternative events.

Table 1–1 Vascular Function

Permeability	→ Leakage
Fragility	→ Rupture
Construction	→ Occlusion

Neural control (sympathetic system)
Local control (temperature, pH, partial carbon dioxide pressure)
Humoral control (Epinephrine, Norepinephrine, ADP, kinins, FDP)

sequent petechiae and purpura, especially in the integument and mucous membranes, large ecchymoses and potential serious deep-tissue hemorrhage. Another important function of the vasculature is that of vasoconstriction, but if this is inappropriately intense, there may be occlusion of the vessel via thrombus formation. Vasoconstriction is under local, neural, and humeral control, the most important of which is humeral. It will be noted in Table 1–1 that those compounds that mediate humeral control of vasoconstric-

tion are primarily released from platelets, including epinephrine, norepinephrine, adenosine diphosphate, (ADP), kinins, and thromboxanes.[33,47,129] Fibrin(ogen) degradation products (FDPs) liberated when the fibrinolytic system acts on a fibrin clot will also modulate vasoconstriction.

Properties of the endothelium are summarized in Table 1–2. Endothelial cells are contractile when stimulated by histamine, serotonin, kinins, or thromboxanes. In addition, the endothelial cell is the major site of high molecular weight Factor VIII biosynthesis (von Willebrand factor or ristocetin cofactor).[28,128] Low molecular weight Factor VIII or Factor VIII coagulant (Factor VIII:C) is synthesized by the hepatocyte and probably at other cellular sites. The endothelial cell also provides one of the two key activation pathways of the fibrinolytic system through the synthesis and release of plasminogen activator activity,[3,62,92] as is protein C activator activity and inhibitor activity.[66] The role of endothelial cell prostaglandin synthesis will be discussed in subsequent appropriate sections.

Properties of the subendothelium are also listed in Table 1–2. Platelet attraction and subsequent activation occurs when basement membrane or collagen is exposed. It should also be noted that subendothelial collagen is capable of the direct activation of Factor XII to Factor XIIa as well as Factor XI to Factor XIa.[134,141] Of course, any of these activation processes could conceivably give rise to a disseminated intravascular coagulation (DIC)-type syndrome or generalized activation of the hemostasis system when a significant amount of endothelial sloughing and a large amount of subendothelial collagen or basement membrane is exposed.

Platelet Function

Platelet function will be discussed, followed by the platelet endothelial interaction. The normal platelet morphologic divisions are somewhat artificial although they serve a discrete purpose (Table 1–3). In general, the platelet can be thought of as being comprised of a peripheral zone, a so-called sol-gel zone, and an organelle zone.[48] The peripheral zone is comprised of an extramembranous glycocalyx inside of which is a plasma membrane that is similar to any other trilamellar cellular plasma membrane, and just under the

plasma membrane of the platelet is an open canalicular system. The sol-gel zone is comprised of microtubules and microfilaments, a dense tubular system that primarily contains adenine nucleotides and calcium and in addition is found the all-important contractile protein, thrombosthenin. Thrombosthenin is similar if not identical to actomyosin. The organelle zone is comprised of dense bodies, alpha granules, mitochondria, and other organelles found in other cellular systems, including lysozymes and endoplasmic reticulum. Alpha granules contain and release fibrinogen and lysozomal enzymes, and dense bodies contain and release adenine nucleotides, serotonin, catecholamines, and platelet factor 4.[31,126,137,138]

Figure 1–8 depicts a transmission electron micrograph of a platelet demonstrating many of these constituents and organelles. The open canalicular system, dense bodies, mitochondria, and lysozymes are apparent.

Table 1–4 summarizes factors that are necessary for normal platelet function. The reader is well acquainted with many or all of these. Firstly, an adequate number of platelets must be present for normal platelet function in vivo and in vitro; this is usually defined as approximately 100,000/mm.^{3} In vitro test results of platelet function with a platelet count of less than 100,000/mm^3 will usually be abnormal. For example, prolonged template bleeding times and abnormal platelet aggregation will usually be noted if the

Table 1–3 Platelet Morphology

Peripheral zone
  Glycocalyx
  Platelet membrane
  Open canalicular system
Sol-gel zone
  Microtubules and microfilaments
  Dense tubular system
  Thrombosthenin
Organelle zone
  Dense granules
  Mitochondria
  Alpha Granules

Table 1–2 Properties of the Endothelium and Subendothelium

Endothelium
  Contraction by histamine, kinins, serotonin and
    thromboxanes
  Synthesis of plasminogen activator activity
  Synthesis of Factor VIII:vW
  Synthesis of protein C inhibitor
Subendothelium
  Platelet activation and attraction
  Factor XII activation
  Factor XI activation

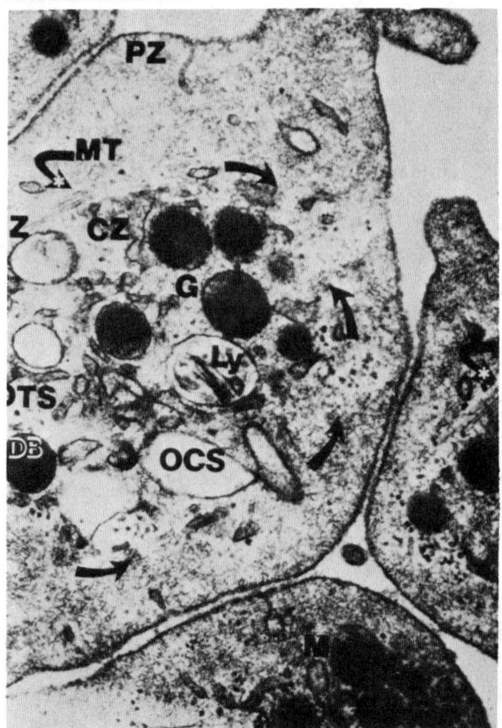

Fig. 1–8. Platelet Morphology DB: dense bodies; MT: mitochondria; Ly: lysozymes; OCS: open canalicular system.

function. Platelet membrane receptors must be present and must be responsive to appropriate stimuli. Platelets require adequate divalent cations, the most important of which is calcium, for normal function and, of course, adequate physical conditions, such as pH and temperature.

Table 1–5 summarizes the common platelet proteins, some of which are not platelet specific, including numerous plasma proteins that are found in or on platelets. Many of the coagulation proteins are found in or on platelets, including Factor XIII or fibrin-stabilizing factor, Factors II, V, VII, VIII, IX, X, XI, and XII.[87,113] In some instances these factors are found in a slightly different form in platelets as opposed to plasma, for example, fibrin-stabilizing factor, but in many instances these are found in the same form in both. Platelet-specific proteins are also present.

Thus far, platelet factors 1 through 7 have been recognized (Table 1–6). The most important of these are platelet factor 3 (or platelet membrane phospholipoprotein, so-called platelet thromboplastin) and platelet factor 4 (antiheparin factor), which has become an important molecular marker of hemostatic activity and platelet reactivity in particular.[26,67,90,127]

Table 1–4 Factors Necessary for Normal Platelet Function

Adequate number of platelets ($>$100,000/mm^3)
Adequate energy metabolism
Adequate number and contents of storage granules
Adequate storage granule release
Adequate cationic proteins
Adequate membrane receptors and responsiveness
Adequate divalent cations (Mg++ and Ca++)
Adequate physical conditions (pH, temperature)

Table 1–5 Platelet Proteins

Nonspecific (plasma) proteins	
Fibrinogen	Albumin
Factors II, V, VII, VIII,	Plasminogen
IX, X, XII, and XIII	Complement components
Specific proteins	
Thrombosthenin	Platelet antiplasmin
Platelet glycoprotein	Cathepsin A
Platelet factors 2 and 4	

platelet count is less than 100,000/mm.^{3} Platelets present must have adequate energy metabolism, and there has to be an adequate number of storage granules present for normal platelet function. Additionally, storage granules must be able to release their contents adequately when appropriate stimuli are present. Adequate cationic proteins, such as thrombosthenin, must also be present for normal platelet

Table 1–6 Platelet Factors

Platelet factor 1: Coagulation Factor V
Platelet factor 2: Thromboplastic material
Platelet factor 3: Platelet thromboplastin (phospholipoprotein)
Platelet factor 4: Antiheparin factor
Platelet factor 5: Fibrinogen coagulant factor
Platelet factor 6: Antifibrinolytic factor
Platelet factor 7: Platelet cothromboplastin

The significance with respect to normal platelet physiology and function of the other platelet factors is as yet unclear.

Table 1–7 summarizes compounds released from platelets. These include the biogenic amines, including serotonin, catecholamines, and histamine; the all-important adenine nucleotides, adenosine monophosphate (AMP), ADP, and adenosine triphosphate (ATP): various enzyme activities, including acid hydrolases; specific ions, including calcium, magnesium, and potassium; and platelet factors, including 3 and 4 and beta-thromboglobulin. Platelet factor 3 is not actually released, but most likely represents a confirmational change in the platelet membrane making available an activity that is referred to as platelet factor 3. In addition, other proteins, including fibrinogen, other clotting factors, albumin, and other compounds are released from platelets during a release reaction.

Many materials will induce a platelet release reaction.[16,18,73,142] These include subendothelial collagen and basement membrane, as previously mentioned. Very potent inducers of a platelet release reaction are thrombin, soluble fibrin monomer, which has been solubilized by complexing with split products, FDPs, especially fragment X, endotoxin: circulating antigen-antibody complex, gamma/globulin coated surfaces: various viruses, ADP, catecholamines,[25,30,80,94] and free fatty acids. Numerous proteolytic enzymes, including trypsin, snake venoms, papain, and elastase are used in vitro to study platelet release; other in vitro release reaction techniques include the use of centrifugation, cold fracture, latex particles, carbon particles, kaolin, and Celite.

Figure 1–9 is a scanning electron micrograph of a moderately activated platelet. As platelets become activated, they begin to contract and form pseudopods. During the process of contraction, the numerous intraplatelet compounds and granules are concentrated at the center of the platelet. Figure 1–10 reveals markedly activated platelets; as activation progresses, platelets become contracted with pronounced pseudopod formation. It is thought that during this event the platelet organelles, including alpha granules and dense bodies, are concentrated at the center of the platelet where organelle membranes disrupt, their contents are released and subsequently transported outside the platelet

Table 1–7 Compounds Released from Platelets

Biogenic Amines	
Serotonin	Histamine
Epinephrine	Norepinephrine
Adenine nucleotides	
ADP	cyclic AMP
ATP	
Cations	
K+	
CA++	
Platelet factors 3 and 4	
Platelet proteins	
Fibrinogen	Albumin
Platelet factor 4	

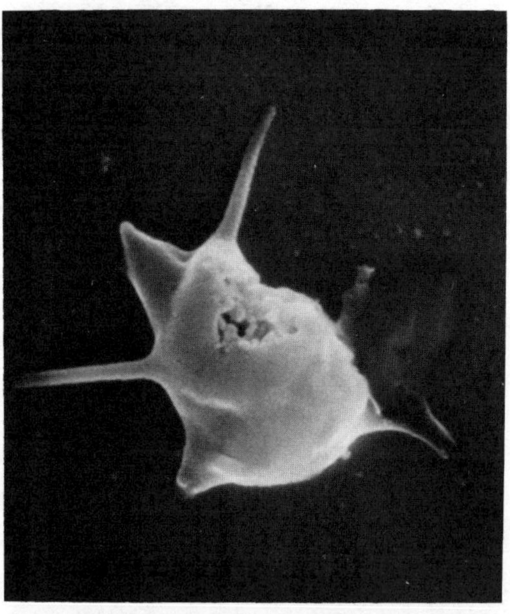

Fig. 1–9. Moderately activated platelet. (Courtesy of Dr. Marion Barnhart.)

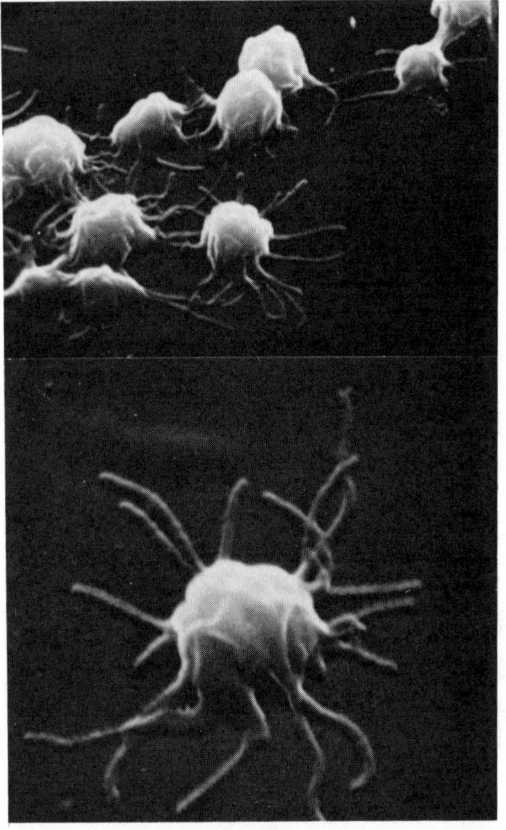

Fig. 1–10. Markedly activated platelets. (Courtesy of Dr. Marion Barnhart.)

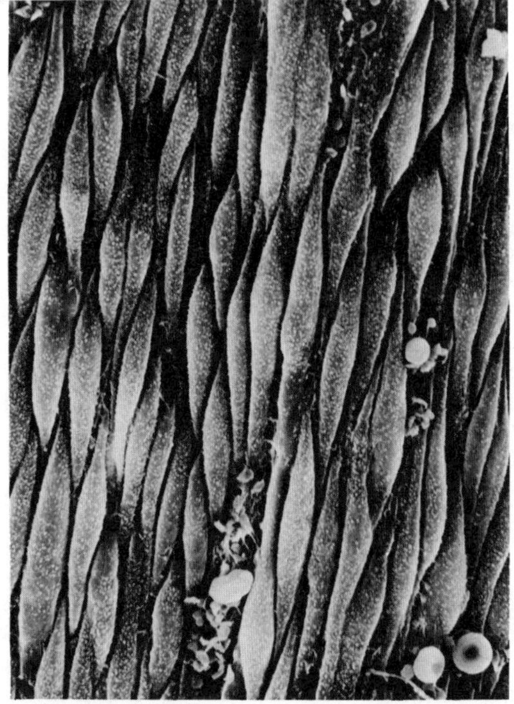

Fig. 1–11. Low-power scanning electron micrograph of hypoxic endothelium. (Courtesy of Dr. Marion Barnhart.)

via the open canalicular system. These compounds then interact with platelet membrane receptors of adjacent platelets, causing further platelet activation in a type of logarhythmic amplification process whereby numerous platelets become activated. In addition, many of these compounds may interact with adjacent endothelium. Pseudopod formation enhances platelet-surface interactions (adhesion) and platelet-platelet interaction (cohesion).

Figure 1–11 shows a low-power scanning electron micrograph of endothelium that has been made hypoxic. There are several areas where endothelial cells are missing. These have been sloughed off because of hypoxia. Figure 1–12 depicts a high-power scanning electron micrographic view of one of these areas, revealing that this endothelial cell gap has been filled by activated platelets (contracted and with marked pseudopod formation). A simplified view of platelet function is presented in Figure 1–13. The first process that occurs during platelet activation is that of platelet adhesion, a process that can occur, for example, with glass beads, other artificial surfaces, or collagen and/or basement membrane. After platelet adhesion, an initial release reaction occurs with the release of intraplatelet ADP. This is a reversible process and accounts for the primary wave on an aggregation pattern

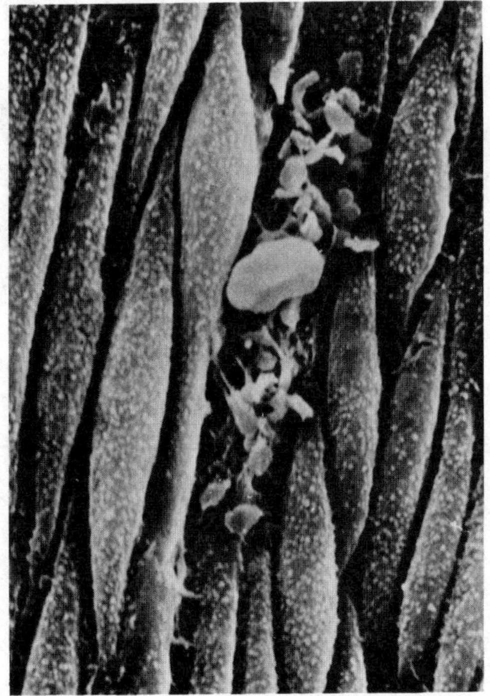

Fig. 1–12. High-power view of Figure 1–11. (Courtesy of Dr. Marion Barnhart.)

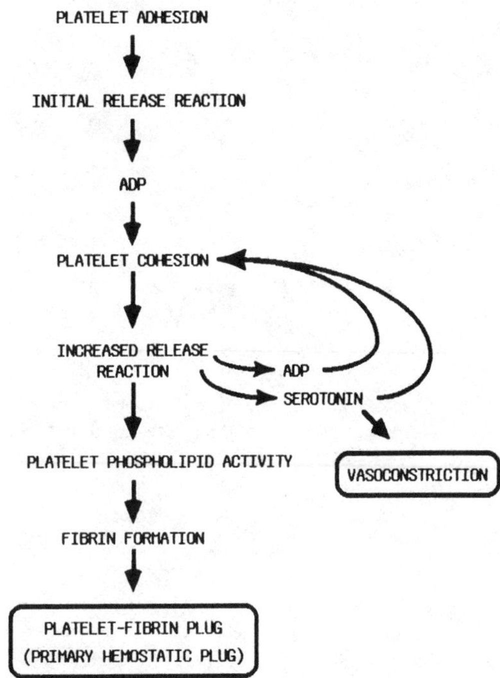

Fig. 1–13. Simplified concept of platelet function.

and is referred to as primary (reversible) aggregaton. As the concentration of ADP increases, a process of platelet cohesion occurs and more and more ADP and other compounds, including serotonin, are released. Serotonin and other platelet release compounds not only act on adjacent platelets, causing further activation, but also begin to induce vascular constriction to prepare for an effective primary hemostatic plug or primary platelet-fibrin plug. During the process of this increased release reaction in which more and more ADP is released, the ADP concentration reaches a critical point at which an irreversible confirmational change occurs in the platelet membrane, making available platelet factor 3 or platelet membrane phospholipid-type activity. This material then serves as a surface for coagulation protein activity with eventual fibrin formation. The process of platelet cohesion, increased release reaction, and the confir-

mational membrane change leading to the availability of platelet factor 3 is an irreversible process and accounts for the secondary wave seen on a platelet aggregation pattern and is referred to as secondary aggregation. The subsequent end result of all of this is the formation of a platelet-fibrin plug, or so-called primary hemostasis plug, again made more efficient by vasoconstriction primarily induced from compounds released from platelets.

Simplified intraplatelet biochemistry is summarized in Figure 1–14. The key modulator of intraplatelet function is cyclic AMP.[17,46,109] The role of platelet cyclic AMP is to combine with a cyclic AMP dependent protein to form a kinase. The role of this kinase is to convert a receptor protein to a phosphorylated receptor protein that then binds calcium. If intraplatelet calcium is bound and is not available to thrombosthenin, the platelet cannot function appropriately and becomes hypoaggregable and hypoadhesable. Alternatively, if there is a high concentration of free ionized calcium in the platelet, the platelet becomes hyperadhesable and hyperaggregable. In reviewing Figure 1–14 note that epinephrine, thrombin, collagen, and serotonin inhibit the enzyme adenylate cyclase. Adenylate cyclase is responsible for the conversion of ATP to cyclic AMP. Thus, if the concentration of adenylate cyclase decreases, cyclic AMP and kinin concentrations will decrease, phosphorylated receptor protein will decrease, causing ionized calcium concentration to increase, and the platelet will become hyperaggregable. The enzyme responsible for biodegrading cyclic AMP into an inactive form is phosphodiesterase.[21,51] One of the mechanisms of action of one popular antiplatelet agent, dipyridamole, is to inhibit phosphodiesterase. Caffeine and papaverine also inhibit this enzyme. When phosphodiesterase is inhibited, the concentrations of cyclic AMP and of kinase will increase, and therefore phosphorylated receptor protein concentration will increase, intraplatelet calcium will become bound, and the platelet will be rendered nonfunctional.

The role of prostaglandins and prostaglandin derivatives in platelet function is summarized in Figure 1–15. Many of these processes occur in most cellular membranes; however, this discussion will be limited to the platelet and endothelial cell membranes. Platelet and endothelial cell membrane phospholipids are converted into arachidonic acid by an enzyme, phospholipase A_2.[36,50,88] Phospholipase A_2 is activated by both thrombin and collagen. Arachidonic acid is converted into prostaglandin intermediates, prostaglandin G_2, and prostaglandin H_2

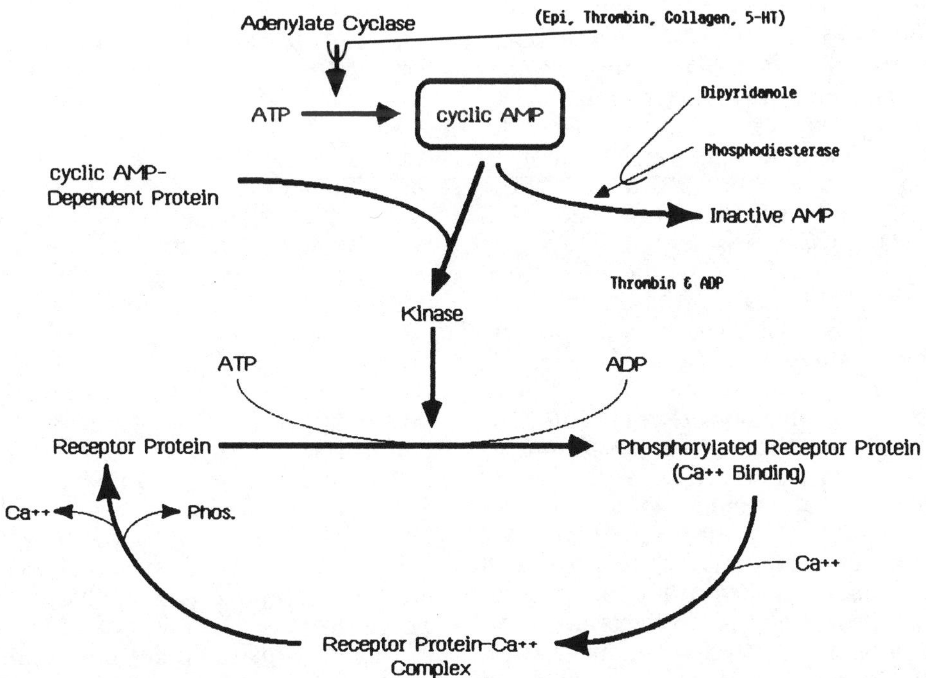

Fig. 1–14. Intraplatelet biochemistry.

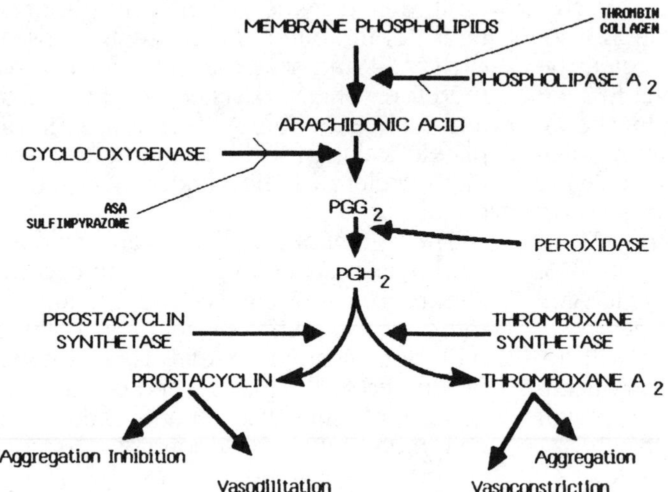

Fig. 1–15. Prostaglandins in platelet or endothelial function.

(PGH$_2$) by the enzyme cyclo-oxygenase. At this point, there is a biologically superb division of labor. In the platelet membrane, and only in the platelet membrane, is found a specific enzyme: thromboxane synthetase. Thromboxane synthetase converts PGH$_2$ into thromboxane A$_2$, one of the most potent aggregating agents yet described. Thromboxane A$_2$ also has very potent vasoconstricting activity. In the endothelial cell, as well as in some subendothelial muscle cells, is found a specific enzyme, prostacyclin synthetase, which converts PGH$_2$ into protascyclin. Prostacyclin has vasodilatory and platelet inhibitor effects that are diametrically opposed to thromboxane A$_2$.[27,42,75] Prostacyclin is being assessed in clinical trials for thromboembolic and vaso-occlusive events.[41,49] Thus, there is a division of labor whereby arachidonic acid and its prostaglandin derivatives are converted into thromboxane in the platelet and will induce vasoconstriction and platelet aggregation; the opposite effects are seen with prostacyclin. Cyclo-oxygenase is inhibited by aspirin and sulfinpyrizone, two popular antiplatelet agents.[20,55,130] Cur-

rent evidence suggests that the selectivity of these two antiplatelet agents is directed approximately 70% toward platelets and only 30% toward the endothelial cell with respect to prostacyclin synthesis. In addition, endothelium continues to synthesize prostaglandins, but platelets do not.

Figure 1–16 summarizes platelet function, including the role of prostaglandins. Attention should be directed to adenylate cyclase, the enzyme converting ATP to cyclic AMP, and again appreciate that cyclic AMP combines with a cyclic AMP-dependent protein to form a kinase. The role of this kinase is to phosphorylate a receptor protein that will then bind calcium. If calcium is bound, it is not available to thrombosthenin and thrombosthenin cannot contract appropriately. The role of prostaglandin derivaties, thromboxane A$_2$, and prostacyclin are depicted at the top of Figure 16. Thromboxane A$_2$ is a potent inhibitor of adenylate cyclase and prostacyclin is a potent stimulator of adenylate cyclase. Therefore the presence of bleeding or thrombosis may depend on the relative concentrations of these two compounds. For example, if there is an enhanced con-

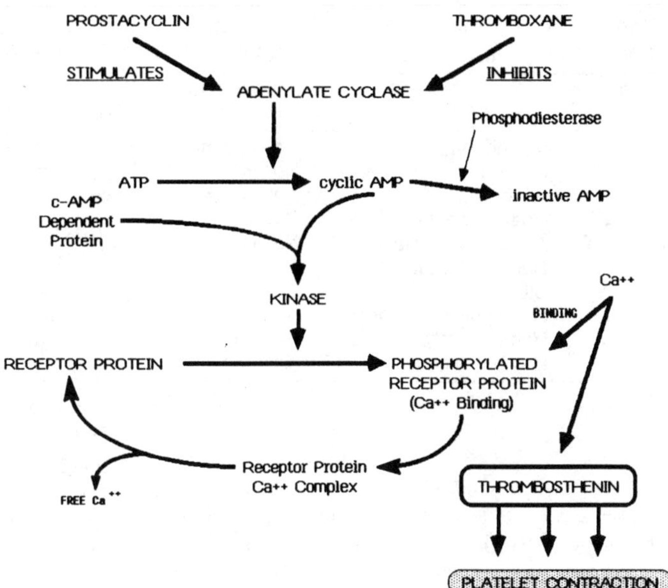

Fig. 1–16. Summary of platelet function.

centration of thromboxane A_2, adenylate cyclase is inhibited, the concentrations of cyclic AMP, kinase, and phosphorylated receptor protein decrease, and free ionized calcium concentration increases and becomes available to thrombosthenin. There is contraction (activation) of the platelet with subsequent release of platelet materials to react with and activate adjacent platelets. Alternatively, with a high concentration of prostacyclin being released from the adjacent endothelium, adenylate cyclase is stimulated, concentrations of cyclic AMP, kinase, and phosphorylated receptor protein increase, calcium becomes bound and is no longer available for thrombosthenin, preventing platelets from contracting or undergoing a release reaction. This represents an exquisite biologic system whereby platelets are synthesizing and releasing into the adjacent milieu a compound (thromboxane A_2) that is inducing platelet aggregation, and alternatively the adjacent endothelium is synthesizing and releasing prostacyclin that keeps platelets away from the endothelium and inhibits aggregation.

Blood Protein Function

Blood protein function in hemostasis comprises numerous systems, the five most important of which are the coagulation protein, the fibrino(geno)lytic, the kinin generating, the complement, and the inhibitors for the first four systems. Kinin and complement generation (activation) are often not appreciated as important in thrombohemorrhagic disorders; however, as shall be discussed subsequently, these systems assume extreme importance, especially in such disorders as DIC. Table 1–8 gives a classically taught concept that is now known to be incorrect and incomplete and our thinking regarding plasma versus serum factors must be modified. The factors present in plasma versus the factors present in serum depend on how they are measured. It is quite true that plasma versus serum factors depicted are correct if assays that depend on the biologic activity of a coagulation (or blood) protein are used. However, this concept is not correct if immunologic or

Table 1–8 Historical Concept of Plasma and Serum Factors (Biologic Function)

Plasma Factors		Serum Factors
I	Fibrinogen	Not present
II	Prothrombin	Not present
V	AC-globulin	Not present
VII	Cothromboplastin	Present
VIII:C	Antihemophilic factor	Not present
IX	Hemophilia B factor	Present
X	Stuart-Prower factor	Present
XI	Hemophilia C factor	Present
XII	Hageman factor	Present
XIII	Profibrinoligase	Not present

other assays that detect the presence or absence of a protein without regard for biologic function are used. The use of immunologic assays or those that detect the presence of a protein in conjunction with those that measure biologic activity are becoming extremely important, since it is now appreciated that almost all forms of hereditary coagulation protein deficiencies are possible in both the absent form or the "dysfunctional" form. Dysfibrinogenemias represent fibrinogens that do not function properly even though they are present; this is in distinction to afibrinogenemia, the absolute absence of fibrinogen. For example, Factor V or accelerator globulin is present in both plasma and serum if measured as a protein or immunologically. However, it is no longer biologically active in serum. The same is true for Factor VIII coagulation activity (Factor VIII:C); it is present in plasma and absent in serum if measured by biologic activity. However, if measured immunologically or by other assays to detect only the protein, independent of biologic activity, there are normal levels of Factor VIII:C activity in serum. Thus, what is found in plasma versus serum will depend on the type of assay used to measure that factor.

Coagulation Proteins

Most readers are familiar with the coagulation factor synonyms; although the Roman numeral system is most widely used and is preferred (Table 1–9). However, in some instances there have been no Roman numerals assigned to factors. Protein C has also been referred to as Factor XIV or autoprothrombin II-A, Fletcher factor is synonymous with prekallikrein, and Fitzgerald factor, also called William's factor, Flaujeac factor, Reid factor, or Fujiwara factor, is a high molecular weight kininogen.[22,43,83]

Coagulation, or the formation of a fibrin clot, is best thought of as consisting of three key reactions listed in Table 1–10. This concept is helpful in making the procoagulant system easily understandable. These three key reactions are of help in remembering the entire coagulation system and the order and interplay of its reactions.

The first key reaction, or the formation of Factor Xa, is exemplified in Figure 1–17. The formation of Factor Xa, like the formation of thrombin, consists of a five component system and requires a substrate, an enzyme, a determiner or cofactor, a surface, and calcium.[53,114] The sub-

Table 1–9 Coagulation Factors and Synonyms

Factor	Synonym
I	Fibrinogen
II	Prothrombin
V	Accelerator-globulin
VII	Prothrombin conversion accelerator
VIII:C	Antihemophilic factor
IX	Christmas factor
X	Stuart-Prower factor
XI	Thromboplastin antecedent
XII	Hageman (contact) factor
XIII	Profibrinoligase
Fletcher factor	Prekallikrein
Fitzgerald factor	High molecular weight kininogen
Protein C	Xa inhibitor

Table 1–10 Coagulation: Formation of a Fibrin Clot
The Three Key Reactions

1. Generation of Factor Xa
2. Generation of thrombin
3. Formation of fibrin

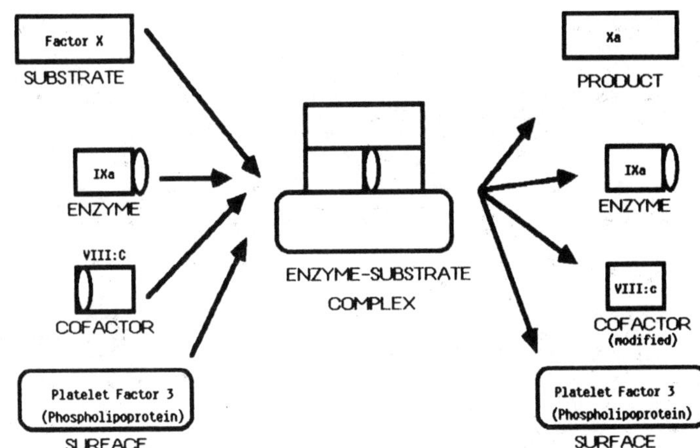

Fig. 1–17. Formation of factor Xa.

strate, enzyme, cofactor, and surface form an enzyme substrate complex that is bound by calcium. The enzyme Factor IXa cleaves a peptide from the substrate with resultant exposure of an active serine site on the substrate, now creating a new enzyme, or Factor Xa, the product of this reaction. There is salvage of the original enzyme (Factor IXa) but the cofactor or determiner has been slightly modified so that it will no longer work as a cofactor or determiner in this reaction. Also, platelet factor 3 or platelet membrane phospholipid surface is salvaged for further enzyme substrate complex formation. In the case of the formation of Factor Xa the substrate is, of course, Factor X, the enzyme is Factor IXa, the determiner or cofactor is Factor VIII:C, and the surface is platelet factor 3 or platelet membrane phospholipoprotein.

The second key reaction is the formation of thrombin. Before discussing the actual mechanism by which thrombin is formed, it is important to realize that thrombin comes from a vitamin K dependent precurser, prothrombin. Prothrombin and the other prothrombin complex factors, Factors II, VII, IX, and X can be synthesized in a normal form or a so-called plasma abnormal form.[29,93,125] The role of vitamin K in synthesizing these prot-

hrombin complex factors is to post-ribosomally attach a calcium-binding prosthetic site to each of the four proteins. In the absence of vitamin K, for example a patient on warfarin-type therapy, these calcium-binding sites are not attached and therefore a complete protein will be synthesized but will be missing calcium-binding sites. This situation is depicted on the left-hand side of Figure 1–18. Normal prothrombin complex factor synthesis is depicted on the right-hand side of the figure, with the calcium-binding prothetic groups being attached postribosomally by vitamin K. Thus, abnormal or normal plasma prothrombin complex factors can be synthesized, depending on the absence or presence of vitamin K. These abnormal prothrombin complex factors are referred to as proteins induced by vitamin K absence or antagonists (PIVKAs).

This all-important calcium-binding prosthetic group, attached to the prothrombin complex factors by vitamin K, is gamma-carboxyglutamic acid, depicted in Figure 1–19. Figure 1–20 summarizes enzyme substrate complex formation for the generation of thrombin. This, like the formation of Factor Xa, is also comprised of a five-component system that requires a substrate, an enzyme, a determiner or cofactor, platelet factor 3 or platelet mem-

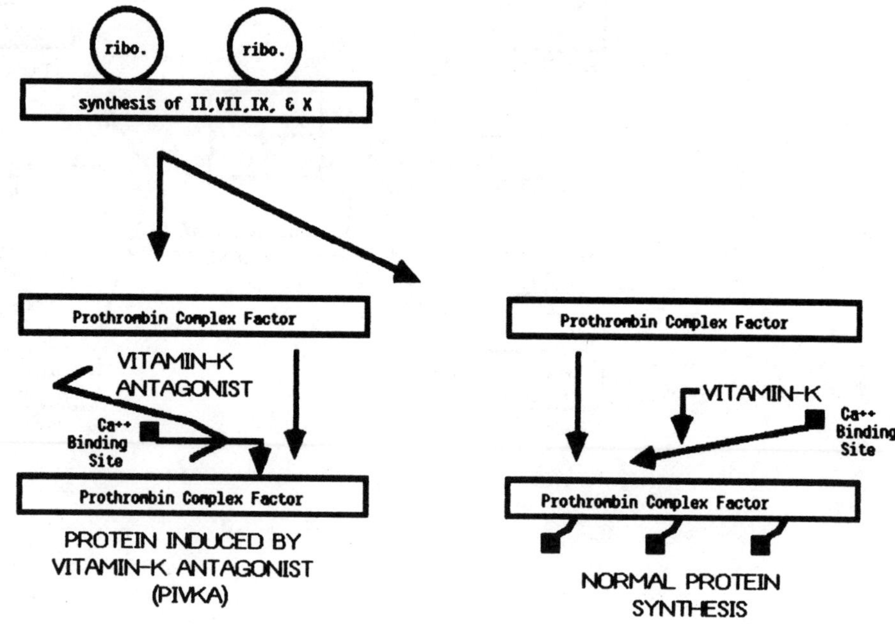

Fig. 1–18. Prothrombin complex factors and PIVKA synthesis.

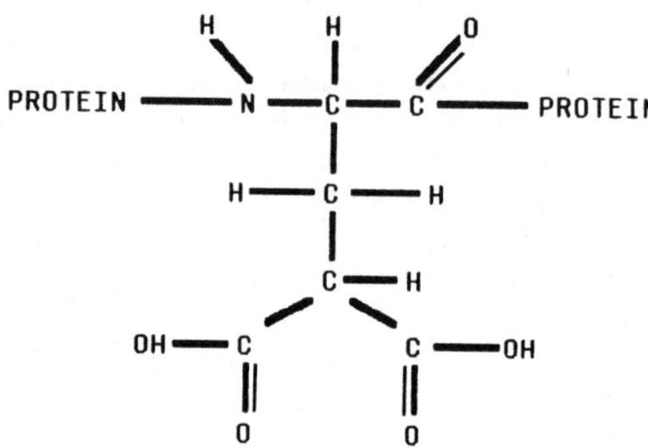

Fig. 1–19. Gamma-Carboxyglutamic acid (calcium-binding group).

brane phospholipoprotein that acts as a surface,[115–117] and calcium. These components form an enzyme substrate complex on the phospholipid or platelet factor 3 surface and a product—thrombin, the new enzyme—is generated. The enzyme used, Factor Xa, is salvaged and returned to the system; Factor V, as for Factor VIII in the previous reaction, is slightly modified and no longer has biologic activity with respect to this particular enzyme substrate complex formation. Again, there is return of platelet factor 3 or platelet membrane phospholipid surface. As depicted in Figures 18 and 19, the role of calcium in attaching these components into an enzyme substrate complex and the role of vitamin K in attaching these calcium-binding sites, gamma-carboxyglutamic acid is all-important. If these calcium-binding sites are missing from the substrate or enzyme, an enzyme substrate complex cannot be formed and the product cannot be generated; the "patient is thus anti-coagulated." To generate thrombin, the substrate is Factor II or prothrombin, the enzyme is Factor Xa (the enzyme made in the first key reaction), the determiner or cofactor is Factor V, and the surface is again platelet factor 3 or platelet membrane phospholipoprotein. The role of the determiner or cofactor is to ensure that the correct enzyme and substrate enter into complex formation. For example, the presence of Factor V enables the

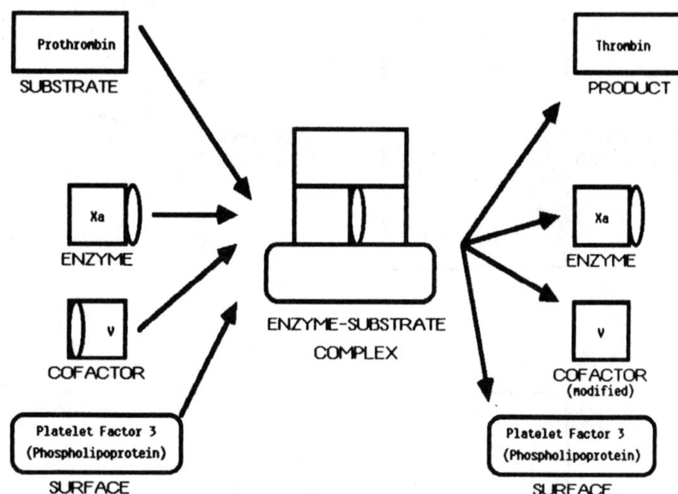

Fig. 1-20. The formation of thrombin.

enzyme Factor Xa to interact with the correct substrate, Factor II, and not with an inappropriate substrate, such as Factor X. Alternatively, in the first key reaction, the role of Factor VIII as a determiner or cofactor is to ensure that the appropriate enzyme, Factor IXa, reacts with the appropriate substrate, Factor X.

Figure 1-21 serves to summarize the first two key reactions, emphasizing that both are similar five-component systems. The first key reaction is the generation of Factor Xa, the enzyme necessary for the second key reaction. The second key reaction is the generation of thrombin, which is necessary for the third key reaction.

Figure 1-22 serves to exemplify the necessity of stoichiometry for these first two reactions. If the amounts of prothrombin (substrate), Factor V concentration, enzyme Factor Xa, or platelet factor 3 or platelet phospholipid available are decreased, then the amount of thrombin generated will also be decreased. Thus,

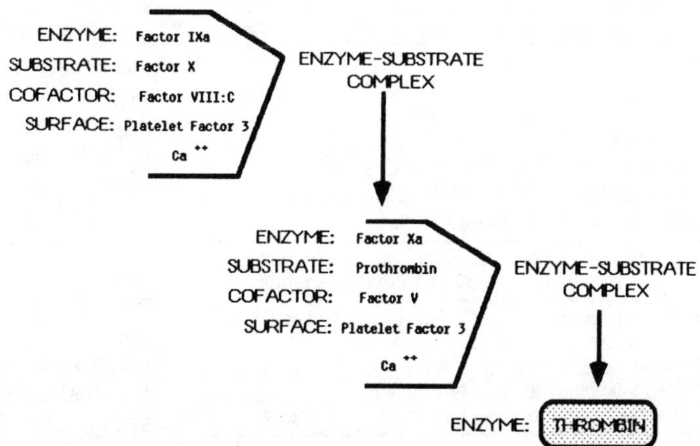

Fig. 1-21. Summary of the first two key reactions, the formation of factor Xa and thrombin.

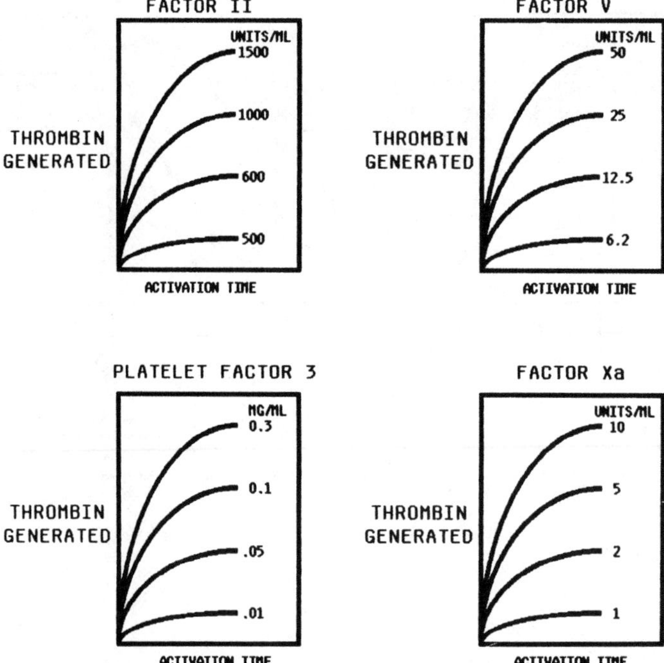

Fig. 1–22. Stoichiometry in coagulation reactions.

for these two first key reactions to occur, all five components must be present in relatively normal concentrations and must be appropriately functional.[118]

Platelet membrane phospholipid or platelet factor 3 has many individual constituents, four of which are selectively active in the first two key reactions; these four constituents and their activities are summarized in Table 1–11.[119] Phosphatidylserine and phosphatidylinositol are active in the second key reaction, or thrombin generation; however, these have no activity in Factor Xa formation.

Alternatively, phosphatidylcholine and phosphatidylethanolamine have no activity in thrombin formation, but are active in the formation of Factor Xa.

The third key reaction is the formation of fibrin. Figure 1–23 summarizes the conversion of fibrinogen to fibrin. The primary role of thrombin, generated in the second key reaction, is to remove two small peptides, fibrinopeptide A and fibrinopeptide B, from fibrinogen; the remaining molecule is referred to as fibrin monomer.[52,135] Fibrin monomer begins to aggregate end-to-end and side-to-side; these aggregates are held together by hypophobic bonds. These fibrin monomer aggregates form soluble fibrin that will dissolve in 5 M urea or 1% monochloroacetic acid, two reagents used in the laboratory to detect the presence or absence of Factor XIII. Both of these reagents will disrupt hydrophobic bonds. The formation of soluble fibrin monomer aggregates, held together only by hydrophobic bonds, is referred to as polymerization I. Another important role of thrombin is to activate Factor XIII, or profibrinolygase,

Table 1–11 Platelet Membrane Phospholipid (Platelet Factor 3) Selectivity in Hemostasis

Phospholipid Component	Factor Xa Generation	Thrombin Generation
Phosphatidylethanolamine	Active	Not active
Phosphatidylcholine	Active	Not active
Phosphatidylinositol	Not active	Active
Phosphatidylserine	Not active	Active

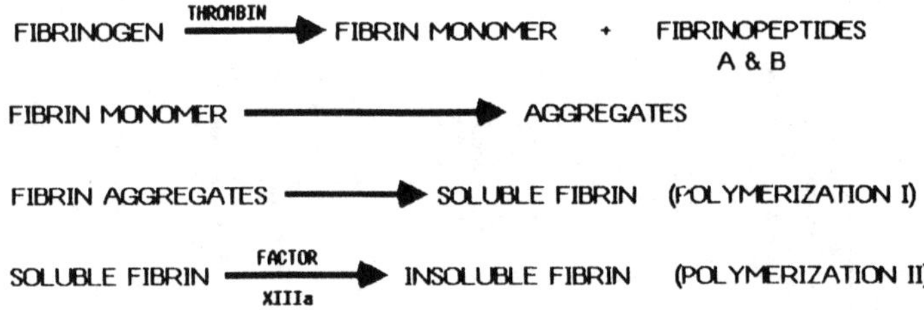

Fig. 1–23. The formation of fibrin.

to Factor XIIIa or fibrinoligase. Fibrinoligase then replaces previously formed hydrophobic bonds with solid peptide bonds; this gives rise to fibrin that will not dissolve in 5 M urea or 1% monochloracetic acid.[1,96] When insoluble fibrin is formed, this is referred to as polymerization II.

Figure 1–24 is a model of fibrinogen. It will be noted that fibrinogen is a dimer, each symmetrical side composed of three polypeptide chains, A-alpha, B-beta, and gamma.[120] The role of thrombin is to proteolytically remove fibrinopeptides A and B by cleaving at specific amino acid sites.

Fibrinopeptide A, consisting of 16 amino acids, is released very rapidly and fibrinopeptide B, consisting of 14 amino acids, is released more slowly. Fibrin monomer aggregation begins as soon as fibrinopeptide A is released, and the B peptide need not necessarily be released for fibrin monomer aggregation to occur. Figure 1–25 illustrates polymerization I, depicting the alpha and gamma chains being held together by hydrophobic bonds before Factor XIII or fibrinoligase,

has become active. Figure 1–26 illustrates polymerization II with Factor XIIIa having replaced hydrophobic bonds with peptide bonds. Assays are available for both fibrinopeptides, A and B, and the importance of their measurements will be discussed in appropriate subsequent chapters.

Contact Activation

The contact activation phase of coagulation begins with the activation of Hageman factor, or Factor XII. There are numerous potential mechanisms by which Factor XII can be activated, and several of these are depicted in Figure 1–27. Phospholipids, collagen, subendothelial collagen, and kallikrein (activated Fletcher factor) are capable of converting Factor XII to Factor XIIa.[56,57,74,97] Active Hageman factor, also a serine protease, then converts Factor XI to Factor XIa. This reaction occurs very quickly in the presence of Fitzgerald factor (high molecular weight kininogen); the reaction occurs very slowly without Fitzgerald factor, thus accounting for a significantly prolonged activated partial

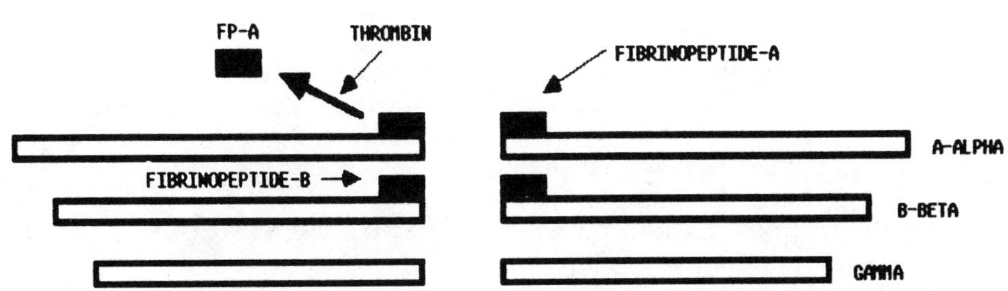

Fig. 1–24. The structure of fibrinogen.

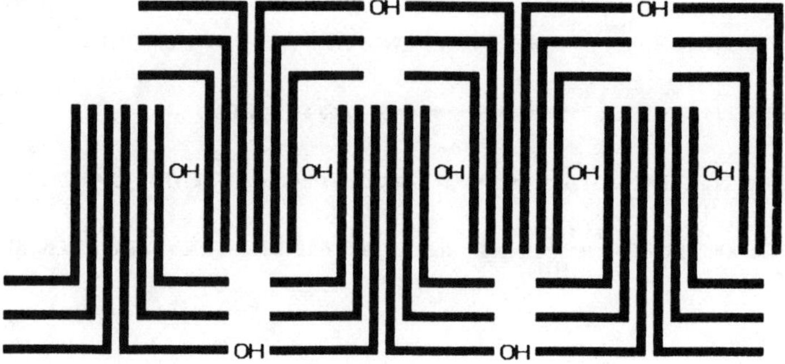

Fig. 1–25. Polymerization I, soluble fibrin.

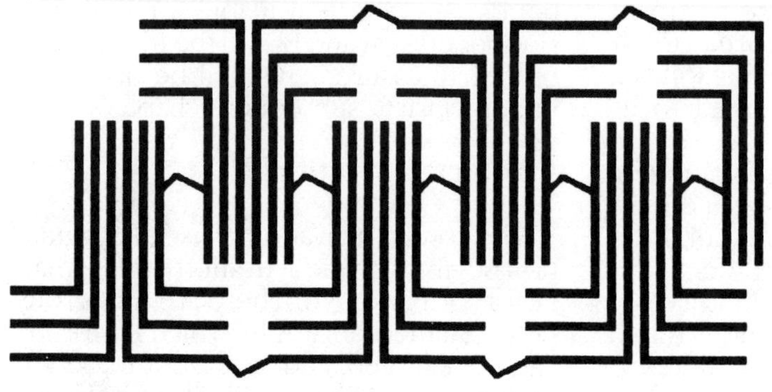

Fig. 1–26. Polymerization II: insoluble fibrin.

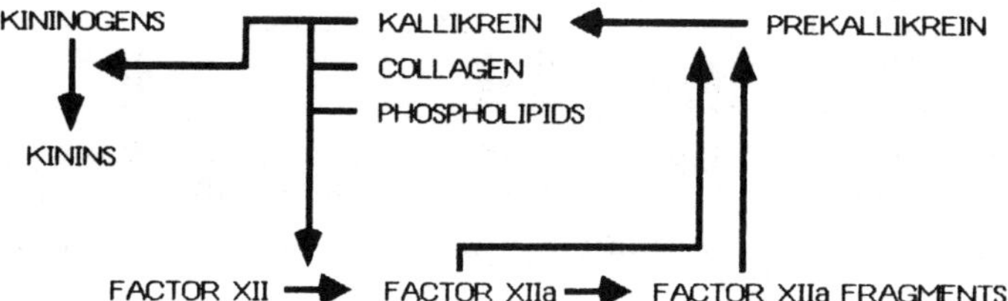

Fig. 1–27. Mechanisms of Factor XII activation.

thromboplastin time in the absence of Fitzgerald factor.[40,139] The role of Factor XIa, also a serine protease, is to convert Factor IX (in the presence of calcium) into Factor IXa. Factor IXa is the enzyme responsible for the first key reaction previously discussed, the generation of Factor Xa. It should also be noted (Fig. 1–23) that Factor XIIa itself is able to convert prekallikrein (Fletcher factor) into kallikrein, which is capable then of converting more Factor XII into Factor XIIa.

Fibrinolytic System

The second blood protein system is the fibrinolytic, which is responsible for the destruction of a fibrin clot. It is generally thought that small amounts of fibrin are constantly and probably systemically being deposited, with subsequent lysis of these fibrin deposits. The presence or absence of hemorrhage or thrombosis, thus, is likely to be dependent on a delicate balance between the procoagulant system and the fibrinolytic system.[11] Figure 1–28 summarizes the physiology of the fibrinolytic system, which consists of a proenzyme, plasminogen (or profibrinolysin), that is converted via numerous mechanisms into the active enzyme, plasmin.[19] Mechanisms of activation will be discussed subsequently. Plasmin, also a serine protease, is not as specific as thrombin. Thrombin is quite specific in its activity; however, plasmin is a very nonspecific proteolytic serine protease and has equal affinity for both fibrinogen and fibrin, degrading both into FDPs.[5] In addition, plasmin may biodegrade Factors V, VIII, IX, and XI, as well as ACTH, growth hormone, insulin, and possibly many other plasma proteins.[12,98,99] There are two primary physiologic (and probably pathophysiologic) activation pathways for the fibrinolytic system. One primary physiologic plasminogen activator is endothelial plasminogen activator activity.[4] A second key physiologic activation pathway is that of Hageman factor activation.[32,58] Active Hageman factor converts a proactivator (plasminogen proactivator) into an activator that then converts plasminogen into plasmin. This proactivator may be a high molecular weight kininogen. There are also numerous poorly characterized tissue activators, and most likely other plasma activators that convert plasminogen into plasmin. In addition, two pharmacologic activators that are currently used and will be discussed in detail in a subsequent chapter are streptokinase and urokinase; both are used for therapeutic thrombolytic therapy.[84] Urokinase has the ability to directly activate, or convert, plasminogen into its active form, plasmin. However, streptokinase must first form a streptokinase-plasminogen complex and the complex then converts plasminogen into plasmin.

Figure 1–29 summarizes the Hageman factor activation pathway for the fibrinolytic system. Numerous materials are able to convert Hageman factor into active Hageman factor, including such endogenous materials as collagen and phospholipids. However, endotoxin, antibody-antigen complex, and other pathologic materials may also initiate this activation pathway and give rise to circulating plasmin.[56,57,74,97] It should be appreciated that plasmin tends to be a self-perpetuating enzyme: a self-feeding loop generating more plasmin once plasmin is generated via the Hageman activation pathway. The conversion of active Hageman factor into Hageman factor fragments by plasmin, will then convert more proactivator to more activator, thus converting more plas-

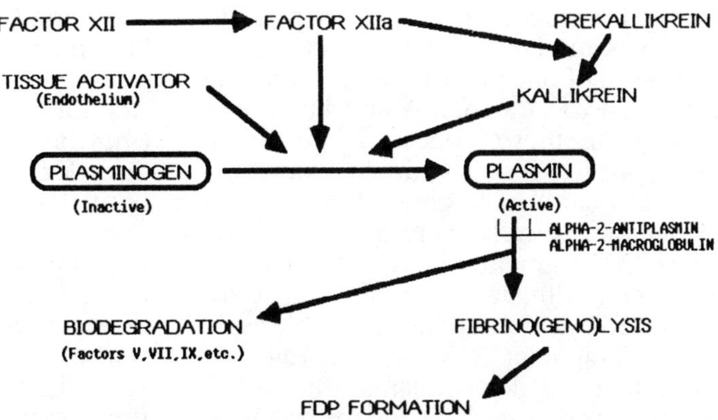

Fig. 1–28. Physiology of the fibrinolytic system.

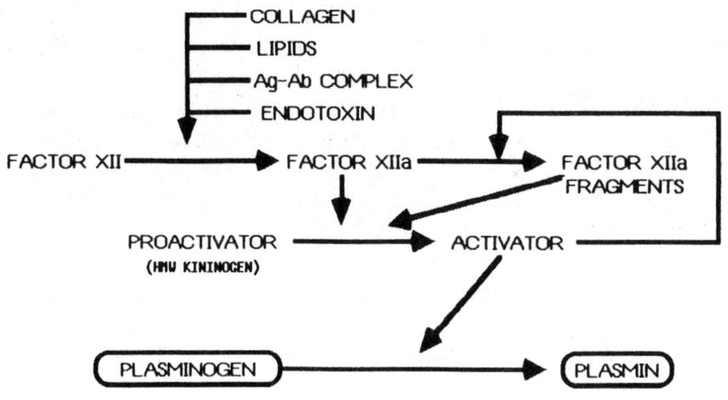

Fig. 1–29. Factor XII-Dependent activation of fibrinolysis.

minogen to plasmin.[37,59] There are two primary inhibitors of the fibrinolytic system. Alpha-2-antiplasmin, a rapid inhibitor of plasmin activity, and alpha-2-macroglobulin, an effective, although slow, inhibitor of plasmin activity.[2,110] As previously discussed, the primary activity of thrombin is to cleave fibrinopeptides A and B from fibrinogen, creating fibrin monomer; however, plasmin begins to biodegrade fibrinogen at the carboxy-terminal end of the A-alpha chain.

Figure 1–30 depicts the clinically significant FDPs. At the top of the figure fibrinogen is depicted as being comprised of the A-alpha, B-beta, and the gamma chains, with the A-peptide and the B-peptide being depicted as small circles. Fibrinogen and fibrin are first degraded into fragment X after plasmin-induced symmetrical cleavage of the carboxy terminal end of the A-alpha chains. Subsequent digestion of fibrinogen and fibrin by plasmin is then asymmetrical, with the amino terminal end of one portion of the molecule giving rise to a fragment Y and a fragment D. After this, there is plasmin digestion of the opposite amino terminal portion, giving rise to another fragment D and a fragment E, or a so-called N-terminal disulfide knot.[61,85] Fragments X, Y, D, and E are those clinically significant FDPs that are measured by commercially available assay kits.[6,68] Fragment E is the last fragment with antigenic determinants; thus products that are digested beyond the fragment

E stage will not be detected in the kits commonly used in which antifibrinogen or anti-FDP latex particles are present. This is of importance in such disorders as DIC and will be discussed in detail in appropriate chapters.

It should be emphasized that in the currently available test kits for FDPs thrombin clot tubes are provided, so that the antifibrinogen or anti-FDP latex particles will only react with the degradation products and not with fibrinogen itself. However, it should be noted that fragment X and fragment Y still contain fibrinopeptide A. Therefore the addition of thrombin will clot out fibrinogen as well as fragment X and fragment Y. The currently used FDP detection kits detect fragments D and E, resulting in situations in which false-negative FDP titers are noted. This is not a criticism of the FDP kits available, but serves to emphasize that in selected circumstances there may be false-negative FDP titers in the presence of significant primary or secondary fibrinolysis. For example, if there is only minimal fibrinolytic system activation in a DIC-type disorder, there may only be degradation of fibrinogen or fibrin to the fragment X stage or some intermediate in between fibrinogen and fragment X. In this instance there is nothing for the test system to detect. Alternatively, in an overwhelming fibrinolytic situation, such as may occur secondary to DIC or one of the primary fibrinolytic system disorders, there may

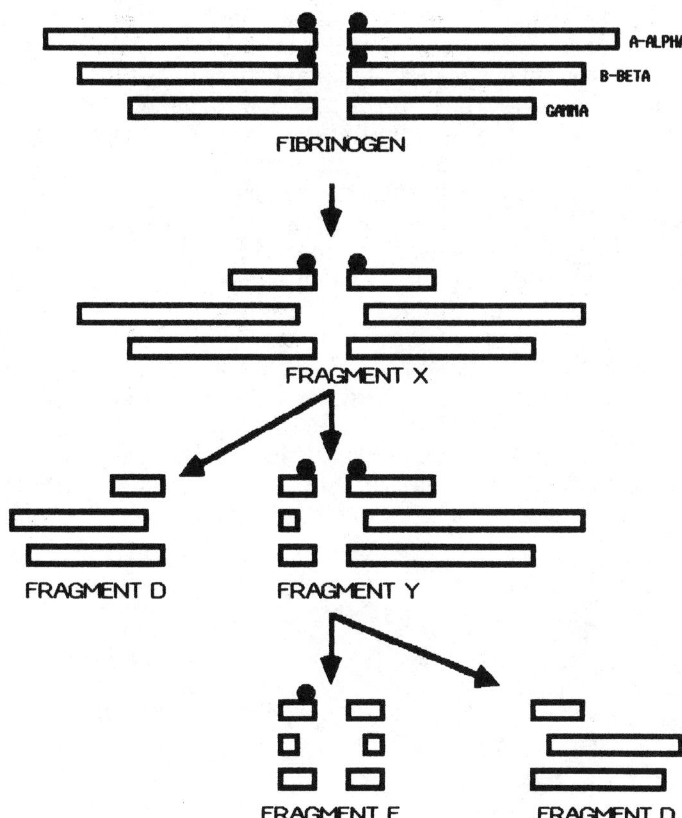

Fig. 1–30. Formation of fibrin(ogen) degradation products.

be degradation past the fragment D and E stage by either plasmin or proteolytic enzymes released from granulocytes monocytes, or other cellular systems, such as elastases or collagenases. In such a case, there are no antigenic determinants present and a negative FDP titer may be noted simply because of digestion to a nonantigenic subspecies of fragments D or E.

It should be noted that the FDPs are named in descending order of molecular weight, with fibrinogen having a molecular weight of approximately 340,000 daltons, fragment X having a molecular weight of approximately 265,000 daltons, fragment Y having a molecular weight of approximately 155,000 daltons, fragment D being approximately 95,000 daltons, and fragment E, the smallest and last of the fragments (with recognizable anti-

genicity), having a molecular weight of approximately 50,000 daltons. The presence of FDPs may seriously compromise hemostasis by interference with fibrin monomer polymerization and platelet function.[13,66,69] This will be discussed in detail in subsequent chapters.

Complement Activation and Hemostasis

The next blood protein system to be discussed is that of complement activation and complement interrelationships with coagulation. Complement activation is often not considered important with respect to the hemostasis system; however, more current concepts assume major importance of complement in many thrombohemorrhagic disorders, such as DIC. The complement system is capable of increasing vascular permeability and this, of course, has important implications with respect to hypotension and shock, common occurrences in the patient with DIC and other thrombohemorrhagic disorders.[104,106] If complement activation proceeds to the C8-9 phase, cell membrane alterations leading to osmotic lysis will occur.[71,82] When considering complement-induced lysis, usually only red cells are thought of; however, equally important to red cell lysis is complement-induced platelet lysis. The lysis and disruption of red cells or platelets will lead to the release of procoagulant material that may accelerate a procoagulant process.

For example, if there is complement-induced red cell lysis, there is the release of membrane phospholipoprotein as well as ADP; both serve as procoagulant or coagulation-accelerating materials. In addition, the lysis of platelets will lead to the release of molecular materials, including ADP, that may also promote clotting activity and act as accelerators to the procoagulant system.

The complement system is a sequential activation pathway system similar to the procoagulation system (Fig. 1–31). It should be recalled that there is a primary activation pathway via activation of C1 and a so-called alternate or properdin activation pathway through the activation of C3.[39,95] The activation of C1 through C5

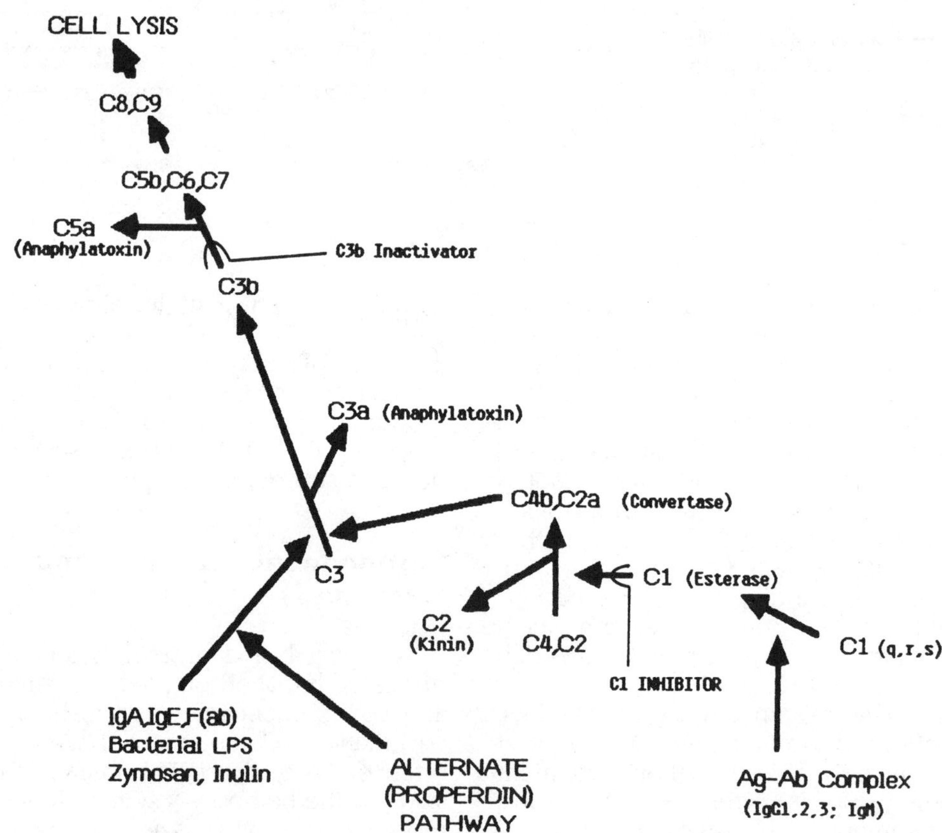

Fig. 1–31. The complement system.

is the activation phase and the activation of C5 through C9 is the attack phase that often leads to osmotic lysis. Figure 1–32 serves to summarize mechanisms of complement activation in the hemostasis system. Attention should be directed to Factor XII or Hageman factor, which is converted into Factor XIIa via numerous mechanisms, including phospholipids, collagen, and kallikrein. Factor XIIa then converts proactivator to activator, which converts plasminogen to plasmin. Plasmin is capable of directly activating C1 or directly activating C3, thereby providing two independent pathways by which plasmin may activate the complement system. In most instances of clinically significant DIC or primary hyperfibrino(geno)lytic syndromes, such as may occur in certain malignancies, some instances of liver disease, and in many instances of cardiopulmonary bypass, there is plasmin-induced activation of the complement system.[14] This may, on occasion, be associated with serious clinical consequences, as previously discussed.

Kinins and Coagulation

The next blood protein system to be discussed is the kinin system. As with the complement system, only recently has the importance of kinin generation during pathologic thrombohemorrhagic phenomena has been realized. Kinins are capable of blood vessel dilation, which may clinically lead to hypotension, shock, and other potential end organ damage.[8,108,131] In addition, kinins increase vascular permeability, with the clinical consequences again being hypotension and shock. Figure 1–33 summarizes mechanisms of kinin activation in the hemostasis system, i.e., the interrelationships between Hageman factor, the fibrinolytic system, and the kinin system. Activation of kinins centers around Hageman factor pathway activation. Active Hageman factor converts prekallikrein (Fletcher factor) into kallikrein and kallikrein directly converts kininogens into kinins. Active Hageman factor (XIIa) is converted to Hageman factor fragments by plasmin, and these fragments also activate prekallikrein to kallikrein and, thus, there is subsequent generation of kinins from precursor kininogens.

Figure 1–34 is quite complicated and simply serves to illustrate the important interrelationships between the coagulation, fibrinolytic, complement, and kinin systems. Hageman factor is converted to active Hageman factor by various compounds, including collagen and phospholipids; active Hageman factor converts proactivator to activator and activator converts plasminogen to plasmin. Plasmino-

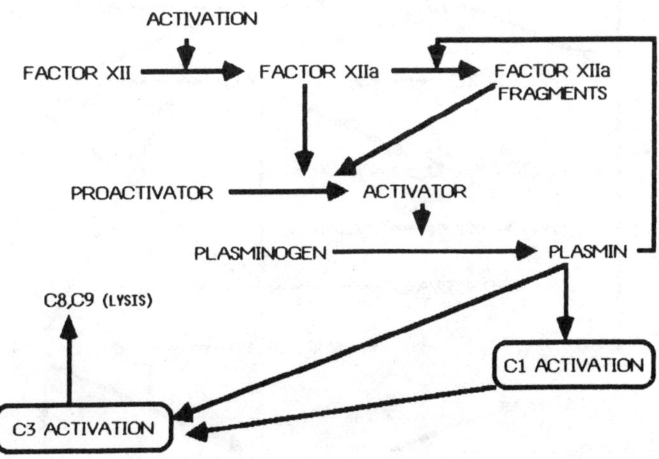

Fig. 1–32. The fibrinolytic system and complement activation.

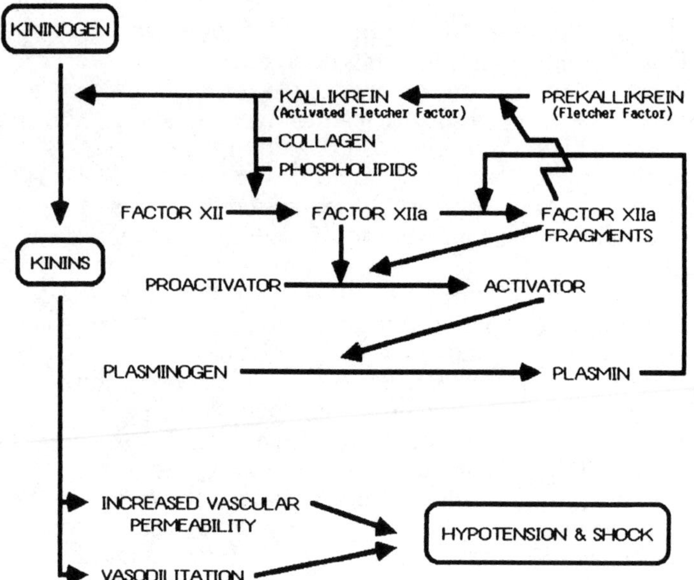

Fig. 1-33. Kinin generation and hemostasis.

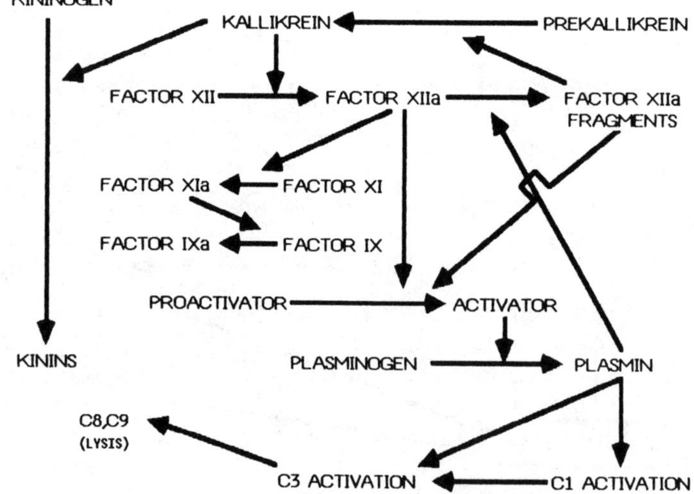

Fig. 1-34. Coagulation, contact activation, complement activation, and kinin generation.

gen activates C1, C3, or both, thereby activating the complement system. Additionally, active Hageman factor (or plasmin-induced Hageman factor fragments) will convert prekallikrein to kallikrein, which will then convert kininogens to kinins. Kinin and complement activation occurs via these pathways in many thrombohemorrhagic disorders. In addition, these activation pathways often lead to serious clinical consequences, which have to be contended with by the physician.

Inhibitor Systems

The most important inhibitor of the procoagulant system is antithrombin III (AT III). Table 1–12 summarizes inhibitory mechanisms in hemostasis. Most of which are important physiologically and some assume major importance in pathophysiology. Firstly, there is inactivation of Factors V and VIII by thrombin as well as by activated protein C (protein Ca).[32,121] In addition, there is inhibition of prothrombin activation as well as fibrin formation by small fragments, which are generated during the conversion of prothrombin to thrombin (profragments 1 and 2). There is inhibition of factor Xa by modified protein C and recent evidence

Table 1–12 Inhibitory Mechanisms in Hemostasis

Inactivation of Factors V and VIII by thrombin and activated protein C
Inhibition of prothrombin activation and fibrin formation by prothrombin fragments
Inhibition of Factor Xa by activated protein C
Inhibition of thrombin or Factor Xa formation by suboptimal "complex" components
Inhibition of thrombin, Factor Xa, IXa, XIa, XIIa, and kallikrein by antithrombin III
Inhibition of thrombin activity by absorbing to fibrin
Inhibition of fibrin monomer polymerization and platelet function by fibrino(geno)lytic degradation products

would suggest that alpha-1-antitrypsin may also be a very important inhibitor of Factor Xa.[111] In addition, the necessity of stoichiometry for the first two key reactions has been discussed. Decreased generation of thrombin formation or Factor Xa formation by less than optimal concentrations of those complex components will occur with inadequate components of these two systems. Additionally, there is major inhibition of the serine proteases, thrombin, Factor Xa, Factor IXa, Factor XIa, Factor XIIa, and kallikrein by AT III.[101,102,122] It is thought that AT III probably accounts for at least 90 to 95% of the total inhibition of the serine protease system.[86] The major inhibitory activity of AT III is directed against Factor Xa and thrombin, with less inhibitory activity against other serine proteases previously mentioned. The inhibitory activity of AT III is markedly enhanced in the presence of heparin.[54,103,123]

As fibrin is formed, it may absorb out thrombin, and thus there is inhibition of thrombin activity by decreasing its concentration by absorbing to already formed fibrin. An additional inhibitory activity is that of inhibition of fibrin monomer polymerization, as well as platelet function by FDPs. If FDPs complex with a fibrin monomer before that fibrin monomer complexes with another fibrin monomer, the fibrin monomer becomes solubilized (stays "in solution") and is unable to polymerize. In addition, the later degradation products, especially D and E fragments, have a high affinity for platelet membranes and render platelets markedly dysfunctional. In some pathologic instances this latter activity can lead to quite significant clinical hemorrhage via an FDP-induced platelet function defect.

Figure 1–35 depicts a popular model of AT III and its inhibitory activity against serine proteases. It is thought that arginine-rich centers in the AT III molecule react irreversibly with the serine centers of serine protease.[102] In this particular figure thrombin is depicted, although Factor Xa, Factor IXa, or other serine proteases could also have been illustrated. It is thought that the serine protease will ir-

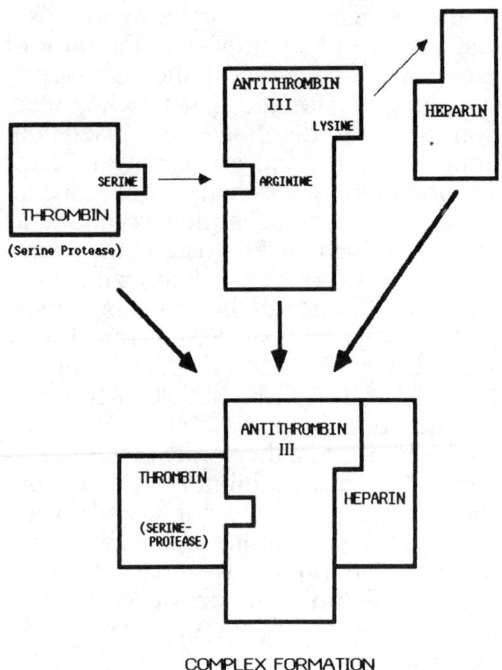

Fig. 1–35. Antithrombin III inhibitory activity.

reversibly react with the arginine-rich center on AT III and the complex is then removed from the circulation. The mechanism of action of heparin as it is currently understood is also illustrated. Heparin is thought to react with lysine sites on the AT III molecule, thereby changing its configuration and making more available the arginine-rich center. Thus, in the presence of heparin, AT III inhibitory activity is markedly enhanced.

Protein C is capable of the inactivation of Factors V and VIII and may also be a competitive inhibitor of Factor Xa.[32,121] Although the mechanism is poorly understood, protein C is able to enhance fibrinolysis by depressing fibrinolytic inhibitors or enhancing activators. Also poorly understood is the relationship of protein C to clot retraction. Interestingly, although the first four activities tend to be inhibitory in nature, the fifth activity of protein C is enhancement of epinephrine-induced platelet aggregation.[121] Figure 1–36 depicts the protein C system.

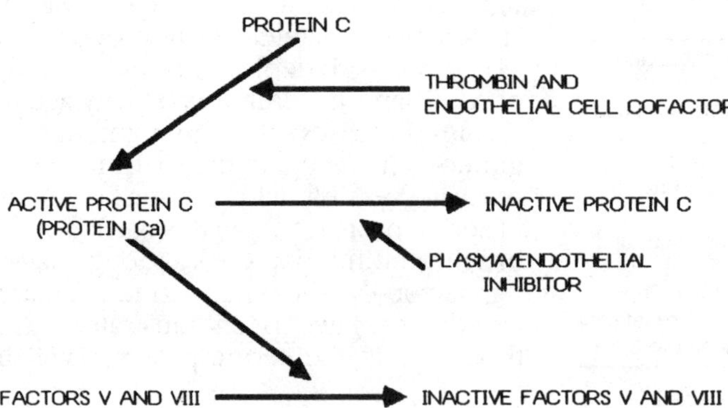

Fig. 1–36. Protein C activity in hemostasis.

Other Interactive Components

Numerous other interactive components of hemostasis, including the vascular proteoglycans, fibronectin, complement derivatives, neutrophils and monocytes, and other as yet unknown components may have important, although poorly understood, roles in modulating hemostasis. With time, it is hoped that the interactive activities of these components will become more and more clear. It can also be anticipated that many other components in the cellular and blood systems may be found to interact and perhaps be very important to hemostasis and thrombosis.

Fibronectin is a high molecular weight glycoprotein that is found in its soluble form in blood.[78] An insoluble form is found in connective tissue and basement membranes.[91] Fibronectin is known to bind to collagen, fibrin, fibrinogen, and intact cells.[35,70,105] It is thought to be synthesized by vascular endothelium and is also found in, and is possibly synthesized by, the alpha granules of platelets.[143] It is known that fibronectin is cleaved by thrombin and trypsin and coprecipitates with fibrin,[76,133] and it is covalently cross-linked to a fibrin clot by Factor XIIIa.[76,133] Additionally, fibronectin is known to be necessary to support cell growth and the cellular migration into a fibrin clot.[77] Fibronectin also provides an extracellular matrix that will eventually replace a fibrin clot. Other activities include the potentiation of plasminogen activators, thus mediating clot lysis and matrix turnover. Fibronectin can also mediate the activation of platelets by damaged tissue and can promote the opsonization of bacteria and may mediate attachment of bacteria to damaged tissues. The fibronectin associated with alpha granules of platelets is known to be released by collagen or thrombin-induced platelet aggregation; after this release, fibronectin binds to the platelet surface. On the platelet surface, it appears that fibronectin mediates collagen-platelet adhesion and seems to stimu-

late further collagen-induced platelet aggregation and platelet release. Other activities of fibronectin include cellular binding, especially to fibroblasts, binding to bacteria, where promotion of opsonization by neutrophils may occur (this requires Factor XIIIa) and inhibiting the endothelial uptake of low-density lipoprotein. Fibronectin interacts intimately with fibrinogen and fibrin. As clot formation occurs, approximately 50% of plasma fibronectin is lost.[79] This is enhanced if clot formation occurs at less than 4°C. This loss is known to be due to cross-linking of fibronectin to the alpha chain of fibrin by Factor XIIIa. Thus, fibronectin will account for approximately 5% of the total protein of a fibrin clot.

Fibronectin is necessary for cryoprecipitation of fibrinogen-fibrin complexes and accounts for the cryoprecipitation seen in DIC. The fibrin-fibronectin complex is also known to be necessary for the migration and adhesion of cells in an area of thrombus formation. Fibronectin is commonly decreased in DIC, in the postoperative state, in patients sustaining major trauma and burns, and in patients with solid tumor metastases.[77] It also interacts with collagen and other vascular proteoglycans, by binding to collagen, which is induced by cross-linking of fibronectin to collagen by Factor XIIIa. It also binds to heparin, endogenous heparan sulfate, hyaluronic acid, and chondroitin sulfate. Heparin may accelerate the binding of fibronectin to both fibrinogen and collagen; however, the binding of heparin to fibronectin does not change the "anticoagulant" nature of the bound heparin. For details, an excellent review is available.[77]

Vascular proteoglycans are a heterogeneous group of high molecular weight protein polysaccharides consisting of carbohydrate polymers (glycosaminoglycans) covalently linked to a protein core.[140] The common vascular proteoglycans are hyaluronic acid, chondroitin-4-sulfate, chondroitin-6-sulfate, dermatan sulfate, keratin sulfate, heparan sulfate, endogenous heparan sulfate, and heparin.

Endogenous heparan sulfate differs from USP heparin in that it is a low-sulfated, D-glucuronic, acid-rich polysaccharide, whereas USP heparin is a highly sulfated, L-iduronic, acid-rich polysaccharide. The amount of each particular type of vascular proteoglycan depends on the type and portion of the vascularture in which it is measured. Most of the vascular proteoglycans are concentrated in the intimal layer of the vessel. The concentration of some of the vascular proteoglycans, especially dermatan and heparan sulfate, correlate closely with antithrombotic activity. In addition, selected vascular proteoglycans inhibit collagen and thrombin-induced platelet aggregation and accelerate AT III inhibitory activity directed against thrombin and Factor Xa. Vascular proteoglycans are also able to induce the release of platelet factor 4. The concentrations of different vascular proteoglycans will change with the development of atherosclerotic plaques. The physiologic role of vascular proteoglycans is thought to consist of supporting vascular integrity, to maintain the viscoelastic properties of vessels, to regulate permeability of macromolecules from the plasma passing through the vessel wall, and regulation of arterial lipid deposition. Vascular proteoglycans are potentially of importance in regulating hemostatic balance by modulating interactions of blood proteins and the vascular wall.

The complement system has been discussed; however, several complement derivatives, especially C3a and C5a, may have importance in the hemostasis system. These components not only regulate vascular tone, but also may induce a neutrophil and monocyte release of elastases and collagenases which may have importance in the degradation of fibrinogen, fibrin, and FDPs.[15] Additionally, complement derivatives may modulate the release of granulocyte and monocyte procoagulant activity and platelet reactivity, and may have activity in the neutrophil and monocyte interaction with fibronectin.[38] Granulocytes and monocytes contain procoagulant activity that may be released under pathologic conditions, such as acute leu-

kemia, and interact with the hemostasis system.[64]

It is to be hoped that the future will reveal with more clarity the nature of these interactive components of hemostasis, and, as previously mentioned, it can be reasonably anticipated that many other components of cellular and blood protein system may be found to interact with, and perhaps to be very important to, the physiology and pathophysiology of hemostasis and thrombosis.

Summary

Subsequent chapters in this book, all of which will deal with specific disease states, will be far more easily understood by mastering the basic mechanisms discussed in this chapter. As mentioned earlier, there are other very important reasons for understanding basic mechanisms of hemostasis and thrombosis. Firstly, one must absolutely have a working knowledge of basic mechanisms of hemostasis and thrombosis in order to be able to interpret appropriately new highly sophisticated testing modalities for the hemostasis system and its components and interrelationships. Secondly, the pathophysiology of most disorders of hemostasis and thrombosis are now well understood, and by understanding their basic mechanisms, the clinician can more firmly understand the basic pathophysiology occurring in the patient. Thirdly, a mastering of basic mechanisms of hemostasis and thrombosis has now allowed for the more specific development of highly specific therapeutic agents for the treatment of thrombohemorrhagic disorders. A good example of this is the development of thrombolytic therapy using urokinase and streptokinase, the development of which required an understanding of the basic mechanisms of the fibrinolytic system. An additional example of this is the new impetus on the part of the pharmaceutical industry to develop specific platelet-inhibiting drugs.

References

1. Alami SY, Hampton JW, Race GH, Speer RJ: Fibrin stabilizing factor (Factor XIII). Am J Med 44:1, 1968.
2. Aoki N, Harpel PC: Inhibitors of the fibrinolytic enzyme system. Semin Thromb Hemost 10:24, 1984.
3. Astrup T: Fibrinolysis: An overview. In Davidson JF, Rowan RM, Samama MM, Desnoyers
4. Bachmann F, Kruithof EKO: Tissue plasminogen activator: Chemical and physiological aspects. Semin Thromb Hemost 10:6, 1984.
5. Bang NU: Physiology and biochemistry of the fibrinolytic system. In Bang NU, Beller KF, Deutch E, Mammen EF (Eds): Thrombosis and Bleeding Disorders. Academic Press, New York, 1971, p 292.
6. Bang NU, Chang ML: Soluble fibrin complexes. Semin Thromb Hemost 2:91, 1974.
7. Barnhart MI, Chen ST: Vessel wall models for studying interaction capabilities with blood platelets. Semin Thromb Hemost 5:112, 1978.
8. Bennett B, Ogston D: Role of complement, coagulation, fibrinolysis, and kinins in normal haemostasis and disease. In Bloom AL, Thomas DP (Eds): Haemostasis and Thrombosis. Churchill-Livingstone, London, 1981, p 236.
9. Bick RL: Basic mechanisms of hemostasis pertaining to DIC. In Bick RL (Ed): Disseminated Intravascular Coagulation and Related Syndromes. CRC Press, Boca Raton, FL, 1983, p 1.
10. Bick RL: Vascular disorders associated with thrombhemorrhagic phenomena. Semin Thromb Hemost 5:167, 1979.
11. Bick RL: The clinical significance of fibrinogen degradation products. Semin Thromb Hemost 8:302, 1982.
12. Bick RL: Disseminated intravascular coagulation. In Bick RL (Ed): Disseminated Intravascular Coagulation and Related Syndromes. CRC Press, Boca Raton, FL, 1983, p 31.
13. Bick RL: The Clinical Significance of Fibrinolytic Degradation Products. Health Sciences Consortium Press, Chapel Hill, NC, 1982, p 15.
14. Bick RL: Alterations of hemostasis associated with surgery, cardiopulmonary bypass surgery, and prosthetic devices. In Ratnoff OD, Forbes CD (Eds): Disorders of Hemostasis. Grune & Stratton, New York, 1984, p 379.
15. Bick RL: Pathophysiology of hemostasis and thrombosis. In Sodeman WA, Sodeman TA, (Eds): Pathologic Physiology: Mechanisms of Disease, 7th ed. W.B. Saunders, Philadelphia, 1985.
16. Born GVR, Cross MJ: The aggregation of blood platelets. J Physiol (Lond) 168:178, 1963.
17. Brodie GN, Bienziger NL, Chase LR: The effects of thrombin on adenylcyclase activity and a membrane protein from platelets. J Clin Invest 51:81, 1972.
18. Bull BS, Zucker MB: Changes in platelet volume produced by temperature, metabolic inhibitors, and aggregating agents. Proc Soc Exp Biol Med 120:296, 1965.
19. Castellino FJ: Biochemistry of human plasminogen. Semin Thromb Hemost 10:18, 1984.
20. Cohen LS: Clinical pharmacology of acetylsalicylic acid. Semin Thromb Hemost 2:146, 1976.
21. Cole B, Robison GA, Hartman RC: Effects of prostaglandin E and theophylline on aggregation and cyclic AMP levels of human blood platelets. Fed Proc 29:316, 1970.
22. Coleman RW, Bagdasarian A, Talmo RC, Scott CF, Seaven W, Guimardes JA, Pierce JV, Kaplan MP: Williams trait: Human kininogen deficiency with diminished levels of plasminogen proactivator and prekallikrein associated with abnormalities of the Hageman factor dependent pathway. J Clin Invest 56:1650, 1975.
23. Crawford T: Blood and lymphatic vessels. In Anderson WAD, Kissane JM (Eds): Pathology. C.V. Mosby, St. Louis, 1977, p 879.
24. Davie WE, Ratnott OD: Waterfall sequence for intrinsic blood clotting. Science 145:1310, 1964.
25. Davis RB, Mecker WR, Bailey WL: Serotonin release after injection of E. coli endotoxin in the rabbit. Fed Proc 20:261, 1961.
26. Day NJ: Stormorken H, Holmsen H: Subcellular localization of platelet factor 3 and platelet factor 4. Proceedings of the 12th Congress of the International Society of Hematology, Mexico City, 1968, p 172.
27. Day CE: On the newly discovered role of prostaglandins in arteries and its implications for the control of atherosclerosis, platelets, and thrombosis. Artery 2:480, 1976.
28. de Los Santos, LW Hoyer: Antihemophiliac factor in tissue: Localization by immunofluorescence. Fed Proc 31:262, 1972.
29. Denson KWE: The levels of Factor II, VII, IX, and X by antibody neutralization techniques in the plasma of patients receiving phenindione therapy. Br J Haematol 20:643, 1971.
30. Des Prez RM, Horowitz HI, Hook EW: Effects of bacterial endotoxin on rabbit platelets. I. Platelet aggregation and release of platelet factors in vitro. J Exp Med 114:857, 1961.
31. Droller MJ: Ultrastructure of the platelet release reaction in response to various aggregating agent and their inhibitors. Lab Invest 29:595, 1973.
32. Esmon CT: Protein-C: Biochemistry, physiology, and clinical implications. Blood 62:1155, 1983.

33. Fareed J, Walenga JM, Bick RL, Bermes EJ, Messmore HL: Impact of automation on the quantitation of low molecular weight markers of hemostatic defects. Semin Thromb Hemost 9:355, 1983.

34. Friedman RJ, Burns ER: Role of platelets in the proliferative response of the injured artery. Prog Hemost Thromb 4:2498, 1978.

35. Fyrand O, Solum ND: Heparin precipitable fraction (HPF) from dermatological patients: Studies on the non-clottable components; identification of cold-insoluble globulin as the major non-clottable component. Thromb Res 8:659, 1976.

36. Gerrard JM, White JG, Prostaglandins and thromboxanes: "Middlemen" modulating platelet function in hemostasis and thrombosis. Prog Hemost Thromb 4:87, 1978.

37. Goldsmith GN, Saito H, Ratnoff OD: The activation of plasminogen by Hageman factor (Factor XII) and Hageman factor fragments. J Clin Invest 21:54, 1978.

38. Goldstein IM, Perez HD: Biologically active peptides derived from the fifth component of complement. Prog Hemost Thromb 5:41, 1980.

39. Gotze O: Proteases of the properdin system. In E Reich, Rifkin DB, Shaw E (Eds): Proteases and Biological Control. Cold Spring Harbor Symposium, Cold Spring Harbor, New York, 1975, p 255.

40. Griffin JH, Cochrane CG: Recent advances in the understanding of contact activation reactions. Semin Thromb Hemost 5:254, 1979.

41. Gryglewski RJ, Szczcklik A, Nizankowski R: Antiplatelet action of intravenous infusion of prostacyclin in man. Thromb Res 13:153, 1978.

42. Gryglewski RJ, Bunting S, Moncada S, Flower RJ, Vane JR: Arterial walls are protected against deposition of platelet thrombi by a substance (prostaglandin X) which they make from prostaglandin endoperoxides. Prostaglandins 12:685, 1976.

43. Habel FM, Movat HZ: Kininogens of human plasma. Semin Thromb Hemost 3:27, 1976.

44. Harker LA, Ross R: Pathogenesis of arterial vascular disease. Semin Thromb Hemost 5:274, 1979.

45. Harker LA, Schwartz SM, Ross R: Endothelium and arteriosclerosis. Clinics in Haematology 10:283, 1981.

46. Haslam RJ: Interactions of the pharmacological receptors of blood platelets with adenylate cyclase. Ser Haematol 6:333, 1973.

47. Henry RL: Platelet function in hemostasis. In Murano G, Bick RL (Eds): Basic Concepts of Hemostasis and Thrombosis. CRC Press, Boca Raton, FL., 1980, p 17.

48. Henry RL: Platelet function. Semin Thromb Hemost 4:93, 1977.

49. Hensby CN, Lewis PJ, Hilgard P, Mofti GP, Hows J, Webster J: Prostacyclin deficiency in thrombotic thrombocytopenic purpura. Lancet 2:748, 1979.

50. Hinman JW: Prostaglandins. Annu Rev Biochem 41:161, 1972.

51. Horlington M, Watson PA: Inhibition of 3′ 5′-cyclic-AMP, phosphodiesterase by some platelet aggregation inhibitors. Biochem Pharmacol 19:955, 1970.

52. Huseby RM: Conformational structure of the fibrinopeptides related during fibrinogen to fibrin conversion. Physiol Chem Phys 5:1, 1973.

53. Irwin JF, Seegers WH, Andary TJ, Fekete LF, Novoa E: Blood coagulation as a cybernetic system: Control of autoprothrombin C (X_a) formation. Thromb Res 6:431, 1975.

54. Jaques LB, McDuffies NM: The chemical and anticoagulant nature of heparin. Semin Thromb Hemost 4:277, 1978.

55. Jobin F: Acetylsalicylic acid, hemostasis, and human thromboembolism. Semin Thromb Hemost 4:199, 1978.

56. Kaplan AJ, Meier HL, Mandle R: The Hageman factor dependent pathways of coagulation, fibrinolysis, and kinin-generation. Semin Thromb Hemost 3:1, 1976.

57. Kaplan AP: Initiation of the intrinsic coagulation and fibrinolytic pathways of man: The role of surfaces, Hageman factor, prekallikrein, high molecular weight kininogen, and Factor XI. Prog Hemost Thromb 4:127, 1978.

58. Kaplan AP:, Austin F: The fibrinolytic pathway of human plasma. Isolation and characterization of the plasminogen proactivator. J Exp Med 135:1378, 1972.

59. Kaplan AP, Austen KF: A prealbumin activator of prekallikrein. II. Derivation of activators of prekallikrein from active Hageman factor by digestion with plasmin. J Exp Med 133:696, 1971.

60. Kowalski E: Fibrinogen derivatives and their biological activity. Semin Hematol 5:45, 1968.

61. Kudryk B, Collen D, Woods KR, Blomback B: Evidence for localization of polymerization sites in fibrinogen. J Biol Chem 249:3322, 1974.

62. Kwaan HC: The role of fibrinolysis in disease states. Semin Thromb Hemost 10:71, 1984.

63. Lie JT, Brown AL: Normal structure of the vascular system and general reactive changes of the arteries. In Fairbairn JF, Ivergens JL, Spittel JA (Eds): Peripheral Vascular Diseases. W.B. Saunders, Philadelphia, 1972, p 45.

64. Lisiewicz J: Mechanisms of hemorrhage in leukemia. Semin Thromb Hemost 4:241, 1978.

65. Macfarland RG: An enzyme cascade in blood clotting mechanisms and its function as a biochemical amplifier. Nature 202:498, 1964.

66. Mammen EF: Inhibitor abnormalities. Semin Thromb Hemost 9:42, 1983.

67. Mammen EF: Physiology and biochemistry of blood coagulation. In Bang NU, Beller FK, Deutsch E, Mammen EF (Eds): Thrombosis and Bleeding Disorders. Georg Thieme Verlag, Stuttgart, 1971, p 1.

68. Marder VJ, Matchett M, Sherry S: Detection of serum fibrinogen and fibrin degradation products. Am J Med 51:71, 1971.

69. Marder VJ, Shulman NR: High molecular weight derivatives of human fibrinogen produced by plasmin: Mechanisms of their anticoagulant activity. J Biol Chem 224:2120, 1969.

70. Matsuda M, Saida T, Hasegawa R: Cryofibrinogen in the plasma of patients with skin ulcerative lesions of the legs: A complex of fibrinogen and cold-insoluble globulin. Thromb Res 9:541, 1976.

71. Mayer MM: The component system. Sci Am 229:54, 1973.

72. McCoy L: Vascular function in hemostasis. In Murano G, Bick RL (Eds): Basic Concepts of Hemostasis and Thrombosis. CRC Press, Boca Raton, FL., 1980, p 5.

73. McLean JR, Veloso N: Changes of shape without aggregation caused by ADP in rabbit platelets at low pH. Life Sci 6:1983, 1967.

74. Meyer KL, Pierce JV, Coleman RW, Kaplan AP, Activation and function of human Hageman factor. J Clin Invest 60:18, 1977.

75. Moncada S, Gryglewski R, Bunting S, Vane JR: A lipid peroxide inhibits the enzyme in blood vessel microsomes that generate from prostaglandin endoperoxides the substance (prostaglandin x) which prevents platelet aggregation. Prostaglandins 12:715, 1976.

76. Moser DF, Schad PE, Kleinman HK: Cross-linking of fibronectin to collagen by blood coagulation Factor XIII. J Clin Invest 64:781, 1979.

77. Moser DF: Fibronectin. Prog Hemost Thromb 5:111, 1980.

78. Mosseson MW: Cold-insoluble globulin (CIg): A circulating cell surface protein. Thromb Haemost 38:742, 1977.

79. Mosseson MW, Umfleet RA: The cold-insoluble globulin of plasma. J Biol Chem 254:5728, 1970.

80. Mueller-Eckhardt C, Luscher EF: Immune reactions of human blood platelets. I. A comparative study on the effects on platelets of heterologous antiplatelet antiserum, antigen-antibody complexes, aggregation gamma-globulin, and thrombin. Thromb Diath Haemorrh 20:155, 1968.

81. Muller-Berghous G: Pathophysiology of generalized intravascular coagulation. Semin Thromb Hemost 3:209, 1977.

82. Muller-Eberhard HJ: Complement. Annu Rev Biochem 44:667, 1975.

83. Murano G: The "Hageman connection," interrelationships of blood coagulation, fibrino-(geno)lysis, kinin generation, and complement activation. Am J Hematol 4:303, 1978.

84. Murano G, RL Bick: Thrombolytic therapy. In Murano G, Bick RL (Eds): Basic Concepts of Hemostasis and Thrombosis. CRC Press, Boca Raton, FL., 1980, p 259.

85. Murano G: The molecular structure of fibrinogen. Semin Thromb Hemost 1:1, 1974.

86. Musumeci V, Lanolfi R, Bizza B: Amidolytic assay of thrombin bound to α-2-macroglobulin in plasma. Hemostasis 6:98, 1977.

87. Nachman RL: Platelet proteins. Semin Hematol 5:18, 1968.

88. Nalbandian RM, Henry RL: Platelet-endothelial cell interactions: Metabolic maps of structure and actions of prostaglandins, prostacycline, thromboxane, and cyclic AMP. Semin Thromb Hemost 5:87, 1979.

89. O'Brian JR: The adhesiveness of native platelets and its prevention. J Clin Pathol 14:140, 1961.

90. Packham MA, Mustard JF: Platelet reactions. Semin Hematol 8:30, 1971.

91. Pearlstein E, Gold LI, Garcia-Pardo A: Fibronectin: A review of its structure and biological activity. Mol Cell Biochem 29:103, 1980.

92. Pechet L: Fibrinolysis. N Engl J Med 273:966, 1965.

93. Pereira M, Couri D: Studies on the site of action of dicoumarol on prothrombin synthesis. Biochim Biophys Acta 237: 348, 1971.

94. Pfueller SL, Luscher EF: The effects of immune complexes on blood and their relationship to complement activation. Immunochemistry 9: 1151, 1972.

95. Pillimer L, Blum L, Lepow IH: The properdin system and immunity. I. Demonstration and isolation of a new serum protein, properdin, and its role in immune phenomena. Science 120: 279, 1954.

96. Ratnoff OD: The molecular basis of hereditary clotting disorders. Prog Hemost Thromb 1:39, 1972.

97. Ratnoff OD, Saito H: coagulation factors and the role of surfaces in their activation. Ann NY Acad Sci 283:88 1977.

98. Ratnoff OD, Naff GB: The conversion of C'1s to C'1 esterase by plasmin and trypsin. J Exp Med 125:337, 1967.

99. Robbins KM: Present status of the fibrinolytic system. In Fareed J, Messmore HL, Fenton J, Brinkhous KM (Eds): Perspectives in Hemostasis. Pergamon Press, New York, 1980, p 53.

100. Roberts WC, Ferrans VJ: The role of thrombosis in the etiology of atherosclerosis (a positive one) and in precipitating fatal ischemic heart disease (a negative one). Semin Thromb Hemost 2:123, 1976.

101. Rosenberg RD: The effect of heparin on Factor XI_a and plasmin. Thromb Diath Haemorrh 33:51, 1975.
102. Rosenberg RD, Damus P: The purification and mechanism of action of human antithrombin-heparin cofactor. J Biol Chem 248:6490, 1973.
103. Rosenberg RD: Biologic actions of heparin. Semin Hematol 14:427, 1977.
104. Rosse WF: Complement. In Williams WJ, Beutler E, Erslev AJ, Rundles RW (Eds): Hematology. McGraw-Hill, New York, 1977, p 87.
105. Ruoslahti E, Vaheri A: Interaction of soluble fibroblast surface antigen with fibrinogen and fibrin: Identity with cold insoluble globulin of human plasma. J Exp Med 141:497, 1975.
106. Ruddy S, Gigli I, Austen KF: The complement system in man. I. Activation, control, and products of the reaction sequences. N Engl J Med 178:489, 1972.
107. Ryan TJ: The investigation of vasculitis. In Microvascular Injury. W.B. Saunders, Philadelphia, 1976, p 333.
108. Ryan JW, Ryan US: Biochemical and morphological aspects of the actions and metabolism of kinins. In Pisano JJ, Austen KF (Eds): Chemistry and Biology of the Kallikrein-Kinin System in Health and Disease. DHEW Pub #76-791, US Department of Health, Education, and Welfare, Bethesda, MD, 1974, p 315.
109. Salzman EW: Cyclic AMP and platelet function. N Engl J Med 286:358, 1972.
110. Schreiber AD: Plasma inhibitors of the Hageman factor dependent pathways. Semin Thromb Hemost 3:43, 1976.
111. Scully MF, Ellis V, Kakkar VV: Studies of anti-X_a activity. Thromb Res 29:387, 1983.
112. Seegers WH: Basic principles of blood coagulation. Semin Thromb Hemost 7:180, 1981.
113. Seegers WH: Prothrombin. Harvard University Press, Cambridge, MA, 1962, p 262.
114. Seegers WH: Enzymes in blood clotting. J Med Enzymol (Jp) 2:68, 1977.
115. Seegers WH: Murano G: Blood coagulation: A cybernetic system. Pol Arch Med Wewn 55:1, 1976.
116. Seegers WH, Hassouna HI, Hewett-Emmett D, Andary TJ: Prothrombin and thrombin: Selected aspects of thrombin formation, properties, inhibition, and immunology. Semin Thromb Hemost 1:211, 1975.
117. Seegers WH, Sakuragawa N, McCoy LE, Sedensky JA, Dombrose FA: Prothrombin activation: Ac-globulin, lipid, platelet membrane, and autoprothrombin c (X_a) requirements. Thromb Res 1:293, 1972.
118. Seegers WH: Prothrombin complex. Semin Thromb Hemost 7:291, 1981.
119. Seegers WH: Platelets, phospholipids, and platelet cofactors. Semin Thromb Hemost 7:270, 1981.
120. Seegers WH: Fibrinogen. Semin Thromb Hemost 7:281, 1981.
121. Seegers WH: Protein C and autoprothrombin II-A. Semin Thromb Hemost 7:257, 1981.
122. Seegers WH: Antithrombin III. Semin Thromb Hemost 7:263, 1981.
123. Seegers WH: Antithrombin-III theory and clinical applications. Am J Clin Pathol 69:367, 1978.
124. Sheppard B, French JE: Platelet adhesion in the rabbit abdominal aorta following the removal of endothelium: A scanning and transmission electron microscopic study. Proc R Soc Lond 176:427, 1971.
125. Stenflo T: Vitamin K, prothrombin, and gamma-carboxy-glutamic acid. N Engl J Med 296:624, 1977.
126. Stuart MJ: Inherited defects of platelet function. Semin Hematol 12:233, 1975.
127. Thomas DP, Niewiarowski S, Ream VJ: Release of adenosine nucleotides and platelet factor 4 from platelets of man and four other species. J Lab Clin Med 75:607, 1970.
128. Todd AS: Histologic localization of fibrinolysis activator. J Pathol Bacteriol 78:281, 1959.
129. Triplett DA: The platelet: A review. In Triplett DA (Ed): Platelet Function. ASCP Press, Chicago, 1978, p 1.
130. Turpie AGG: Antiplatelet therapy. Clin Haematol 10:497, 1981.
131. Van Arman CG, Bohidar HR: Role of the kallikrein-kinin system in inflammation. In Pisano JJ, Austen KF (Eds): Chemistry and Biology of the Kallekrein-Kinin System in Health and Disease. DHEW Publ #76-791, US Department of Health, Education and Welfare, Bethesda MD, 1974, p 471.
132. Vennerod AM, Kaake K: Prekallikrein and plasminogen proactivator. Absence of plasminogen proactivator in Fletcher factor deficient plasma. Thromb Res 8:519, 1976.
133. Wagner DD, Hynes RO: Doman structure of fibronectin and its relationship to function. J Biol Chem 254:6746, 1979.
134. Walsh P: The effect of collagen and kaolin on the intrinsic coagulation activity of platelets. Evidence for an alternative pathway in intrinsic coagulation not requiring Factor XII. Br J Haematol 22:393, 1972.
135. Walz DA, Seegers WH, Reuterby J, McCoy LE: Proteolytic specificity of thrombin. Thromb Res 4:713, 1974.
136. Wessler S, Yin ET: On the mechanism of thrombosis. Prog Hematol 4:201, 1969.
137. White JG: Identification of platelet secretion in the electron microscope. Series Haematologia 6:429, 1973.
138. White JG: Interaction of membrane systems in blood platelets. Am J Pathol 66:295, 1972.
139. Wiggins RC, Bouma BN, Cochrane CG, Griffin JH: Role of high-molecular weight kininogen

in surface-binding and activation of coagulation Factor XI and prekallikrein. Proc Natl Acad Sci (USA) 74:4636, 1977.

140. Wight TN: Vessel proteoglycans and thrombogenesis. Prog Hemost Thromb 5:1, 1980.

141. Wilner GD, Nossel HL, LeRoy EL: Activation of Hageman factor by collagen. J Clin Invest 47:2608, 1968.

142. Zucker MB, Peterson J: Serotonin, platelet factor 3 activity and platelet aggregating agent released by adenosine diphosphate. Blood 30:556, 1967.

143. Zucker MB, Mosesson M, Broekman M, Kaplan KL: Release of platelet fibronectin (cold-insoluble globulin) from alpha granules induced by thrombin or collagen: Lack of requirement for plasma firbronectin in ADP-induced platelet aggregation. Blood 54:8, 1979.

2
Clinical Approach to the Patient with Hemorrhage

Disorders of hemostasis are numerous and penetrate all areas of pathophysiology and clinical medicine; in addition, although many disorders of hemostasis are straightforward and simple, many are multifaceted and extremely complex in pathophysiology, diagnosis, and management. Disorders of hemostasis can be conveniently compartmentalized into hereditary and acquired, with acquired defects being much more common than hereditary defects. All hereditary and acquired defects can further be compartmentalized into defects of the vasculature, platelets, or coagulation proteins. In general, the inherited defects of hemostasis tend to be simple, confined to one hemostasis compartment, and commonly to one coagulation protein, especially in most cases of coagulation protein disorders. In constrast, acquired disorders of hemostasis tend to be multifaceted in etiology and in pathophysiology and involve more than one coagulation factor and in many instances tend to involve several or all of the hemostatic compartments. With a patient with a bleeding disorder or a bleeding history, a systematic and logical approach to diagnosis is imperative. My approach is outlined in this chapter.

History Taking

In obtaining a medical history from the patient the chief complaint is traditionally elicited first by asking the patient to summarize the reasons for referral. In addition, exactly who found this condition and the date the condition was found is imperative. It is also important to find out if any therapy was rendered for the condition; often a patient will be sent for evaluation of a hemostatic problem after having recently been transfused with whole blood, fresh frozen plasma, or other blood components, thus altering laboratory manifestations. Therefore the initial encounter with the patient should involve briefly describing the problems in as precise a manner as possible. Next, the patient should be queried about any and all other medical conditions that have been diagnosed and are currently being treated. Especially a specific drug history is of extreme importance and all drugs (and doses) that are regularly or previously ingested by the patient should be elicited and recorded. Specific attention should be paid to aspirin, aspirin-containing compounds, antihypertensives, cough medications, digitalis preparations, hormones, cortisone, diabetic medications, thyroid medications, narcoleptics, analgesics, weight-reducing medications, anticoagulants, phenytoin, diuretics, antibiotics, barbiturates, tranquilizers, oral contraceptives, or any type of antidepressant.

A thorough medical history should be taken, including childhood illnesses, such as mumps, measles, chickenpox, rheumatic fever or scarlet fever, as well as other illnesses such as coronary artery disease, heart disease of any type, hypertension, diabetes, emphysema, recurrent bronchitis, recurrent pneumonia, asthma, tuberculosis, herpes zoster, hepatitis, peptic ulcer disease, liver disease, jaundice, renal disease, hives, venereal disease, anemia, seizures, or mental disease. In addition, a thorough history should be taken with respect to the type of past bleeding the patient has experienced, especially if it has occured spontaneously. For example, careful inquiries should be instituted regarding the development of petechiae or purpura, to find out if bruises are spontaneous or accounted for, and to find out if there has been a childhood history of epistaxis, umbilical stump bleeding, gingival bleeding with toothbrushing, or easy and spontaneous bruising during earlier years. A thorough surgical history should also be taken and in this context the association of bleeding or the necessity of blood transfusions should be elicited for each surgical procedure. Information regarding dental extraction and associated bleeding or the necessity of transfusions should be elicited. When obtaining this history the patient should also be specifically questioned regarding a transfusion reaction or any type of untoward experience occuring with respect to transfusions. It may be anticipated that the patient, if truly demonstrating a bleeding problem, may require some type of transfusion in the future. The patient should be asked about serious injuries or accidents, especially those that have required hospitalization and the presence of, and nature of, any particular associated bleeding. The patient should be subjected to a careful allergic history, especially allergies to any medications.

Next, a specific review of systems should be obtained, including the type, site, and severity of any type of bleeding problems , and the development of any mucosal membrane bleeding, such as gastrointestinal bleeding, genitourinary bleeding, hemoptysis, or blood-tinged sputum. A past history of any type of deep tissue bleeding, including intracranial hemorrhage, intra-articular or deep muscle bleeding, is obtained. The patient should also be asked about complaints of generalized weakness, chills, drenching night sweats, weight loss, loss of appetite, unexplained fevers, unexplained skin rashes, with an exact description of any rashes, poorly healing sores, or enlarging moles. The patient should be asked about frequent, recurrent, or localized headaches, dizziness, or the loss of consciousness. A history regarding blurred vision, double vision, or persistent scotomata, tinnitus, hearing loss or sore tongue is also important. Additionally, the patient should

be asked about the wearing of dentures, frequent upper respiratory infections, difficulty in swallowing, or any unexplained hoarseness. A history of cervical pain, supraclavicular or cervical adenopathy, chronic cough, coughing spells, shortness of breath, paroxysmal nocturnal dyspnea, orthopnea, angina-type chest pain, the presence of intermittent or persistent tachycardia and palpitations, and the presence of or persistence of ankle edema should be noted. A history of preprandial or postprandial epigastric distress, epigastric pain, nausea, emesis, hematemesis, melena, hematochezia, or any changes in bowel habits within the past 6 months should be recorded. A history of hematuria, pyuria, frequency, urgency, renal disease, renal stones, or port wine colored urine is also obtained. The presence or absence of joint pain, back pain, or bone pain should be documented and the precise areas noted.

In the female patient, the age of beginning menstruation, the age of first pregnancy, and the presence or absence of continued menses and of menopause, including the year menopause occurred, should be recorded. A careful history with respect to the degree and length of menstrual periods is of key importance. The prior ingestion of oral contraceptives, the presence or absence of excessive vaginal discharge, recurrent vaginal infections, intramenstrual bleeding, or the noting of nodules, discharge, or irritation of the breasts should also be elicited. The number of pregnancies and any potential or real bleeding problems in any of her children that may have been manifested at childbirth, spontaneously, or in association with surgery should be elicited at this point. In addition, the patient should be asked if she bled unusually during delivery and whether blood transfusions were required. In the male patient, a history of difficulty in urination, history of prostatic disease, and of circumcision, including the presence or absence of unusual bleeding with circumcision, should be noted.

With respect to a personal history, it is of obvious importance to ask the patient about the use of tobacco, and the amount and form of tobacco use. An ethanol history is also often difficult to take, but needs to be defined precisely in the patient with a potential or real disorder of hemostasis. This should include the type of alcohol and the daily amount ingested. Questions regarding special diets or food fadism should also be carefully elicited because the patient may be potentially nutritionally deficient, including vitamin K deficiency. A careful occupational history, especially with respect to exposure to radiation, industrial toxins, pesticides, benzene, carbon tetrachloride, lead, or any other potentially marrow-damaging agents should be recorded.

A very careful family history including the birth date, birthplace, status of health of the parents or, if dead, the age they died and the cause of death should be recorded. In addition, the patient should be carefully asked about any bleeding tendencies in the mother, father, or any siblings. Since many inherited disorders are sex-linked and may skip several generations, a careful history regarding bleeding tendencies in maternal and paternal grandparents, aunts, uncles, and cousins should also be obtained. If married, the general health of the spouse should be recorded. Of more importance, however, is to inquire regarding the general health of the patient's children. If the bleeding history in children is negative, the patient should be specifically asked if any of the children have been stressed by surgery or trauma. A family history of cerebrovascular disease, hypertension, tuberculosis, diabetes mellitus, thyroid disease, gout, arthritis, coronary artery, heart, pulmonary, peptic ulcer and renal disease, chronic inflammatory conditions, or anemia should be elicited. It is again stressed that the clinician should carefully query the patient about any type of bleeding tendency in any immediate or remote family members. At the end of eliciting a complete history, the clinician should summarize and ask the patient if there are any additional points of information that the patient wishes to impart.

Physical Examination

Once the history is obtained, a careful and thorough physical examination is performed; at times the physical examination will be preferentially directed by data elicited in the history. First, the vital signs of the patient should be noted and recorded, including the right brachial blood pressure, pulse rate and regularity, respiratory rate, temperature, weight, height, and body surface area. During this time, a careful general inspection of the patient is performed to obtain a clue regarding the general health. A general inspection of the patient will usually immediately demonstrate changes associated with chronic illness, including sallow skin, tenting of the skin, loss of subcutaneous supportive tissue, or symmetrical muscle wasting. In addition, careful examination of the entire integumentary system should occur, carefully searching for petechiae, purpura, ecchymoses, nonpulsatile, pinpoint, or nodular telangiectasia, and other signs of a systemic bleeding disorder. In particular, a careful examination of the nail beds, perioral areas, and the sublingual areas are imperative.

Examination of the eyes should include a careful inspection of the vasculature and looking for arteriovenous fistulae, vascular conjunctival abnormalities, bulbar and palpebral conjunctival erythema, petechiae, purpura, telangiectasia, or the presence of bulbar conjunctival icterus. A careful funduscopic examination should also be performed, looking carefully at the vasculature for signs of hemorrhages, exudates, or the formation of arteriovenous fistulae or other abnormalaties. The oral and nasal mucosa should be carefully inspected for signs of localized vascular defects, or the presence of petechiae, purpura, or telangiectasia, patients should also always be asked to remove dentures. It is important to note the presence or absence of lateral papillae and to look under the tongue for sublingual telangiectasia and to inspect the gums for hyperplasia or the presence of petechiae, purpura, or hemorrhagic bullae. In addition, the circumoral area should be inspected for the presence or absence of perioral telangiectasia. Weber and Rinne tests should be done to assess hearing, and the auditory canal should likewise be inspected for any signs of blood or abnormal vascular malformations or the presence of petechiae, purpura, or telangiectasia. The presence or absence of supraclavicular, cervical, and axillary adenopathy as well as epitrochlear, inguinal, and deep iliac adenopathy should next be searched for. Following this, the presence or absence of sternal, cervical, thoracic, or lumbosacral spine tenderness should be assessed.

The chest is next examined to ascertain if it is clear to percussion and auscultation, to demonstrate the presence or absence of rhonchi, localized wheezing or rales, and to document the presence of adequate diaphragmatic excursion bilaterally. Palpation and auscultation of the heart need to be performed carefully, especially listening for murmurs, which may be indicative of a chronic underlying anemia secondary to a hemorrhagic tendency. The carotid and femoral arteries as well as the abdominal aorta should be palpated and auscultated for the presence or absence of bruits. The carotid, brachial, radial, ulnar, femoral, dorsalis pedis, and posterior tibial pulses should be assessed.

The abdominal examination should include careful percussion and palpation of the liver and spleen as well as an attempt to elicit hepatic or splenic tenderness and to auscultate the left upper quadrant for splenic rubs. In addition, bowel sounds should be recorded, the entire abdomen palpated for evidence of any masses, aortic aneurysm, and the presence or absence of direct or indirect inguinal hernias. An examination of the genitalia and rectal examination should be performed in any adult patient with a real or imagined potential bleeding disorder, and the stool should be examined and tested for occult blood.

The extremities are next carefully evaluated, looking for changes in the integument, including petechiae, purpura, or telangiectasia, which may, in some instances, be pinpoint-sized and require the use of a magnifying glass. While inspecting the integument, the fingernail and toenail beds should be carefully inspected for underlying petechaie, purpura, (splinter hemorrhages) and telangiectasia. Any vascular malformations of the skin should likewise be noted and recorded. While inspecting the extremities and integument, the presence or absence of muscle wasting, chronic hemosiderin deposits, especially in the lower extremities, or any changes compatible with varicosities, or chronic venous insufficiency, including the presence or absence of ankle edema, should be noted. The presence of chronic hemosiderin deposits should alert one to the potential presence of a chronic longstanding extravasation of blood from the vasculature, which is suggestive of a potential of simple chronic venous insufficiency or, alternatively, a longstanding quantitative or qualitative platelet defect, or a vascular defect affecting either the small or large vessels, or both.

The neurologic examination is usually performed last and should consist of a general assessment of the cerebrum and cerebellum as well as the eliciting of the presence of biceps, triceps, brachioradialis, patellar, and Achilles tendon reflexes. Vibratory sensation, two point sensation and pinpoint sensation of the lower extremities should be tested. Information regarding function or dysfunction of cranial nerves II through XII will have been gathered in previous portions of the examination.

Often, the presence or absence of a disorder of hemostasis can be documented with at least 90% accuracy with the presence of a careful history and physical examination, which should allow for categorization of the type of defect present before subjecting the patient to selected laboratory testing procedures. Once the type of bleeding is carefully delineated, the clinician will usually have a specific diagnosis or several diagnoses in mind, and numerous others will have been ruled out. Also, at this time, the clinician will have a relatively good idea as to whether this is a hereditary or acquired hemostasis disorder, and whether the disorder involves the vasculature, the platelets, or the blood protein system, or alternatively, is a multiple hemostatic compartment defect (for example, DIC-type syndromes). With this clinical impression the clinician then orders appropriate laboratory tests.

Laboratory Tests

Laboratory testing should always be strongly directed by the initial clinical impression or impressions. Laboratory tests of hemostasis are not only numerous, but also extremely expensive and a tremendous amount of time, money, and effort can be wasted unless the laboratory investigation of a disorder of hemostasis is directed by initial clinical impressions and the working diagnosis. In this capacity, laboratory screening tests for compartmentalizing a specific type of defect can be performed using five simple tests: a platelet count, template bleeding time evaluation of the peripheral blood smear, a prothrombin time, and a partial thromboplastin time. Often all of the screening tests will not be needed and only tests appropriate to one particular hemostatic compartment will be necessary. If these are negative, of course, other hemostatic compartments are then evaluated. In the vast majority of situations the eliciting of a careful history and the performance of a careful physical examination and then the conceptualization of a working diagnosis followed by the ordering of specific laboratory tests to confirm or rule out the diagnosis will almost always lead to a correct diagnosis and to define the severity of the defect suspected.

Thus, it should be strongly emphasized that the approach to a patient with a potential or real bleeding disorder must be logical, sequential, and preceded by a careful clinical evaluation of the patient rather than the haphazard ordering of numerous laboratory tests of hemostasis. If a strong working diagnosis is not suggested by the history or physical examination, the aforementioned laboratory screening tests may be needed to define carefully the hemostatic compartment or compartments housing the defect. If a vascular or platelet defect is present, the template bleeding time will usually be prolonged. The finding of a prolonged template bleeding time or aspirin tolerance test with a normal platelet count suggests platelet or vascular dysfunction. The aspirin tolerance test will help distinguish between a questionable or borderline template bleeding time when there is a strongly suggestive history. In addition, a careful examination of the blood smear, often neglected by clinicians, is paramount and may reveal findings suggestive of an associated blood dyscrasia, including leukemia, leukocytosis, schistocytosis, reticulocytosis, or other underlying conditions to account for the hemostatic defect. In this regard it must be recalled that up to 50% of patients with acute leukemia may initially present with easy and spontaneous bruising and petechiae and purpura. In addition, during a careful evaluation of the blood smear, platelet morphology and number should be noted. If the template bleeding time is prolonged, and the platelet count is normal, one cannot differentiate between a platelet function defect and a vascular defect; therefore a platelet aggregation or lumiaggregation test should be performed to differentiate between a platelet function defect and a vascular defect. If a clinically significant coagulation protein abnormality is present, either the prothrombin time, activated partial thromboplastin time, or both, will be prolonged. In multiple compartment defects, such as disseminated intravascular coagulation with secondary fibrinolysis, numerous tests of hemostasis may be abnormal, including the prothrombin time, the partial thromboplastin time, the template bleeding time, the platelet count, and platelet aggregation. Primary fibrinolytic syndromes will present with the same findings, except that platelets may be normal in number. More sophisticated techniques for establishing specific differential diagnoses from the laboratory standpoint are found in appropriate chapters.

Bleeding due to a vascular disorder may require a very careful clinical and laboratory evaluation to uncover an underlying primary disease, such as Cushing's syndrome, scurvy, an allergic vasculitis, or malignant paraprotein disorder. If no primary disease can be found, the template bleeding time, and platelet function studies will help to define the vascular nature of a disorder. In this regard it should be noted that the template bleeding time should never be performed when there is obvious bleeding or obvious thrombocytopenia, since unnecessary bleeding may occur. Since the template bleeding time and aspirin tolerance test may be abnormal in other than vascular disorders, further studies are necessary to establish the diagnosis and specifically to differentiate a vascular disorder from a platelet function defect. When initial screening tests suggest a platelet disorder, a platelet count must be performed. If low, the bone marrow should next be examined if the cause of thrombocytopenia is not obvious. If the platelet count is normal, however, platelet aggregation studies need to be performed to help define the qualitative abnormalities of platelets that are most likely present.

As previously mentioned, clinically significant coagulation factor abnormalities are almost always diagnosed from the initial prothrombin time or partial thromboplastin time. The ability to perform these assays by totally automated instrumentation utilizing premeasured small amounts of reagents has greatly enhanced their accuracy and convenience for use by physicians in private practice as well as in outpatient facilities. Reagents, however, should be carefully chosen. Several recent comparative studies have shown that some commercial reagents do not perform adequately as screening tests of hemostasis. The interpretation of abnormal laboratory parameters is discussed in appropriate chapters along with each disease category in this text.

Comments

A simple and workable approach to a patient with a bleeding disorder is always to think of the hemostasis system as being comprised of three compartments: the vasculature, the platelets, and the coagulation proteins. Generally, for normal hemostasis to occur all three of these compartments must be intact. Platelets must be normal in both number and function and coagulation proteins must be quantitatively and qualitatively normal. Often a defect in only one hemostatic compartment can be corrected by overcompensation of the other two compartments and clinically significant bleeding may or may not ensue. For example, disruption of the vasculature, as in minor trauma or surgery, may not lead to pathologic bleeding if platelet number and function and coagulation proteins are intact and function to overcome this insult. Commonly, abnormalities in two of the three hemostatic systems must be present for significant pathologic bleeding to occur. It should be recalled that persons with hemophilia often do not bleed (coagulation protein abnormality) unless another of the hemostatic compartments is disrupted, for example, the vasculature is interrupted by surgery or trauma, thus, inducing a defect in two of the three hemostatic compartments. Once one can discern which compartment or combination of compartments contains a defect, a thorough evaluation of this compartment can then be carried out from both the clinical and laboratory standpoint.

If the patient has petechiae and purpura, one can assume that the vasculature or platelets (either number or function) are at fault. Petechiae and purpura almost never arise from coagulation protein disorders alone. Thus, platelet function defects, thrombocytopenia, and vascular defects are most commonly characterized by petechiae and purpura, easy and spontaneous bruising, gingival bleeding with toothbrushing, and mild to moderate mucosal membrane bleeding. Alternatively, single or multiple coagulation protein abnormalities are usually manifested by deep tissue bleeding including intra-muscular, intra-articular, and intracranial bleeding in association with moderate to severe mucosal membrane bleeding and the development of large subcutaneous ecchymoses. A careful history should pinpoint a family or personal history of bleeding, and the type, site, and severity of bleeding that has occurred. Obviously, patients should be thoroughly questioned about drugs for the detection of drug-induced platelet dysfunction, thrombocytopenia, or vascular defects. Drugs interfering with these functions are listed in detail in appropriate chapters.

Probably no area of laboratory medicine is more confusing to the clinician than the field of hemostasis. Rapid growth in the understanding of hemostasis and blood proteins involved with hemostasis, the superfluity in terminology, the potpourri of techniques purported to measure the same factors, and the mystique of reagents used, such as "thromboplastin" and "activators," serve to compound this confusing state of affairs. Even to the present time, there is still no general agreement on such a routine procedure as a prothrombin time, despite more than three decades of international committee meetings. Tables 2–1, 2–2, and 2–3, classify the bleeding disorders according to pathogenetic mechanisms and outline laboratory screening procedures that will permit a systematic approach to the categorization of most bleeding disorders. Although a bleeding disorder can usually be defined without the aid of laboratory screening tests—only a careful history and physical examination—the diagnosis needs to be confirmed and the severity of the defect delineated by the use of appropriate laboratory testing modalities. However, the selection and interpretation of these tests should always be predicated on the basis of major clinical data solicited by the history and physical examination. Although a complete history should be taken, particular emphasis should be directed toward the family history, and drug ingestion (obvious or surreptitious).

A history of obstetrical and surgical events associated with unusual bleeding requires a search for defects in hemostasis. Vascular defects are usually asso-

Table 2–1   Classification of Bleeding Disorders

Vascular Disorders
Hereditary
Acquired
Drug-induced
Platelet defects
Quantitative
Hereditary
Acquired
Qualitative
Hereditary
Acquired
Drug-induced
Coagulation factor disorders
Hereditary
Single factor
Multiple factors (rare)
Acquired
Single factor (rare)
Multiple factors
Multiple compartment defects
Disseminated intravascular coagulation-type syndromes
Primary fibrinolysis syndromes
Hypercoagulability and thrombosis
Usually multiple causes

Table 2–2   Screening Tests of Hemostasis

Platelet count
Blood smear evaluation
Template bleeding time
Prothrombin time
Activated partial thromboplastin time

Aspirin Tolerance test.

ciated with easy and spontaneous bruising, petechiae, and purpura, which are usually dependent and mild to moderate bleeding from mucous membranes. Alternatively, platelet defects although also associated with easy and spontaneous bruising and mild to moderate mucosal membrane bleeding, are usually associated with petechiae and purpura that are symmetrical rather than dependent. In contrast, the blood protein defects rarely, if ever, present as petechiae and purpura, but are usually associated with large subcutaneous ecchymoses, moderate to severe mucosal membrane hemorrhage, and deep tissue bleeding. Thrombocytopenias, hereditary or acquired, are discussed in Chapter 4 and may be due to

Table 2–3 Screening Test Result Versus Compartment at Fault

	Vascular Function	Platelet Function	Platelet Number	Coagulation Proteins
Platelet Count	Normal	Normal	Abnormal	Normal
Template Bleeding Time	Abnormal	Abnormal	Abnormal	Normal
Prothrombin Time	Normal	Normal	Normal	Normal or abnormal
Activated partial thromboplastin time	Normal	Normal	Normal	Normal or abnormal

bone marrow failure, maturation or metabolic defects, and peripheral platelet loss. However, it should also be recognized that more commonly bleeding may be due to platelet dysfunction, either hereditary or acquired. Coagulation protein abnormalities whether hereditary or acquired may result from absent, decreased, or abnormal synthesis of a clotting factor, or the development of antibodies against these factors.

In liver disease or a suspected drug-induced bleeding (particular antibiotics) a therapeutic trial of vitamin K may prove useful in selected patients. In life-threatening situations, specific hemotherapeutic agents may be necessary to establish the diagnosis as well as to manage the hemorrhage. For example, the use of prothrombin complex concentrates in selected clinical situations in which a diagnosis is strongly suspected but not yet confirmed and bleeding is so severe that laboratory confirmatory evidence cannot be waited for.

The recognition of inhibitors to specific clotting factors has increased in recent years, and these are discussed in appropriate sections of this text. These may develop in up to 10% of hemophiliac patients but also occur in postpartum females, in autoimmune disorders, and in association with other well-defined disease entities. Occasionally they may occur spontaneously with no obvious associated condition. Patients with most acquired defects, including both disseminated intravascular coagulation type syndromes and primary fibrinolytic syndromes, and with chronic liver disease will harbor multiple coagulation factor abnormalities as well as multiple hemostatic compartment-type defects. After knowing the underlying disease process, the laboratory evaluation of such patients should be guided by knowing the type of hemorrhagic syndromes that occur in selected clinical disorders. Additionally, in our decade of polypharmacy, drug-induced bleeding must be considered, the classic example being aspirin ingestion. However, a host of other drugs, alone or in combination, may induce bleeding tendencies and not always by the same mechanisms. Drugs should be suspected when one or more defects can be demonstrated, without other obvious cause, and should especially be suspected when the discontinuation of medication causes hemostasis tests to return to normal.

Summary

Careful initial clinical evaluation of the patient, including a carefully solicited history and a carefully performed physical examination, are the mainstay of diagnosis in the patient with a suspected or real hemorrhagic disorder. After this is performed, an initial clinical impression or working diagnosis is formulated and is usually correct in up to 90% of patients. After the formulation of a working diagnosis or initial impression, laboratory testing procedures, carefully selected and based on the logical and sequential clinical evaluation of the patient, are selectively ordered to document the presence or absence of the defect and to delineate its severity. In this regard a simple screening battery to assess all hemostasis compartments consists of a peripheral blood smear evaluation, platelet count, template bleeding time, prothrombin time, and activated partial thromboplastin time.

3

Vascular Disorders Associated with Thrombohemorrhagic Phenomena

Petechiae and purpura are hallmark findings of vascular disorders (Table 3–1). In addition, patients with vascular disorders may complain of mild to moderate mucosal membrane bleeding, often manifested as bilateral epistaxis, gastrointestinal bleeding, or genitourinary bleeding. Patients will usually relate a history of easy and spontaneous bruising as well as gingival bleeding with toothbrushing. Many normal individuals experience occasional gingival bleeding with toothbrushing; however, if the gums bleed almost daily with toothbrushing, a vascular or platelet defect is highly likely. An additional clinical clue to the presence of a vascular disorder is the finding of petechiae and purpura that are dependent, i.e., primarily found on the extremities and absent from the torso. This is usually, but not always, a characteristic of vascular bleeding; platelet defects are typically associated with symmetrical petechiae and purpura found on the extremities and torso.[7–9] Figure 3–1 demonstrates an individual with marked petechiae and purpura.

The presence of a vascular disorder is usually documented in the hemostasis laboratory; however, once established, a definitive diagnosis usually requires other types of laboratory procedures, such as special biopsies and staining.[26,27] The primary laboratory screening test for a vascular disorder or a platelet function defect is the standardized template bleeding time, which has replaced the Rumpel-Leede tourniquet test, a once popular test that had too many false positive results. A standardized template bleeding time is usually not performed in young individuals, especially infants and children younger than 15 years; a normal range has not been established for this age group and undue scar formation may be ex-

pected in this population. In addition, prolonged bleeding times in children are common and therefore difficult, if not impossible, to interpret. In these instances the petechiometer test should be resorted to; the petechiometer will be discussed in subsequent sections.

If an individual demonstrates a borderline template bleeding time, i.e., in the 10 to 12 minute range in conjuction with a positive or suggestive history, the aspirin tolerance test is then performed.[10] This test consists of giving a patient 600 mg of aspirin and repeating the template bleeding time in the opposite antecubital fossa 2 hours later. The results in normal persons will be prolonged by approximately 2 to 3 minutes; however, the ingestion of aspirin will unmask an underlying vascular or platelet function defect and render a bleeding time approximately three times the baseline reading, usually 20 to 30 minutes. Once an abnormal template bleeding time, abnormal petechiometer test, or an aspirin tolerance test has been noted in the appropriate clinical setting, with a normal platelet count, the differential diagnosis is then between a platelet function defect or a vascular defect. To make this differential diagnosis, platelet function testing must be performed. Platelet adhesion was advocated in the past, but is no longer used in most modern laboratories. Platelet retention (adhesion) by the glass bead column technique is of historical interest, but of doubtful clinical relevance.[38,57] Therefore the best testing modality is platelet aggregation to numerous aggregation reagents, as will be discussed. Once an abnormal template bleeding time or abnormal petechiometer test has been noted, in conjunction with a prolonged aspirin tolerance test when appropriate, with normal platelet function

Table 3–1 Clinical Findings of Vascular Disorders

Petechiae
Purpura
Mucosal membrane bleeding
  Epistaxis
  Gastrointestinal
  Genitourinary
History of easy and spontaneous bruising
Gingival bleeding with toothbrushing
Petechiae and purpura usually dependent

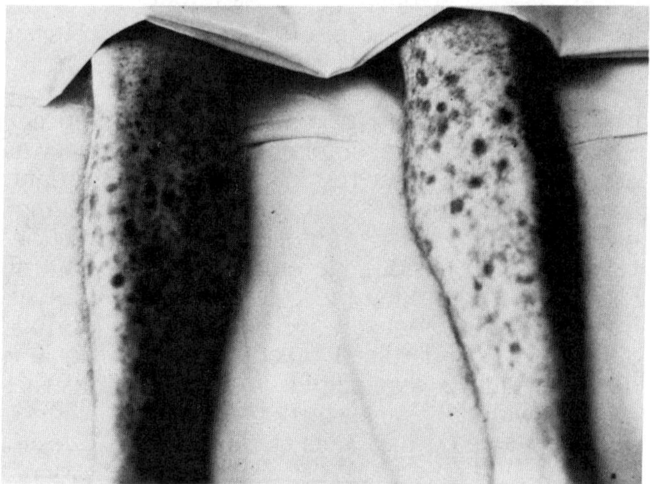

Fig. 3–1. Petechiae and purpura.

as defined by platelet aggregation, a vascular disorder is most likely. Once a vascular defect has been documented, more definitive tests, including an evaluation for autoimmune disease, paraprotein disorders, possibly a connective tissue or vascular biopsy, or other similar modalities will often be needed to make a definitive diagnosis.

Laboratory Findings in Vascular Defects

Table 3–2 summarizes the laboratory evaluation of vascular defects, including both older and newer methods.[11] The Duke bleeding time, the Ivy bleeding time (nonstandardized Ivy bleeding time) and

Table 3–2 Laboratory Evaluation of the Vasculature

Old Methods	New methods
Duke bleeding time	Template bleeding time
Ivy bleeding time	Aspirin tolerance test
Tourniquet test	Petechiometer test (children)
Definitive tests	
Platelet lumiaggrega-tion	Cryoglobulins
Autoimmune investi-gation	Cold Agglutinins
	Thromboxane assays
Paraprotein investi-gation	Prostacyclin assays
	Tissue plasminogen-activator assay
Vascular biopsy and immunofluorescent staining	

the tourniquet test have been abandoned by most laboratories. Newer methods available are the standardized template bleeding time,[52] and aspirin tolerance test[66] (which is only performed when there is borderline or a slightly prolonged template bleeding time, in the presence of a suggestive history), or alternatively the petechiometer test in younger individuals. More definitive tests needed after documenting the probable presence of a vascular disorder are platelet aggregation to rule out a platelet function defect as the cause of a prolonged bleeding time.

Figure 3–2 depicts the popular Simplate II or double-bladed standardized template bleeding time device commonly used. Figure 3–3 illustrates the template as originally described by Mielke and co-workers;[52] this device consists of a blade holder (right) holding two no. 11 Bard-Parker blades, and the template (left). The device is built so that resultant cuts are exactly 1 mm deep and 9 mm long. I have given up the use of these autoclavable devices, because residue develops in the template wells making the cuts less and less deep. I now exclusively use the Simplate II standardized bleeding time device, which is less painful and is associated with less scar formation than the nondisposable devices. Cuts made by the

Simplate II are shown in Figure 3–4. The cuts should always be made cephalocaudad and should never be made horizontally, or across the arm. There are several reasons for this; most clinical studies establishing normal and abnormal ranges for the standardized template bleeding time have utilized cuts made in the cephalocaudad direction. In addition, the natural skin lines are cephalocaudad, and consequently if cuts are made across the arm, prolonged template bleeding times may result and more scar formation will occur. Many laboratories have been reluctant to perform template bleeding times because of the invasive nature of the test and potential scar formation. Significant scar formation can easily be avoided with attention to proper technique. Attention must be directed to correct bandaging for prevention of scars. After completion of the template bleeding time, a butterfly bandage should be placed over the cuts (Figs. 3–5 and 3–6), barely opposing the two cut edges and being careful not to pinch the skin, and the patient is instructed to remove the dressing 24 hours later. The patient should always be questioned about a family or personal history of keloid formation and if present a template bleeding time should not be performed, or the potential scars accepted. In summary, with correct technique and correct bandaging, after the template bleeding time test, very few adult patients will be left with significant scars.

The petechiometer is an alternative to template bleeding times in children, older individuals, or patients with a personal or family history of keloid formation. A popular petechiometer is shown in Figure 3–7. This device applies a defined amount of suction to the skin, petechiae develop, and the number of petechiae formed are then recorded. Figure 3–8 depicts an easy manner in which the petechiae can be counted after being created by the suction device. This is accomplished by laying a glass microscope slide over the suction area. Zero to 10 petechiae per cm^2 after 50 cm vacuum for 60 seconds are considered normal. When more than 10 petechiae per cm^2 develop, there is strong evidence for a vascular (or platelet) defect.

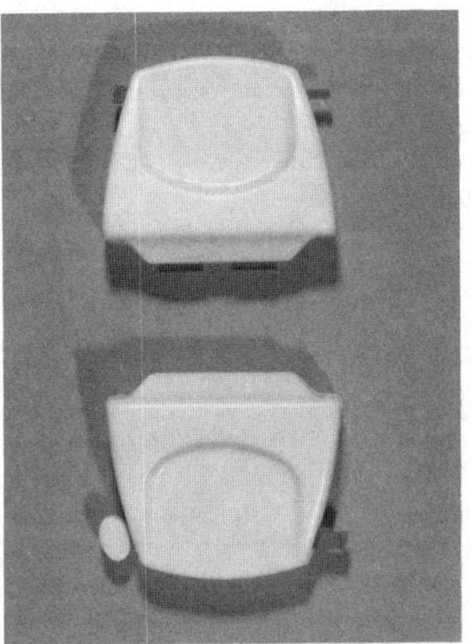

Fig. 3–2. The Simplate II standardized template bleeding time.

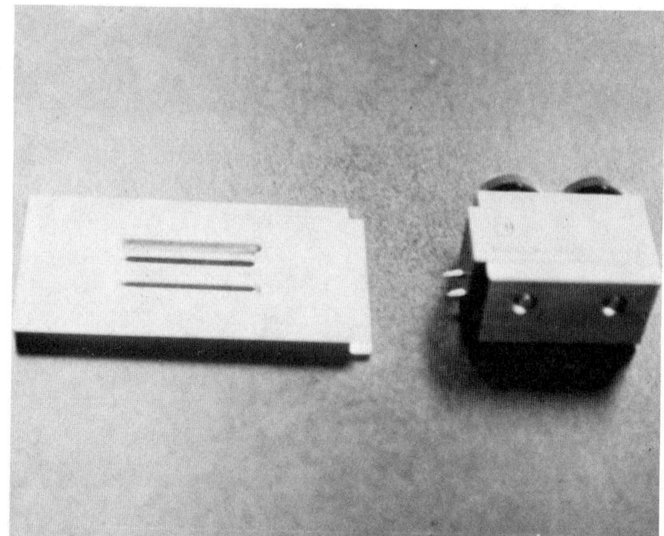

Fig. 3–3. Autoclavible non-disposable template bleeding time.

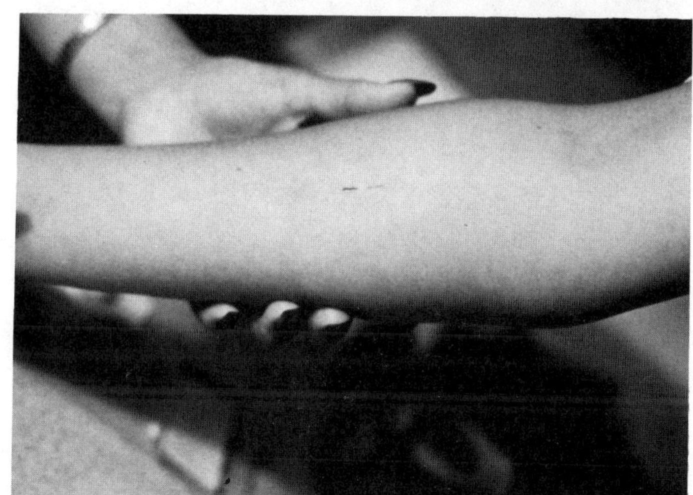

Fig. 3–4. Duplicate cuts made by the Simplate II device.

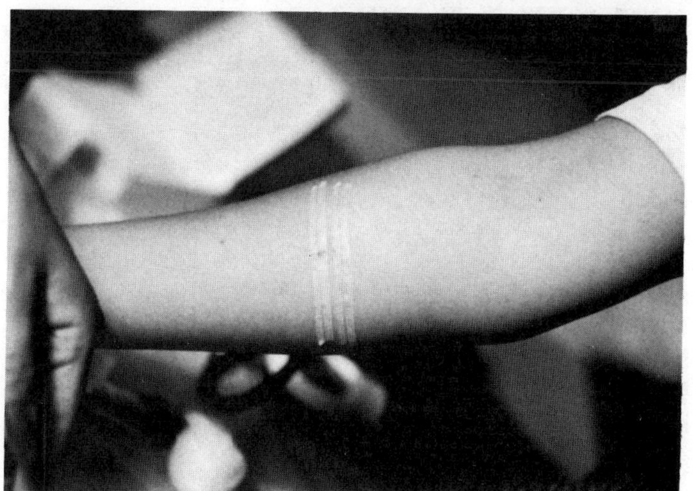

Fig. 3–5. Initial dressing of the template bleeding time cuts.

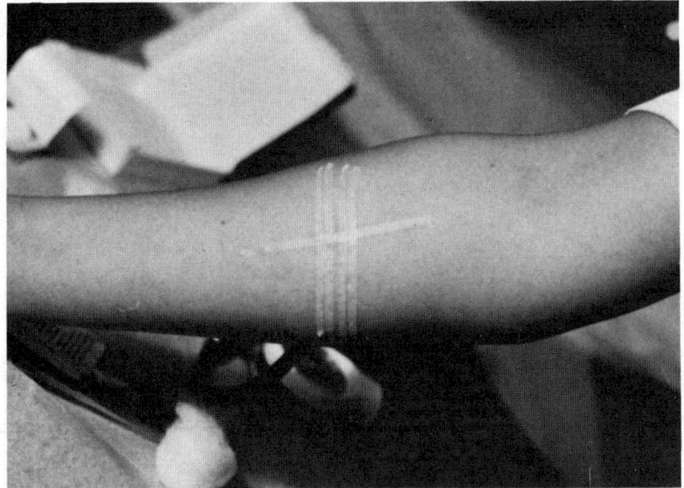

Fig. 3–6. Final dressing of the template bleeding time cuts.

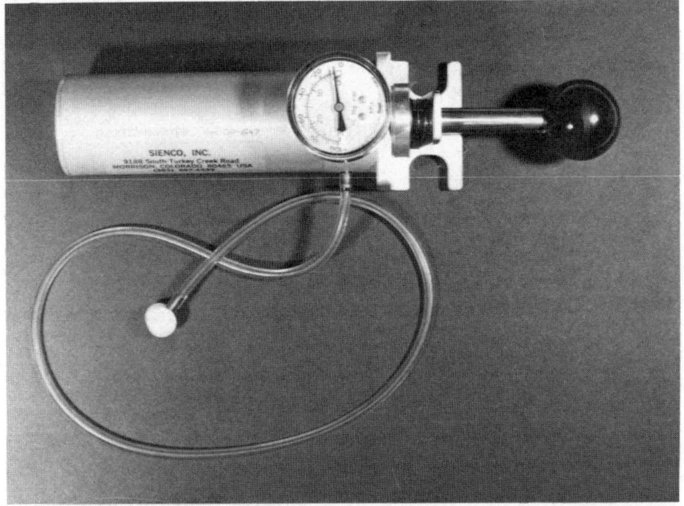

Fig. 3–7. A popular petechiometer.

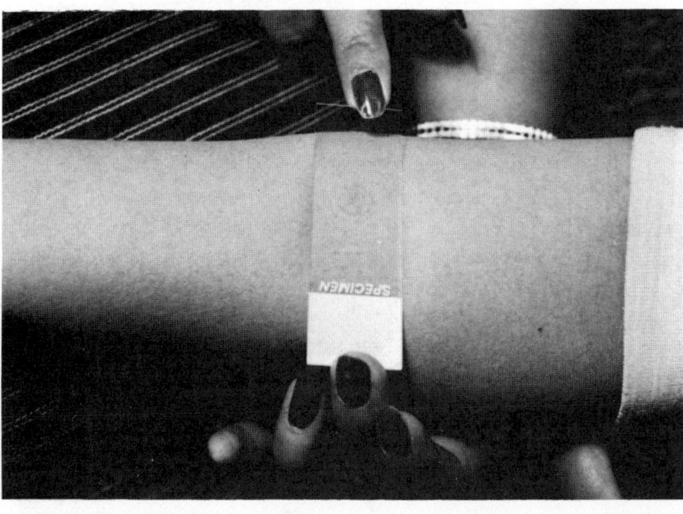

Fig. 3–8. Reading of the petechiometer test results.

Clinical Aspects of Vascular Disorders

Vascular disorders are best categorized as the hereditary vascular disorders, the acquired vascular disorders, and drug-induced vascular disorders, (Table 3–3). The hereditary vascular disorders primarily consist of the hereditary collagen vascular diseases and most are clinical oddities. The one exception to this rarity is that of Osler-Weber-Rendu disease, or hereditary hemorrhagic telangiectasia (HHT) which is quite common. Alternatively, the acquired vascular disorders are very common and all clinicians should be familiar with them. The importance of becoming familiar with acquired vascular disorders is severalfold: When a patient presents with dependent petechiae and purpura, and easy or spontaneous bruising, the patient should be evaluated for any one of the acquired vascular disorders. In addition, if the patient has one of the acquired disorders associated with vascular defects and is going to be subjected to surgery or sustains trauma, it should be assumed the patient has a systemic vascular disorder that may lead to clinically significant thrombohemorrhagic problems.

Vascular disorders may present in bizarre and varied ways. Determinants of varied clinical presentations are summarized in Table 3–4. Firstly, there are numerous potential host responses to a vascular disorder. For example, there may be simply an antigenic response, there may be activation of the coagulation system only, activation of the fibrino(geno)lytic system only, activation of kinins only, activation of complement only, or any combination of these activation pathways may occur. In addition, there are varied severities of a vascular insult, injury, or disorder. A mild vascular insult or disorder will usually lead to serum effusion only, which will clinically be interpreted as bullae and erythema. However, if the insult is more moderate, serum and blood may effuse from the vasculature, giving rise to bullae, erythema, and wheals in association with petechiae and purpura. If the insult is severe, there will not only be effusion of blood, but also endothelial cell death, and petechiae and purpura and gross hemorrhage, often in the form of large ecchymoses in association with small or large vessel thrombosis, will be noted. When the host responses to a vascular disorder overlap with the degree of severity of the vascular disorder or insult, it is appreciated how many seemingly similar vascular disorders may present with such varied clinical findings.

Table 3–3 Vascular Disorders

Hereditary vascular disorders
  Ehlers-Danlos syndrome
  Marfan's syndrome
  Osteogenesis imperfecta
  Pseudoxanthoma elasticum
  Cystathionine beta-synthase deficiency
  Hereditary hemorrhagic telangiectasia
Acquired vascular defects
  Collagen vascular disease
  Cushing's syndrome
  Macroglobulinemia
  Multiple myeloma
  Amyloidosis
  Allergic purpuras
  Circulating immune complex
  Autoerythrocytic sensitization
  Drug-induced vascular defects

Table 3–4 Determinants of Clinical Manifestations in Vascular Disorders

Host response to vascular disorder or injury
  Antigenic response
  Activation of coagulation
  Activation of fibrinolysis
  Activation of kinins
  Activation of complement
  Activation of other enzymes
  Leukocyte migration
Severity of vascular disorder or injury
  Mild
    Serum effusion: bullae and erythema
  Moderate
    Serum and blood effusion: bullae, erythema, wheals, and petechiae and purpura
  Severe
    Effusion of blood and endothelial cell death: petechiae and purpura
    Gross hemorrhage
    Thrombosis

Hereditary Vascular Disorders

The hereditary vascular disorders will be discussed separately (Table 3–5). The following are the most common hereditary vascular (or collagen-vascular) disorders that may present as thrombotic, hemorrhagic, or mixed disorders of hemostasis and thrombosis.

Ehlers-Danlos Syndrome

The Ehlers-Danlos (ED) syndrome is a rare connective tissue disorder that is inherited by autosomal dominance.[42] Interestingly, one of the earliest descriptions of this syndrome may have concerned the violin virtuoso Paganini, in that this disorder was thought to contribute to his remarkable dexterity and talent. The ED syndrome is characterized by extreme vascular fragility, skin fragility, hypermobile joints, and molluscoid pseudotumors of the knees and elbows. Bleeding may be highly variable; however, easy and spontaneous bruisability is a hallmark of this syndrome. Patients commonly have gingival bleeding with toothbrushing and undue bleeding after dental extraction. Also, petechiae, purpura, gastrointestinal bleeding, and hemoptysis are often present. The bleeding diathesis may be severe enough to suggest hemophilia. In addition, some patients may have associated platelet function defects as well as the characteristic vascular defects.[71] Other characteristics commonly noted in this syndrome are blue sclerae and angioid streaks. In addition, aortic insufficiency and the "floppy" mitral valve syndrome often occur. The common laboratory findings are a positive Rumpel-Leede tourniquet test, prolonged template bleeding times, and in many instances abnormal platelet aggregation if the patient has an associated platelet function defect. Basic pathologic of the ED syndrome is poorly understood but appears to represent a decrease in collagen and an increase in elastic tissue. In addition, the collagen from these patients is thought to have an abnormal amino acid composition.[64] A prolonged template bleeding time is classically present. Characteristics of ED syndrome are summarized in Table 3–6.

Marfan's Syndrome

This syndrome is well described and is the most popularized of the hereditary collagen vascular disorders. It is inherited as an autosomal dominant trait and is characterized by skeletal defects (markedly long extremities and arachnodactyly), cardiovascular abnormalities (ascending aortic aneurysm or dissection) and ocular defects, primarily manifested as ectopia lentis.[2,32] In addition, hyperextensible joints are present. Of all the hereditary collagen vascular disorders, Marfan's syndrome is least characterized clinically by a hemorrhagic diathesis. However, many patients have easy and spontaneous bruisability, and some may demonstrate a poorly characterized platelet function defect as

Table 3–5 Hereditary Vascular Disorders

Ehlers-Danlos syndrome
Marfan's syndrome
Osteogenesis imperfecta
Pseudoxanthoma elasticum
Cystathionine beta-synthase deficiency (homocystinuria)
Giant cavernous hemangiomas (Kasabach-Merritt syndrome)
Hereditary hemorrhagic telangiectasia

Table 3–6 Ehlers-Danlos Syndrome

Clinical Features	Laboratory Features
Autosomal dominant	Prolonged template
Vascular fragility	bleeding time
Skin fragility	
Easy bruising	
Spontaneous bruising	Some with abnormal
Gingival bleeding	platelet function
Dental bleeding	(storage pool)
Petechiae and purpura	
Gastrointestinal hemorrhage	
Hemoptysis	
Blue sclerae	
Angioid streaks	
Molluscoid pseudotumors	
Aortic insufficiency	
Floppy mitral value syndrome	

well. A prolonged template bleeding time may be present (Table 3–7).

Osteogenesis Imperfecta

Osteogenesis imperfecta (brittle bones and blue sclerae) is also one of the more common hereditary collagen vascular disorders and is inherited as an autosomal dominant trait. The disorder is characterized by a patchy lack of bone matrix. However, the matrix that does exist undergoes normal calcification. Osteogenesis imperfecta is clinically manifested as deformed and brittle bones that fracture easily. In addition, skin and subcutaneous hemorrhages are characteristic.[2] Death commonly occurs in childhood, due to intracranial hemorrhage caused by an abnormal calvarium coupled with a vascular hemorrhagic diathesis. Easy and spontaneous bruisability, hemoptysis, epistaxis, and intracranial bleeding are common in osteogenesis imperfecta. An abnormal template bleeding time and a positive Rumpel-Leede tourniquet test are characteristic.[75] In addition, many cases have been described with abnormal platelet function as defined by aggregation studies. The basic pathophysiology of osteogenesis imperfecta appears to be related to the inability of reticulin to mature into collagen. In addition, the collagen present demonstrates an abnormal amino acid composition. Characteristics of this syndrome are summarized in Table 3–8.

Table 3–7 Marfan's Syndrome

Clinical Features	Laboratory Features
Autosomal dominant	Prolonged template
Easy bruising	bleeding time
Spontaneous bruising	
Ectopia lentis	
Hyperextensible joints	Some with abnormal
Ascending aortic	platelet function
aneurysm	(storage pool)
Dissecting aortic	
aneurysm	
Arachnodactyly	
Systemic clinical bleed-	
ing very rare	

Table 3–8 Osteogenesis Imperfecta

Clinical Features	Laboratory Features
Autosomal dominant	Prolonged template
Easy bruising	bleeding time
Spontaneous bruising	
Skin and subcutaneous	
hemorrhage	Some with abnormal
Epistaxis	platelet function
Hemoptysis	(storage pool)
Intracranial hemor-	
rhage	
Death common at birth	
from central nervous	
system bleeding	
Patchy lack of bone	
matrix	
Deformed and brittle	
bones	

Pseudoxanthoma Elasticum

Pseudoxanthoma elasticum, unlike the other hereditary vascular diseases, often does not become manifest until the second or third decade in life.[65] This very rare disorder is inherited as an autosomal recessive trait. This syndrome is commonly characterized by significant hemorrhage, since abnormal elastic fibers affect the entire arterial system. Hemorrhage can occur in any organ, most commonly the skin, eyes, kidneys, and gastrointestinal tract. These patients have a marked tendency to easy and spontaneous bruisability and commonly are noted to have petechiae and purpura and a marked predisposition to thrombosis, especially cerebrovascular thrombosis, acute myocardial infarction, and peripheral vascular occlusion, with resultant gangrene and loss of extremities. Other clinical characteristics include relaxed, inelastic, and redundant skin in facial, neck, axillary, orbital, and inguinal areas. Hyperkeratotic plaques develop in these areas and subcutaneous calcinosis is also common. Death is frequently caused by gastrointestinal hemorrhage. Excessive uterine bleeding and intra-articular bleeding with formation of characteristic hemarthroses are common. The basic vascular pathologic state of this disorder is poorly understood, but is thought to be due to metabolic (enzyme) defects in elastic fibers (Table 3–9).

Homocystinurea

Homocystinurea is a rare inborn error of metabolism, inherited as an autosomal recessive and demonstrating molecular heterogeneity.[54] Patients have decreased levels of cystathionine beta-synthase leading to characteristic homocystinemia, methioninemia, and homocystinuria. Patients characteristically demonstrate ectopia lentis, varying degrees of mental retardation, and skeletal deformities, including osteoporosis with resultant biconcave vertebrae, scoliosis, and pes cavus.[82] Striking and unusual vascular changes are noted. Histologically, significant fibrosis of the intima and frayed muscle fibers in the media of arteries are found. Additionally, venous changes include fibrous changes as well. Clinically, patients demonstrate arterial and venous thrombi, with carotid artery thrombosis being a common occurrence. Both large and small arteries and veins may be involved with thrombosis and resultant occlusions. In addition, widespread atheromatous changes occur in patients at an early age.[20]

Table 3–9 Pseudoxanthoma Elasticum

Clinical Features	Laboratory Features
Autosomal recessive	Prolonged template
Significant hemorrhage	bleeding time
Mucosal membrane bleeding	
Intraocular hemorrhage	
Intra-articular hemorrhage	Some with abnormal platelet function (storage pool)
Petechiae and purpura	
Easy bruising	
Spontaneous bruising	
Death most common from gastrointestinal hemorrhage	
Becomes manifest in 2nd to 3rd decade	
Relaxed, inelastic, redundant skin in facial, neck, axillary and inguinal areas	
Hyperkeratotic plaques	
Subcutaneous calcinosis	

Homocystine-induced endothelial cell toxicity with resultant patchy endothelial cell sloughing and subsequent platelet-induced intimal proliferation of smooth muscle media cells, thus leading to atheroma formation, is the proposed pathophysiologic mechanism. The disease may be managed, and complications somewhat aborted, by treatment with large doses of pyridoxine; thrombotic manifestations have been successfully controlled with combination platelet suppressive therapy consisting of dipyridamole and aspirin.

Giant Cavernous Hemangiomas and the Kasabach-Merritt Syndrome

Hemangiomas are usually congenital, although they may not become clinically obvious until the patient is several years old. They are more common in females and may be of three types: capillary, cavernous, or capillary-cavernous mixtures.[19] Cavernous forms are less common than capillary types, but are more often associated with systemic thrombohemorrhagic problems. Cavernous hemangiomas are benign vascular tumors consisting of dialated thin wall vessels and sinuses lined by endothelium that is most likely abnormal. The most common sites of involvement are the gastrointestinal tract, bones, liver, and integument of the face and neck as well as various mucosal membrane surfaces, including the oral mucosa.[1] Hemangiomas of the extremities may often involve the skin, subcutaneous tissue, and adjacent bone. Numerous thrombi may form in these cavernous hemangiomas; however, of more importance, many of these individuals will develop a local or disseminated intravascular coagulation syndrome (DIC). The association of giant cavernous hemangiomas and DIC is referred to as the Kasabach-Merritt syndrome, after two investigators who originally noted this association.[43] The DIC may be chronic, but frequently progresses to an acute form.[41] Some patients develop a life-threatening acute DIC with attempted surgical resection of these hemangiomatous masses.

Other patients develop DIC spontaneously.

DIC can often be controlled with heparin, usually delivered subcutaneously; however, occasionally local radiation therapy or injections of sclerosing agents have been reported to be beneficial.[25] Steroids may also be of benefit in decreasing the size of hemangiomatous lesions. When seeing patients with giant cavernous hemangiomas, appropriate laboratory evaluation to determine the presence or absence of DIC (chronic or acute) should be instituted, because the occurrence of DIC may significantly alter morbidity or mortality and the clinician may wish to consider appropriate prophylactic therapy for chronic DIC, in the form of low-dose heparin or platelet suppressive therapy. Certainly any patient with giant cavernous hemangiomatous lesions who is being considered for corrective surgery should be evaluated for DIC, and the DIC syndrome corrected before surgery is performed. Additionally, these patients should be carefully monitored for DIC postoperatively. A patient with the Kasabach-Merritt syndrome is shown in Figure 3–9. This patient developed a fulminant DIC in association with attempts to resect bothersome areas of the hemangiomatous lesions. In this particular individual, the use of subcutaneous heparin controlled life-threatening hemorrhage.

Hereditary Hemorrhagic Telangiectasia

HHT (Osler-Weber-Rendu disease) is a relatively common disorder and, in fact, is the most common hereditary vascular disorder leading to a hemorrhagic diathesis.[36,59,60] The disorder is inherited as an autosomal dominant but only 70% of individuals have a positive family history. The homozygous state is thought to be lethal. In addition, there is evidence that the gene responsible for HHT is somehow linked to blood group O. The hallmark characteristic of this disease is epistaxis, which may be profuse and usually begins in early childhood. The classic telangiectatic lesions of HHT may not appear until later in life, commonly the second or third decade. The classic diagnostic triad of HHT is: a hereditary basis, telangiectasia, and bleeding from telangiectatic lesions. Chronic blood loss, commonly from the gastrointestinal or genitourinary tracts, is often severe enough to be manifested as a significant iron deficiency anemia of unknown etiology.

The telangiectatic lesions of HHT can be of three types: pinpoint, nodular, and spiderlike.[61] Unlike telangiectasia associated with chronic liver disease, those of HHT are nonpulsatile. Telangiectasia and bleeding usually increase with advancing age, although epistaxis often de-

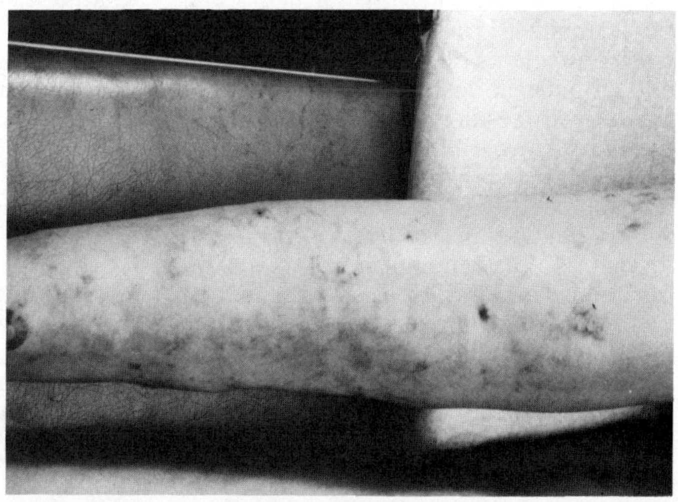

Fig. 3–9. The Kasabach-Merritt syndrome.

creases with age. The bleeding of HHT may be occult, but common causes are gastrointestinal hemorrhage, genitourinary hemorrhage, hemoptysis, or heavy menstrual flow, and approximately 20% of patients develop arteriovenous fistulae of the lungs.[39] In addition, there is an inordinately high incidence of Laennec's type cirrhosis occurring in these patients. Hamartomas of the liver and spleen may also be associated with HHT.[28] The basic pathophysiology of this disorder is poorly understood. Most studies have shown that elastic fibers are missing from the vascular walls. There are few characteristic laboratory findings in HHT. The tourniquet test and template bleeding time may be normal or abnormal, depending on the integrity of the vascular wall in the particular area where the test is performed. The diagnosis is suggested by a history of recurrent bilateral epistaxis, occult gastrointestinal bleeding, and the noting of pinpoint, nodular, or spiderlike telangiectasia, most commonly found in the skin, in sublingual areas, in the buccal mucosa, under the nails, or perioral.

HHT appears to be closely associated with other defects in hemostasis, such as abnormal platelet function.[12,67] A poorly defined defect in the fibrinolytic system may also occur in these patients.[49,73] Of major importance, and often unrecognized, is that many patients with HHT have an associated classic DIC type of syndrome. This is usually present in a chronic form but periodically may become acute. This is found in approximately 40 to 50% of patients with HHT, if searched for.[13,14] In some patients bleeding may be severe enough that spontaneous intra-articular bleeds with resultant hemarthroses may develop. Thus, HHT may be somewhat similar to the syndrome of giant cavernous hemangiomas and DIC, resulting in a "mini-Kasabach-Merritt syndrome," although, as already mentioned, this is often not recognized. When this occurs, treatment should be aimed at acute or chronic DIC. Characteristics of HHT are listed in Table 3-10.

Therapy of uncomplicated HHT depends on the particular clinical situation and the age of the patient. Localized epistaxis can often be controlled with local supportive measures and vasoconstrictive nasal sprays. However, electrocauterization may become necessary. Most instances of troublesome bleeding in HHT, such as gingival bleeding with toothbrushing, spontaneous bruising, and gastrointestinal or genitourinary bleeding, can often be controlled with carbazochrome.[80] This agent is usually used in a dosage of 5 to 10 mg orally every 3 to 4 hours during waking hours and is without significant toxicity. High-dose estrogens may be used to scarify telangiectatic lesions and control bleeding. However, this modality should be used as a last resort, especially in younger patients.[45]

Specific therapy for significant bleeding associated with congenital vascular defects, other than HHT, is generally not satisfactory and depends primarily on supportive measures and control of the underlying disease process. A patient with HHT and typical lesions in shown in Figure 3-10. Figure 3-11 depicts a biopsy of a nodular telangiectatic lesion; note the dialated thin-walled vessels. The hereditary collagen vascular disorders are depicted in Table 3-5.

Table 3-10 Hereditary Hemorrhagic Telangiectasia

Clinical Features	Laboratory Features
Autosomal dominant	Template bleeding
70% with family history	time variable
Epistaxis in childhood	
Occult bleeding	
common	Findings of DIC in 50%
Classic triad of	
Telangiectasia	
Hereditary	Platelet dysfunction
Hemorrhage	in 50%
Hamartomas of liver	
and spleen	
Pulmonary arteriovenous fistulae	
Laennec's-type	
cirrhosis	
Bleeding improves	
with age	
Telangiectasias increase with age	
Platelet dysfunction	
in 50%	
Chronic DIC in 50%	

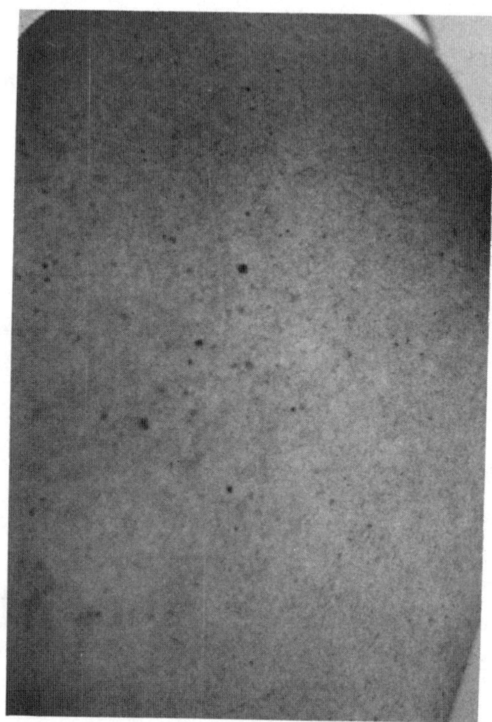

Fig. 3–10. Hereditary hemorrhagic telangiectasia.

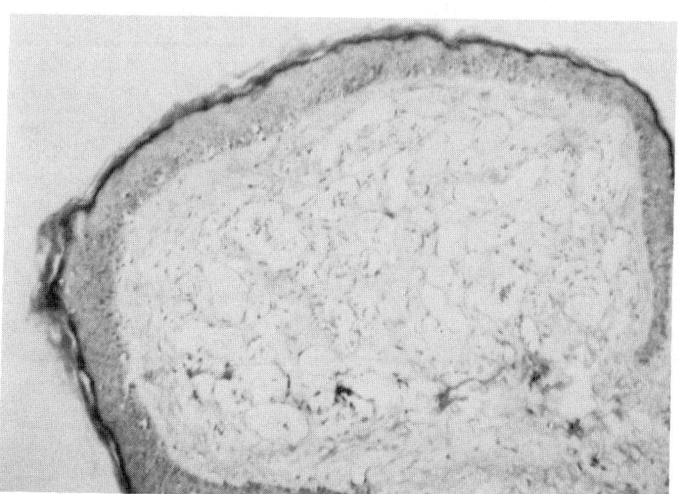

Fig. 3–11. Biopsy of a nondular telangiectatic lesion.

Acquired Vascular Defects

The common acquired vascular defects are summarized in Table 3–11. It is important to be familiar with these because they are quite common. A patient presenting with easy and spontaneous bruising, petechiae, and purpura, especially dependent, and other suggestive historical and physical findings should be suspected of having, and be evaluated for, the disorders associated with an acquired vascular defect. Alternatively, if a patient has one of these disorders and is going to have surgery or is involved in trauma, it can be assumed that a vascular defect is likely to be present and significant thrombotic or hemorrhagic problems may be encountered. The common acquired diseases that are associated with systemic vascular problems and that may lead to systemic hemorrhagic problems include the collagen vascular disorders, circulating immune complex disorders, multiple myeloma, Waldenstrom's macroglobulinemia, cryoglobulinemia, amyloidosis, Cushing's syndrome, diabetes mellitus, the allergic (Henoch-Schönlein) purpuras, numerous infectious agents, and drug-induced vascular defects.

Table 3–12 depicts several of the mechanisms whereby these vascular defects occur. In the collagen vascular disorders

Table 3–11 Acquired Vascular Disorders

Collagen Vascular Disorders
  Systemic lupus
  Polyarteritis
  Scleroderma
  Rheumatoid Arthritis
  Dermatomyositis
Paraprotein Disorders
  Multiple myeloma
  Macroglobulinemia
  Amyloidosis
  Cryoglobulinemia
Immune complex disorders
Cushing's syndrome
Diabetes mellitus
Allergic purpuras
Infectious agents
Drug-induced

Table 3–12 Mechanisms of Acquired Vascular Disorders

Collagen diseases
  Collagen or connective tissue abnormalities in vascular tissue and perivascular supportive tissue
Cushing's syndrome
  Loss of mucopolysaccharides in perivascular tissue leading to poor vascular support
Paraprotein disorders
  Coating of endothelium by paraprotein, and occlusion of vasa vasorum
Allergic vasculitis
  Immune complex-induced vascular and perivascular damage
Autoerythrocytic sensitization
  Chronic subcutaneous extravasation of red blood cells and eventual allergic reaction to red blood cells
Diabetes mellitus
  Basement membrane thickening with increased porosity, decreased proteoglycans, and increased lipohyaline deposits

the vascular hemorrhagic defect is thought to be due to poor vascular support from the intrinsic collagen abnormality. In Cushing's syndrome it is thought that the vascular disorder and typical hemorrhage occur because of abnormal mucopolysaccharides in the perivascular supporting tissue. In the paraprotein disorders all of the paraproteins, including immunoglobulins A, M, and G (IgA, IgM, IgG), appear to have an affinity for attachment to the vasculature (endothelium) and thus lead to a vascular hemorrhagic problem. This is most commonly noted with IgM and IgG_3 paraproteins. In addition, it is thought that these paraproteins may occlude the vasa vasorum of affected vasculature, again leading to hemorrhagic difficulties. Aspirin is commonly regarded as a platelet function inhibitor; however, aspirin is also a very effective inhibitor of acetylcholine esterase, which leads to a vascular bleeding problem.[68] If a patient is ingesting aspirin and trauma (or microtrauma in the form of a template bleeding time) ensues, vascular bleeding may occur. The usual vascular response to trauma is constriction. With vascular trauma, acetylcholine esterase breaks down the acetylcholine that keeps the vessel dialated; trauma-induced release of catecholamines will then constrict the vessel. If the patient is taking aspirin and the vasculature is severed, acetylcholine esterase is inhibited, acetylcholine cannot be degraded, and inadequate vascular constriction will result. Indeed prolongation of the template bleeding time after the ingestion of aspirin may be due to the vascular rather than platelet inhibitory effect.

Malignant Paraprotein Disorders and Amyloidosis

The numerous thrombotic or hemorrhagic tendencies in patients with malignant paraprotein disorders and amyloidosis, be they primary or secondary, are well recognized. In addition, these disorders can present with a wide spectrum of hemorrhagic or thrombotic tendencies, depending on the host response, size, and site of the vasculature involved, and response of the particular end organ. There have been numerous proposed mechanisms for the vascular complications of malignant paraprotein disorders and only the salient features of most of these mechanisms are discussed here. It has been proposed that increased circulating levels of IgG and IgM, which are complement fixing and thus may lead to histamine release, chemotaxis of leukocytes, and platelet aggregation, may thus lead to increased vascular permeability, serum or blood effusion, and in some instances small vessel thrombosis. Hyperviscosity in the malignant paraprotein disorders is a well-known cause of stasis, with resultant ischemia and acidosis. This will lead to increased vascular permeability, the consequences of which may be retinal hemorrhage and exudates, epistaxis, and petechiae and purpura, as well as hemorrhage into other organs, including vital organs. Frank necrotizing vasculitis may occur via unclear mechanisms in the malignant paraprotein disorders.

Obviously, the clinical manifestations, whether they be thrombosis or hemorrhage, will depend on the site and severity of the necrotizing vasculitis. When the malignant paraprotein disorders are associated with cryoglobulinemia (IgG and IgM paraprotein disorders), paraprotein is commonly found in the walls of the small vessels, which may lead to a frank vasculitis; again, the clinical manifestations obviously range from effusions, bullae, petechiae and purpura, or frank end organ damage (especially glomerulonephritis) to ischemia, cellular death, and end organ failure. In all of the malignant paraprotein disorders there is a high incidence of thrombosis as well, especially manifested as diffuse recurrent deep vein thrombosis, thromboembolism, pulmonary emboli, and renal vein thrombosis.[15,47] The mechanisms leading to this remain unclear, but need not be related to the development of hyperviscosity except in cases of retinal vein thrombosis.[77]

DIC is also often seen in patients with malignant paraprotein disorders. Whether this is due to endothelial damage by paraprotein or by other unexplained mechanisms remains unclear. In addition, the fibrino(geno)lysis that occurs in many individuals with malignant paraprotein disorders is initiated via as yet undefined mechanisms. This may represent fibrinolysis secondary to DIC or to endothelial damage, or alternatively may be due to deranged endothelial plasminogen activator activity.[16]

Amyloidosis further complicates the vascular changes of malignant paraprotein disorders, and thus leads to an increased incidence of hemorrhage and/or thrombosis via disruptions of the vasculature. Classically, primary amyloidosis is associated with an unknown etiology or one of the malignant paraprotein disorders. Primary amyloidosis characteristically involves the skin, tongue, heart, and gastrointestinal tract, whereas secondary amyloidosis is seen with chronic inflammatory or infectious diseases and characteristically involves the liver, spleen, kidney, and adrenal glands. However, many "cross-overs" and mixtures of the two are commonly seen and, in fact, one cannot often precisely define amyloidosis as being primary or secondary. There are numerous proposed mechanisms for vasculitis in patients with primary and secondary amyloidosis, but the precise mechanisms remain unclear. Hemorrhage due to a vascular defect is a classic hallmark of amyloidosis, especially manifested as petechiae and purpura, ecchymoses, easy and spontaneous bruising, along with spontaneous hemorrhage into lymph nodes, recurrent hematuria, and spontaneous hemorrhage into other vital organs. Several proposed pathophysiologic events leading to generalized vasculitis have included antigen-antibody complex-induced endothelial damage or deposits of amyloid on the endothelium as well as in the perivascular areas.[78] Endothelial and perivascular amyloid deposits seem to be more commonly noted in the secondary forms, especially in arterioles. This then leads to a hemorrhagic as well as a thrombotic tendency. In secondary amyloidosis, amyloid deposits are noted along the endothelium, and intimal deposits are noted to start in the intima and to progress to the media, with amyloid being deposited in parallel with reticulum fibers rather than around the collagen fibers, as is more commonly seen in primary amyloidosis. In addition, in primary amyloidosis the deposits are usually seen along the collagen with progression from the adventia to the media of arterioles and veins. The same process appears to occur in veins, thus possibly accounting for the thrombotic tendencies seen in these patients. In some patients with systemic amyloidosis a selective acquired Factor X deficiency has been reported.[33,34,40,46,50,81]

In two patients similarly affected an acquired combined deficiency of Factors IX and X was noted.[50] Furie and associates[31] investigated the mechanisms of Factor X deficiency in such cases by use of ^{131}I-labeled Factor X. It was discovered that a triphasic plasma clearance pattern occurred, so that 85% of the labeled Factor X cleared in less that 30 seconds, about 10% in less than 90 seconds, and the remaining 5% in 10½ hours. Subsequent surface scanning of the patients 24 hours after the labeled infusion showed high concentrations in hepatic and splenic regions. This observation, coupled with the rapid clearance of the label on initial transit in the circulation, led these investigators to conclude that the Factor X is deposited in some cases of systemic amyloidosis at prior tissue sites of amyloid. At first glance, it may seem that these cases

should respond to therapeutic infusions with Factors II, VII, IX, and X concentrates. However, Krause[46] has reported only a transient correction by such preparations of Factor X-deficient cases of amyloidosis. The wide variability of hemorrhagic and thrombotic manifestations in patients with paraprotein disorders and amyloidosis will depend on the particular end organ involved and the degree of vascular permeability or occlusion.

In summary, patients with malignant paraprotein disorders and amyloidosis may develop a diffuse vascular disease that may be manifested as hemorrhage or thrombosis, or both. A high variability of end organ damage may be seen. In dealing with this patient population it is important to recognize that patients may experience significant vascular bleeding, as well as bleeding from obvious other causes when subjected to surgery or trauma. Alternatively, when seeing a patient with a vascular disorder presenting as hemorrhage or thrombosis, malignant paraprotein defects or amyloidosis should be considered in the differential diagnosis. When a selective acquired Factor X deficiency in an adult is found, underlying systemic amyloidosis should be strongly suspected.

Autoimmune Disorders Associated with Thrombohemorrhagic Phenomena

Immunologic diseases associated with circulating immune complexes, especially those associated with circulating cryoglobulins, are of paramount importance as disorders associated with a diffuse vasculitis and resultant thrombosis or hemorrhage. At least three potential mechanisms by which circulating immune complexes, circulating cryoglobulins, or circulating antibodies may lead to vasculitis have been described: the production of an antibody that is directed specifically against the endothelium,[79] which is probably the least common mechanism operative; the production of a nonspecific antibody or immune complex that nonspecifically attacks and damages endothelium as well as other cellular systems;[24] and the generation of an antibody or immune complex that attaches to and damages perivascular tissues (including basement membrane), and secondarily causes endothelial damage and increased vascular permeability. The vascular response and clinical manifestations will depend on severity, duration, and degree of repetition of the endothelial or periendothelial insult and damage.[48] If the attack is mild, then increased vascular permeability, fibrin deposition, and a fibrinolytic response will occur. This will lead to minimal hemorrhage and thrombosis. If, however, the insult is persistent, then there will be excessive endothelial damage, depletion of fibrinolytic enzymes and endothelial fibrinolytic activators, increased fibrin and platelet deposition, more pronounced thrombosis or hemorrhage, and, as a second feature, more enhanced and perpetuated endothelial damage. In yet more severe attacks on the endothelium or surrounding tissue by antibody, immune complex, or cryoglobulins, endothelial death, sloughing, and more severe thrombosis, hemorrhage, and end organ damage may ensue.

As previously mentioned, an antibody directed specifically against the endothelium is a rare mechanism of autoimmune-induced vasculitis and is limited to the allergic purpuras (Henoch-Schönlein) and polyarteritis nodosum.[79] However, further immunologic investigations may, in the future, define other disorders in this class. The other two mechanisms of immune complex-induced vasculitis are much more common and are seen in a wide variety of "autoimmune disorders." In many of these diseases, circulating immune complexes (IgG and IgM) attach to the endothelium, fix complement, and induce migration of leukocytes, which may disintegrate and destroy the vessel.[22] For example, all are familiar with the results of antistreptococcal antibody attaching to the glomerular endothelium or basement membrane, thus giving rise to subsequent renal vascular damage.[30] An extension of this is, of course, Goodpasture's syndrome, in which case antibody or immune complexes are directed against both renal and pulmonary basement membrane with associated resultant endothelial damage and thrombohemorrhagic manifestations.

Many infectious agents are known to be associated on rare occasions with vasculitis and the attendant clinical manifestations aforementioned. These include numerous bacterial, viral, and mycoplasma infections. The mechanisms, when known, include the induction of nonspecific antiendothelial antibody by the invading organism, the inducement of specific antiendothelial antibody by the invading microorganism, and the development of circulating immune complexes.[62-64] These mechanisms were previously described. Table 3–13 lists the most common infectious agents known to be associated with a vasculitis.

In most circulating immune complex diseases the injury is nonspecific and not only the endothelium but many other cellular systems are damaged. Diseases with circulating antibody, immune complex, or cryoglobulin-induced vasculitis are highly varied and include the collagen vascular disorders, drug reactions, serum sickness, and a large group of seemingly unrelated disorders. Table 3–14 summarizes pathophysiologic mechanisms and Table 3–15 lists the most common disorders that fit into this category of acquired diseases associated with circulating immune complex, resultant endothelial damage, vasculitis, and clinical thrombohemorrhagic problems.

Table 3–13 Infectious Agents Associated with Vascular Disorders

Bordetella pertussis
Clostridium tetani
Corynebacterium diphtheriae
Escherichia coli
Pseudomonas aeruginosa
Salmonella typhi
Staphylococcus
Streptococcus
Subacute bacterial endocarditis
Mycobacteria
Coccidioidomycosis
Leprosy
Syphilis
Tuberculosis
Malaria
Chlamydia trachomatis
Cytomegalovirus
Epstein-Barr virus
Hepatitis B virus
Influenza virus

Table 3–14 Pathophysiology of Vascular Damage by Immunologic Mechanisms

Development of a specific antiendothelial cell antibody

Immune complex (IgG and IgM) attachment to endothelium, followed by complement fixation, migration of leukocytes, and disintegration of the vessel

Attachment of immune complex or antibody to perivascular tissue or basement membrane, thus increased vascular permeability or induction of other vascular damage

Table 3–15 Immune Complex Disorders Associated with Vascular Thombohemorrhagic Findings

Collagen vascular diseases
    Lupus erythematosus
    Rheumatoid arthritis
    Dermatomyositis
    Scleroderma
    Polyarteritis
Cryoglobulinemia
Sjögren's syndrome
Glomerulonephritis (proliferative)
Lymphoreticular disorders
Chronic infection or inflammation
Viral infections
Malignant hypertension
Allergic vasculitis
Subacute bacterial endocarditis
Drugs

Malignant Hypertension, Eclampsia, Cushing's Syndrome and Diabetes Mellitus Associated with Thrombohemorrhagic Manifestations

Patients with malignant hypertension, advancing age, or diabetes mellitus deposit lipohyaline material in the subendothelium of arteries and arterioles. In malignant hypertension, fibrinoid necrosis is an additional characteristic feature. As constant unrelenting damage occurs, the vessels eventually develop increased vascular permeability with plasma seepage and fibrin deposition. This leads to thrombosis and thromboembolism, a common clinical manifestation of these disorders.[3] The resultant downstream capillary stasis leads to the development of chronic purpura and local hyperpig-mentation of the skin. The reader is referred to authoratative reviews for more complete pathophysiologic events in these disorders.[27,44,72] The findings in eclampsia are similar to those previously described, with the development of hypertension and localized intravascular coagulation (fibrin deposition) in the placental and renal microcirculation.[53,70] Some women develop classic findings of either chronic or acute DIC with any or all of the attendant clinical manifestations of this secondary syndrome.[17]

The vascular changes of Cushing's syndrome remain poorly defined, but they include loss of subcutaneous elastic tissues leading to poor endothelial cell support, increased vascular permeability and fragility, and the loss of elastic tissue in the vascular walls. In addition, advanced atherosclerotic changes occur in larger vessels in these patients.[29] All are aware of the easy and spontaneous bruising seen in the vast majority of patients with Cushing's syndrome and the marked increase of thrombosis and thromboembolic disease in this patient population. Many patients with Cushing's syndrome may have profuse bleeding when subjected to surgery or trauma.

Behçet's Syndrome

Behçet's syndrome is an ill-defined disorder characterized by a typical triad of aphthous stomatitis, genital ulcerations, and iritis.[5,35] In addition, many patients develop recurrent deep vein thrombosis of unexplained pathophysiologic origin, usually involving large veins, the saphenous veins, and the superior and inferior vena cava.[57] Many of these patients develop a widespread, poorly defined arteritis.[37] Several patients have demonstrated fibrinoid necrosis of the arterial tree.[74] Numerous case reports have documented impaired fibrinolysis and some patients have responded to thrombolytic therapy.[21] With the exception of the finding of impaired endothelial fibrinolytic activity, thus far the pathophysiologic mechanisms for recurrent deep vein thrombosis, arteritis, and hemorrhage, usually manifested as petechiae and purpura, have remained undefined.

Vascular Defects Associated with Cardiopulmonary Bypass

Poorly understood defects in the vasculature may occur during or after cardiopulmonary bypass surgery. A syndrome of mild to moderate nonthrombocytopenic purpura, accompanied by splenomegaly and atypical lymphocytosis following bypass has been noted.[6] In this syndrome, purpura is usually benign, selflimiting, and frequently manifested only after discharge from the hospital. One patient has been reported who developed classic glomerular nephritis of the type seen with the allergic vasculitities. In addition, fatal purpura fulminans may also occur after cardiopulmonary bypass.[18] Thus, an inflammatory vasculitis may be associated with cardiopulmonary bypass; however, the mechanisms remain totally unclear.

Drug-Induced Vasculitis

Drug-induced vasculitis is a common occurrence in clinical medicine, and very often neglected as a cause of petechiae and purpura, skin necrosis, or frank gangrene. There are numerous mechanisms by which drugs may induce vasculitis, and most of these do not significantly differ from the mechanisms depicted when discussing circulating immune complex disorders. In many instances, however, the precise mechanisms by which drugs induce vasculitis are poorly understood. There are at least three mechanisms by which drugs may induce a vascular defect. These include the development of a specific antivessel antibody,[79] the development of circulating immune complexes, in some instances associated with cryoglobulinemia,[23] and, more rarely, drug-induced independent changes in vascular permeability. A characteristic, catastrophic, and well-characterized vasculitis due to warfarin anticoagulants should be familiar to all.[55-58] This particular and common hemorrhagic skin vasculitis is manifested as hemorrhagic skin infarction and in some instances has been associated with intravascular coagulation.[56,58] Virtually all warfarin derivatives

have been incriminated: 90% of cases have been women and gangrene of the breast has occurred in at least 25% of cases reported in the literature. Nalbandian and co-workers[56] have described the histologic features of this syndrome quite well, showing perivascular accumulations of inflammatory cells involving predominantly the venules, with extensive thrombosis of the draining veins and with little or no invasion of arterioles. Typically, the clinical picture develops 3 to 10 days after starting therapy and bears little relationship to the prothrombin time. The proposed mechanism is thought to be a direct toxic effect on the endothelium by warfarin and its derivitives. Many patients are noted to respond to heparin therapy.[56] The most common drugs causing vascular problems are listed in Table 3–16.

Laboratory Testing Modalities

The laboratory screening for a vascular defect is simple and straightforward, although the precise definition of a vascular defect is difficult and often beyond the scope of a hematology-hemostasis laboratory. Table 3–3 depicts older methods, newer methods, and definitive tests available for assessing vascular defects. The older methods, which are no longer used, and the newer methods have been discussed previously. However, it should

Table 3–16 Common Drugs Causing Vasculitis

Acetylsalicylic acid	Iodine
Allopurinol	Isoniazid
Arsenicals	Meprobamate
Chloramphenicol	Methyldopa
Chlorothiazide	Piparazine
Chlorpropamide	Quinidine
Coumadin	Quinine
Digoxin	Reserpine
Estrogens	Sulfonamides
Furosemide	Tolbutamide
Gold salts	Warfarin
Indomethacin	

again be emphasized that the newer tests will not distinguish between a vascular and a platelet function defect. To make this differential diagnostic distinction, platelet aggregation should be performed. If platelet aggregation is normal, with an abnormal template bleeding time, aspirin tolerance test, or petechiometer test, it may be assumed that a vascular defect is present. After this evaluation, the hemostasis laboratory must usually defer the workup to other departments of the laboratory where other tests are considered, such as an autoimmune or paraprotein investigation, possibly a vascular biopsy including immunofluorescent staining, tests for cryoglobulins, cold agglutinins, prostacyclin, and other prostaglandin derivatives, or histochemical evaluations for endothelial fibrinolytic system activators or components. Recently, synthetic substrate assays for tissue (endothelial) plasminogen activator activity have become available.[4,69,83]

Summary

This chapter has summarized the more important disease entities that may be accompanied by or lead to a disorder of hemostasis or thrombosis via alterations of the vasculature. It is to be emphasized that the vascular component of hemostasis is often overlooked by clinicians caring for patients with disorders of hemostasis and thrombosis. It should be appreciated that the vasculature is intricately related to the coagulation protein system and to platelets when involved in a thrombohemorrhagic diatheses.

References

1. Allen PW, Enzinger FM: Hemangiomata of skeletal muscle: analysis of 89 cases. Cancer 28:8, 1972.
2. Anderson M, Pratt-Thomas RH: Marfan's syndrome. Am Heart J 46:911, 1953.
3. Ashton N: The eye in malignant hypertension. Trans Am Acad Ophthalmol Otolaryngol 76: 17, 1972.
4. Bachmann F, Kruithof EKO: Tissue plasminogen activator: Chemical and physiological aspects. Semin Thromb Hemost 10:6, 1984.
5. Behçet H: Uber die rezidivierende Apthose durch ein Virus verursachte geschwure am Mund, am Auge und an den Genitalien. Dermatol Wochenschr 105:1152, 1937.
6. Behrendt PM, Epstein SE, Marrow AG: Postperfusion nonthrombocytopenic purpura: An uncommon sequel of open heart surgery. Am J Cardiol 22:631, 1968.
7. Bick RL: Vascular disorders associated with thrombohemorrhagic phenomena. Semin Thromb Hemost 5:167, 1979.
8. Bick RL: A systemic approach to the diagnosis of bleeding disorders. In Murano G, Bick RL (Eds): Basic Concepts of Hemostasis and Thrombosis. CRC Press, Boca Raton, FL, 1980, p 81.
9. Bick RL: Vascular disorders. In Murano G, Bick RL (Eds): Basic Concepts of Hemostasis and Thrombosis. CRC Press, Boca Raton, FL, 1980, p 89.
10. Bick RL, Adams T, Schmalhorst WR: Bleeding times, platelet adhesion, and aspirin. Am J Clin Pathol 65:65, 1976.
11. Bick RL: Clinical hemostasis practice: The major impact of laboratory automation. Semin Thromb Hemost 9:139, 1983.
12. Bick RL, Fekete LF: Hereditary hemorrhagic telangiectasia and associated defects in hemostasis. Blood 52:179, 1978.
13. Bick RL: Hereditary hemorrhagic telangiectasia and disseminated intravascular coagulation: A new clinical syndrome. Ann NY Acad Sci 370:851, 1981.
14. Bick RL: Hereditary hemorrhagic telangiectasia and disseminated intravascular coagulation. Vasc Surg 15:394, 1981.
15. Bick RL: Acquired circulating anticoagulants and defective hemostasis in malignant paraprotein disorders. In Murano G, Bick RL (Eds): Basic Concepts of Hemostasis and Thrombosis. CRC Press, Boca Raton, FL, 1980, p 205.
16. Bick RL, Klein CA, Fekete LF, Wilson WL: Alterations of hemostasis associated with malignant paraprotein disorders. Trans Am Soc Hematol, p 63, 1976.
17. Bick RL: Disseminated intravascular coagulation. In Murano G, Bick RL (Eds): Basic Concepts of Hemostasis and Thrombosis. CRC Press, Boca Raton, FL, 1980, p 31.
18. Bick RL, Arbegast NR, Comer TP: Fatal purpura fulminans following total cardiopulmonary bypass. J Cardiovasc Surg 14:569, 1973.
19. Burbank MK, Spittell JA: Tumors of blood and lymph vessels. In Juergens JL, Spittell JA, Fairbairn JF (Eds): Peripheral Vascular Diseases. W.B. Saunders, Philadelphia, 1980, p 679.
20. Carey MC, Donovan DE, Fitzgerald O, McAuley

FD: Homocystinuria. I. A Clinical and pathologic study of nine subjects in six families. Am J Med 45:17, 1968.

21. Chajek T, Fainard M: Behcets disease with decreased fibrinolysis and superior vena caval occlusion. Br Med J 1;782, 1973.

22. Cochrane CG: Mediators of the arthus and related syndromes. Prog Allergy 11:1, 1967.

23. Criep LH, Cohen CG: Purpura as a manifestation of penicillin sensitivity. Ann Intern Med 34:1219, 1951.

24. Dixon FJ, Vazques JJ, Weigle WD, Cochrane CG: Pathogenesis of serum sickness. Arch Pathol 65:18, 1958.

25. Edgerton MT: The treatment of hemangiomas: With special reference to the role of steroid therapy. Ann Surg 183:517, 1976.

26. Fairbairn JF: Clinical manifestations of peripheral vascular disease. In Fairbairn JF, Juergens JL, Spittell SA (Eds): Peripheral Vascular Diseases. W.B. Saunders, Philadelphia, 1980, p 3.

27. Farber EM, Hines EA, Montgomery H, Craig W: Arterioles of skin in essential hypertension. J Invest Dermatol 9:215, 1947.

28. Fitz-Hugh T: Splenomegaly and hepatic enlargement in hereditary hemorrhagic telangiectasia. Am J Med Sci 181:261, 1931.

29. Forsham PH: The adrenal cortex. In Williams RL (Ed): Textbook of Endocrinology. W.B. Saunders, Philadelphia, 1968, p 287.

30. Freedman P, Meister NP, Lee HJ, Smith EA, Co BS, Midas BD: The renal response to streptococcal infections. Medicine (Baltimore) 49:433, 1970.

31. Furie B, Green E, Furie BC: Syndrome of acquired Factor X deficiency and systemic amyloidosis. N Engl J Med 297:81, 1977.

32. Futcher PH, Southworth H: Arachnodactyly and its medical complications. Arch Intern Med 61:693, 1938.

33. Galbraith PA, Sharma N, Parker WL, Kilgour JM: Acquired Factor X deficiency. Altered plasma antithrombin activity and association with amyloidosis. JAMA 230:1658, 1974.

34. Glenner GG: Factor X deficiency and systemic amyloidosis. N Engl J Med 297:108, 1977.

35. Haim S, Sobel JD, Freidman-Birnbaum R: Thrombophlebitis and a cardinal symptom of Behcets syndrome. Acta Derm Venereol (Stockh) 54:299, 1974.

36. Hans FM: Multiple hereditary telangiectasia causing hemorrhage (hereditary hemorrhagic telangiectasia). Bull Johns Hopkins Hosp 20:63, 1909.

37. Hills EA: Behcets syndrome with aortic aneurysms. Br Med J 4:152, 1967.

38. Hirsh J: Laboratory diagnosis of thrombosis. In Colman RW, Hirsh J, Marder VJ, Salzman EW (Eds): Hemostasis and Thrombosis: Basic Principles and Clinical Practice. J.B. Lippincott, Philadelphia, 1982, p 789.

39. Hodgsum CH, Kaye RL: Pulmonary arteriovenous fistula and hereditary hemorrhagic telangiectasia. Dis Chest 43:449, 1963.

40. Howell M: Acquired Factor X deficiency associated with systematized amyloidosis—report of a case. Blood 21:739, 1963.

41. Inceman S, Tangun Y: Chronic defibrination syndrome due to a giant hemangioma associated with microangiopathic hemolytic anemia. Am J Med 46:997, 1969.

42. Johnson SA, Falls EF: Ehler-Danlos syndrome: A clinical and genetic study. Arch Dermatol (Suppl) 60:82, 1949.

43. Kasabach HH, Merritt KK: Capillary hemangioma with extensive purpura. Am J Dis Child 59:1016, 1940.

44. Kazmier FJ, Didisheim P, Fairbanks VF, Ludwig J, Payne WS, Bowie EJW: Intravascular coagulation and arterial disease. Thromb Diath Haemorrh (Suppl) 36:295, 1969.

45. Koch HJ, Escher GL, Lewis JS: Hormonal management of hereditary hemorrhagic telangiectasia. JAMA 149:1376, 1952.

46. Krause JR: Acquired Factor X deficiency and amyloidosis. Am J Clin Pathol 67:170, 1977.

47. Lachner H: Hemostatic abnormalities associated with paraprotein abnormalities. Semin Hematol 10:125, 1973.

48. Markowitz AS, Lang CF: Streptococcal related glomerulonephritis. J Immunol 92:565, 1964.

49. McDervitt TJ, Toh AS: Epistaxis: Management and prevention. Laryngoscope 47:1109, 1967.

50. McPherson RA, Onstad JW, Vgoretz RT, Wolf PL: Coagulopathy in amyloidosis: Combined deficiency of Factor IX and X. Am J Hematol 3:225, 1977.

51. Meyer D, Zimmerman TS: von Willebrand's disease. In Coleman RW, Hirsh J, Marder VJ, Salzman EW (Eds): Hemostasis and Thrombosis: Basic Principles and Clinical Practice. J.B. Lippincott, Philadelphia, 1982, p 64.

52. Mielke CH, Kaneshiro MM, Maher LA, Rappaport SI: The standardized normal Ivy bleeding time and its prolongation by aspirin. Blood 34:204, 1969.

53. Morris RN, Vassalli P, Beller FK, McCluskey RT: Immunofluorescent studies of renal biopsies in the diagnosis of toxemia of pregnancy. Obstet Gynecol 24:32, 1964.

54. Mudd SH, Levy HL: Disorders of transsulfuration. In Stanbury JB, Wyngaarden JB, Fredrickson DS, Goldstein JL, Brown MS (Eds): The Metabolic Basis of Inherited Disease. McGraw-Hill, New York, 1983, p 522.

55. Nalbandian RM, Mader IJ, Barrett JL, Pierce JF, Rupp EC: Petechiae, ecchymoses, and necrosis of skin induced by coumarin cogeners. JAMA 192:603, 1965.

56. Nalbandian RM, Beller FK, Hamp AK, Henry RL, Wolf PL: Coumarin necrosis of the skin treated successfully with heparin. Obstet Gynecol 38:395, 1971.
57. Nazzarro P: Cutaneous manifestations of Behcets disease: Clinical and histological findings. Proceedings of the International Symposium on Behcets Disease. S. Karger, Basel, 1966, p 15.
58. Nudelman HL, Kempson RL: Necrosis of the breast: A rare complication of anticoagulant therapy. Am J Surg 111:728, 1966.
59. Osler W: On multiple hereditary telangiectasia with recurrent hemorrhages. Q J Med 1:53, Oct., 1907.
60. Osler W: On telangiectasia circumscripta universalis. Bull Johns Hopkins Hosp 12:33, 1901.
61. Osler W: On a family form of recurrent epistaxis associated with telangiectasia of the skin and mucous membranes. Bull Johns Hopkins Hosp 12:333, 1901.
62. Parish WE: Studies on vasculitis: I. Immunoglobulins, beta-1-C, C-reactive protein, and bacterial antigens in cutaneous vasculitis lesions. Clin Allergy 1:95, 1971.
63. Parish WE: Studies on vasculitis: II. Some properties of complexes formed of antibacterial antibodies from persons with or without cutaneous vasculitis lesions. Clin Allergy 1: 111, 1971.
64. Pinnell SR, Krane SM, Kenzora J, Glincher MJ: A new heritable disorder of connective tissue with hydroxylysine-deficient collagen. N Engl J Med 286:1013, 1972.
65. Polimer IJ: Pseudoxanthoma elasticum and gastrointestinal hemorrhage. J Maine Med Assoc 58:76, 1967.
66. Quick AJ: Salicylates and bleeding: The aspirin tolerance test. Am J Med Sci 252:265, 1966.
67. Quick AJ: Telangiectasia. In Quick AJ (Ed): Hemorrhagic Diseases and Thrombosis. Lea & Febiger, Philadelphia, 1966, p 285.
68. Quick AJ: Hemostasis then and now. In Quick AJ (Ed): The Hemorrhagic Diseases and the Pathology of Hemostasis. Charles C Thomas, Springfield, IL, 1974, p 3.
69. Ranby M, Norrman B, Wallen P: A sensitive assay for tissue plasminogen activator. Thromb Res 27:743, 1982.
70. Robboy SJ, Mihm MC, Coleman RW, Minna JD: The skin in disseminated intravascular coagulation: Prospective analysis of 36 cases. Br J Dermatol 88:221, 1973.
71. Roberts HR, Kroncke FG: Tests of platelet activity: Application to clinical diagnosis. In Brinkhous KM, Shermer RW, Mostofi FK (Eds): The Platelet. Williams & Wilkins, Baltimore, 1971, p 365.
72. Ryan TJ: The investigation of vasculitis, In Ryan TJ (Ed): Microvascular Injury. W.B. Saunders, Philadelphia, 1976, p 333.
73. Ryan AJ: Control of bleeding in familial telangiectasia. Meriden Hosp Bull 7:1, 1958.
74. Sakuri M, Miyaji T: Behcets disease from the point of view of vascular pathology. Folia Ophthalmol Jpn 22:903, 1971.
75. Seibel BM, Briedman IA, Schwartz SO: Hemorrhagic disease in osteogenesis imperfecta: Studies of platelet function defect. Am J Med 22:315, 1957.
76. Snapper I: Neurological complications. In Snapper I, Kahn A (Eds): Myelomatosis. University Park Press, Baltimore, 1971, p 226.
77. Snapper I: Amyloidosis. In Snapper I, Kahn A (Eds): Myelomatosis. University Park Press, Baltimore, 1971, p 238.
78. Stefanini M, Mednicoff IB: Snapper I: Amyloidosis. In Snapper I, Kahn A (Eds): Myelomatosis. University Park Press, Baltimore, 1971, p 238.
79. Stefanini M, Mednicoff IB: Demonstration of antivessel antibodies in serum of patients with anaphylactoid purpura and polyarteritis nodosa. J Clin Invest 33:967, 1954.
80. Stitch MH: Carbazochrome salicylate therapy in hereditary hemorrhagic telangiectasia. NY State J Med 59:2725, 1959.
81. Triplett DA, Bang NU, Harms CS, Benson MD, Miletich JP: Mechanisms of acquired Factor X deficiency in primary amyloidosis. Blood 50:285, 1977.
82. Valle D, Pai GS, Thomas GH, Pyeritz RE: Homocystinuria due to cystathionine beta-synthetase deficiency: Clinical manifestations and therapy. Johns Hopkins Med J 146:110, 1980.
83. Wiman B, Mellbring G, Ranby M: Plasminogen activator release during venous stasis and exercise as determined by a new specific assay. Clin Chim Acta 127:279, 1983.

4
Platelet Defects

The common clinical findings of qualitative or quantitative platelet defects are petechiae and purpura, mild to moderate mucosal membrane bleeding, and a history of easy and spontaneous bruisability.[34] In addition, gingival bleeding with toothbrushing is a common clinical manifestation of platelet dysfunction or thrombocytopenia.[35] As was emphasized in Chapter 3, gingival bleeding with toothbrushing can be a normal finding if it occurs occasionally; however, if a patient reports gingival bleeding with toothbrushing numerous times per week, then the platelet function defect, thrombocytopenia, or vascular defect is likely. In platelet function defects or thrombocytopenia, petechiae and purpura are usually symmetrical, i.e., found throughout the integumentary system on the extremities as well as the torso. This is in distinction to the noting of dependent petechiae and purpura, which are more commonly associated with vascular disorders.[36] Clinical findings of platelet defects are summarized in Table 4–1. Typical petechiae and purpura are depicted in Figure 4–1.

Table 4–2 lists traditional tests of platelet number and function, especially the older tests. New methods of assessing molecular markers of platelet reactivity and other modalities to assess platelet function will be discussed. Firstly, and extremely important in assessing platelets, is careful evaluation of a peripheral blood smear for a quantitative estimation of the number of platelets present and an evaluation of platelet morphology. This is an often neglected simple modality performed in the hemostasis laboratory, and certainly the peripheral blood smear should be carefully evaluated in patients presenting with easy or spontaneous bruising or petechiae and purpura. Many clinical clues may be obtained from an evaluation of platelet morphology, such as noting abnormal granularity in the gray platelet syndrome, the large platelets and borderline thrombocytopenia of Bernard-Soulier syndrome, or the noting of many "large bizarre platelets" or young platelets indicative of rapid platelet turnover and decreased platelet survival. An examination of a peripheral blood smear may actually lead to the specific diagnosis accounting for petechiae and purpura or easy bruising, for example, an acute or chronic leukemia. In addition, a quantitative platelet count should always be performed, for only with a normal platelet count can a platelet function defect be defined.[35] In the past, platelet adhesion in glass bead columns by a wide variety of techniques has been utilized to assess platelet function. However, experience with this technique has been far less than satisfactory and the procedure should not be used, for although of clinical curiosity and historical interest, it is unreliable and has no clinical relevance.[174,248]

The standardized template bleeding time is the primary screening test for platelet function and vascular function[37,251] (Fig. 3–2). Once a normal platelet count is documented with a suggestive or positive history, consisting of a history of petechiae, purpura, easy and spontaneous bruising, the differential diagnosis is between a vascular defect and a platelet function defect, both of which will usually cause prolongation of the standardized template bleeding time.[35,38,250] The reasons for using the standard petechiometer in children were discussed in Chapter 3 (Fig. 3–7). Thus, template bleeding times are used to screen for a platelet function or vascular defect in adults and the petechiometer test is used

Table 4–1 Clinical Findings in Platelet Defects

Petechiae
Purpura
Mucosal membrane bleeding (epistaxis, gastrointestinal, genitourinary)
History of easy and spontaneous bruisability
Gingival bleeding with toothbrushing
Symmetric petechiae and purpura (usually)

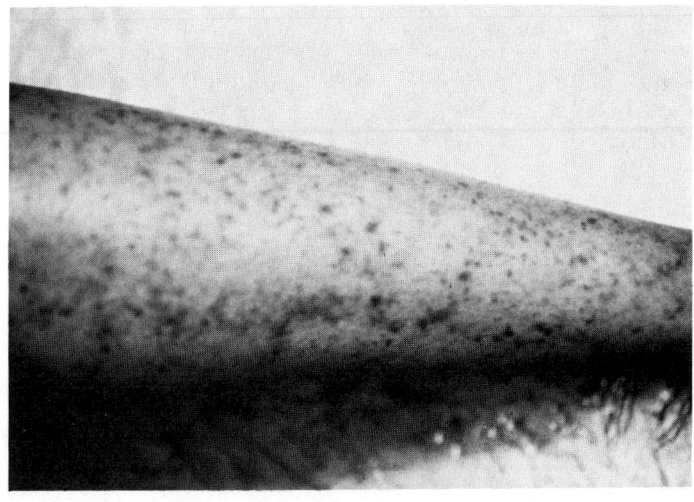

Fig. 4–1. Typical petechiae and purpura.

Table 4–2 Traditional Tests of Platelet Function

Blood smear for estimation of number and morphology
Quantitative platelet count
Template bleeding time
Aspirin tolerance test
Tourniquet test
Clot retraction
Prothrombin consumption test
Platelet factor 3 availability
Platelet Aggregation

in children. These two tests are only done when there is a normal platelet count and positive or suggestive history.[38]

Figure 4–2 depicts a standardized aggregometer for assessing platelet function. The aggregometer is a standardized photometer; platelet-rich plasma is added to a photometric well, to which is then added various aggregating reagents.[5, 164,171] As platelets aggregate, increasing levels of light are allowed through the photometric chamber; the change in light density (percent transmission) is then recorded on a strip recorder, giving rise to typical platelet aggregation "patterns."[287] Figure 4–3 gives normal platelet aggregation patterns as seen on a standardized platelet aggregometer. The usual aggregating agents used are adenosine diphosphate (ADP), epinephrine, ristocetin, collagen, arachidonic acid, and serotonin. The patterns depicted in Figure 4–3 were elicited by the addition of each of these reagents to platelet-rich plasma in the aggregometer. It will be noted that a monophasic (all or none) curve is elicited with ADP; the bottom of the curve represents platelet-poor plasma after aggregation has occurred. A biphasic curve is usually elicited with epinephrine. Ristocetin also usually induces a monophasic curve, with the change in light density going from the very top, or platelet-rich plasma, to the very bottom, representing platelet-poor plasma. This is also true for arachidonic acid.[190] Collagen characteristically demonstrates a lag-phase, followed

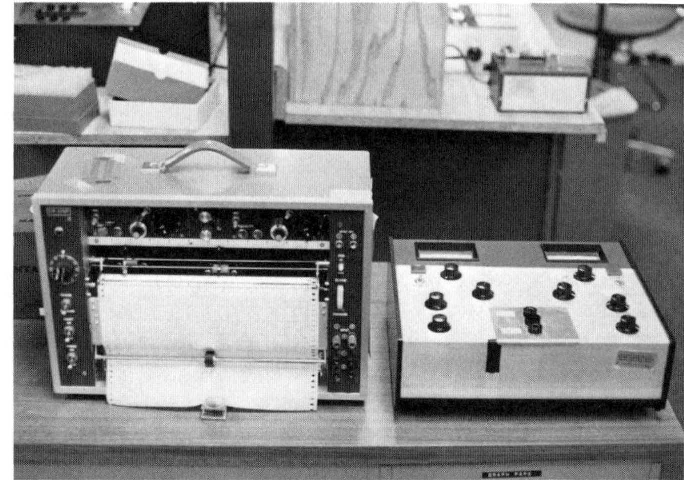

Fig. 4–2. A standard popular (Payton) platelet aggregometer.

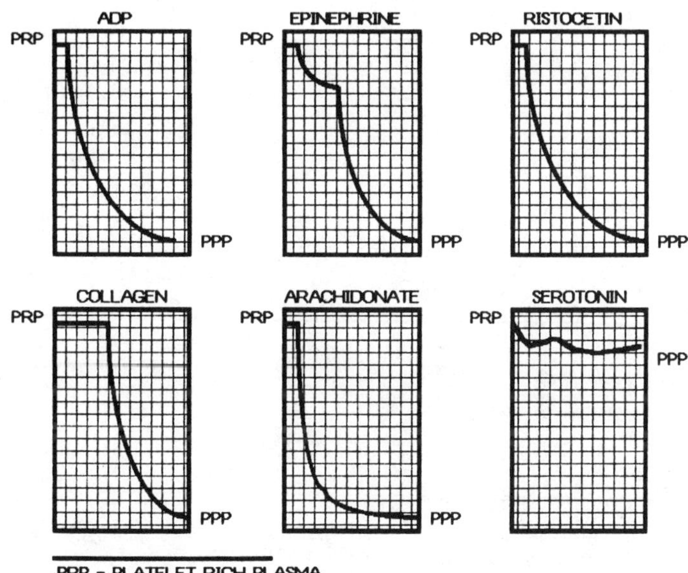

Fig. 4–3. Normal platelet aggregation patterns. PRP: platelet-rich plasma; PPP: platelet-poor plasma.

by complete aggregation to platelet-poor plasma. The slight curve seen with serotonin is a normal pattern of the platelet aggregation curve.

A much newer refinement of aggregation to assess platelet function is that of lumiaggregation;[130,131,254] and Figure 4–4 demonstrates a popular lumiaggregation instrument. This instrument utilizes both a photometric and a fluorometric well. The use of firefly lucipherase (ATPase) in the fluorometric well allows the measure-ment of simultaneous ATP release while measuring aggregation in the photometric well. Thus, aggregation and simultaneous release can be studied with the use of this instrument. In fact in our laboratory almost all aggregation or platelet workups are done exclusively with lumi-aggregation. Figure 4–5 demonstrates a typical lumiaggregation pattern with the aggregating agent epinephrine. The bottom curve going upward represents the typical biphasic aggregation pattern induced by

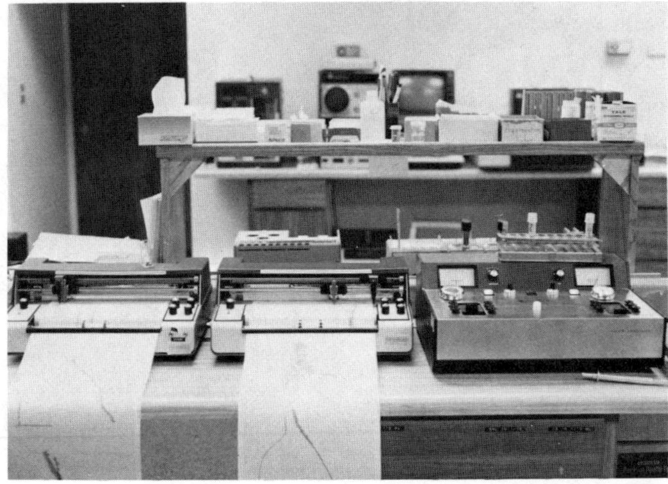

Fig. 4-4. A popular (Payton) lumiaggregation instrument.

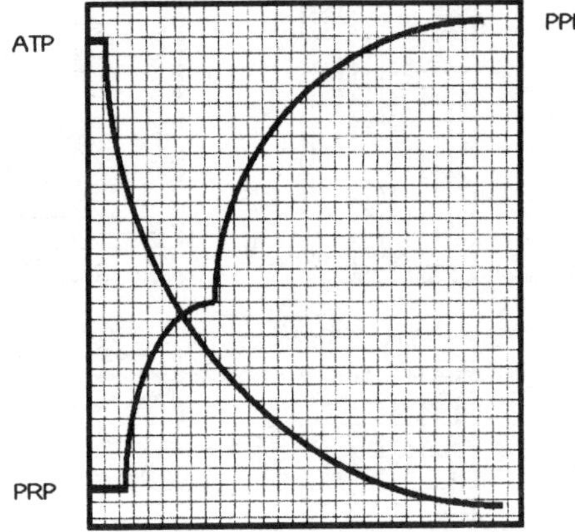

PRP = PLATELET RICH PLASMA
PPP = PLATELET POOR PLASMA
ATP = ATP RELEASE

Fig. 4-5. Platelet lumiaggregation induced by epinephrine. PRP: platelet-rich plasma; PPP: platelet-poor plasma; ATP: adenosine triphosphate release.

epinephrine. The top line coming down to the bottom represents the simultaneous release of adenosine triphosphate (ATP). Figure 4-6 summarizes normal lumiaggregation patterns generated by the aggregating reagents depicted. The aggregation curves are now read upside down compared with the aggregation curves seen in Figure 4-3. The aggregating pattern is on the bottom; for example, in Figure 4-6 the lag phase typically seen with collagen goes from platelet-rich plasma on the bottom to platelet-poor plasma on the top; simultaneous ATP release is seen from top to bottom. The typical biphasic epinephrine curve goes from platelet-rich plasma on the bottom to platelet-poor plasma at the end of the curve. Ristocetin commonly causes only partial ATP release, usually about 35%.[182] Thus, lumiaggregation has added a significant new dimension to assessment of platelet function, allowing observation of simultaneous release and aggregation.

Types of Platelet Defects

Platelet defects are most easily divided into those that are quantitative and those that are qualitative. The qualitative disorders, platelet function defects, are further divided into those that are hereditary and those that are acquired. Quantitative defects are best divided into (1) thrombocytopenia due to decreased production and metabolic or maturation defects, including the hereditary, congenital, and infantile thrombocytopenias associated with decreased platelet production, the acquired platelet production defects, and drug-induced nonimmune thrombocytopenias; (2) acquired thrombocytopenia

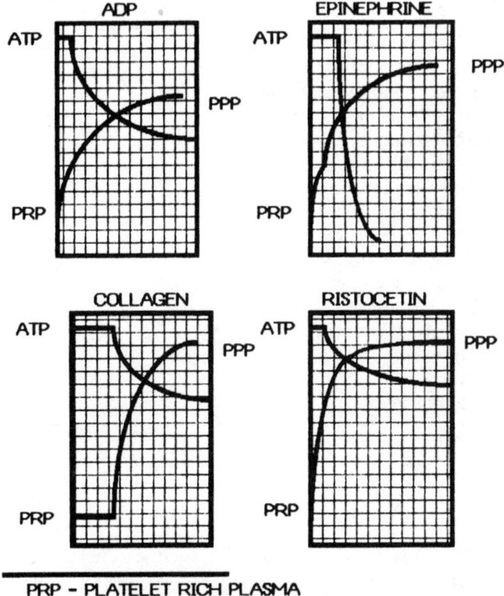

Fig. 4–6. Normal platelet lumiaggregation patterns. ADP: adenosine diphosphate; ATP: adenosine triphosphate release; PPP: platelet-poor plasma; PRP: platelet-rich plasma.

Table 4–3 Platelet Disorders

Qualitative
  Hereditary
    Adhesion defects
    Aggregation defects
    Factor deficiencies
    Miscellaneous
Acquired
    Associated with other diseases
    Drug-induced
Quantitative (thrombocytopenias)
  Hereditary
    Megakaryocytic
    Amegakaryocytic
    Drug-induced
  Acquired
    Megakaryocytic
    Amegakaryocytic
    Drug-induced
Quantitative (thrombocytosis and thrombocythemia)

due to increased destruction, increased consumption, or peripheral loss; and (3) thrombocytosis, thrombocythemia, and hyperactive platelets associated with, or formed as a consequence of, hypercoagulability and thrombosis.

Table 4–3 summarizes platelet defects, divided into those that are qualitative (functional) versus those that are quantitative, i.e., thrombocytopenia, thrombocytosis, and thrombocythemia. There is little use in instituting an expensive and laborious platelet function workup until normal platelet counts have been documented. Attempting to study platelet function in thrombocytopenia is usually a fruitless endeavor.[39] As with vascular defects, the hereditary forms are clinical oddities and extremely rare. However, the acquired forms are very common and, as shall be seen, are associated with many common acquired diseases.

Platelet Function Defects

Hereditary Platelet Function Defects

The hereditary platelet function defects are summarized in Table 4–4. These are divided into those of (1) platelet adhesion, typified by the Bernard-Soulier syndrome; (2) defects of primary aggregation, characterized by Glanzmann's thrombasthenia; and (3) defects of secondary aggregation characterized by storage pool diseases as well as other more rare defects.[232] In addition, there have been described patients with an isolated deficiency of platelet factor 3, and patients with very severe plasma coagulation protein deficiencies may have an associated platelet function defect. This is especially noted in severe afibrinogenemia, severe hemophilia A, and severe hemophilia B. The accompanying platelet function defect seen in these patients serves to exemplify the importance of blood coagulation proteins for normal platelet function. Although the division of hereditary platelet function defects into those of adhesion, primary aggregation, or secondary aggregation is somewhat artificial, it provides a convenient way to

Table 4–4 Hereditary Platelet Function Defects

Adhesion defects
  Bernard-Soulier syndrome
  Impaired adhesion to collagen
Aggregation defects: primary
  Glanzmann's thrombasthenia
  Essential athrombia
Aggregation defects: secondary
  Storage pool diseases
  Aspirin-like defect
  Release reaction defects
Isolated platelet factor 3 deficiency
  Afibrinogenemia
  Factor VIII:C deficiency
  Factor IX:C deficiency

Table 4–5 Bernard-Soulier Syndrome

Clinical findings
  Autosomal inheritance
  Heterozygotes often asymptomatic
  Easy bruising
  Spontaneous bruising
  Petechiae and purpura
  Epistaxis
  Mucosal membrane bleeding
Laboratory findings
  Giant platelets
  Thrombocytopenia (mild to moderate)
  Prolonged template bleeding time
  Abnormal adhesion to collagen
  Abnormal aggregation to ristocetin
Therapy
  Platelet concentrates

categorize the defects and to recall the laboratory manifestations.

Table 4–5 summarizes characteristics of the Bernard-Soulier syndrome, which typifies a disorder of platelet adhesion. It is important to recall the Bernard-Soulier syndrome because superficially this syndrome can be mistaken for von Willebrand's disease. The clinical features are those of easy bruising, epistaxis, hypermenorrhagia, and petechiae and purpura,[30,372] which may also suggest von Willebrand's disease. During laboratory assessment, these patients demonstrate abnormal adhesion as well as abnormal ristocetin-induced aggregation, and if only adhesion and ristocetin aggregation are performed one would think the patient has von Willebrand's disease rather than the Bernard-Soulier syndrome. The difference is made by examining a peripheral smear, which will usually demonstrate giant platelets and borderline thrombocytopenia in most, but not all patients.[60,181] In addition, if von Willebrand's disease were suspected, Factor VIII coagulation activity (Factor VIII:C), Factor VIII-related antigen (Factor VIII:RAg), and ristocetin cofactor activity (Factor VIII:RCo) would also be performed, leading to the correct diagnosis. Thus, it is important to recall the Bernard-Soulier syndrome, its clinical and laboratory features, its superficial resemblence to von Willebrand's disease and that this syndrome is manifested as a hereditary adhesion defect of platelets.

Primary aggregation disorders are Glanzmann's thrombasthenia[135,144] and an even rarer disorder, essential athrombia.[185] Glanzmann's thrombasthenia is extremely rare. The clinical features are those usually expected with platelet dysfunction; easy and spontaneous bruising, subcutaneous hematomata, and petechiae are characteristics.[107,144] Rare patients have been reported to have intra-articular bleeding with hemarthroses. The bleeding tendency tends to decrease in severity with age, as is the case with many of the hereditary defects. The clinical and laboratory diagnostic features are depicted in Table 4–6.[77,78] All of these abnormalities are also noted for the even rarer related disorder, essential athrombia. However, in essential athrombia clot retraction is normal.[185] Therapy for these disorders, is the infusion of platelet concentrates as needed for serious or life-threatening bleeding. My general approach is to infuse platelet concentrates until bleeding stops rather than to rely on empirical monitoring of aggregation or the template bleeding time. The vast majority of patients with a hereditary platelet function defect of any type will stop bleeding abruptly with the appropriate use of platelet concentrates.[40]

Secondary aggregation disorders are more common than primary aggregation disorders and are summarized in Table 4–7. Among all of the hereditary platelet function defects, storage pool disease type disorders are by far the most com-

Table 4–6 Glanzmann's Thrombasthemia and Essential Athrombia

Clinical findings
  Autosomal recessive
  Petechiae and purpura
  Easy bruising
  Spontaneous bruising
  Mucosal membrane bleeding
  Large hematomas
  Intra-articular bleeding (rare)
  Decreasing severity with age
Laboratory findings
  Prolonged template bleeding time
  Abnormal or absent primary aggregation with
    ADP
    Epinephrine
    Thrombin
    Collagen
  Abnormal platelet factor 3 release
  Clot retraction
    Glanzmann's, abnormal
    Essential athrombia, normal
Therapy
  Platelet concentrates

Table 4–7 Secondary Aggregation Defects

Storage pool disease
  Isolated defect (most common presentation)
  Associated with (less common)
    TAR baby syndrome
    Hermansky-Pudlak syndrome
    Chédiak-Higashi syndrome
    Wiskott-Aldrich syndrome
Aspirin-like defect
  Cyclo-oxygenase deficiency
  Thromboxane synthetase deficiency
Release reaction defects
  Hereditary collagen disorders
  Glycogen storage disease
  May-Hegglin anomaly
  Hurler's syndrome
  Hunter's syndrome

mon.[176,288] In rare instances, storage pool defects are seen in patients with other rare clinical oddities, including the Wiskott-Aldrich syndrome,[152] the thrombocytopenia absent radii syndrome (TAR baby syndrome),[110] the Hermansky-Pudlak syndrome,[318] and the Chédiak-Higashi syndrome.[71] Most patients with these rare clinical syndromes have an associated storage pool defect. However, it should be noted that the majority of patients who present with a hereditary storage pool defect have no such associated disease and are otherwise perfectly normal.[389] The clinical features of secondary aggregation disorders are those expected with a platelet function defect and consist of mucocutaneous hemorrhages, hematuria, and epistaxis.[390] For unexplained reasons, petechiae are less common than in other disorders. Easy and spontaneous bruising are common complaints. During laboratory evaluation, patients with storage pool defects have absent epinephrine- and ADP-induced secondary aggregation waves, although the primary waves are present. Collagen-induced aggregation is absent or markedly blunted, and normal ristocetin-induced aggregation is typically noted.[258,391] A prolonged standardized template bleeding time is uniformly seen. The mainstay of therapy is the use of platelet concentrates if the patient bleeds. The clinical and laboratory features of hereditary storage pool disease are summarized in Table 4–8.

Figure 4–7 summarizes platelet aggregation findings in hereditary storage pool disease. In this Figure is noted a small primary wave induced by epinephrine, an essentially normal serotonin-induced curve, primary aggregation induced by ADP, followed by disaggregation, and a markedly blunted collagen-induced aggregation curve. These findings are classic for hereditary storage pool defects.

Table 4–8 Hereditary Storage Pool Disease

Clinical findings
  Variable inheritance
  Petechiae, uncommon
  Purpura, uncommon
  Mucosal membrane bleeding
  Epistaxis
  Easy bruising
  Spontaneous bruising
  Hematuria, common
Laboratory findings
  Abnormal template bleeding time
  Abnormal adhesion to collagen
  Absent aggregation to collagen
  Absent second aggregation curve to
    ADP
    Epinephrine
  Normal ristocetin aggregation
  Normal arachidonate aggregation (usually)
Therapy
  Platelet concentrates

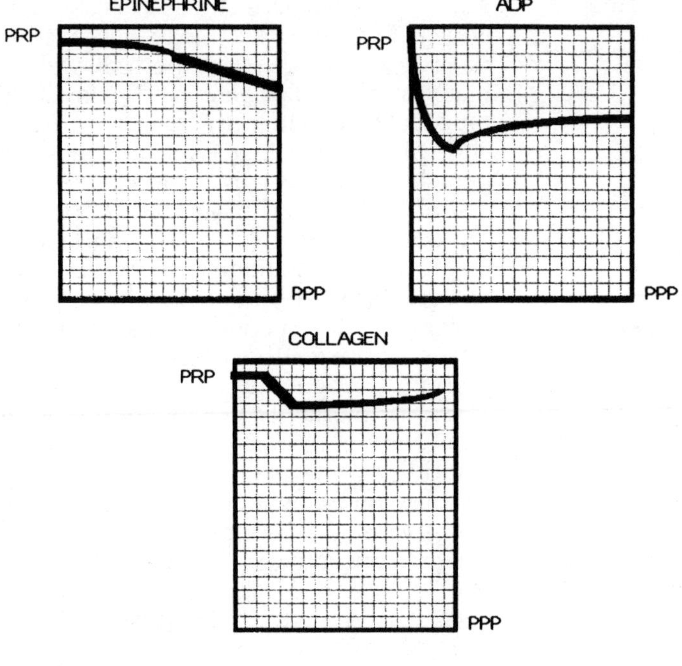

Fig. 4–7. Hereditary storage pool disease: aggregation defects.

The patterns in Figure 4–9 came from the mother of a patient who had initially presented to an Emergency Room with uncontrollable bilateral epistaxis. As soon as aggregation was performed, a diagnosis of storage pool disease was made. She was infused with platelets and her profuse epistaxis ceased immediately. Following this, the mother and two siblings were evaluated and found to have the same defect.

Another secondary aggregation defect is that of the aspirin-like effect that is inherited as an autosomal dominant.[363] This disorder is extremely rare, with very few cases having been described.[7,19,333,392] The clinical features are similar to other platelet function defects and consist of easy and spontaneous bruising, occasional spontaneous bleeding from mucosal membranes, epistaxis, hypermenorrhagia, petechiae, and purpura. From the laboratory standpoint, these patients demonstrate a prolonged template bleeding time, an absent secondary wave to epinephrine, and absent collagen-induced aggregation; therefore they resemble a patient who has ingested aspirin or other cyclo-oxygenase inhibitor.[393] This defect is due to either a hereditary deficiency of the enzyme cyclo-oxygenase or a hereditary deficiency of the enzyme thromboxane synthetase.[177,216,236] Therapy, when clinically significant bleeding occurs, is to infuse platelet concentrates. Some patients have improved with the use of steroids.[418] The features of this heterogeneous syndrome are summarized in Table 4–9. Aggregation findings in the aspirin-like effect are seen in Figure 4–8.

Hereditary storage pool diseases are the most common of the rare hereditary function defects and are usually not associated with one of the other rare clinical syndromes, such as Chédiak-Higashi or Wiskott-Aldrich. The other hereditary platelet function defects mentioned are extremely rare and are best classified as true clinical oddities.

Table 4–9 Hereditary Aspirin-like Defect

Clinical findings
  Easy bruising
  Spontaneous bruising
  Mucosal membrane bleeding
  Epistaxis
Laboratory findings
  Prolonged template bleeding time
  Abnormal adhesion to collagen
  Absent secondary aggregation curves to
    ADP
    Epinephrine
  Absent aggregation to collagen
  Absent aggregation to arachidonate
  Absence of cyclo-oxygenase or thromboxane
    synthetase
Therapy
  Platelet concentrates
  Possibly steroids

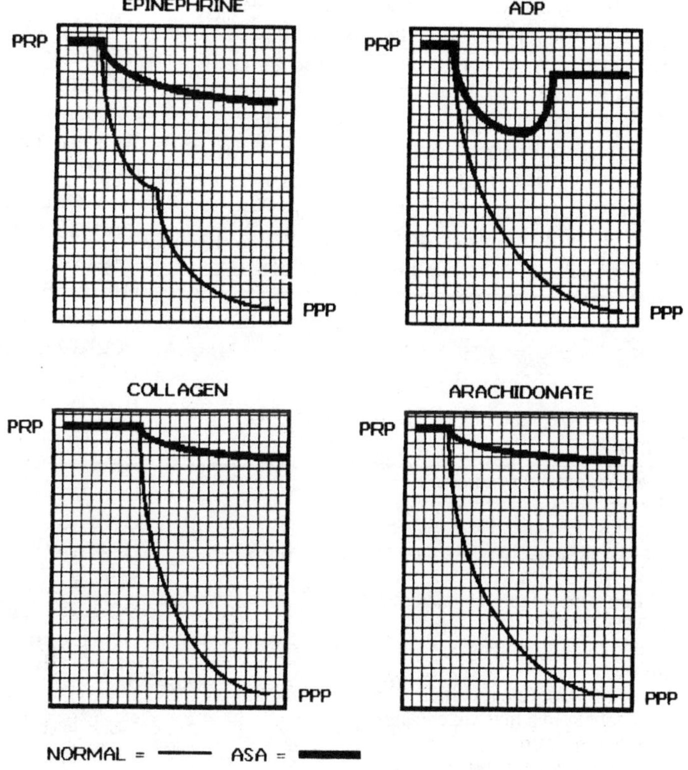

Fig. 4–8. Aspirin-induced platelet aggregation abnormalities.

Acquired Platelet Function Defects

The very common acquired platelet defects are summarized in Table 4–10. Many of these are of significant clinical concern and will be discussed in detail. Acquired platelet function defects are commonly seen in all of the myeloproliferative syndromes,[6,41,367] especially essential thrombocythemia, agnogenic myeloid metaplasia, paroxysmal nocturnal hemoglobinuria, polycythemia rubra vera, patients with chronic myelogenous leukemia, refractory anemia and excessive blasts (RAEB syndrome), or preleukemic syndromes, and the sideroblastic or sideroacrestic anemias. In addition, all are familiar with the almost universal finding of a platelet function defect in patients who are uremic.[221,308] In uremic patients it is thought that circulating guanidinosuccinic[178,179] or hydroxyphenolic acids[309] interfere with platelet function by eradicating platelet factor 3 activity. Both of these compounds are dialyzable, and dialysis will often correct or improve platelet function. Other mechanisms of altered platelet function in uremia, including altered prostaglandin metabolism, have also been proposed.[125,192,314,315,337]

Table 4–10 Acquired Platelet Function Defects

Myeloproliferative syndromes
   Essential thrombocythemia
   Agnogenic myeloid metaplasia
   Paroxysmal nocturnal hemoglobinuria
   Polycythemia vera
   Chronic myelogenous leukemia
   RAEB syndrome
   Sideroblastic anemia
Uremia
Malignant paraproteinemias
   Waldenstrom's macroglobulinemia
   Multiple myeloma
   Leukemic reticuloendotheliosis
Autoimmune disorders
   Collagen vascular diseases
   Antiplatelet antibodies
Presence of fibrin(ogen) degradation products
   Disseminated intravascular coagulation
   Primary fibrinolysis
Anemia
   Severe iron deficiency
   Severe folate or vitamin B_{12} deficiency
Drug-induced

Figure 4–9 demonstrates lumiaggregation patterns in a uremic patient. Many patients with malignant paraprotein disorders, including multiple myeloma, Waldenstrom's macroglobulinemia, or other monoclonal gammopathies will demonstrate a platelet function defect.[42,43,215,228] This is due to the coating of platelet membrane by paraprotein and does not depend on the type of paraprotein and occurs with immunoglobulins A, M, G (IgA, IgM, IgG). Almost all patients with paraprotein disorders will demonstrate significant platelet dysfunction manifested by clinically significant bleeding as well as noting abnormal platelet function by aggregation on lumiaggregation testing. Lumiaggregation patterns before and after plasmapheresis therapy in a patient with IgA myeloma are depicted in Figure 4–10. Patients undergoing cardiopulmonary bypass demonstrate the severest of platelet function defects.[44–46] Typical mid-bypass and postbypass lumiaggregation patterns are seen in Figures 4–11 and 4–12. This will be discussed in detail in Chapter 9.

Acquired platelet function defects are also seen in autoimmune disorders, including systemic lupus erythematosus, rheumatoid arthritis, scleroderma, and others.[312,414] The presence of fibrin(ogen) degradation products (FDPs) very often induces a clinically significant platelet function defect.[47,48,208] The FDPs can be of any origin, including disseminated intravascular coagulation (DIC) or primary hyperfibrino(geno)lytic syndromes.[49–51] The later degradation products, especially fragments D and E, appear to have a high affinity for the platelet membrane, attach to the membrane, and produce a very severe and clinically significant acquired platelet function defect. Patients with severe iron deficiency or severe folate or vitamin B_{12} deficiency may also demonstrate a platelet function defect that may or may not lead to clinically significant hemorrhage.[186,219] Drug-induced platelet function defects are very commonly noted, are a common cause of easy and spontaneous bruising, petechiae and purpura, and bleeding after surgery or trauma.[373] Drug-induced defects will be discussed subsequently. Unlike the rare

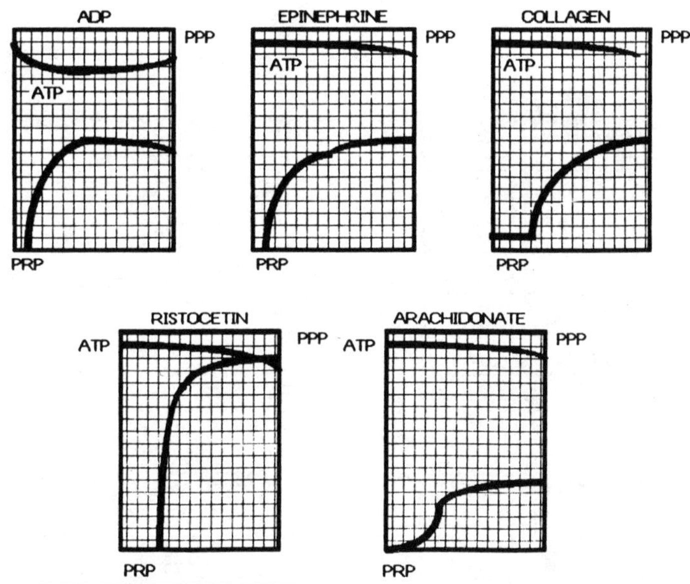

Fig. 4–9. Platelet function in uremia: Lumiaggregation. ADP: adenosine diphosphate; ATP: adenosine triphosphate release; PPP: platelet-poor plasma; PRP: platelet-rich plasma.

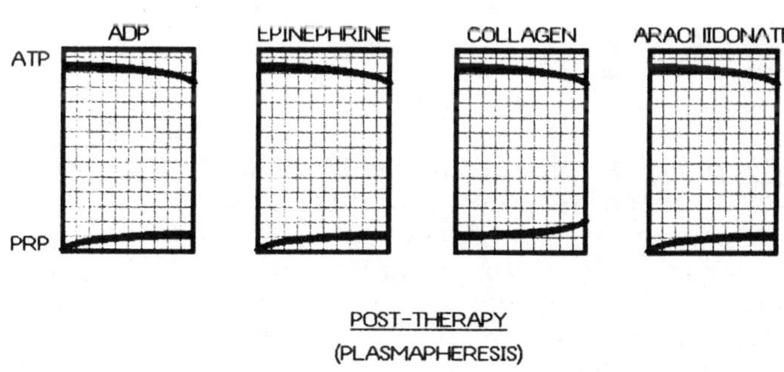

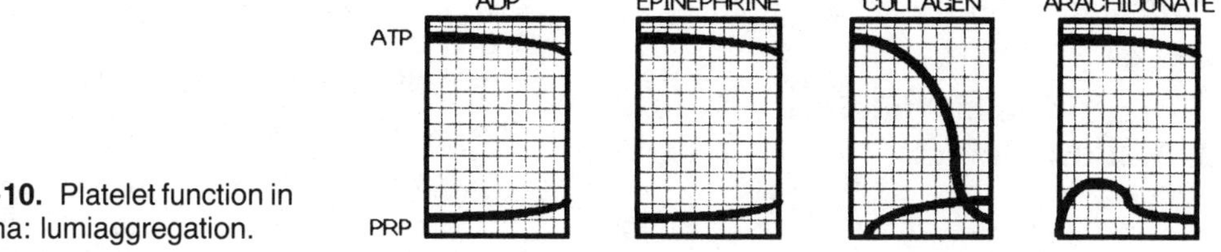

Fig. 4–10. Platelet function in myeloma: lumiaggregation.

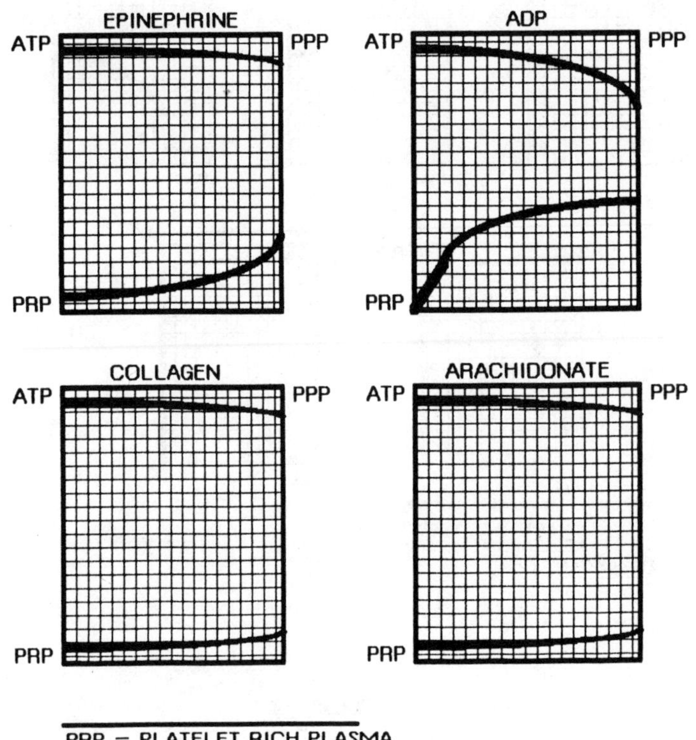

Fig. 4–11. Cardiopulmonary bypass surgery: lumiaggregation patterns. ATP: adenosine triphosphate release; PPP: platelet-poor plasma; ADP: adenosine diphosphate; PRP: platelet-rich plasma.

hereditary platelet function defects, the acquired defects do not demonstrate typical aggregation abnormalties when patterns are studied. For example, one can study many patients with chronic myelogenous leukemia and all will likely have abnormal aggregation patterns. However, many different varieties of abnormalities will usually be noted.

Drug-Induced Platelet Function Defects

The common clinical drugs that may cause a clinically significant platelet function defect and hemorrhage are numerous. The number of drugs interfering with platelet function as defined by laboratory tests (aggregation) is much more extensive.

This review will be restricted to commonly used drugs that reportedly cause clinically significant hemorrhage in patients. The three most common mechanisms by which drugs interfere with platelet function, in descending order of relevance, are drug interference with the platelet membrane receptor sites, with prostaglandin synthetic pathways, and with phosphodiesterase activity.[374,394] The most common drugs interfering with platelet membrane function or receptors are amitriptyline,[255] imipramine,[327] doxepin,[395] thorazine,[256] cocaine,[359] lidocaine,[277] isoproterenol,[278] propanolol,[398] cephalothin,[269] ampicillin,[86] carbenicillin,[67] penicillin,[68] diphenhydramine,[279] Phenergan,[340] and alcohol.[105] Other drugs inducing platelet dysfunction by this mechanism are phentolamine,[75] phenoxybenzamine,[75] reserpine,[62]

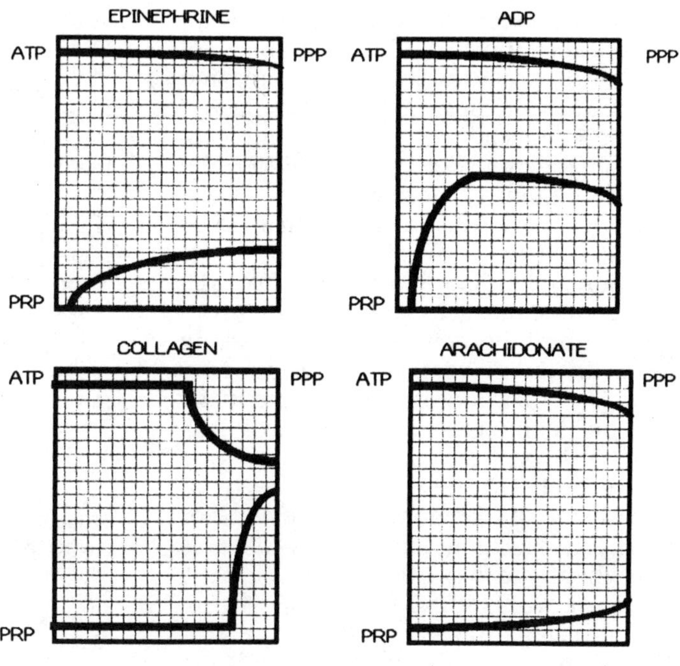

Fig. 4–12. Cardiopulmonary bypass surgery: lumiaggregation defects.

dihydroergotamine,[257] norpramine,[327] nortriptyline,[327] trifluoperazine,[402] procaine,[16] dibucaine,[16] nitrofurantoin,[324] nafcillin,[10] moxalactam,[25] ticarcillin,[69] dextran,[126] and hydroxyethyl starch.[148]

The most common drugs interfering with platelet prostaglandin synthetic pathways are aspirin,[94] indomethacin,[207] phenylbutazone,[419] ibuprofen,[274] naproxen,[312] sulfinpyrazone,[406] furosemide,[325] and verapamil.[8] Less commonly used drugs that share this mechanism of inducing platelet dysfunction are hydralazine,[73] quinacrine,[409] fenoprofen,[394] mefenamic acid,[280] tocopherol,[361] hydrocortisone,[145] methylprednisolone,[299] and cyclosporine.[272]

The most common drugs interfering with platelet phosphodiesterase activity and inducing platelet dysfunction are caffeine,[249] dipyridamole,[311] aminophylline, theophylline, and papaverine.[18,24,410] Vinblastine, vincristine,[403] and colchicine interfere with the platelet contractile[357] protein, thrombosthenin.

Acetazolamide,[417] ethacrynic acid,[417] chlortetracycline, hydroxychloroquine,[83] dicumarol,[358] nitroprusside,[331] cyproheptadine,[313] glycerol guaiacolate,[351] and heparin[281,330,400,420] interfere with platelet function by unclear mechanisms. Nitroglycerine induces platelet dysfunction by interference with platelet cyclic adenosine monophosphate (AMP).[332] Anti-inflammatory drugs are common offenders; aspirin, colchicine, ibuprofen, indomethacin, and sulfinpyrazone are the most common. Sulfinpyrazone and aspirin are used to suppress platelet function and have the same mode of action; both drugs inhibit cyclo-oxygenase, thereby inhibiting the eventual platelet synthesis of thromboxane A_2. Psychiatric drugs may also inhibit platelet function. The phenothiazine-related drugs, including chlorpromazine and trifluoperazine may inhibit platelet function and lead to a clinically significant platelet function defect. In addition, the tricyclic amines interfere with platelet function. Numerous cardiovascular drugs are also known to interfere with platelet function including clofibrate, dipyridamole, nicotinic acid, papaverine, propranolol, and the newer calcium-blocking drugs, including verapamil. This category is of particular importance because many patients deemed candidates for cardiopulmonary bypass surgery will be on one or several of these agents, such as papaverine, propranolol, theophylline or a calcium-blocking agent. These patients may therefore have enhanced bleeding risk with bypass surgery due to a drug-induced platelet function defect.

Antibiotics are also common inducers of platelet dysfunction. Most of the penicillin derivatives, including nafcillin, ampicillin, carbenicillin, and ticarcillin, are capable of interfering with platelet function; this is most commonly seen with carbenicillin. Carbenicillin will also commonly cause thrombocytopenia. Gentamicin is also capable of interfering with platelet function. Various anesthetics, including the local anesthetics, cocaine, and procaine, as well as the volatile gaseous anesthetics may interfere with platelet function and lead to clinically significant hemorrhage. Miscellaneous drugs interfering with platelet function are the antihistamines, the most common offenders being diphenhydramine and Actifed, the dextrans, furosemide (Lasix), glycerol guaiacolate (the base of many common cough syrups), nitroprusside, and vincristine or vinblastine. Categories of common drugs capable of causing a clinically significant platelet function defect are listed in Table 4–11. The mechanism of action, where known, is also depicted. Table 4–12 lists common drugs containing aspirin.[217,343]

The clinical importance of drug-induced platelet function defects is exemplified by the following case presentation.

Case 1. A 21-year-old male was involved in a minor motorcycle accident and presented to an Emergency Room with fractures of the left second, third, and fourth ribs anteriorly. He also had a costrochondral separation and adjacent to this, a lung contusion was noted on chest roentgenography. In the Emergency Room the patient was noted to be mildly lethargic. He was seen in consultation by

Table 4–11 Drug-Induced Platelet Dysfunction

Cardiovascular and respiratory	Anesthetics
Aminophylline*	Cocaine[†]
Clofibrate[†]	Dibucaine[†]
Dibenzyline[†]	Procaine[†]
Dicoumarol[‡]	Lidocaine[†]
Dihydroergotamine[†]	Anti-inflammatory drugs
Dipyridamole*	Sulfinpyrazone[§]
Heparin[‡]	Aspirin[§]
Hydralazine[§]	Colchicine[¶]
Isoproterenol[†]	Ibuprofen[§]
Nitroglycerine[‖]	Indomethacin[§]
Nitroprusside[‡]	Fenoprofen[§]
Papaverine*	Naproxen[§]
Propanolol[†]	Phenylbutazone[§]
Phentolamine[†]	Mefenamic acid[§]
Reserpine[†]	Diuretics
Theophylline*	Acetazolamide[‡]
Verapamil[§]	Ethacrynic acid[‡]
Antibiotics	Furosemide[§]
Ampicillin[†]	Miscellaneous drugs
Chlortetracycline[‡]	Alcohol[†]
Carbenicillin[†]	Diphenhydramine[†]
Nitrofurantoin[†]	Caffeine*
Gentamicin[†]	Cyclosporin A[§]
Cephalothin[†]	Dextran[†]
Moxalactam	Glycerol guaiacolate[‡]
Nafcillin[†]	Hydroxyethyl starch[†]
Piperacillin[†]	Hydrocortisone[§]
Hydorxychloroquine[‡]	Methylprednisolone[§]
Quinacrine[§]	Cyproheptadine[‡]
Psychiatric drugs	Promethazine[†]
Nortriptyline[†]	Methysergide maleate[‡]
Amitryptyline[†]	Tocopherol[§]
Desipramine[†]	Vinblastine[¶]
Doxepin[†]	Vincristine[¶]
Trifluoperazine[†]	
Chlorpromazine[†]	
Imipramine[†]	

* Interference with phosphodiesterase.
[†] Interference with membrane or membrane receptors.
[‡] Unknown mechanism of action.
[§] Interference with prostaglandin synthesis.
[‖] Interference with platelet cyclic-amp.
[¶] Interference with thrombosthenin.

Table 4–12 Drug-Induced Platelet Dysfunction

Common Drugs Containing Aspirin

Alka-seltzer	Empiral
Anacin	Empirin
Anahist	Empirin with codeine
APC	Emprazil
APC with codeine	Emprazil-C
APC with demerol	Equagesic
ASA	Excedrin
ASA compound	Excedrin PM
ASA compound with	Fiorinal
codeine	Fiorinal with codeine
Aspergum	Fizrin
Aspirin (USP)	4-Way cold tablets
Aspirin (childrens)	Liquiprin
Bayer	Measurin
Bayer (childrens)	Midol
Bayer timed-release	Norgesic
Bufferin	PAC Compound
Calurin	PAC Compound with
Cama inlay	codeine
Cope	Percodan
Coricidin	Robaxisal
Coricidin "D"	Robaxisal-PH
Coricidin Demilets	Sine-Off
Coricidin Medilets	St. Joseph's
Darvon with ASA	St. Joseph's for children
Darvon-N with ASA	Super-Anahist
Darvon Compound	Synalgos
Dolene	Synalgos-DC
Dristan	Triaminicin
Ecotrin	Vanquish

a neurologist, and a computed tomography (CT) scan was ordered. The neurologic examination and CT scan of his central nervous system (CNS) were completely within normal limits. It was decided to admit him for observation because of these findings and because of his mild lethargy. His admission laboratory data consisted of a white cell count of $22,500/mm^3$ with a very mild shift, a hemoglobin of 14.4 g/dL, a hematocrit of 44%, and a platelet count of $250,000/mm^3$. A urinalysis was within normal limits.

On the second hospital day, the patient was noted by the physicians and nursing staff to be much improved, a chest roentgenogram was repeated, revealing general improvement in his pulmonary contusion, and his lethargy had also improved. Laboratory tests were repeated and found to be unchanged. Early on day three, the patient was found by nursing staff to be unarousable. Evaluation re-

vealed no localized neurologic findings. However, he was noted to have mild hematuria and his initial ecchymoses from his accident were increasing in size. The physician was called and a diagnosis of "probable hypoxia" was made; a chest radiograph was repeated, revealing continued improvement, and a repeat CT scan revealed massive diffuse intracranial hemorrhage. The patient was subjected to a craniotomy on day 3.

During attempted craniotomy diffuse CNS bleeding was noted and the neurosurgeon was unable to close due to profuse, nonlocalized hemorrhage. During the craniotomy the nursing staff noted that the patient had developed gross hematuria and during surgery the patient began passing bright red blood per rectum. Hematology consultation was obtained and an evaluation was ordered and revealed the findings summarized in Table 4–13. The slight elevation of the FDPs was compatible with surgery or minor trauma. Since the template bleeding time was greater than 45 minutes, an aggregation test was ordered, and as soon as the blood was drawn, platelet concentrates were infused. Figure 4–13 shows the aggregation patterns found. The epinephrine-induced aggregation curve revealed only a slight primary wave, ADP-induced aggregation curve demonstrated a primary wave followed by disaggregation, markedly blunted collagen-induced aggregation was noted and totally absent arachidonic acid-induced aggregation was present and, ristocetin aggregation was normal.

Table 4–13 Hemostasis Evaluation of Case 1

Laboratory findings
  Prothrombin time: 19.0 seconds
  Activated partial thromboplastin time: 23.0 seconds
  Fibrinogen: 340 mg/dL
  FDP: >10>40
  Antithrombin III: 91%
  Protamine sulfate test: negative
  Template bleeding time: >45 minutes
Repeat laboratory findings (after platelets given)
  Prothrombin time: 11.0 seconds
  Activated partial thromboplastin time: 26.0 seconds
  Template bleeding time: 7 minutes

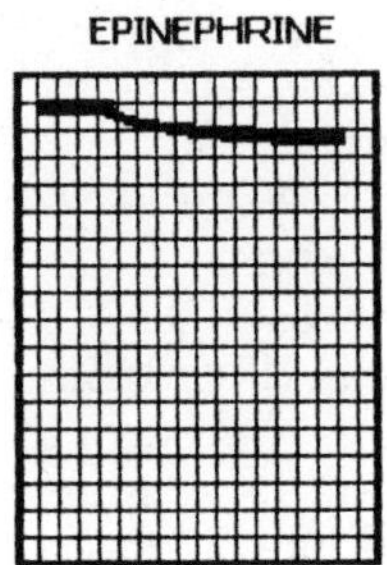

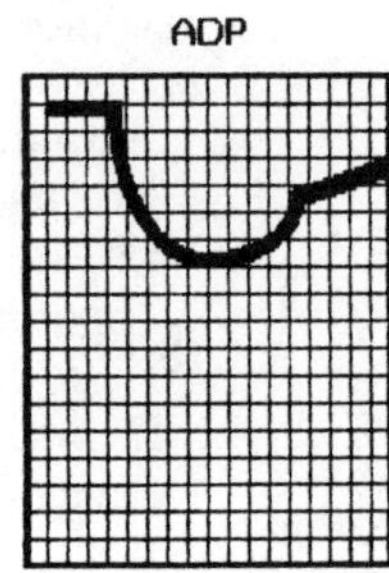

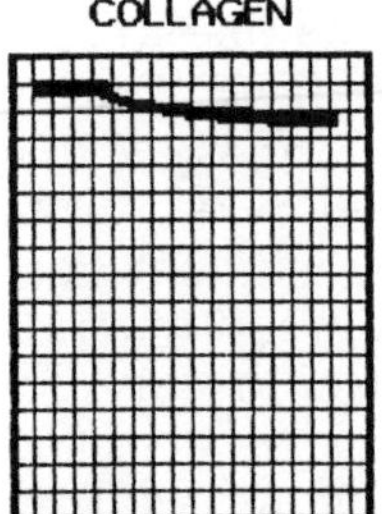

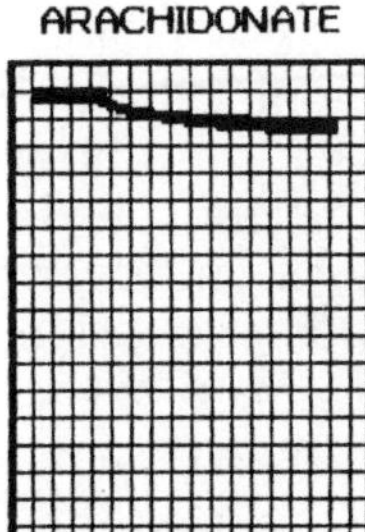

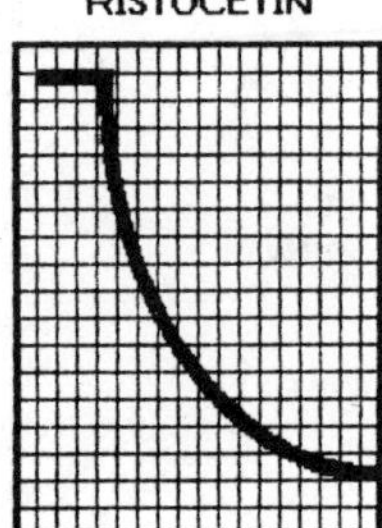

Fig. 4–13. Aggregation pattern for case 1.

As soon as these aggregation patterns were seen, it was clear that the patient had a platelet function defect associated with the ingestion of aspirin or some type of cyclo-oxygenase inhibitor. The family was questioned and stated that the patient had ingested no aspirin and, in fact, had taken no drugs for the 10 days following admission. While awaiting the return of these laboratory studies, the patient was given 30 mg of phytonadione, 4 U of fresh frozen plasma, 10 U of platelets twice daily for 24 hours. As soon as the initial platelets and the plasma were infused, laboratory work was repeated (Table 4–13). At this point, the patient also ceased bleeding clinically. While these were being done, the chart was reviewed, which showed that at the time of admission an order was written to give the patient aspirin suppositories 650 mg every 3 hours as needed, and the patient had been given a total of 6 g of aspirin before the intracranial bleeding.

In this case a quick search of the chart, after seeing aggregation patterns and a prolonged template bleeding time, rendered the correct diagnosis. Of course, the infusion of platelet concentrates immediately stopped the clinical bleeding, however, the patient died approximately 3 months later with irreversible brain damage, the third case of death due to aspirin ingestion that I have seen. Thus, this case serves to exemplify that drug-induced platelet function defects can be a very significant clinical reality and must always be considered when seeing patients with clinically significant hemorrhage and appropriate suggestive aggregation patterns.

Laboratory Evaluation of Platelet Function Defects

The laboratory evaluation of platelet function defects, including both older and newer methods available for the evaluation of platelet function, are summarized in Table 4–14. Of the older manual methods, the platelet count is paramount to rule out thrombocytopenia in patients with petechiae and purpura, mucosal membrane bleeding, and other suggestive historical findings. Both the Duke bleeding time and nonstandardized Ivy bleed-

Table 4-14 Laboratory Evaluation of Platelet Function

Old methods	New methods
Manual	Manual
Platelet count	Template bleeding time
Duke bleeding time	Platelet aggregation to
Ivy bleeding time	Ristocetin
Platelet aggregation to	Arachidonate
ADP	Lumi-aggregation for
Epinephrine	release reaction
Collagen	Automated
Thrombin	Platelet count
Serotonin	Platelet factor 4
Platelet factor 3	Beta-thromboglobulin
Clot retraction	Thromboxane assay
Prothrombin consumption	Cyclo-oxygenase

ing time have been abandoned with availability of the newer standardized template bleeding time. Platelet aggregation to the aggregating agents ADP, epinephrine, serotonin, thrombin, and collagen have been generally available for greater than a decade.[63] In addition, numerous methods to assess platelet factor 3 release have been generally available for many years.[305,396]

Of the newer methods available the automated molecular markers may be of some value in assessing platelet function defects. However, thromboxane B_2 assays, representing the immediate breakdown product of thromboxane A_2, and assays for platelet factor 4 and beta-thromboglobulin may be of more value in assessing hyperaggregable or hypercoagulable states than in assessing platelet function defects. These molecular markers will be discussed in appropriate subsequent sections.

Thrombocytopenia

Pseudothrombocytopenia

Pseudothrombocytopenia is a laboratory artifact that may occur via several mechanisms and should be investigated thoroughly in the asymptomatic patient before embarking on an extensive workup for thrombocytopenia.

Platelet autoagglutinins are usually IgG or IgM.[377] These may induce spontaneous autoagglutination of platelets, or in some instances, IgG and IgM autoagglutination activity may be enhanced by the anticoagulant ethyline diaminetetraacetic acid (EDTA).[283] Additionally, there may be adherence of platelets to granulocytes (platelet satellitism) that may also be mediated by EDTA or platelet membrane IgG.[204,415] If unexplained thrombocytopenia is seen with automated platelet counters, the smears should be carefully observed for platelet clumps (autoagglutination) or platelet satellitism. Pseudothrombocytopenia may also be noted in patients with a significantly expanded plasma volume, such as patients with marked fluid overload or patients with hyperviscosity syndromes. Pseudothrombocytopenia may also be seen if a small platelet-trapping clot forms in the collection tube.[289] Instances of unexplained spontaneous platelet aggregation may occur, presumably from the presence of "hyperactive" or partially activated platelets that may aggregate in vivo or in vitro, giving rise to pseudothrombocytopenia. Unless pseudothrombocytopenia is suspected and investigated, an expensive and laborious evaluation of the patient may be unnecessarily instituted. Additionally, a misdiagnosis may be made, and inappropriate or unnecessary therapy rendered. Cases of unnecessary splenectomy have been performed when pseudothrombocytopenia is present, thinking the patients had steroid-resistant idiopathic thrombocytopenic purpura (ITP).[292] Although EDTA-induced clumping of platelets is the most common cause of pseudothrombocytopenia, other causes are listed in Table 4-15. When pseudothrombocytopenia is suspected, the

Table 4-15 Causes of Pseudothrombocytopenia

Ethylene diaminetetraacetic acid induced platelet autoagglutination
IgG or IgM-induced platelet autoagglutination
Platelet satellitism
Expanded plasma volume
Collection tube clot formation
Spontaneous platelet aggregation (in vivo or in vitro)

platelets should be evaluated on a peripheral smear after blood collection in EDTA and the platelet count should be repeated by finger-stick technique with an ammonium oxalate unipette and counting by phase microscopy.[289]

Thrombocytopenia Due to Decreased Platelet Production

Congential and Neonatal Platelet Production Defects

Fanconi's syndrome is a rare disorder inherited as an autosomal recessive and comprised of congenital aplastic anemia with multiple congenital abnormalties[23,284] (Table 4–16). Thrombocytopenia may precede the development of granulocytopenia and anemia; however, macrocytic anemia is the most pronounced hematologic feature noted. Bone marrow hypoplasia is almost always seen. Other defects include hypermelanosis of the skin, strabismus, nystagmus, and numerous varied skeletal abnormalities.[273] The hematologic abnormalities usually occur after the age of 4 years and almost always are present be-

fore the early teenage years. Splenectomy may increase the platelet count to nonbleeding levels; however, the most common cause of death in patients with Fanconi's syndrome is intracranial or gastrointestinal hemorrhage. Life-threatening hemorrhages should be treated with appropriate numbers of platelet transfusions; single donor platelets are preferable, because these patients are candidates for numerous platelet transfusions throughout their lifetime. In some instances, a moderate response to the thrombocytopenia has been seen with androgens; however, the rise in platelet count often takes several months.

The TAR baby syndrome (thrombocytopenia and absent radii) is an autosomal recessive trait and is associated with severe thrombocytopenia due to marked deficiency of marrow megakaryocytes.[118,157] Bilateral aplasia of the radii is the most common associated abnormality, but cardiac and renal abnormalities may also be present (Table 4–17). Infections with rubella have been incriminated in some cases.[28] More than 50% of patients die of intracranial hemorrhage before reaching 1 year of age.[157] Splenectomy and/or androgens usually do not correct thrombocytopenia, but a few responses to these modalities have been noted.[342] The syndrome is differentiated from Fanconi's syndrome by the earlier onset and absence of granulocytopenia and anemia. When life-threatening bleeding occurs, platelet concentrates, preferably single donor, should be infused to control bleeding. Single donor platelets are preferable

Table 4–16 Salient Features of Fanconi's Syndrome

Clinical findings
Autosomal recessive
Usually manifested after age 4 years
Petechiae and purpura
Gastrointestinal hemorrhage
Intracranial hemorrhage
Hypermelanosis
Microcephaly
Mental retardation
Hyperactive deep tendon reflexes
Deafness
Ocular ptosis
Skeletal deformaties
Dwarfism
Congenital heart defects
Laboratory findings
Bone marrow hypoplasia
Aplastic anemia
Macrocytic anemia
Granulocytopenia
Thrombocytopenia
Therapy
Platelet concentrates
Androgens ?

Table 4–17 Characteristic Features of the TAR Baby Syndrome

Clinical findings
Autosomal recessive
Petechiae and purpura
Intracranial hemorrhage (50%)
Absence of radii, bilaterally
Congenital cardiac defects
Congenital renal defects
Laboratory findings
Thrombocytopenia
Deficiency of marrow megakaryocytes
Therapy
Platelet concentrates

because long-term platelet concentrate use can usually be anticipated.

The Wiskott-Aldrich syndrome is a rare sex-linked recessive disorder characterized by severe eczema, increased susceptibility to infections, and severe thrombocytopenia[9,296] (Table 4–18). Circulating platelets are classically small and demonstrate a decreased mean platelet volume (MPV) when evaluated by electronic particle counters with this capability.[262] Severe bleeding usually is manifested in the first 6 months of life, and then it may, like many other hereditary hemostasis defects, tend to improve. However, patients who survive bleeding episodes in their early childhood commonly die of overwhelming pyogenic infections or a malignancy, usually lymphoma.[296] Cellular and humoral immune defects are noted.[102,282,411] Patients usually demonstrate decreased IgM levels with normal IgG and IgA levels. Steroids are usually not effective, even though some investigators have postulated that the thrombocytopenia of the Wiskott-Aldrich syndrome is due to IgG-induced immune mechanisms.[201,230] However, splenectomy has been successful in selected patients,[231] although this places them at an even greater risk of infection because of the already compromised cellular and humoral immune defects. Patients undergoing splenectomy for thrombocytopenia associated with Wiskott-Aldrich syndrome should either be placed on prophylactic antibiotic therapy or should be followed carefully for observation and as soon as suggestive symptoms appear cultures should be obtained rapidly and appropriate antibiotic therapy should be instituted.

Several cases of "congenital thrombopoietin deficiency" have been reported.[222,339] These cases were characterized by severe thrombocytopenia with the presence of adequate marrow megakaryocytes. Patients have not responded to steroids or splenectomy, but the infusion of plasma or whole blood, presumably providing thrombopoietin, induced an increase in platelet counts. In the few cases thus far reported, patients also demonstrated a microangiopathic hemolytic anemia and features suggestive of the hemolytic-uremic syndrome (HUS). Thus, it may be disputed that some of these patients, in fact, have HUS or thrombotic thrombocytopenic purpura (TTP) rather than congenital thrombopoietin deficiency.

The May-Hegglin anomaly is inherited as an autosomal dominant trait and is a rare clinical oddity[146] (Table 4–19). The

Table 4–18 Features of the Wiskott-Aldrich Syndrome

Clinical findings
  Sex-linked recessive
  Severe thrombocytopenia
  Severe hemorrhage
  Bleeding improves with age
  Severe eczema
  Pyogenic infections
Laboratory findings
  Severe thrombocytopenia
  Small platelets
  Decreased MPV
  Decreased IgM
  IgG and IgA usually normal
  Cellular immune defects
  Humoral immune defects
Therapy
  Platelet concentrates
  Splenectomy ?

Table 4–19 Features of May-Hegglin Anomoly and Alport's Syndrome

May-Hegglin Anomoly
  Clinical findings
    Autosomal dominant trait
    Severe hemorrhage rare
  Laboratory findings
    Thrombocytopenia in 50%
    Giant platelets
    Increased MPV
    Bizzare morphology of platelets
    Hypergranularity of platelets
    Marrow megakaryocytes normal
    Döhle bodies in granulocytes
  Therapy
    Platelet concentrates
Alport's syndrome
  Clinical findings
    Autosomal dominant trait
    Microscopic or gross hematuria common
    Bleeding from other sites, uncommon
    Deafness
  Laboratory findings
    Thrombocytopenia
    Increased MPV
    Platelet function defect
    Sclerosing glomerular lesions
    Interstitial nephritis

disorder is characterized by giant platelets and a greatly increased MPV when platelet counts are performed by electronic particle counters.[141] In addition, large Döhle bodies are seen in peripheral and marrow granulocytes, and most patients have a mild neutropenia but no significant increased susceptability to infection.[70] Approximately 50% of patients have severe thrombocytopenia, but life-threatening hemorrhage is rare. In those individuals who are significantly thrombocytopenic, marrow megakaryocytes appear normal in number. The platelets of the May-Hegglin anomaly are not only enlarged, but many tend also to display bizarre morphology and hypergranularity.

Alport's syndrome is inherited as an autosomal dominant trait and is clinically characterized by proliferative and sclerosing glomerular nephritis and associated interstitial nephritis with fibrosis; deafness is also usually present[31] (Table 4–19). Thrombocytopenia with an increased MPV is characteristically present; in addition, platelets display a poorly defined platelet function defect.[90,121] Clinical hemorrhage is usually manifested as microscopic or gross hematuria. However, significant nonrenal hemorrhage may also occur. Significant or life-threatening hemorrhage should be treated with, and usually responds to, platelet concentrates.

The gray platelet syndrome is a rare disorder that is inherited as an autosomal dominant and is characterized by large platelets and an increased MPV on electronic particle counters[310] (Table 4–20). The platelets are either markedly hypogranular or agranular.[142] The thrombocytopenia is usually pronounced and severe hemorrhage may occur. The hypogranularity or agranularity is due to an absence or marked reduction of alpha granules; thus, although adenine nucleotide pools remain normal, these platelets lack beta-thromboglobulin and platelet factor 4.[404] However, platelet function, as defined by aggregometry, is usually normal despite the absence of granularity and the large size of these platelets. If significant bleeding occurs, the thrombocytopenia can usually be normalized by splenectomy. If indicated, platelet concentrates should be

Table 4–20 Features of the Gray Platelet Syndrome

Clinical findings
Autosomal dominant trait
Petechiae and purpura
Ecchymoses
Severe hemorrhage may occur
Laboratory findings
Thrombocytopenia
Large gray platelets
Increased MPV
Platelets agranular or hypogranular
Absence of alpha granules
Decreased platelet factor 4
Decreased beta-thromboglobulin
Platelet nucleotides normal
Platelet aggregation normal
Therapy
Platelet concentrates
Splenectomy

used to control life-threatening hemorrhage.

The Bernard-Soulier syndrome was discussed in detail previously under platelet function defects; however, it should be reemphasized that this is inherited as an autosomal recessive disorder and that platelets are markedly enlarged, demonstrate a significantly elevated MPV, and have shortened survival. The degree of thrombocytopenia is moderate to severe. In some individuals, however, thrombocytopenia is periodic or absent. Since the Bernard-Soulier platelet classically does not aggregate to ristocetin, the disorder can be easily superficially confused with von Willebrand's variant associated with thrombocytopenia unless platelet morphology is carefully examined and definitive laboratory tests are performed for von Willebrand disease. In significantly thrombocytopenic patients with Bernard-Soulier syndrome, splenectomy is usually not of benefit and thus not indicated.

One report of thrombocytopenia in a von Willebrand variant has been noted.[365] von Willebrand's disease and its variants are discussed in Chapter 5. Hereditary thrombocytopenias of unclear pathophysiologic mechanisms have been described and many types of inheritance have been noted in these disorders.[141,211,263,267,344,381] These disorders may be inherited as autosomal dominants and can be divided into those with normal and those with shortened platelet survival. A rare hereditary thrombocytopenia of sex-linked inheritance, some with an associated elevation of IgA, but without other characteristics of Alport's syndrome, has been described; hereditary thrombocytopenia with autosomal recessive inheritance has been described.[154] In many of these individuals it may be impossible to distinguish them from patients with ITP, especially if shortened platelet survival is documented.

The most commonly seen congenital marrow infiltrative processes leading to significant thrombocytopenia are the congenital leukemias and the congenital reticuloendothelioses. Thrombocytopenia with and without associated myeloid and erythroid depression occurs in children with numerous infiltrative disorders, including leukemia, lymphoma, solid tumors, myelofibrosis, Gaucher's disease, Niemann-Pick disease, and the mucopolysaccharidoses.[198,209,328] Infiltrative thrombocytopenia may also be seen with granulomatous diseases. A so-called leukoerythroblastic reaction may be seen in these clinical settings and the noting of thrombocytopenia in association with tear-drop red cells, nucleated red cells, marked anisopoikilocytosis, and polychromatophilia in some neonates and infants should suggest thrombocytopenia due to a marrow infiltrative process.

The maternal ingestion of ethanol, thiazides, chlorpropamide and tolbutamide, or steroids, especially prednisone and estrogens, may lead to significant thrombocytopenia in the newborn.[167,199,290,307,322,334] In addition, if the mother is ingesting cytotoxic chemotherapeutic drugs that are capable of crossing the placenta, neonatal thrombocytopenia may result. Other nonimmune (marrow suppressive) drug-induced thrombocytopenias seen in infants as well as adults will be discussed later.

Maternal infections with cytomegalovirus, hepatitis, varicella, or rubella may lead to congenital thrombocytopenia in the newborn; additionally, recent maternal vaccinations (rubella or rubeola) may lead to neonatal thrombocytopenia.[103,158,202,385] Although these appear to be the most common, many other maternal viral infestations may also lead to congenital throm-

bocytopenia.[199] Congenital and neonatal decreased platelet production defects are summarized in Table 4–21.

Acquired Production Defects

Aplastic anemia is often associated with severe thrombocytopenia,[138] but an in-depth discussion of aplastic anemia and its causes are beyond the scope of this text. However, thrombocytopenia may precede the myeloid and erythroid decreases by weeks to months in patients who are developing aplastic anemia, and in this instance a bone marrow examination may demonstrate an absence of megakaryocytes only.[223] In addition, thrombocytopenia associated with aplastic anemia may lag many months behind the recovery of myeloid and erythroid elements in recovering patients. In many patients who regenerate erythroid or myeloid elements in aplastic anemia, thrombocytopenia may never abate. The symptoms of thrombocytopenia, primarily petechiae, purpura, and hemorrhage, may often lead the patient to the clinician and thus to a diagnosis of aplastic anemia. The circulating platelets in thrombocytopenia associated with aplastic anemia are usually associated with a decreased MPV.[32] Common causes of

Table 4–21 Causes of Congenital and Neonatal Thrombocytopenia

Alport's syndrome
Bernard-Soulier syndrome
Congenital thrombopoietin deficiency
Fanconi's syndrome
Gray platelet syndrome
May-Hegglin anomoly
TAR Baby syndrome
Wiskott-Aldrich syndrome
Congenital marrow infiltration
  Congenital leukemias
  Congenital reticuloendothelioses
  Congenital mucopolysaccharidoses
  Congenital granulomatous diseases
Maternal drug ingestion
  Ethanol
  Thiazides
  Tolbutamide
  Steroids (estrogen and prednisone)
Maternal infections
  Cytomegalovirus
  Hepatitis
  Rubella
  Varicella

acquired platelet production defects are summarized in Table 4–22.

Isolated selective megakaryocyte marrow aplasia is an extremely rare condition.[362] This finding may, in some instances, herald the future development of an autoimmune disorder, such as systemic lupus erythematosus, a preleukemic state, or may represent a toxic effect from a drug, toxin, or infectious agent that was forgotten by the patient and therefore not related to the clinician. However, if vacuolated megakaryocytes are noted on bone marrow examination, a preleukemic state, or a drug or toxin, or infection should be strongly suspected and the patient appropriately evaluated and followed.[198,209,328] Patients with selective megakaryocytic marrow aplasia may have normal numbers of megakaryocytes; however, decreased megakaryocytes are more commonly noted. Patients with normal

Table 4–22 Acquired Causes of Platelet Production Defects

Aplastic anemia
Isolated megakaryocyte aplasia (rare)
Marrow infiltrative diseases
  Leukemia
  Lymphoma
  Hodgkin's disease
  Metastatic carcinoma
  Myelofibrosis
  Myelosclerosis
  Gaucher's disease
  Niemann-Pick disease
  Mucopolysaccharidoses
  Infiltrative infections
    Coccidioidomycosis
    Tuberculosis
    Toxoplasmosis
    Histoplasmosis
    Various bacteria
    Various viruses
Drug-induced marrow suppression
  Cytotoxic chemotherapy
  Thiazides
  Ethanol
  Gold
  Anti-inflammatory drugs
  Tranquilizers
  Anticonvulsants
Cyclic thrombocytopenia
Renal failure
Myeloproliferative syndromes
Maturation or metabolic defects
  B_{12} deficiency
  Folate deficiency

numbers of megakaryocytes may be difficult, if not impossible, to distinguish from those with ITP.

Decreased platelet production due to marrow infiltration (myelophthisis) may occur from chronic or acute leukemias, lymphomas, Hodgkin's disease, or metastatic carcinoma, the latter most commonly occurring from metastatic lung, breast, or prostatic carcinoma.[276] Myelofibrosis and myelosclerosis may also present with selective peripheral thrombocytopenia. In addition, marrow infiltration by Gaucher's disease, Niemann-Pick disease, mucopolysaccharidoses, and disseminated tuberculosis, coccidioidomycosis, histoplasmosis, toxoplasmosis, brucellosis, and malaria may induce marrow myelophthisis and subsequent peripheral thrombocytopenia.[65,89,113,114,123,151,354,380]

Thrombocytopenia due to marrow suppression from the administration of chemotherapy is usually not selective, but is often seen in combination with granulocytopenia and, less commonly, anemia. The drug that is most likely to cause selective thrombocytopenia from interference with megakaryocyte production is cytosine arabinoside. Other drugs that cause severe thrombocytopenia are nitrogen mustard, melphalan, busulfan, chlorambucil, the nitrosoureas, and vinblastine.[166] Intermediate degrees of marrow toxicity with associated megakaryocyte insult and resultant peripheral thrombocytopenia include cyclophosphamide, 5-fluorouracil, 6-mercaptopurine, methotrexate, procarbazine, and actinomycin D, assuming DIC does not occur with this last agent.[166] Mild degrees of megakaryocyte toxicity and peripheral thrombocytopenia are seen with vincristine, blenoxane, L-asparaginase, cisplatin, and hormones, including diethylstibesterol and prednisone.[166] Thrombocytopenia may also be induced by the antiestrogen drug, tamoxifen; however, this is rare. Estrogens may occasionally cause thrombocytopenia by decreased production; more commonly estrogens and estrogen derivatives as well as dexamethasone are not only associated with an increased risk of thrombosis and thromboembolism, but may also cause thrombocytopenia by inducing in vivo platelet aggregation or in vitro platelet aggregation after a blood sample has been drawn for platelet counting. Degrees of thrombocytopenia associated with chemohormonal therapy are summarized in Table 4–23.

Grades of thrombocytopenia associated with marrow (megakaryocyte) suppression have been developed by the University of California, Los Angeles and consist of the following platelet counts: Grade 0: approximately 100,000/mm^3; Grade 1: 75,000 to 99,999/mm^3; Grade 2: 50,000 to 74,999/mm^3; Grade 3: 25,000 to 49,999/mm^3, and Grade 4: less than 25,000/mm^3.[166] With initiation of radiation therapy, platelet suppression occurs after several days; however, megakaryocytes are less susceptible to radiation than myeloid and erythroid precursors. Radiation may also lead to rare, although often catastrophic, severe myelofibrosis, and resultant, usually irreversible, severe thrombocytopenia.[127]

Many drugs and chemicals are capable of inducing severe and, uncommonly, irreversible thrombocytopenia by nonimmune marrow suppression or production mechanisms. The drug or chemical may act at the promegakaryocyte stem cell stage or directly on the megakaryocyte or, more rarely, the circulating platelet.

Thiazide diuretics are the most common etiologic agents, but ethanol, anti-inflammatory drugs, tranquilizers, and anticonvulsants are also common offenders.[88,105,212,307,407] Unlike drug and chemical immune-mediated thrombocytopenia, the thrombocytopenia associated with drug- or chemical-induced marrow suppression is gradual in onset, requiring from weeks to several months to become manifest, and megakaryocytes are usually decreased rather than increased, as is commonly seen in immune-induced thrombocytopenia. When the offending drug is removed, the platelet count is slow to return to normal in comparison to most instances of immune-mediated drug-induced thrombocytopenia in which recovery is usually more rapid. If the drug or chemical exposure is continued for a long period of time, however, irreversible thrombocytopenia and aplastic anemia may ensue. A list of the common drugs and chemicals causing thrombocytopenia by nonimmune marrow suppression mechanisms is provided in Table 4–24.

Cyclic thrombocytopenia of unclear mechanisms has been noted in females and in older males.[95,119,353] The average cycle or nadir of thrombyocytopenia is approximately 30 days. Thrombocytopenia may be severe enough that significant or life-threatening hemorrhage may occur. Splenectomy and prednisone therapy have been without significant benefit

Table 4–23 Intensity of Thrombocytopenia with Antineoplastic Chemotherapy

Mild thrombocytopenia
  L-Asparaginase
  Bleomycin
  Cisplatin
  Vincristine
  Diethylstilbesterol
  Prednisone
  Tamoxifen
Moderate thrombocytopenia
  Actinomycin D
  Cyclophosphamide
  5-Fluorouracil
  6-Mercaptopurine
  Methotrexate
  Procarbazine
Severe thrombocytopenia
  Busulfan
  Chlorambucil
  Cytosine arabinoside
  Melphalan
  Nitrogen mustard
  Nitrosourea compounds
  Vinblastine

Table 4–24 Common Drugs Causing Decreased Platelet Production

Acetaminophen	Furosemide
Acetazolamide	Gold
Allopurinol	Indomethacin
Amphotericin	Mephenytoin
Aspirin	Meprobamate
Benzene	Oxyphenbutazone
Chloramphenicol	Phenylbutazone
Chlordiazepoxide	Prednisone
Chlorpromazine	Primidone
Chlorpropamide	Pyrimethamine
Chlorthalidone	Quinacrine
Cimetidine	Streptomycin
Colchicine	Sulfamethoxazole
Diazepam	Sulfisoxazole
Diethylstilbestrol	Sulfonamides
Diphenylhydantoin	Thiazides
Estrogens	Tolbutamide
Ethanol	

and thus, platelet transfusions, preferrably single donor platelets, remain the treatment of choice.

Infections associated with decreased production of platelets include numerous viral, bacterial, and fungal agents. Disseminated tuberculosis, coccidioidomycosis, brucellosis, and toxoplasmosis were previously discussed. The megakaryocytes provide an ideal cell for bacterial and viral invasion and replication, thereby interfering with platelet production.[92,93,124] When this occurs, morphologic changes in the megakaryocytes can usually be noted on marrow examination, the most common being cytoplasmic vacuolization and nuclear degeneration. Megakaryocytes may also be decreased in number. Viral invasion of megakaryocytes with resultant viral replication and subsequent megakaryocyte degeneration and associated decreased platelet production occurs in measles, including persons receiving live measles vaccinations, infectious mononucleosis, herpes simplex and herpes zoster, cytomegalovirus infection, and hepatitis.[11,79,84,87,141,285] Other viruses known to be associated with thrombocytopenia due to marrow-suppressive mechanisms are adenovirus, enteroviruses, mumps virus, and variola.

Bacterial infections, especially septicemia, are often associated with thrombocytopenia.[96] However, it is often difficult, if not impossible, to incriminate marrow suppression alone as the mechanism. In many instances, DIC secondary to sepsis may be involved, bacterial-platelet complexes may cause splenic removal of platelets (peripheral loss), and antibiotic use may also contribute to thrombocytopenia via several mechanisms. In gram-negative sepsis, endotoxin may induce platelet release and subsequent thrombocytopenia. Thus, in patients with bacterial infections, especially with septicemia, the often associated thrombocytopenia is usually a clinical summation of numerous pathophysiologic mechanisms. Since the mechanisms are unclear and often impossible to define clinically, significant or life-threatening hemorrhage is treated with 6 to 8 U of platelet concentrates every 6 to 12 hours, depending on the site and severity of hemorrhage. However, in septicemia, especially if due to gram-negative organisms, the patient should first be started on intravenous hydrocortisone succinate at 15 mg/kg intravenous push followed by 7 mg/kg intravenous push every 6 hours for at least 24 hours. The platelets can be given after the first intravenous dose of hydrocortisone succinate; this will often blunt any immune-induced component of the septicemia-associated thrombocytopenia.

Renal failure may be associated with defective platelet production; the mechanism or mechanisms remain totally unclear. Other causes for thrombocytopenia also occur in patients with renal disease, including splenomegaly and associated hypersplenism, circulating immune complex-mediated thrombocytopenia, and, at times, other mechanisms that may be a direct consequence of the underlying disease leading to renal failure.[221,308] The platelet function defect seen in renal failure is a much more common cause of significant bleeding in patients with renal disease than is thrombocytopenia. Effective treatment of the underlying disease process leading to renal failure or vigorous hemodialysis will usually correct, or partially correct, both the quantitative and qualitative platelet defects seen in these patients.

Unexplained thrombocytopenia may herald the development of several of the myeloproliferative syndromes, especially paroxysmal nocturnal hemoglobinuria (PNH).[165] However, it should be recalled that thrombocytosis may also be seen with many myeloproliferative disorders, including chronic myelogenous leukemia, essential thrombocythemia, and polycythemia rubra vera.[80,387] The primary exception being PNH and myelofibrosis with agnogenic myeloid metaplasia, in which case significant thrombocytopenia is seen in 30% of patients. Although defective platelets are produced in PNH,[20] the basic defect is a characteristic abnormality of red cells manifested as increased sensitivity to complement-mediated osmotic lysis, with activation by the primary or alternate (properdin) complement activation pathway. The disease is clearly a clonal stem cell disorder, since not only are erythrocytes and megakaryocytes defective, but also granulocytes. Thus, the presumably neoplastic clonal change occurs in a stem cell precursor common to the erythroid, myeloid, and megakarocytic maturation stages. Little is known of the megakaryocyte or platelet defect in PNH; however, platelets, like red cells, demonstrate increased sensitivity to complement-mediated lysis. The noting of pancytopenia, a decreased leukocyte alkaline phosphatase score, and a history of hemoglobinuria should prompt an acid hemolysis and sucrose hemolysis test for PNH. Thrombocytopenic bleeding is best treated with appropriate platelet concentrates, but this may induce further platelet lysis if complement is infused with the small amount of plasma present in platelet concentrates.

Maturation and Metabolic Defects

Severe iron deficiency may be associated with thrombocytosis or thrombocytopenia.[264] The mechanisms of decreased platelet production remain unclear, but may be related to the need for iron in platelet production by megakaryocytes. Iron therapy will usually induce prompt correction of thrombocytopenia. Significant bleeding and the need for platelet transfusions are extremely rare in severe iron deficiency anemia.

Patients with severe vitamin B_{12} or folate deficiency may present with hemorrhage due to thrombocytopenia.[219,356] Thrombocytopenia may be quite pronounced and is primarily due to ineffective megakaryopoiesis; however, other mechanisms are also operative, including absence of megakaryocytes from the marrow and a reduced platelet survival. The thrombocytopenia in severe folate or severe vitamin B_{12} deficiency usually is corrected promptly with appropriate hematinic therapy.

Thrombocytopenia Due to Increased Consumption or Destruction

Neonatal Increased Platelet Destruction or Consumption

Maternal ingestion of drugs or agents known to induce immune-mediated thrombocytopenia may cause immune thrombocytopenia in the newborn if these agents are capable of crossing the placenta. Thus, the maternal ingestion of quinine, quinidine, hydralazine, or selected antibiotics known to induce immune-mediated thrombocytopenia may result in congenital immune-mediated thrombocytopenia.[241,290,307,322,334,405] Thrombocytopenia in these neonates usually abates rapidly and only rarely does severe or fatal hemorrhage occur.

A more serious neonatal thrombocytopenia can arise from a maternal immune reaction to fetal platelet antigens (PLA) that have been inherited from the father.[291] Transplacental passage of the maternal antibody (usually an IgG) may create a severe thrombocytopenia in the neonate in utero.[345] This usually occurs when the mother has PLA[1] negative platelets and the fetus has inherited PLA[1] positive platelets from the father.[291,382] In other instances, anti-HLA antibodies have been incriminated.[382,383] Infants with this type of alloimmune neonatal thrombocytopenia may be covered with petechiae and purpura or may demonstrate more severe hemorrhage at the time of birth, or may appear normal at delivery and then manifest severe bleeding within the first week of birth. The thrombocytopenia usually abates within 1 month. Since approximately 30% of these infants may die of CNS hemorrhage, cesarean sections have been advocated to avoid the trauma of childbirth if a prenatal diagnosis has been made.[202] Other successful modes of therapy have been the use of platelet transfusions, exchange transfusions, and steroids in the severely thrombocytopenic infant.[17,247,345] Prenatal administration of corticosteroids to the mother may also be of benefit. Splenectomy does not appear to be useful, since the disorder is self-limiting and the other modalities of therapy just mentioned will usually control significant hemorrhage.

Neonatal infestation with toxoplasmosis, rubella, cytomegalovirus, herpes, or syphilis may cause an immune-mediated increased platelet destruction. However, the mechanisms remain poorly understood and poorly defined.[355,401]

Other causes of neonatal thrombocytopenia due to increased platelet consumption or destruction include neonatal thrombocytopenia in association with maternal ITP which will be discussed later. In addition, neonatal thrombocytopenia may occur in women who are preeclamptic, or develop frank toxemia of pregnancy.[143] This topic will be addressed more thoroughly in Chapter 6. Causes of neonatal increased platelet consumption or destruction are summarized in Table 4–25.

Acquired Increased Platelet Destruction or Consumption

Nonimmune Mechanisms.

Hemolytic-Uremic Syndrome. HUS is a poorly understood platelet consumptive disease first described in 1955,[384] which may be related to TTP or DIC with respect to pathophysiology. However, unlike TTP or DIC, this disease is almost always organ specific with respect to endothelial damage and thrombus formation. The disorder is more common in children but may

Table 4–25 Common Causes of Increased Platelet Destruction or Consumption In the Neonate

Maternal drug ingestion
Quinine
Quinidine
Hydralazine
Antibiotics
Alloimmune neonatal thrombocytopenia
Neonatal infection
Toxoplasmosis
Syphilis
Rubella
Herpes
Cytomegalovirus
Maternal immune thrombocytopenia purpura
Maternal preeclampsia
Maternal eclampsia

be seen in adults.[163] Many of the clinical and laboratory findings seen in childhood and adult HUS are similar; however, some striking differences are also noted. The common clinical features are moderate to severe thrombocytopenia, a microangiopathic hemolytic anemia, renal failure, and hypertension, which, at times, may be severe.[147] In children, males, and females are equally affected, but in adults, females develop the syndrome three times as commonly as males.[91,259] In childhood HUS there is commonly a prodrome of a viral or bacterial febrile illness often associated with gastroenteritis or a pneumonia-type syndrome.[304] Adult HUS, however, is almost never preceded by this type of syndrome, but is often associated with complications of pregnancy, including preeclampsia, frank toxemia of pregnancy, obstetric accidents, or a seemingly normal postpartum state.[338] Adult HUS may also be associated with renal transplantation rejection or the use of oral contraceptives.[134,169] Children and adults usually present with the usual clinical findings of anemia, petechiae, purpura, and, at times, more severe bleeding. Additionally, patients usually present with hematuria, renal failure, hypertension, and neurologic symptoms. The neurologic symptoms may be mild, including slurred speech and dull mentation, or may be very severe, including coma and frank seizures. However, neurologic complaints are less common than in TTP or DIC. The neurologic symptoms may be due to renal failure and severe hypertension or may be due to CNS microvascular damage or thrombosis or intracranial hemorrhage. A definite familial tendency has been noted in both children and adults with HUS and some have suggested this to be due to an inherited deficiency of a plasma prostacyclin-stimulating factor.[191] Tissue biopsy or autopsy examination usually reveals platelet and fibrinlike material in renal afferent arterioles and glomerular capillaries and in subendothelial spaces.[116,320] In some instances, especially fatal cases, these same findings may be noted systemically in multiple end organs.

Laboratory findings are those of a microangiopathic hemolytic anemia, manifested as schistocytes, thrombocytopenia with "large bizarre platelets" (young forms) usually obvious on a peripheral smear, and the usual findings of azotemia, hematuria, and proteinuria.[116,147] Coagulation abnormalities, besides thrombocytopenia, are usually limited to an almost universal elevation of FDPs. In occasional cases, however, typical laboratory findings of DIC may also be present.

Steroids, heparin, and antiplatelet agents are usually ineffective in childhood HUS.[147] However, the use of washed packed red cells, plasma exchange, and prompt dialysis have reduced the mortality to about 10%, and only 10 to 15% of surviving patients retain impaired renal function.[66] Unlike children, adults may respond to heparin or the use of antiplatelet agents (aspirin plus dipyridamole) in conjunction with dialysis, prompt control of hypertension, and infusion of washed packed red cells to control anemia.[66,316] Two other modes of therapy that deserve further investigation in adult HUS are plasma exchange and intravenous prostacyclin therapy.[399] The mortality in adults is much higher than in children and approaches 50% despite vigorous therapy. The clinical and laboratory findings of HUS are listed in Table 4–26.

Other Renal Diseases. Renal transplant rejection may be preceded or accompanied by moderate to severe thrombocytopenia, microangiopathic hemolytic anemia, and elevated serum or urine FDPs.[74,300] The thrombocytopenia is thought to be due to interactions between the platelets and damaged renal endothelium.[226] These findings in the renal transplant patient should prompt reinstitution or enhancement of immunosuppressive therapy, or, if clinically warranted, consideration of prompt retransplantation. Severe thrombocytopenia may also be seen in association with poststreptococcal glomerulonephritis. However, the mechanisms are unclear, and it is not known if this is a platelet-destructive process from platelet-renal vascular or glomerular interactions or is due to an immune complex mediated platelet destructive process.[193]

TTP is a disorder in which the etiology, pathophysiology, diagnosis, and management are controversial, confusing and difficult to define.[268] Since TTP is extremely

Table 4–26 Clinical and Laboratory Findings in the Hemolytic-Uremic Syndrome

Common clinical findings
  Anemia
  Thrombocytopenia
  Petechiae and purpura
  Hypertension
  Renal failure
  Hematuria
  Neurologic
  Familial tendency
Pediatric differences
  More common than in adults
  Prodrome of fever and infection
  Female to male ratio, 1:1
Adult differences
  Less common than in children
  Prodrome of
    Eclampsia
    Obstetrical accidents
    Oral contraceptive use
    Renal transplant rejection
    Normal postpartum state
  Female to male ratio, 3:1
Laboratory findings
  Microangiopathic hemolytic anemia
  Schizocytes
  Thrombocytopenia
  Large "young" platelets
  Elevated fibrin(ogen) degradation products
  DIC-type laboratory findings are rare
  Hematuria
    Microscopic
    Gross
  Proteinuria
  Azotemia

rare, investigators often do not acquire any significant clinical experience with this disease. Diagnostic criteria for TTP are so nonspecific that many proposed therapeutic modalities for true cases of TTP will appear to be ineffective when inappropriately applied to cases that simulate TTP, and, conversely, effective therapy may be viewed unfavorably when it does not correct a situation thought incorrectly to represent TTP.[268] TTP is difficult to distinguish from other similar conditions, especially HUS and DIC.[21,225,368] Table 4–27 summarizes conditions and diseases similar to TTP. The universal finding in tissue sections taken from biopsies or autopsy examination of patients with TTP includes the presence of microthrombi, which segmentally involve small arterioles and capillaries with a notable absence of inflammation; these microthrombi are noted in virtually any and

Table 4–27 Conditions Similar to Thrombotic Thrombocytopenic Purpura

Autoimmune hemolytic anemia
Disseminated intravascular coagulation
Eclampsia
Evan's syndrome
Hemolytic-uremic syndrome
Malignant hypertension
Microangiopathic hemolytic anemia
Paroxysmal nocturnal hemoglobinuria
Pediatric respiratory distress syndrome
Polyarteritis nodosa
Rocky Mountain spotted fever
Systemic lupus erythematosus
Vasculitis

Table 4–28 Typical Findings in Thrombotic Thrombocytopenic Purpura

Pathology
  Microthrombi segmentally involve subendothelium, vessel lumen, precapillary arterioles, capillaries, and postcapillary veins
  Arteriocapillary aneurysmal dilations
  Endothelial proliferation with a notable absence of inflammation or fibrinoid necrosis
  Microthrombi can be found in any organ system
Signs and symptoms
  Prodrome of fatigue, pallor, and nausea
  Petechiae, purpura, and ecchymoses
  Epistaxis
  Retinal hemorrhages
  Gastrointestinal bleeding
  Fever
  Jaundice
  Neurologic deficits
  Abdominal pain
  Hepatomegaly
  Splenomegaly
Laboratory
  Schizocytes
  Anemia
  Thrombocytopenia
  Reticulocytosis
  Hematuria
  Leukocytosis
  Elevated fibrin(ogen) degradation products
  DIC-type laboratory findings usually absent
  Coomb's test usually negative
  Proteinuria
  Azotemia
  Indirect hyperbilirubinemia

every organ system of the body (Table 4–28).[106,132] Characteristically hyaline microthrombi, absence of lysis at the periphery of microthrombi, and the absence of fibrinoid necrosis or vasculitis are noted. However, these are not pathognomonic lesions and can be found in tissue biopsies of many of the conditions that simulate TTP, listed in Table 4–27.

The initial lesion of TTP is thought to be caused by some undetermined injury to discontinuous segments of the endothelium of small arteries and capillaries. This insult gives rise to a prethrombotic subendothelial deposit consisting of platelets and fibrin.[149] These lesions are eventually replaced by hyaline microthrombi that may occlude the involved vascular segment.[14] If vasculitis or fibrinoid necrosis is noted, TTP can be excluded.[268] Kwaan and associates[213] have shown that injured endothelial cells in TTP, in contrast to normal endothelial cells, contain no plasminogen activator activity. However, TTP patients with active disease retain plasminogen activator activity in uninvolved vascular segments.[213] This is distinguished from the endothelial cells of vessels involved in DIC in which plasminogen activator activity is uniformly present.[268] Interestingly, the only other condition noted with altered endothelial plasminogen activator activity is scleroderma.[137] Thus, the hyaline microthrombi of TTP may be the result of disseminated intravascular platelet aggregation occurring segmentally at the endothelial site.[270]

On rare instances, a DIC syndrome may develop in a patient with TTP; however, this is probably an independent event and serves only to complicate the course of TTP. Pathologic findings in TTP are summarized in Table 4–28. The pathophysiology of DIC and TTP are quite different. For example, the fibrin seen in occlusive lesions is thought to be platelet derived in TTP as opposed to thrombin mediated in DIC. In addition, the lesion is pathogenically distinct and different from those produced in thrombin-mediated type syndromes. As a consequence of the endothelial injury in the microcirculation, a disordered prostaglandin metabolism is anticipated in TTP.[189,317] This is manifested by potential absence of prostacyclin derivatives, such as 6-keto-PGF$_1$. In addition, thromboxane A$_2$ activity is usually increased, as measured by the metabolic end product thromboxane B$_2$. The therapeutic approach recently advanced by Byrnes and Lian[76] is compatible with these observations; the objective of plasma transfusion is the replacement of a missing platelet aggregation factor inhibitor. This factor is thought to be missing in TTP and present in normal plasma. Platelet inhibitors, including aspirin, may have a major ancillary role in the therapy of TTP, as noted from clinical experience.[268]

Clinically, TTP has been defined in a variety of ways. As a triad, it consists of microangiopathic hemolytic anemia, thrombocytopenia, and fluctuating neurologic abnormalities.[268] When defined as a pentad or quintad, fever and renal abnormalities are added. Sixty percent of patients with TTP are females between the ages of 10 and 40 years, with a peak incidence occurring in the third decade. Within 2 to 3 months of the onset of TTP, 80% of patients are dead. There is almost always evidence of hemorrhage, including petechiae, purpura, ecchymoses, retinal hemorrhage, gastrointestinal hemorrhage, and epistaxis. The typical signs, symptoms, and physical and laboratory findings of TTP are found in Table 4–28. The classic laboratory findings of DIC are usually absent in patients with TTP. When a case fulfills the laboratory diagnostic findings of TTP and has some, but not all, of the laboratory features of DIC, such a case should be regarded as TTP with additional complications. Usually, normal or near normal levels of fibrinogen are noted and no evidence of thrombin activity (as determined by the protamine sulfate test or assays for fibrinopeptide A) and no reduction of antithrombin III levels or other evidence of concomitant DIC findings are present. The one consistent finding in TTP that is reminiscent of DIC and is often confusing to clinicians is an elevated FDP level. When suspecting TTP, available assays for prostaglandin derivatives should be considered.[268] A schistocytosis is almost always present; however, this finding also is only suggestive and certainly not diagnostic.

Therapy for TTP remains controversial and confusing. The rationale for plasma transfusion in TTP is to restore the missing Byrnes-Lian plasma factor and thus inhibit platelet aggregation.[76,268] Plasmapheresis, since it removes TTP plasma and replaces it with fresh plasma containing plasma aggregation inhibitor factor and reduces the level of unopposed platelet aggregating factor in TTP plasma, is a rational approach.[72,139] Blood transfusions will hypothetically deliver to the TTP patient quantities of the Byrnes-Lian factor, but appear to be less effective than plasma exchange. The role of hemodialysis in TTP is minimal, since it does not supply significant amounts of plasma containing the proposed platelet aggregation inhibitor factor of Byrnes-Lian.

Numerous therapeutic modalities have been proposed for the therapy of TTP, and these are summarized in Table 4–29. However, it appears that the Byrnes group has proposed the most rational therapeutic approach to the patient with TTP, that of plasma infusion or plasma exchange. The use of platelet suppressive therapy should be encouraged.[12,15,268] Plasma exchange or plasma infusion in conjunction with platelet suppressive therapy should enhance prostacyclin synthetase activity, depress thromboxane synthetase activity, increase intraplatelet cyclic AMP levels, and inhibit platelet phosphodiesterase activity. It should again be mentioned that, based on current theories of TTP pathophysiology, heparin does not have a rational therapeutic role, since the occlusive lesions are mediated entirely by platelets and not by thrombin or DIC-type mechanisms. If a complicating DIC process is coincidentally present in a patient with TTP, appropriate heparin therapy should be used to control the DIC. Urokinase or streptokinase may be useful as supplementary therapeutic modalities in lysing the platelet-derived fibrin component in

Table 4–29 Proposed Therapeutic Modalities for Thrombotic Thrombocytopenic Purpura

Plasmapheresis
Plasma transfusions
Blood transfusions
Exchange transfusions
Splenectomy
Platelet suppressant therapy
Steroid therapy
Heparin therapy
Dextrans
Urokinase
Streptokinase
Prostacyclin infusion

the occluding microthrombi. When injury to endothelial cells is marginal or the duration of the occlusion short, lysis and dislocation of the microthrombi may be of possible value. However, since the lesions are variable in age and severity in numerous organ systems producing functionally deficient and physically absent endothelial cells at numerous points, massive tissue hemorrhage may be a potentially disastrous consequence of restoring patency to injured vessels with thrombolytic therapy. A new era of therapy in TTP may come about with the possible use of prostacyclin. Although prostacyclin has a very short half-life when infused, the beneficial effects of platelet suppression by this agent may be highly desirous in TTP patients.

In summary, TTP remains a diagnostic and therapeutic challenge; however, if strict clinical and laboratory diagnostic features are applied, the syndrome can be distinguished from HUS as well as DIC-related syndromes.[268,301] Therapeutic management is markedly different from that for DIC-type syndromes, and it appears that the most effective therapy at present is plasma exchange or plasma infusion to supply the TTP patient with platelet aggregation factor inhibitor and the adjuvant use of platelet suppressive therapy in the form of aspirin and dipyridamole. Thorough and provocative reviews regarding the theory, etiology, pathophysiology, diagnosis, and management of TTP have recently been published.[237–239]

Hypersplenism. Splenomegaly and associated hypersplenism can be of numerous etiologies and may not only cause pancytopenia, but also moderately severe to severe thrombocytopenia. Those conditions commonly associated with hypersplenism are listed in Table 4–30. The mechanism of thrombocytopenia in hypersplenism is thought to be due to the pooling of a large percentage of the total body platelet population within the spleen.[120] Normally the spleen contains approximately one third of the total body platelet population at any given time.[22] Intravenous epinephrine causes a marked increase in platelet counts in hypersplenic patients, but only a moderate increase in normal persons, thus supporting the con-

Table 4–30 Common Causes of Hypersplenism

Amyloidosis
Autoimmune disorders
   Systemic lupus erythematosus
   Rheumatoid arthritis
Gaucher's disease
Hemolytic anemias
Hodgkin's disease
Idiopathic splenomegaly
Infections
Inflammatory diseases
Leukemia
Lymphoma
Metastatic carcinoma
Multiple myeloma
Myeloproliferative syndromes
Niemann-Pick disease
Portal hypertension
Thalassemia
Waldenstrom's macroglobulinemia

cept of splenic sequestration in hypersplenism.[224] In addition, large numbers of platelets can be extruded from an enlarged spleen removed during splenectomy.[295] It appears that splenic pooling of platelets in hypersplenism is brought on by the very slow passage of platelets through the spleen as a result of a "percolating" effect causing platelets to take a tortuous and slow course through the splenic sinusoids, thus allowing contact and resultant cohesion between platelets and splenic macrophages and endothelial cells.[120] The noting of increasing platelet counts after an infusion of epinephrine in the patient with hypersplenism may be an indication that the patient will most likely respond to splenectomy if the procedure is clinically indicated.[52]

The clinical manifestations of thrombocytopenia secondary to hypersplenism are usually related to the disorder initially causing the hypersplenism or splenomegaly.[120] In this regard it should be noted that the vast majority of individuals with hypersplenism do have splenomegaly; however, hypersplenism may occur in the presence of a normal-sized spleen. The most common cause of hypersplenism and associated thrombocytopenia is that associated with congestive splenomegaly due to portal hypertension secondary to chronic liver disease.[13] The degree of thrombocytopenia appears to correlate reasonably well with the degree of the splenic enlargement.

The management of thrombocytopenia secondary to hypersplenism is dependent on the underlying disease process giving rise to hypersplenism. Splenectomy is rarely indicated, but when indicated, the efficacy of splenectomy may be inferred by the presplenectomy infusion of epinephrine and noting significant elevation of the peripheral platelet count.[52] Portacaval shunting may be indicated in selected disease states and radiation of the spleen is occasionally useful in patients who have splenomegaly and hypersplenism in association with leukemia, lymphoma, Hodgkin's disease, or related disorders. Even though this is a non-immune cause of thrombocytopenia, the use of steroids to blunt splenic reticuloendothelial function may also be useful if the patient has significant persistent thrombocytopenia. In addition, in severe or life-threatening hemorrhage the use of platelet concentrates should be considered.

DIC and related syndromes, which will be discussed in detail in appropriate subsequent chapters, are almost uniformly associated with significant thrombocytopenia due to nonimmune consumption or destruction of platelets.

Infections and Drugs Directly Toxic to Platelets. Thrombocytopenia may be associated with numerous bacterial,[93,170] viral,[369] fungal,[113] and protozoan infections. The mechanisms may be extremely complex and the thrombocytopenia noted is often a clinical summation of many pathophysiologic events in the patient. Nonimmunologic mechanisms of thrombocytopenia in the patient with infection may include direct platelet destruction by interaction of the infectious agent with platelets, in vivo platelet aggregation induced by bacteria or bacterial products, the development of infection-induced DIC with resultant consumption of platelets, the release of thromboxane A_2 by infectious agents or their products, or the interaction of platelets with endothelium, which has sustained significant damage by the infectious agent.[93,113,170,271,369]

Thrombocytopenia often occurs early in the course of septicemia, and the noting of thrombocytopenia in a febrile patient should prompt early suspicion of the development of septicemia, commonly due to meningococcus, other gram-negative organisms (especially those that produce endotoxin), or staphylococcal organisms.[408] In addition, the febrile patient with thrombocytopenia should be thoroughly investigated for the possibility of subacute bacterial endocarditis.[150] Thrombocytopenia is seen much more commonly in gram-negative than in gram-positive septicemia.[408] Up to 60% of patients with sepsis will have some degree of thrombocytopenia.

Thrombocytopenia associated with infections usually abates with control or resolution of the infectious process. However, if significant or life-threatening hemorrhage occurs or is thought to be impending, platelet concentrates should be readily used. If there is felt to be an immune complex component to the infectious-associated thrombocytopenia, intravenous hydrocortisone succinate, or oral prednisone should precede the use of platelet concentrates. Infections causing nonimmune-mediated thrombocytopenia are listed in Table 4–31.[11,79,84,87,89,113,114,123,141,285,354]

Table 4–31 Common Infections Causing Nonimmune Thrombocytopenia

Brucellosis
Coccidioidomycosis
Cytomegalovirus
Diphtheria
Disseminated herpes
Hepatitis
Histoplasmosis
Infectious mononucleosis
Many gram-negative organisms
Meningococcus
Mumps
Protozoan infections
Rocky Mountain spotted fever
Septicemia
Staphylococcus
Subacute bacterial endocarditis
Toxic shock syndrome
Tuberculosis
Typhoid fever
Varicella

Selected drugs appear to be directly toxic to platelets, causing increased platelet destruction by nonimmunologic mechanisms. The most popular of these is ristocetin, an antibiotic that was removed from clinical use because of inducing in vivo platelet aggregation or agglutination. The mechanism appears to be the ability of ristocetin to promote binding of Factor VIII to a platelet receptor.[140] Bleomycin and other selected chemotherapeutic agents may also cause direct injury to platelets.[173] In the case of bleomycin, it has been suggested that platelets are destroyed after interacting with endothelium previously damaged by this drug.[173] Heparin-induced thrombocytopenia may result in a severe and life-threatening situation and will be discussed in detail in Chapter 14. It remains controversial as to whether this is a direct toxic effect by heparin or whether this is an immune mediated phenomena.[27]

Gold-induced thrombocytopenia occurs in many patients receiving gold therapy. The most serious side effect of gold therapy is that of aplastic anemia; however, thrombocytopenia is the single most common hematologic complication from gold therapy and occurs in approximately 3% of patients.[200] The exact mechanism is unclear, but the early onset of thrombocytopenia, decreased platelet survival, and normal or increased megakaryocytes in the marrow suggest that peripheral platelet destruction is operative. Treatment is immediate discontinuation of gold; other therapy of potential benefit are the use of chelating agents and prednisone.[360] Despite these therapeutic modalities, many patients remain persistently thrombocytopenic after discontinuation of gold.

Protamine sulfate may be associated with rapid development of thrombocytopenia; however, the effect is usually transient, does not often lead to serious or life-threatening hemorrhage, and is thought to be due to the induction of protamine-induced platelet sequestration in the liver.[172] Valproic acid has become popular as an antepileptic agent and is associated with t hrombocytopenia.[99] The mechanism is thought to be due to valproic acid interaction with platelets leading to increased peripheral destruction; however, immunologic mechanisms have also been suggested.

Cardiovascular Diseases and Increased Platelet Consumption/Destruction.

Aortic and mitral valvular disease, especially the types seen in association with rheumatic fever, have been associated with increased platelet consumption or destruction.[187,364] Mild thrombocytopenia commonly occurs in patients with severe aortic stenosis; in addition, patients with mitral disease, associated with left atrial thrombosis or peripheral vascular embolization may have thrombocytopenia.[187,321] Thrombus formation and associated platelet consumption are relatively common in patients with prosthetic valves; the incidence of platelet consumption is significantly lower in patients with tissue than with nontissue valves; however, porcine valves have been associated with platelet consumption and thrombocytopenia.[85,97,234,321] Circulating platelet aggregates are seen in patients with severe coronary artery disease and the presence of many circulating platelet aggregates may be associated with peripheral thrombocytopenia.[229,329] Peripheral arterial disease, especially if associated with significant claudication and gangrene or thromboembolism may also be associated with increased consumption and mild, moderate, or severe thrombocytopenia.[235] Extensive deep vein thrombosis, especially involving the inferior vena cava, or iliofemoral system, but also calf thrombosis and especially that associated with pulmonary embolism, may be associated with significant platelet consumption and resultant thrombocytopenia.[53,375] Thrombocytopenia is a frequent accompaniment of cardiopulmonary bypass surgery, which will be discussed in detail in Chapter 9. Mechanisms on nonimmune-mediated increased consumption or destruction of platelets are summarized in Table 4–32.

Immune-Induced Platelet Destruction.

The common immune-mediated causes of thrombocytopenia are summarized in Table 4–33. Acute ITP occurs primarily in children, but may also be seen

Table 4-32 Causes of Nonimmune Increased Platelet Destruction or Consumption

Cardiovascular disorders
Cardiopulmonary bypass surgery
Disseminated intravascular coagulation
Drugs
Eclampsia
Hemodialysis
Hemolytic-uremic syndrome
Hypersplenism
Infections
Prosthetic devices
Renal diseases
Thrombotic thrombocytopenic purpura

Table 4-33 Causes of Immune-Mediated Increased Platelet Destruction or Consumption

Congenital/neonatal
  Maternal drug ingestion
  Alloimmune neonatal thrombocytopenia
  Neonatal infection
  Maternal immune thrombocytopenia purpura
Acquired
  Acute immune thrombocytopenia purpura
  Chronic immune thrombocytopenia purpura
  Drug-induced immune thrombocytopenia
  Post-transfusion purpura

in adults.[233,246] In acute ITP there is almost always a prodrome of an acute viral illness occurring from 1 week to 1 month before the rapid onset of thrombocytopenia in approximately 80% of patients.[98] The most common viral illnesses noted to precede acute ITP are chickenpox, rubeolla, rubella, or undefined, nonspecific upper respiratory infections.[233,242] However, acute ITP has also been noted after vaccination with live virus for measles, mumps, chickenpox, and smallpox.[81,233,242,246] In many children, spontaneous recovery will occur in several months. The mechanisms thought to be responsible for the abrupt onset of thrombocytopenia is the binding of a viral-induced immune complex to platelets and megakaryocytes.[203] These platelets are thus removed by the reticuloendothelial system, primarily the spleen but also the liver and possibly the bone marrow. Megakaryopoiesis is also compromised because of immune complex binding. Since the disease usually occurs

well after the viremia has abated, presumably the immune response against the initial virus gives rise to an immune complex that then binds to platelet membrane Fc receptors.[203,297] In this respect it has been noted that immune complexes isolated from patients with ITP will not bind to platelets of patients with Glanzmann's thrombasthenia; thus, the immune complexes may be directed toward Fc receptors of platelet membrane glycoproteins IIb or III, missing from Glanzmann's platelets.[205] Significantly increased levels of platelet-associated IgG (PAIgG) are noted to be present in the vast majority of cases.[203] The recent observation that infusions of intravenous gamma globulin will reverse the Fc receptors of phagocytic cells and subsequently reverse the thrombocytopenia provides some evidence that viral antigens may be absorbed onto the platelet membrane surface, followed by immune complex formation.[82,184]

Acute ITP usually occurs before the teenage years, but may also occur in adults. Clinical symptoms of petechiae, purpura, ecchymoses, and mucosal membrane bleeding from the gastrointestinal tract, genitourinary tract, gingiva, or epistaxis usually begin abruptly.[98,203,233,246] Hemorrhagic bullae may be noted on examination of the oral mucosa. Mild adenopathy is usually found, but hepatosplenomegaly is found in less than 10% of patients with acute ITP. Recovery occurs in the vast majority of patients despite the mode of therapy used, if any. Recovery is usually within 2 months, but some patients may not recover for 6 to 12 months.[98,203,233,246,260] Very few patients have recurrences if recovery occurs. The risk of significant hemorrhage is greatest at the onset and appears to abate with initiation of steroid therapy. My general approach is to start prednisone immediately at 2 mg/kg/day in two doses, each dose with 30 mL of a liquid antacid. This may abort a serious or life-threatening hemorrhage, including an intracranial bleeding episode. Patients are also cautioned about restricted activity until the platelet count is greater than 50,000/mm^3, and the patient and family are strictly cautioned regarding the use of any drug known to interfere with platelet function. Platelet transfusions are of minimal efficacy because transfused donor platelets are also affected by the immune complex-containing recipient blood and are thus rapidly consumed by the reticuloendothelial system, primarily the spleen, and therefore they should only be used to abort intracranial or life-threatening hemorrhage. According to limited experience, therapeutic plasma exchange, infusions of fresh frozen plasma, and infusions of intravenous gamma globulin also are effective.[82,139,184,275]

Approximately 10% of children fail to respond to any mode of therapy. If no response is noted by 6 months, or the child becomes unduly cushingoid or cannot tolerate other modes of therapy, I usually recommend splenectomy, followed by extremely slow prednisone taper. The prednisone is decreased by 5 mg/week. Children who fail to respond to these modalities in a reasonable period of time (6 to 12 months) are usually those who had no prodrome of a viral illness, have low levels of IgA, and are only moderately thrombocytopenic, in other words, those who actually have chronic ITP. Only 60% of these individuals will have significant bleeding, which can be controlled with low to moderate doses of prednisone or azathioprine. If splenectomy is performed in children with acute or chronic ITP, it should be followed by pneumococcal vaccine. The salient features of acute ITP are summarized in Table 4–34.

Chronic ITP usually occurs in adults, and females predominate three to one.[305] Although there is not a prodrome of viral illness in chronic ITP, it is also an immune complex disorder in which the immune complex attaches to platelets, leading to destruction by the spleen, bone marrow, or liver, in descending order of importance. Immune complex attachment to the megakaryocyte leading to ineffective platelet production is also operative in chronic ITP.[160,243,413] Women with chronic ITP give birth to thrombocytopenic children in 50 to 80% of cases.[122,168] PAIgG is elevated in 90% of patients, and serum tests for this same antibody are positive in 50% of patients.[203,244] All four classes of IgG may be responsible, but IgG 1 has been the predominate type.[203] It has been speculated that chronic ITP is a disorder of

Table 4–34 Acute Immune Thrombocytopenia Purpura

Clinical findings
Common in children, usually before 12 years of age
Uncommon in adults
Frequent prodrome of viral disease
Spontaneous recovery common
Abrupt onset of hemorrhage
Petechiae and purpura
Ecchymoses
Epistaxis
Gastrointestinal hemorrhage
Genitourinary hemorrhage
Shoddy adenopathy is common
Less than 10% with hepatosplenomegaly
Recurrence is very rare
Therapy
Prednisone, 2.0 mg./kg./day and slow taper
Platelet concentrates: minimal efficacy
Minimal experience
Plasma exchange
Infusion of fresh frozen plasma
Intravenous gamma globulin
Therapy failure (10%):
Splenectomy indicated

immunoregulation; several studies have demonstrated decreased suppressor cell activity.[203,371] The often rapid increase in platelet counts and decrease in PAIgG after splenectomy suggest the spleen to be both the primary site of platelet destruction as well as the major organ of pathologic immunoglobulin synthesis in chronic ITP. In those patients failing to respond to splenectomy, the IgG may originate from the bone marrow or possibly the liver. Like acute ITP, the Fc receptor mechanism appears important; platelet destruction in ITP may occur via splenic (or other reticuloendothelial) phagocytosis with or without complement activation.[203,244] In fact, the role of complement activation in platelet destruction remains unclear. However, as pointed out previously, the blockade of Fc receptor activity will cause rapid rise in the platelet count in the limited experience thus far noted.

Unlike acute ITP, chronic ITP usually begins insidiously, and a syndrome of easy and spontaneous bruising usually precedes other more serious hemorrhagic manifestations that eventually lead the patient to seek medical attention [244] (Table 4–35). Epistaxis and gingival bleeding are common, and petechiae and ecchymoses are usually noted on examination. Oral

Table 4–35 Chronic Immune Thrombocytopenia Purpura

Clinical findings
  Common in adults
  Rare in children
  Female to male ratio, 3:1
  No prodrome of viral illness
  If maternal ITP, neonate has 50% to 80% chance of
    ITP at delivery
  PAIgG found in 90%
  Serum antibody found in 50%
  Insidious onset:
    Easy bruising
    Spontaneous bruising
    Epistaxis
    Gingival bleeding
    Petechiae and purpura
  Mild splenomegaly in 30%
Therapy
  Prednisone: 2.0 mg./kg./day given twice daily, each
    dose with 30 mL liquid antacid
  70% will respond
  After counts normalize for 2 weeks, slow prednisone
    taper at 5 mg./kg./week
  Steroid failure: splenectomy followed by slow pred-
    nisone taper; 70% will respond
  Splenectomy failure
    Long-term prednisone
    Azathioprine
    Vincristine
    Intravenous gamma globulin
    Combinations of above

mucosal petechiae and purpura are also common; however, hemorrhagic bullae of the oral mucosa are only noted in severe cases. Mild splenomegaly is noted in approximately 30% of cases.[244,245] The finding of marked hepatosplenomegaly in association with thrombocytopenia should alert the clinician to consider a malignant lymphoreticular disorder, autoimmune disorder, carcinomatosis, or tuberculosis.

Bone marrow examination, as in acute ITP, usually reveals normal or increased megakaryocytes that have basophilic hypogranular cytoplasm and are without appreciable "platelet budding."[199] Typical marrow findings in ITP are shown in Figures 4–14 and 4–15. These findings suggest a population of less mature megakaryocytes with premature platelet release, which is simply a response to peripheral thrombocytopenia. The mainstay of therapy of chronic ITP is that of prednisone. My approach is to use prednisone at 2 mg/kg/day in two doses, each dose to be taken with 30 mL of liquid antacid. Seventy percent of patients will respond to this mode of therapy. Significant bleeding risk usually abates immediately after institution of prednisone therapy. After the platelet count has remained normal for 1 to 2 weeks, prednisone is tapered extremely slowly at 5 mg/kg/week.

Those patients whose platelet count decreases with steroid tapering may be considered steroid failures and are candidates for splenectomy. Of those patients subjected to splenectomy, 70% will respond with no recurrence of the disease and 30% will fail to respond. After splenectomy, steroid tapering should be extremely slow, and my approach is again to taper prednisone at 5 mg/kg/week. In those patients who require splenectomy oral prednisone therapy is continued until the day before the operation. The night before the patient is given long-acting dexamethasone acetate intramuscularly and the morning of surgery the dose (8 to 12 mg) is repeated. In addition, just before the operation the patient is infused with 100 mg of hydrocortisone, and this dose is repeated that evening. In addition, intramuscular dexamethasone acetate is continued twice daily until the patient is able to take oral medications, and then prednisone is reinstituted and a very slow taper, as defined previously, is begun. If this sequence of events is followed, clearly 70% of patients will respond to splenectomy without relapse.[214] Those patients who have a drop in platelet count with steroid tapering after splenectomy may be considered splenectomy failures. In these individuals long-term prednisone or azathioprine, or a combination of both, will usually be needed to control significant thrombocytopenia. However, many patients remain only borderline thrombocytopenic and will not have significant bleeding consequences.

Plasma exchange and intravenous gamma globulin have also been used with limited success in patients with chronic ITP, both before and after splenectomy. More experience is needed with these modalities of therapy.[82,139,184,275] As with acute ITP, the role of platelets is somewhat limited; infused platelets are destroyed as rapidly as the patient's platelets, and thus

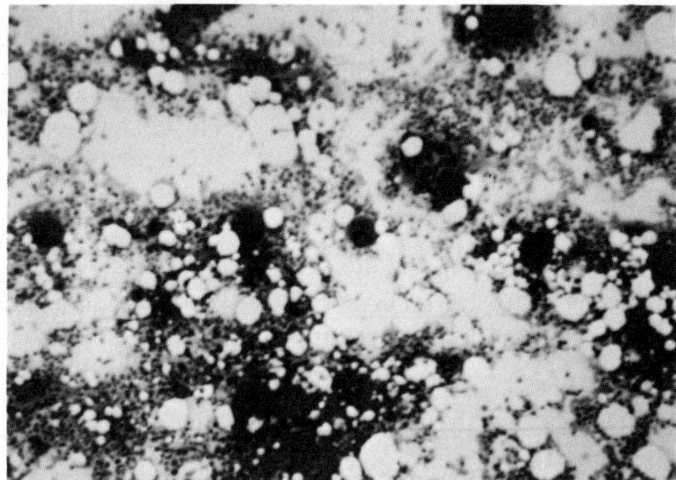

Fig. 4–14. Typical marrow findings in ITP.

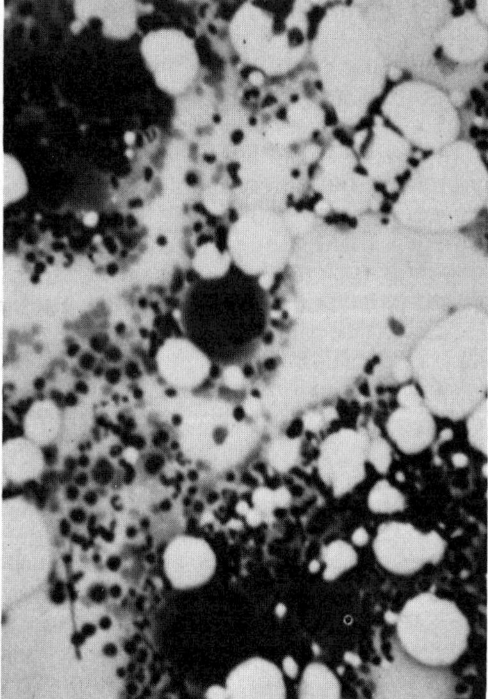

Fig. 4–15. Typical marrow findings in ITP.

platelet infusion should be reserved to abort life-threatening or intracranial hemorrhage. Some patients with chronic ITP may develop an autoimmune hemolytic anemia; this combination is referred to as Evan's syndrome.[293,306,386]

Drugs constitute a major cause of immune thrombocytopenia, which may be associated with a large number of drugs, but is most commonly seen with quinidine, quinine, gold, heparin, sulfonamides, indomethacin, and thiazide diuretics.[156,251] Table 4–36 lists the drugs most commonly associated with immune-mediated thrombocytopenia in descending order of prevalence.[33,64,101,108,109,111,115,155,156,180,183,194,218,245,251–253,388] Table 4–37 lists less common drugs causing immune thrombocytopenia. The first incidence of drug-induced thrombocytopenia was reported in 1895, being noted after quinine ingestion.[378] Ackroyd[2–4] was the first to carefully study drug-induced thrombocytopenia and was able to demonstrate the immune-mediated nature of apronalide-induced thrombocytopenia. Subsequently, numerous studies have confirmed the immune nature of thrombocytopenia induced by quinine, quinidine, and sulfonamides.[156,245,251,252] There are several postulated mechanisms by which drug-induced immune thrombocytopenia are thought to occur. Ackroyd initially thought that the drug became bound to platelet membrane and, following this, antibody was formed against a platelet membrane-drug complex. This mechanism is depicted in Figure 4–16. An alternate mechanism, which appears to be operative for many drugs,

Table 4–36 Common Drugs Causing Immune Thrombocytopenia*

Gold	Phenylbutazone
Heparin	Alpha methyl DOPA
Quinidine	Bleomycin
Quinine	Carbamazepine
Sulfonamides	Acetazolamide
Indomethacin	Ampicillin
Arsenicals	Fenoprofen
Aspirin	Isoniazide
Heroin	Mercurial diuretics
Valproic acid	Nitrofurantoin
Chlorothiazide	Pertussis vaccine
Chlorthalidone	Tolbutamide
Furosemide	Trimethoprim
Rifampicin	Antazoline
Digitalis derivatives	Barbiturates
Diphenylhydantoin	Cephalothins
Para-amino salicylate	Clinoril
Cimetidine	Diazoxide
Acetaminophen	Oxytetracycline
Chlorpropamide	Penicillin
Oxyphenbutazone	Procaine amide

* Listed in descending order of prevalence.

Table 4–37 Less Common Drugs Causing Immune Thrombocytopenia*

Allopurinol	Niroglycerin
Antipyrine	Novobiocin
Cephalexin	Paramethadione
Chlordiazepoxide	Penicillamine
Chlorpheniramine	Pentamidine
Clonazepam	Phenytoin
Copper Sulfate	Primidone
Diazepam	Prochlorperazine
Disulfiram	Propylthiouracil
Gentamicin	Sodium salicylate
Imipramine	Spironolactone
Iopanoic acid	Streptomycin
Levamisole	Tetanus toxoid
Levo-DOPA	Tetraethylammonium
Lidocaine	Thioguanine
Lincomycin	Thiouracil
Meprobamate	Tobramycin
Methicillin	

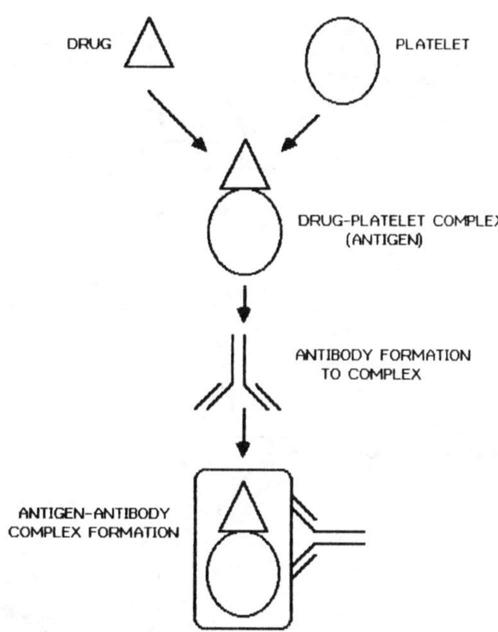

Fig. 4–16. Drug-induced immune thrombocytopenia, Ackroyd mechanism.

is the so-called innocent bystander theory initially advanced by Schulman.[346–349] In this instance the drug interacts with an endogenous plasma protein or other endogenous plasma compounds and the antibody subsequently produced is directed against this drug-plasma-protein complex; thus the drug is acting as a classic hapten. This resultant antibody plus drug-plasma-protein (antigen) complex is then absorbed onto the platelet surface by Fc or C-3 receptors. This mechanism appears operative in quinidine- and quinine-induced thrombocytopenia and is depicted in Figure 4–17.

In most instances IgG antibody is produced in drug-induced immune thrombocytopenia; however, several cases of IgM-mediated thrombocytopenia have also been reported. Studies of the Bernard-Soulier syndrome show that platelets, which are missing platelet membrane glycoproteins IB and IS, do not agglutinate when incubated with drug plus serum from patients with immune-induced thrombocytopenia. This suggests that platelet glycoproteins IB and IS are the receptors for immune complex-mediated drug-induced thrombocytopenia.[156,245,251]

Drug-induced immune thrombocytopenia usually appears with the rapid onset of petechiae and purpura and profound thrombocytopenia. The patient may have been ingesting the drug for only a short period of time or may have been taking the offending agent for months, or in some instances, years. This is in distinction

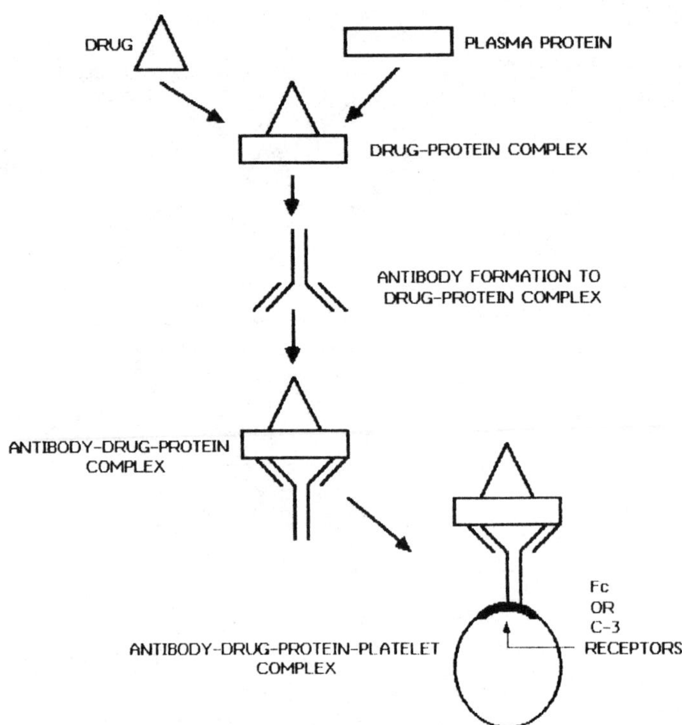

Fig. 4–17. Drug-induced immune thrombocytopenia, innocent bystander mechanism.

to nonimmune drug-induced thrombocytopenia; in this instance the platelet count drops very slowly and returns to normal slowly after withdrawal of the offending drug. Although the integument is the most common site of hemorrhage, bleeding from other sites, including any mucosal membrane surface, may be seen. Catastrophic intracranial hemorrhage is uncommonly seen and is usually the cause of death in fatal cases. Fatality of drug-induced immune thrombocytopenia is approximately 5%. Many patients develop systemic symptoms as well; these usually consist of fever, chills, headaches, generalized malaise, nausea, and emesis. Occasionally, severe abdominal cramping and generalized arthralgias may occur.

The diagnosis is made by noting the sudden onset of petechiae and purpura associated with thrombocytopenia in a patient ingesting one or more drugs. In this regard, a careful drug history is mandatory in thrombocytopenic patients, including a history for any compounds containing aspirin, and any over-the-counter medications or home remedies that may contain quinine. Laboratory confirmation is best made by documenting the presence of PAIgG plus the noting of control platelet agglutination when incubated with patient serum plus the offending drug. Numerous techniques for these tests have been devised and have recently been extensively reviewed.[61,156,203,220,251,265, 335,366,379]

The mainstay of therapy for drug-induced immune thrombocytopenia consists of withdrawal of all suspected drugs, hospitalization of the patient, avoidance of any drug or compound known to interfere with platelet function, and careful observation for suggestions of the potential for significant hemorrhage. Steroids, in the form of oral prednisone or intravenous hydrocortisone succinate may be of benefit in warding off life-threatening hemorrhage; this effect probably comes about via a beneficial effect on the vasculature rather than steroid-induced cessation or blunting of the immune mechanism. Patients who are suspected of developing a life-threatening hemorrhage, especially intracranial, who present with an existing serious hemorrhage, or who have platelet counts of less than 10,000/mm^3 should be infused with platelet concentrates. Although infused platelets will demonstrate a shortened platelet life span, they usually are of benefit in achieving some degree of hemostasis and thus warding off fatal hemorrhage. They may also be of benefit by complexing with and thus enhancing the removal of the offending circulating immune complex.

Post-Transfusion Purpura. Post-transfusion purpura is a rare event and occurs approximately 1 week after transfusions in a patient who is PLA^1 negative.[341] Ninety-eight percent of the population is PLA^1 positive; thus, the transfused patient who is PLA^1 negative has a high risk of receiving incompatible platelets.[341] The vast majority of cases are seen in females who are PLA^1 negative and have been previously sensitized by either transfusion or pregnancy.[416] A few cases have occurred in PLA^1 positive patients and a few have also been noted in nonsensitized individuals, suggesting that in rare instances other platelet antibodies must be involved.[376] Patients with Glanzmann's thrombasthenia are lacking platelet glycoprotein IIIA and are PLA^1 negative; thus, it appears that the PLA^1 antigen site may be associated with platelet membrane glycoprotein IIIA. The clinical course is typically a sudden onset of petechiae, purpura, and mucosal membrane hemorrhage in association with thrombocytopenia approximately 1 week after transfusions. Some patients demonstrate a mild reaction consisting of chills and fever at the time of the transfusion[1] (Table 4–38). In most cases, anti-PLA^1 antibody can be easily demonstrated in the laboratory. In the majority of patients the thrombocytopenia will spontaneously abate in 2 weeks to 2 months, but in rare instances a protracted course occurs. Platelet transfusions should not be used because further isoimmunization of the patient may occur.[1,205,298] Steroids are of questionable benefit, but may ward off serious hemorrhage in some patients by the beneficial, but undefined, effect on the vasculature. If severe thrombocytopenia is present (platelet count less than 10,000/mm^3) or if significant hemorrhage is seen or sus-

pected to be impending, the patient should be treated with plasmapheresis to remove the anti-PLA^1 antibody. This mode of therapy has almost always been successful and is the treatment of choice in high-risk patients.

Thrombocytosis and Thrombocythemia

Thrombocytosis refers to a benign secondary reactive increase in the platelet count. Thrombocytosis is usually associated with increased platelet production or interferance with splenic pooling of platelets, such as postsplenectomy thrombocytosis, thrombocytosis after epinephrine infusion, or the use of large doses of steroids. Thrombocythemia, on the other hand, refers to a primary, uncontrolled (malignant) increase in platelet counts; this may accompany any of the myeloproliferative syndromes, especially polycythemia vera and chronic myelogenous leukemia, or may represent a malignant transformation of the megakaryocyte or stem cell precursor of the megakaryocyte; this latter myeloproliferative disorder is referred to as "essential thrombocythemia."

Thrombocytosis

Thrombocytosis is usually benign and asymptomatic and is commonly associated

Table 4–38 Features of Post-Transfusion Purpura

Clinical findings
Occurs 1 week post-transfusion
Most patients are PLA^1-negative
Most are females previously sensitized by transfusion or pregnancy
Sudden onset of petechiae, purpura, and ecchymoses
Some have chills and fever at time of transfusion
Usually abates spontaneously in 2 weeks to 2 months
Laboratory findings
Thrombocytopenia-usually severe
Anti-PLA^1 antibody in most patients
Therapy
Plasmapheresis
Steroids ?
Platelets containdicated

with acute or chronic inflammatory disorders, including collagen vascular disorders, recovery from acute infections, sarcoidosis, cirrhosis, tuberculosis, and others.[26,161,175,188,240] Reactive thrombocytosis is also commonly associated with acute hemorrhage, malignancy, hemolytic anemia, and severe iron deficiency.[112,336,370] A reactive thrombocytosis is also often noted after treatment and subsequent recovery from a thrombocytopenic disorder (termed "rebound thrombocytosis"), such as ITP or drug-induced immune thrombocytopenia. Thrombocytosis usually occurs after splenectomy and may persist for several weeks or up to 3 months[227] (Table 4–39). In thrombocytosis, platelets usually display normal morphologic features and usually function normally; this is in opposition to thrombocythemia in which platelet morphology and platelet function are commonly abnormal.

Patients with thrombocytosis are usually asymptomatic and require no therapy. Impaired hemostasis, manifested as increased risk of thrombosis, or hemorrhage, is usually not associated with thrombocytosis. An increased risk of thrombosis is seen in two selected instances of reactive thrombocytosis, the first is postsplenectomy thrombocytosis in the presence of anemia of any etiology[175] and the second is associated with severe iron deficiency.[206] In both of these prophylactic anticoagulant therapy in the form of subcutaneous heparin or antiplatelet therapy in the form of aspirin plus dipyridamole is warranted. Additionally, the reactive thrombocytosis associated with iron deficiency anemia

Table 4–39 Common Causes of Thrombocytosis

Acute infections (recovery phase)
Collagen vascular disorders
Chronic inflammatory or infectious diseases
Hemolytic anemias
Malignancy
    Lymphoma
    Hodgkin's disease
    Metastatic Carcinoma
Myeloproliferative syndromes
Rebound phase of thrombocytopenia
Splenectomy

will usually promptly cease within 1 week of initiating appropriate iron therapy. However, in the reactive thrombocytoses of other than these two etiologies, there is no indication for therapy unless an actual thrombotic event occurs.

Reactive thrombocytosis is often associated with laboratory findings of hyperkalemia, hypercalcemia, and, occasionally, decreased oxygen partial pressure levels due to increased platelet consumption by the increased platelet population. In general, these laboratory findings can be considered to be occurring in vitro in the test tube collection system, but not necessarily in the patient. In addition, increased markers of platelet release, platelet factor 4 levels, and beta-thromboglobulin levels are often increased, but template bleeding times and aggregation patterns typically remain normal.

Thrombocythemia

Essential thrombocythemia is one of the myeloproliferative syndromes and is characterized by uncontrolled megakaryocyte and platelet production, selected biochemical and bone marrow abnormalities, a sustained elevated platelet count with a peripheral platelet population comprised of platelets demonstrating bizarre morphology, a clinical course commonly associated with hemorrhage or thrombosis, splenomegaly, and abnormal platelet function generally leading to thrombohemorrhagic phenomena.[136,153,264,352] The disorder is clearly a clonal stem cell disease, similar to the other myeloproliferative syndromes, as demonstrated by studies of female patients with essential thrombocythemia who demonstrate heterozygosity of glucose-6-phosphate dehydrogenase isoenzymes A and B. In these individuals the malignant platelet population will contain only one isoenzyme subspecies.[133] Essential thrombocythemia is the least common of the myeloproliferative syndromes and like the others may progress into a different and often more serious myelodysplastic disorder. Approximately 5% will eventually develop acute myeloblastic leukemia, 5% will develop chronic myelogenous leukemia, 5% will develop myelofibrosis with agnogenic myeloid metaplasia, and approximately 5% will eventually be indistinguishable from polycythemia rubra vera.[264] In this latter instance it is likely that these patients actually had early quiescent polycythemia vera associated with thrombocythemia.

The diagnosis of essential thrombocythemia is one of exclusion; a reactive thrombocytosis is usually easy to exclude, but differentiation from polycythemia vera may be difficult. The primary differential points between essential thrombocythemia and polycythemia vera are normal marrow iron stores and normal blood volume studies (red cell mass) in patients with essential thrombocythemia. To aid in distinguishing between these two disorders, the Polycythemia Vera Study Group has devised strict differential diagnostic criteria.[29,266] The diagnosis of essential thrombocythemia is made by noting a platelet count approximating 1,000,000/mm^3 with no identifiable cause of thrombocytosis, a normal red cell mass, iron present in the bone marrow, or if absent a 1 month trial of oral iron therapy resulting in an increase of the hemoglobin level of no more than 1 gm/dL an absence of collagen fibrosis on bone marrow biopsy, and absence of the Philadelphia chromosome in bone marrow aspirates. In addition, the leukocyte alkaline phosphatase score is usually normal or elevated in patients with essential thrombocythemia, the vitamin B$_{12}$ binding protein is elevated in 30% of patients, and other biochemical abnormalities are also commonly noted, as is typical of other myeloproliferative syndromes.[54,55,286] Approximately 55% of patients will be hyperuricemic, 50% will demonstrate elevated urinary or serum lysozyme levels, almost all will demonstrate elevated lactate dehydrogenase (LDH) levels, and more than 80% will demonstrate elevated alkaline phosphatase levels.[54,55,159,286] Sixty percent of patients will present with hemorrhage, approximately 20% will present with thrombosis, 10% will present with hemorrhage and thrombosis, and approximately 20% are diagnosed in an asymptomatic state without thrombohemorrhagic phenomena yet becoming manifest.[54,55]

Thrombotic events may involve the arterial or venous system and peripheral arterial occlusion as well as peripheral venous occlusion, most commonly demonstrated in the lower extremities, is quite common. The noting of erythema, cyanosis, or pregangrenous changes should immediately suggest the high probability of small vessel involvement and necessity of definitive therapy.[264] The types of hemorrhage that can occur are varied. Most patients present with a history of easy and spontaneous bruising and many have bilateral epistaxis. Bleeding from the gastrointestinal tract is extremely common and patients may also develop other types of mucosal membrane bleeding and may be noted to have petechiae and purpura, as well as large subcutaneous hematomas or bleeding into other organs.[54,55,159,264,286] A few instances can be associated with intra-articular bleeds.[56,57] Sixty percent of patients will present with a mild leukocytosis, usually with a shift to immature forms; this usually is corrected promptly with myelosuppressive therapy. In addition, more than 50% of patients will have prolonged template bleeding times at presentation; the template bleeding time also tends to be corrected after myelosuppressive therapy.[54,55] The hyperuricemia, lysozyme levels, and LDH levels also tend to be corrected with hydroxyurea therapy; however, the leukocyte alkaline phosphatase score usually does not change after myelosuppressive therapy.[54,55] Biochemical abnormalities in essential thrombocytopenia before and after therapy are depicted in Figure 4–18.

Platelet aggregation abnormalities are noted in the vast majority of patients and up to 100% of patients will demonstrate abnormalities to ADP, approximately 60% will demonstrate abnormalities to epinephrine, 50% to collagen, 40% to arachidonic acid, and 30% to ristocetin-induced aggregation.[54,55] ATP release is also significantly abnormal in the vast majority of patients, and ATP release induced by ADP and epinephrine is abnormal in 90% of patients, that induced by collagen is abnormal in 30% of patients, that induced by arachidonic acid is abnormal in 80% of patients, and that induced by ristocetin is abnormal in 70% of patients.[54,55] As

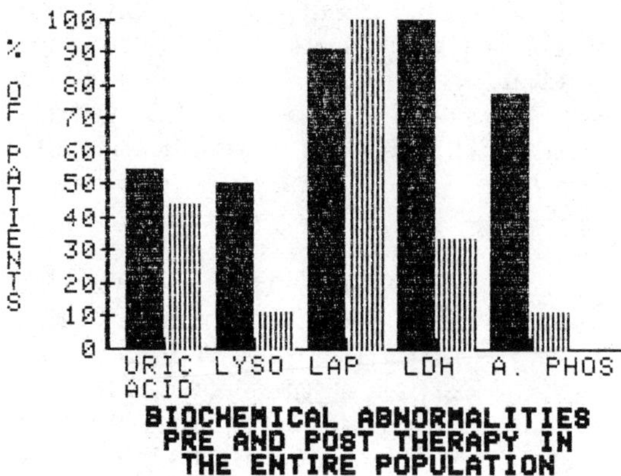

Fig. 4–18. Biochemical abnormalities in essential thrombocythenia. LYSO: lysozyme; LAP: leukocyte alkaline phosphatase; LDH: lactate dehydrogenase; A. PHOS: alkaline phosphatase.

noted in Figure 4–19 there may be significant improvement in aggregation after therapy with hydroxyurea and normalization of the platelet count; however, only moderate correction of release reaction abnormalities is noted after therapy with hydorxyurea, as is seen in Figure 4–20.

Examination of the bone marrow in patients with essential thrombocythemia reveals the marrow to be typically hypercellular, with a striking increase in megakaryocytes that are large, bizarre appearing, and often noted to be engulfing erythroid and myeloid precursors via active phagocytosis.[199] Large islands of platelet aggregates are usually noted throughout the marrow smears. Myeloid and erythroid hyperplasia is usually evident, and marrow iron stores are usually normal. The megakaryocyte volume is clearly increased as opposed to patients with chronic myelogenous leukemia who typically have decreased megakaryocytic volumes.[264] Evaluation of a peripheral smear will also reveal a striking increase in platelets that are usually large and demonstrate bizarre morphology. In addition, megakaryocyte fragments and large platelet aggregates are commonly noted on a peripheral smear. The leukocytosis and the increase in immature forms is usually also obvious. Typical marrow findings in essential thrombocythemia are shown in Figures 4–21, 4–22 and 4–23.

The mainstay of therapy is to keep the platelet count below 700,000/mm^3, since this usually eradicates the thrombotic or hemorrhagic complications of essential thrombocythemia. Rapid lowering of the platelet count in the patient sustaining hemorrhage, thrombosis, or in preparation for surgery can be easily accomplished by cytoreductive plateletpheresis. If the patient is asymptomatic, the platelet count can be effectively lowered by the use of numerous myelosuppressive agents including, busulfan, mel-

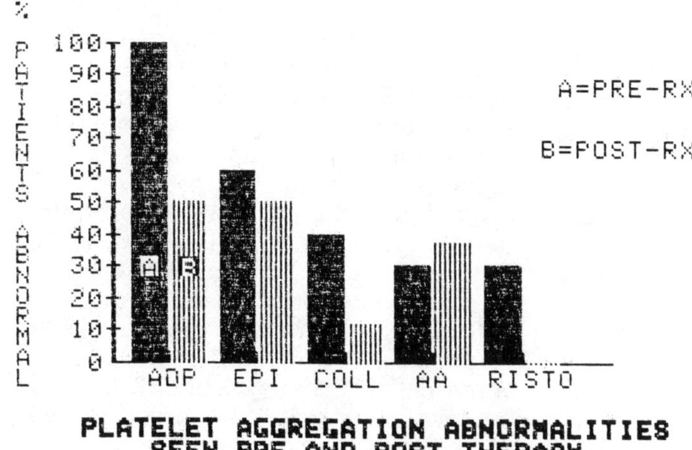

Fig. 4–19. Platelet aggregation patterns in essential thrombocythemia. EPI: epinephrine; COLL: collagen; AA: arachidonic acid; RISTO: ristocetin.

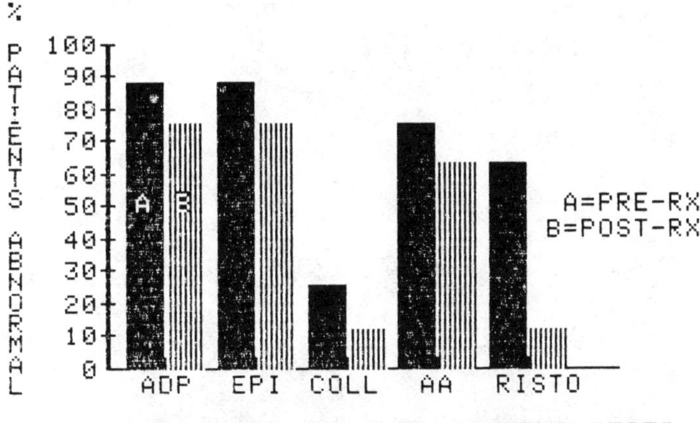

Fig. 4-20. Platelet ATP release patterns in essential thrombocythemia. EPI: epinephrine; COLL: collagen; AA: arachidonic acid; RISTO: ristocetin.

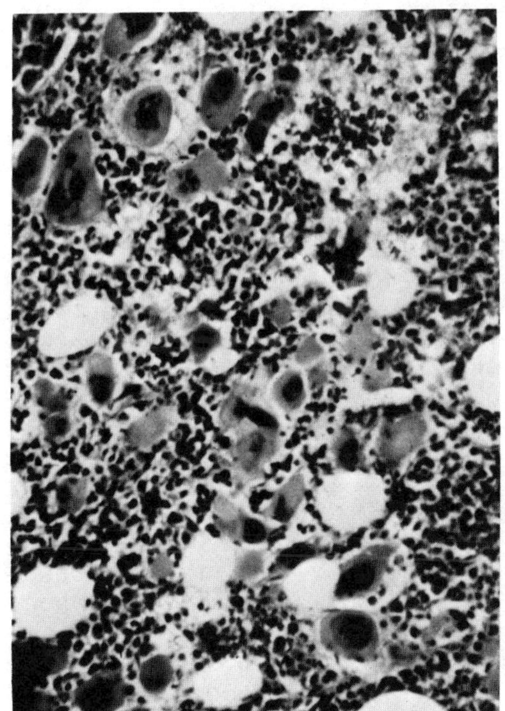

Fig. 4-21. Typical marrow findings in essential thrombocythemia.

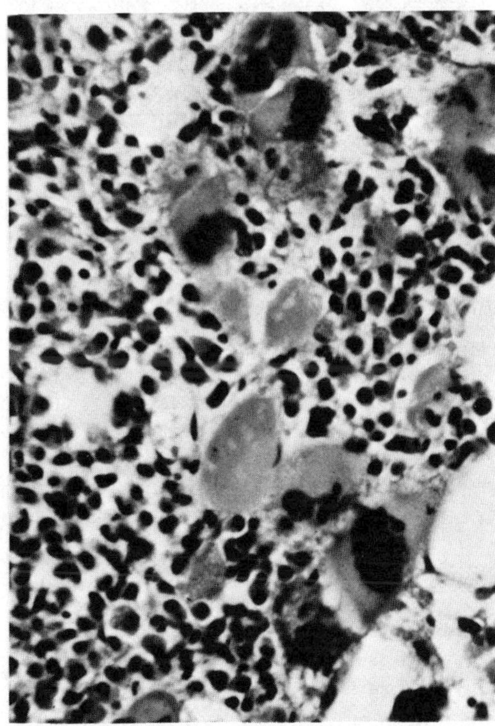

Fig. 4-22. Typical marrow findings in essential thrombocythemia.

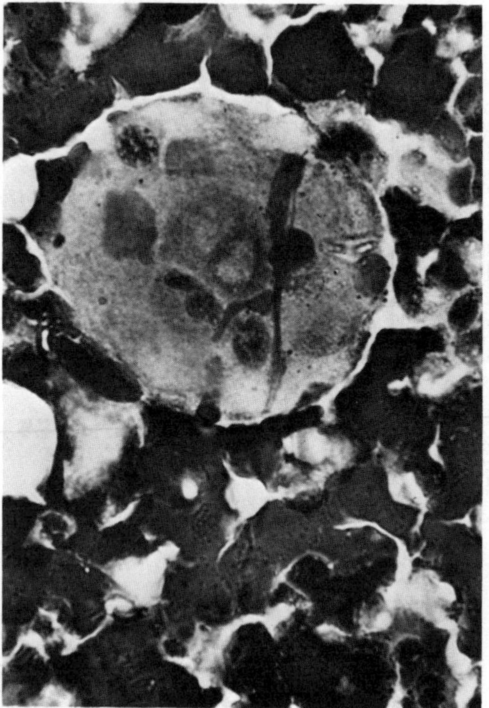

Fig. 4–23. Megakaryocyte phagocytosis of red cells and white cells in essential thrombocythemia.

choice is, again, hydroxyurea given at a dose to maintain the platelet count at less than 700,000/mm^3. The choice of this agent over other myelosuppressive agents was previously discussed. Figure 4–24 and 4–25 depict platelet lumiaggregation patterns in a patient both before and after therapy with hydroxyurea demonstrating significant, but not total, correction of platelet aggregation and release abnormalities. The saliant clinical and laboratory features of essential thrombocythemia are summarized in Table 4–40.

Hyperactive Prethrombotic Platelets

Large "bizarre" platelets are commonly seen in hypercoagulable patients, and in patients undergoing frank clinical or subclinical thrombotic episodes, Figure 4–26 depicts a so-called large "bizarre" platelet. It has been demonstrated that large platelets represent the young and presumably hemostatically more active platelets.[195,210] Therefore, in individuals undergoing thrombotic disorders manifested as increased fibrin deposition with the entrapment of platelets, one would expect concomitant consumption of platelets, a rapid platelet turnover, and decreased platelet survival.[162,196] Thus, in this type of situation there should be a greater than usual number of young platelets or large platelets, or hemostatically more active platelets, in the peripheral blood. This, indeed, has been noted by numerous investigators.[195,210] Thus, in a patient undergoing a thrombotic event, be it subclinical or obvious, such as a deep vein thrombosis, a pulmonary embolus, or acute arterial thromboembolus, an increase in the percentage of young or large platelets in the peripheral smear would be expected.[196,294] This assumption is only valid in the presence of a normal bone marrow and absence of hypersplenism.

phalan, and hydroxyurea. My choice of therapy is to use hydroxyurea at 15 to 20 mg/kg/day, which will usually result in prompt lowering of the platelet count. This agent is chosen because it is not associated with prolonged pancytopenia and is not generally associated with mutagenicity when given over a long period of time.

If the patient has sustained a thrombotic episode or if the platelet count is decreasing only very slowly, the addition of antiplatelet therapy in the form of aspirin and dipyridamole may be warranted until the platelet count is less than 700,000/mm^3, at which point the antiplatelet therapy is usually not warranted because thrombohemorrhagic manifestations usually cease at this level and there is usually correction of the template bleeding time, which appears to correlate reasonably well with clinical hemorrhage in this disorder. Most patients will require long-term myelosuppressive therapy and my

Platelet indicies, including the platelet crit, the platelet distribution width (PDW), and calculation of the percent large platelets, the percent normal platelets, and the percent small platelets circulating in

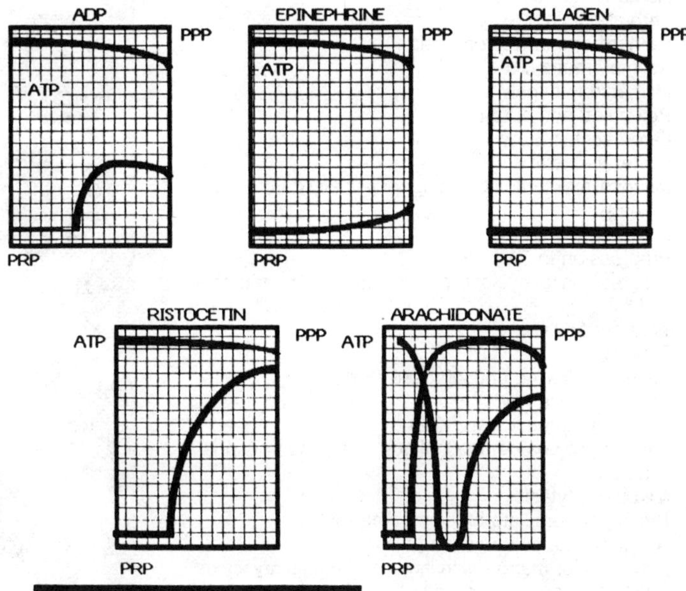

Fig. 4–24. Platelet function in essential thrombocythemia, lumiaggregation (pretherapy). ADP: adenosine diphosphate; ATP: adenosine triphosphate release; PPP: platelet-poor plasma; PRP: platelet-rich plasma.

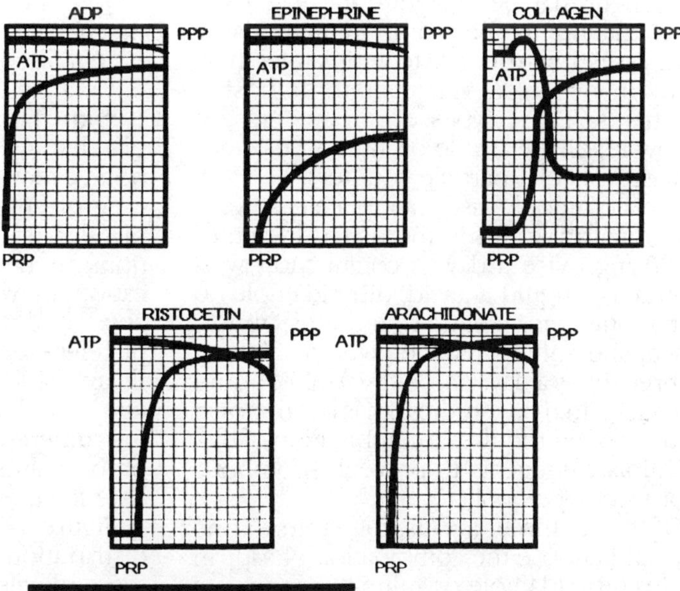

Fig. 4–25. Platelet function in essential thrombocythemia, lumiaggregation (post-therapy). ADP: adenosine diphosphate; ATP: adenosine triphosphate release; PPP: platelet-poor plasma; PRP: platelet-rich plasma.

Table 4–40 Salient Features of Essential Thrombocythemia

Clinical findings
  Hemorrhage (60%)
  Thrombosis (20%)
  Hemorrhage and thrombosis (10%)
  Asymptomatic (20%)
  Mild splenomegaly
  Petechiae and purpura
  Large ecchymoses
  Bilateral epistaxis
  Mucosal membrane bleeding (especially gastrointestinal)
  Progression to AML (5%)
  Progression to CML (5%)
  Progression to myelofibrosis and myeloid metaplasia (5%)
Laboratory findings
  Elevated LDH (90%)
  Elevated alkaline phosphatase (60%)
  Hyperuricemia (55%)
  Elevated muramidase (50%)
  Elevated or boarderline leukocyte alkaline phosphatase
  Mild leukocytosis
  Prolonged template bleeding time (50%)
  Abnormal platelet function (>90%)
  Hypercellular marrow with increased megakaryocytes with "bizzare" morphology
  Numerous platelet "lakes" in marrow
Therapy
  Hydroxyurea, busulfan, or alkeran
  Cytoreductive plateletpheresis
  Platelet suppressive drugs (combination)

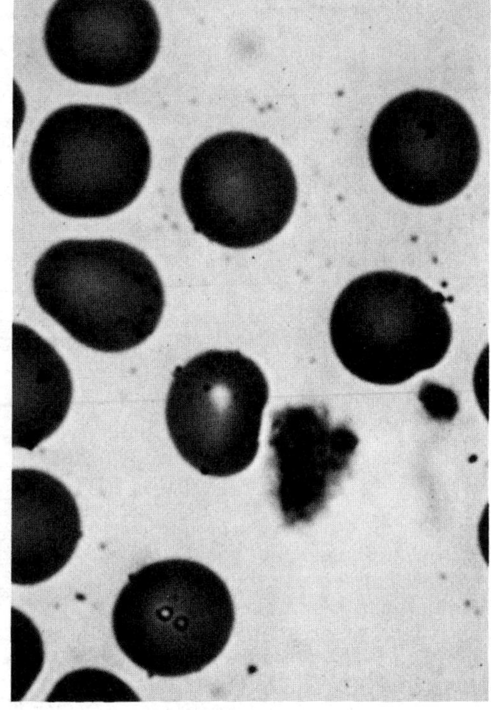

Fig. 4–26. Large "bizarre" platelet, a young platelet.

a patient may be of significant diagnostic benefit and may be an important modality for assessing response to antiplatelet therapy in hypercoagulable or thrombosing patients. These types of parameters are now readily available on numerous automated platelet particle counters.[104,323,326] The commonly used antiplatelet agents are aspirin, given in the usual dosage of 600 mg twice a day in conjunction with 30 mL of liquid antacid, dipyridamole 50 mg four times a day being the usual dosage, and sulfinpyrazone given as 200 mg three times a day, also with 30 mL of liquid antacid. In many studies it has been shown that it often requires a combination of two antiplatelet agents to prevent thrombotic or thromboembolic events.[53,58,59,302,319,397] Of these three agents, of course, one would choose the combination of aspirin plus dipyridamole or sulfinpyrazone plus dipyridamole, since aspirin and sulfinpyrazone have the same mechanism of action and dipyridamole has a differing mechanism of action; therefore these two potential combinations block two different platelet biosynthetic pathways.

With the current trend of using antiplatelet agents as prophylaxis for thrombotic events, modalities to assess the efficacy of antiplatelet therapy are needed; platelet indicies and platelet size distributions often give a reasonable clinical indication of response to antiplatelet therapy.[53,59,117,197] These indicies as well as platelet size distribution profiling is readily available with common particle counters, including the Baker and the Coulter instruments. We have done these studies on both and found them to be quite suitable for these types of studies.[53]

Figure 4–27 depicts the type of platelet distribution curve that is generated by these platelet particle counters. Along the X-axis are the aperture sizes. What is defined as a normal platelet size will depend

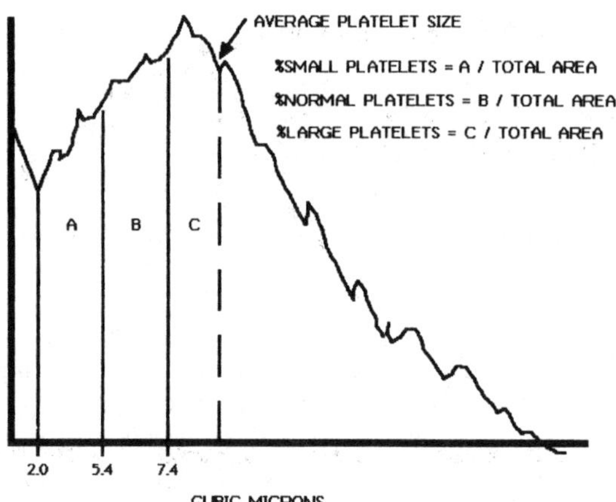

Fig. 4–27. Platelet size distribution profile.

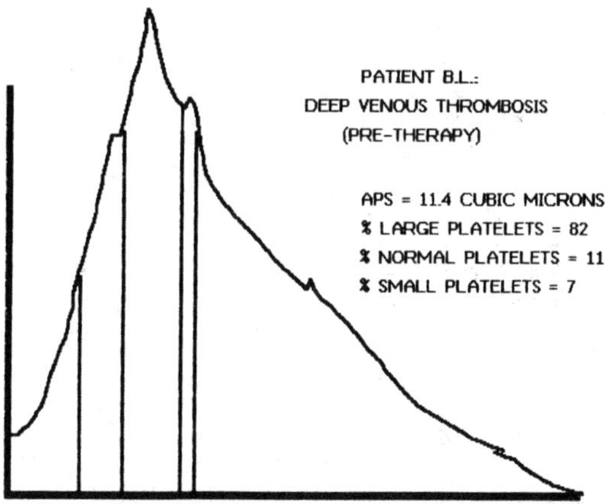

Fig. 4–28. Platelet size distribution profile in thrombosis (pretherapy).

on the instrument and standard used; this particular distribution curve was generated on the Coulter ZBI Channelyzer System. Area A represents the platelets that are between 2 and 5.4 μ^3. Therefore, the area under A divided by the total area represents the percent of small platelets, 16% in the patient demonstrated here. Area B represents the platelets that are between 5.4 and 7.4 μ^3, and area B is also 16% in this patient. Area C represents the percent of large platelets, and is 66%, which is a significant increase above normal. The calculated average platelet size in this patient is 9.6 μ^3; by this particular technique the average platelet size should be approximately 6.4 μ^3. Thus, this patient demonstrates a decrease in the percent of small platelets, a marked increase in the percentage of large platelets, which should be approximately 30%, and an increase in average platelet size. This combination of findings is suggestive of increased platelet turnover and decreased platelet survival.

Figure 4–28 demonstrates the platelet size distribution curve generated in a patient with deep vein thrombosis. Pretherapy this patient had an average platelet size that was increased to 11.4 μ^3. The percent large platelets (young platelets) was markedly increased, representing 82% of the total platelet population, 11% were normal platelets and only 7% were small platelets, thus suggesting increased platelet turnover and decreased platelet

survival. The patient was started on antithrombotic therapy in the form of aspirin plus dipyridamole, and 24 hours later the average platelet size had decreased to 5.4 μ^3, the percent large platelets decreased to 35%, the percent normal platelets were then found to be 20%, and the percent small platelets had increased to 46% (Fig. 4–29). This major shift in the platelet size distribution profile is strong evidence that the initiation of antiplatelet therapy has stopped or markedly blunted the consumption of platelet, and concomitantly increased fibrin deposition has been achieved.

Figure 4–30 summarizes changes in the MPV in 40 patients with deep vein thrombosis compared with a normal population

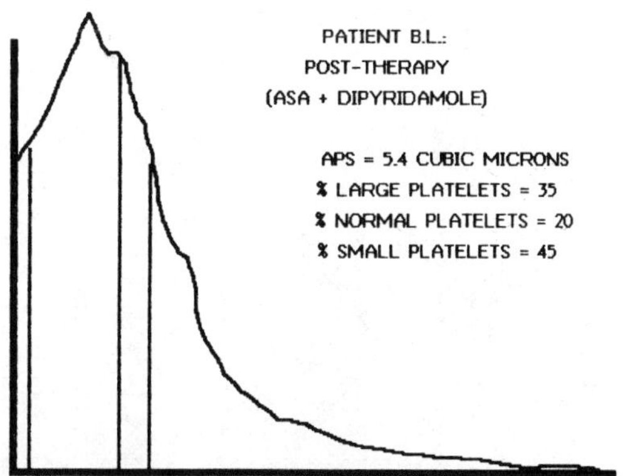

Fig. 4–29. Platelet size distribution profile in thrombosis (post-therapy).

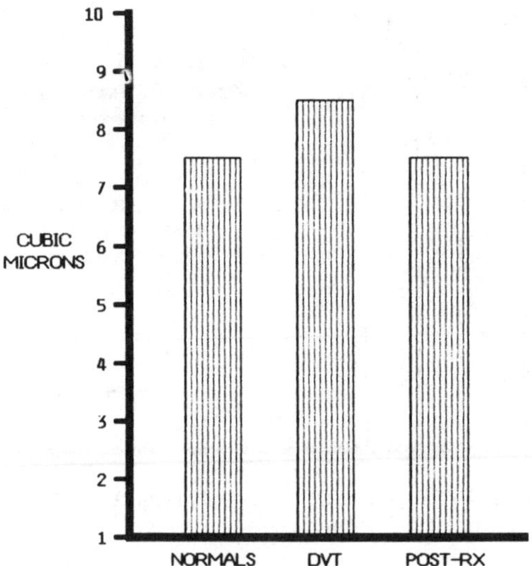

Fig. 4–30. Changes in mean platelet volume with deep vein thrombosis.

(Baker 810) At 24 hours after aspirin and dipyridamole, there was a decrease in MPV. Figure 4–31 depicts a thrombosis-type profile, again performed in 40 patients with deep vein thrombosis, compared with normal individuals. Figure 4–32 depicts the rather marked changes in platelet crit in patients sustaining thrombosis, which is not due to an increase in platelet counts, but to an increase in percentage of large, young platelets in the systemic circulation. This is another indication of increased platelet turnover and decreased platelet survival.

Table 4–41 summarizes changes in platelet indicies and platelet size distribu-

tion profiles in patients with thrombosis and in patients with thrombosis post-therapy. Modalities potentially available for the evaluation of antiplatelet therapy or platelet suppressive therapy are listed in Table 4–42. The petechiometer test and platelet aggregometry are older methods, but are still useful. Prolongation of a bleeding time after the institution of antiplatelet therapy may not truly indicate that the intravascular thrombotic event or hypercoagulable state has actually been eradicated or even blunted. The same can be said of the petechiometer test and the tourniquet test. Noting changes or specific abnormalities in platelet aggregation patterns after the initiation of antiplatelet therapy does not necessarily indicate that a process has been blunted or stopped. The only information abnormal aggregation patterns reveal is that the drug has induced platelet dysfunction; this is not evidence that a hypercoagulable state or actual increased fibrin deposition and platelet consumption have been clinically irradicated.

Newer methods available, most of which are amenable to full automation, are also depicted in Table 4–42 and consist of platelet size distribution profiling as well as molecular markers of platelet reactivity.[59,117,128,129] We find platelet distribution profiling to be the easiest way clinically to assess efficacy of antiplatelet therapy in patients with acute thrombosis or subclinical microvascular thrombosis. When noting abnormalities in platelet size distribution profiles and platelet indicies in acute thrombosis or a hypercoagulable

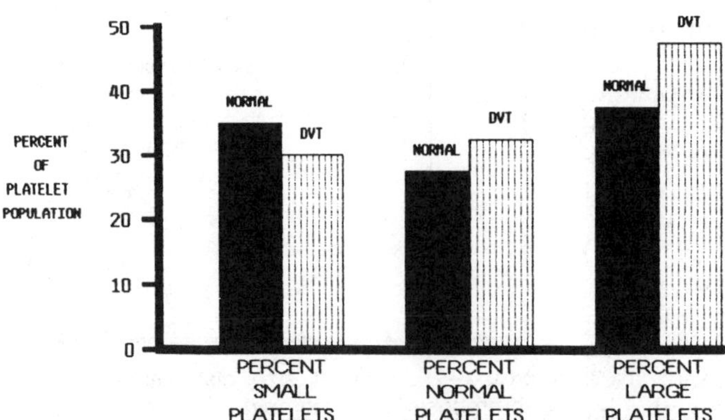

Fig. 4–31. Platelet size distribution profiles: normals versus deep vein thrombosis.

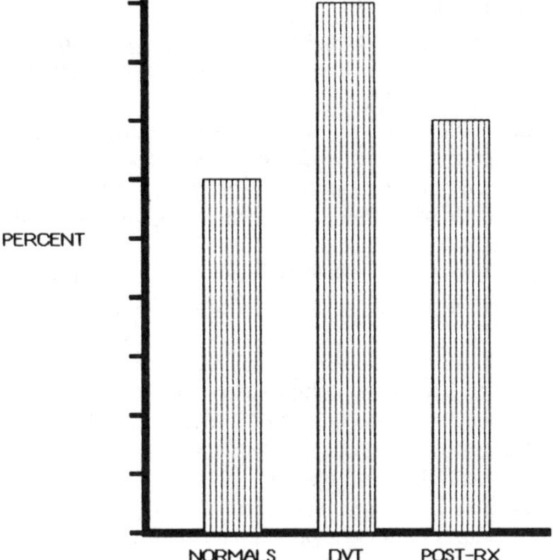

Fig. 4–32. Changes in platelet crit with deep vein thrombosis. Measurements were made 24 hours after the institution of aspirin plus dipyridamole therapy (POST-RX).

Table 4–41 Changes in Platelet Distribution Profiles and Platelet Indices in Acute Thrombosis

Parameter	Thrombosis	Post-therapy
Mean platelet volume	Increase	Decrease
Average platelet size	Increase	Decrease
Platelet crit	Increase	Decrease
% large platelets	Increase	Decrease
% normal platelets	No change	No change
% small platelets	Decrease	Increase
Platelet distribution width	Decrease	Increase

Table 4–42 Laboratory Evaluation of Platelet Suppressive Drug Therapy

Older Methods	Newer Methods
Duke bleeding time	Platelet survival (PSDP)*
Ivy bleeding time	Platelet factor 4
Tourniquet test	Beta-thromboglobulin
Platelet aggregation ?	Thromboxane B_2
Petechiometer	6-Keto-PGF-1-alpha
	Cyclo-oxygenase
	Arachidonate aggregation
	Lumiaggregation
	Fibrinopeptide A
	Antithrombin III

* PSDP: platelet size distribution profile.

state and then noting their near normalization after the institution of antiplatelet therapy is reasonable assurance that the event has been blunted or stopped. Noting decreases in platelet factor 4 levels or beta-thromboglobulin levels after the institution of antiplatelet therapy may also be indicative of clinical efficacy with respect to stopping or blunting increased fibrin deposition.[117,128,129] The diagnostic roles of thromboxane B_2 measurements, prostacyclin derivative measurements (6-keto-PGF_1) and cyclo-oxygenase appear promising, but remain to be established. Arachidonic acid aggregation and lumiaggregation lack specificity and only indicate that the drug has induced platelet dysfunction.

Another modality that may be quite effective for monitoring the efficacy of antiplatelet or other antithrombotic therapy is the radioimmunoassay of fibrinopeptide A.[128,129] If this molecular marker is significantly elevated in a thrombotic event or a hypercoagulable state and is noted to be normal after the institution of antiplatelet drugs, heparin, or other types of antithrombotic therapy, good evidence is provided that the intravascular fibrin deposition or hypercoagulable state has been arrested. In addition, if low antithrombin III levels are noted at the time of diagnosis of a hypercoagulable state or a thrombotic event, and if there is normalization or near normalization of antithrombin III levels after the initiation of antithrombotic therapy, whether it be antiplatelet therapy or heparin therapy, this also is evidence that the intravascular thrombotic event of the hypercoagulable state has been controlled to some degree.[49,50]

The help of Dr. Robert Nalbandian and Dr. Ray Henry in preparing the section on thrombotic thrombocytopenic purpura is gratefully acknowledged.

References

1. Abramson N, Eisenberg PD, Aster RH: Post-transfusion purpura: Immunologic aspects and therapy. N Engl J Med 291:1163, 1974.

2. Ackroyd JF: The pathogenesis of thrombocytopenic purpura due to hypersensitivity to Sedormid (allylisopropil-acetyl-carbamide). Clin Sci 8:249, 1949.

3. Ackroyd JF: The cause of thrombocytopenia in Sedormid purpura. Clin Sci 8:269, 1949.

4. Ackroyd JF: The immunological basis of purpura due to drug hypersensitivity. Proc R Soc Med 55:30, 1962.

5. Adams GA: In vivo and in vitro platelet function testing. Plasma Ther Transfusion Technol 3:265, 1982.

6. Adams T, Schultz L, Goldberg L: Platelet function abnormalities in myeloproliferative disorders. Scand J Haematol 13:215, 1974.

7. Adashi E, Farber M, Mitchell GW: Congenital release thrombocytopathy. Pathophysiology and management. Obstet Gynecol 48:403, 1976.

8. Addonizio VP, Fisher CA, Strauss JF, Edmunds LH: Inhibition of human platelet function by verapamil. Thromb Res 28:545, 1982.

9. Aldrich RA, Steinberg AG, Campbell DC: Pedigree demonstrating a sex-linked recessive condition characterized by draining ears, eczematoid dermatitis, and bloody diarrhea. Pediatrics 13:133, 1954.

10. Alexander DP, Russo ME, Gohram DF, Rothstein G: Nafcillin-induced platelet dysfunction and bleeding. Antimicrob Agents Chemother 23:59, 1983.

11. Alter HJ, Scanlon RT, Schechter GP: Thrombocytopenic purpura following vaccination with attenuated measles virus. Am J Dis Child 115:111, 1968.

12. Amir J, Krauss S: Treatment of thrombotic thrombocytopenic purpura with antiplatelet drugs. Blood 42:27, 1973.

13. Amir-Ahmadi H, McGray RS, Martin F, Mitch W, Kantrowitz P, Zamcheck N: Reassessment of massive upper gastrointestinal hemorrhage on the wards of the Boston City Hospital. Surg Clin North Am 49:715, 1969.

14. Amorosi EL, Ultmann JE: Thrombotic thrombocytopenic purpura: Report of 16 cases and review of the literature. Medicine (Baltimore) 45:139, 1966.

15. Amorosi EL, Karpatkin S: Antiplatelet treatment of thrombotic thrombocytopenic purpura. Ann Intern Med 86:102, 1977.

16. Anderson ER, Foulkes JG, Godin DV: The effect of local anaesthetics and antiarrhythmic agents on the responses of rabbit platelets to ADP and thrombin. Thromb Haemost 45:81, 1981.

17. Andrew M, Barr RD: Increased platelet destruction in infancy and childhood. Semin Thromb Hemost 8:248, 1982.

18. Ardlie NG, Glew G, Shultz BG, Schwartz CJ: Inhibition and reversal of platelet aggregation by methylxanthines. Thromb Diath Haemorrh 18:670, 1968.

19. Arkel YS: Evaluation of platelet aggregation in disorders of hemostasis. Med Clin North Am 60:881, 1976.

20. Aster HP, Enright SE: A platelet and granulocyte membrane defect in paroxysmal nocturnal hemoglobinuria: Usefulness for the detection of platelet antibodies. J Clin Invest 48:1199, 1969.

21. Aster RH: TTP: New clues to the etiology of an enigmatic disease. N Engl J Med 297:1400, 1977.

22. Aster RH: Pooling of platelets in the spleen: Role in the pathogenesis of "hypersplenic" thrombocytopenia. J Clin Invest 45:645, 1964.

23. Babior BM: Folate and aplasia of bone marrow. N Engl J Med 298:506, 1978.

24. Ball G, Brereton GG, Fulwood M, Ireland DM, Yate P: Effect of prostaglandin E, alone and in combination with theophylline or aspirin on collagen-induced platelet aggregation and on platelet nucleotides including adenosine 3':5'-cyclic monophosphate. Biochem J 120:709, 1970.

25. Bang NU, Tessler SS, Heidenreich RO, Marks CA, Mattler LE: Effects of moxalactam on blood coagulation and platelet function. Rev Infect Dis 4:546, 1982.

26. Bean RHD: Thrombocytosis in auto-immune diseases. Bibl Haematol 23:43, 1965.

27. Bell WR, Royall RM: Heparin-induced thrombocytopenia: A comparison of three heparin preparations. N Engl J Med 303:902, 1980.

28. Berge T, Brunnhage F, Nisson LR: Congenital thrombocytopenia in rubella embryopathy. Acta Paediatr Scand 52:349, 1963.

29. Berlin NI: Diagnosis and classification of the polycythemias. In Berlin NI, Jaffe ER, Miescher PA (Eds): Polycythemia. Grune & Stratton, New York, 1975, p 5.

30. Bernard J, Soulier JP: Sur une nouvelle variete dystrophic thrombocytaire hemorrhagipase congenitale. Paris, 24:3217, 1948.

31. Bernheim J, Dechavanne M, Bryon PA, Lagarde M, Colon S, Pozet N, Traeger J: Thrombocytopenia, macrothrombocytopathia, nephritis, and deafness. Am J Med 61:145, 1976.

32. Bessman JD, Williams LJ, Gilmer PR: Platelet size in health and hematologic disease. Am J Clin Pathol 78:150, 1982.

33. Bettman JW: Drug hypersensitivity purpuras. Arch Intern Med 112:840, 1963.

34. Bick RL, Shanbrom E: A systematic approach to the diagnosis of bleeding disorders. Med Counterpoint 6:27, 1972.

35. Bick RL: A systematic approach to the diagnosis of bleeding disorders. In Murano G, Bick RL (Eds): Basic Concepts of Hemostasis and Thrombosis. CRC Press, Boca Raton, FL, 1980, p 81.

36. Bick RL: Vascular disorders associated with thrombohemorrhagic phenomena. Semin Thromb Hemost 5:167, 1979.

37. Bick RL, Adams T, Schmalhorst WR: Bleeding times, platelet adhesion, and aspirin. Am J Clin Pathol 65:65, 1976.

38. Bick RL: Modern concepts of hemostasis and thrombosis. ASCP Manual # 5548. American Society of Clinical Pathology, Chicago, 1979.

39. Bick RL: Difficult diagnostic problems in hemostasis and thrombosis. ASCP Manual # 5549. American Society of Clinical Pathology, Chicago, 1979.

40. Bick RL: Pathophysiology of hemostasis and thrombosis. In Sodeman WA, Sodeman TM (Eds): Pathologic Physiology: Mechanisms of Disease. W.B. Saunders, Philadelphia, 1985.

41. Bick RL: Alterations of hemostasis associated with malignancy. IN Murano G, Bick RL (Eds): Basic Concepts of Hemostasis and Thrombosis. CRC Press, Boca Raton, FL, 1980, p 213.

42. Bick RL: Acquired circulating anticoagulants and defective hemostasis in malignant paraprotein disorders. In Murano G, Bick RL (Eds): Basic Concepts of Hemostasis and Thrombosis. CRC Press, Boca Raton, FL, 1980, p 205.

43. Bick RL: Alterations of hemostasis associated with malignancy: Etiology, pathophysiology, diagnosis, and management. Semin Thromb Hemost 5:1, 1978.

44. Bick RL: Alterations of hemostasis associated with cardiopulmonary bypass: Pathophysiology, prevention, diagnosis, and management. Semin Thromb Hemost 3:59, 1976.

45. Bick RL, Schmalhorst WR, Arbegast NR: Alterations of hemostasis associated with cardiopulmonary bypass. Thromb Res 8: 285, 1976.

46. Bick RL: Alterations of hemostasis associated with surgery, cardiopulmonary bypass surgery, and prosthetic devices. In Ratnoff OD, Forbes CD (Eds): Disorders of Hemostasis. Grune & Stratton, New York, 1984, p 379.

47. Bick RL: The clinical significance of fibrinogen degradation products. Semin Thromb Hemost 8:302, 1982.

48. Bick RL: Primary fibrino(geno)lytic syndromes. In Murano G, Bick RL (Eds): Basic Concepts of Hemostasis and Thrombosis. CRC Press, Boca Raton, FL, 1980, p 181.

49. Bick RL: Disseminated intravascular coagulation and related syndromes: Etiology, pathophysiology, diagnosis, and management. Am J Hematol 5:265, 1978.

50. Bick RL: Disseminated intravascular coagulation. In Bick RL (Ed): Disseminated Intravascular Coagulation and Related Syndromes. CRC Press, Boca Raton, FL, 1983, p 31.

51. Bick RL: Syndromes associated with hyperfibrino(geno)lysis. In Bick RL (Ed): Disseminated Intravascular Coagulation and Related Syndromes. CRC Press, Boca Raton, FL, 1983, p 105.

52. Bick RL: Treatment of bleeding and thrombosis in the patient with cancer. In Nealon TF (Ed): Management of the Patient with Cancer. W.B. Saunders Company, Philadelphia, 1976, p 48.

53. Bick RL, McClain BJ: Deep venous thrombosis: A laboratory evaluation of 118 consecutive patients. Thromb Haemost 50:305, 1983.

54. Bick RL: Essential (hemorrhagic) thrombocythemia: A clinical and laboratory study of 13 patients. Thromb Haemost 50:216, 1983.

55. Bick RL, Wilson WL: Essential (hemorrhagic) thrombocythemia: A clinical and laboratory study of 14 patients. Am J Clin Pathol 81:799, 1984.

56. Bick RL, Lewis M, Don Michael TA: Essential thrombocythemia presenting as intra-articular hemorrhage of the knee and thrombosis of the sino-atrial artery. Thromb Haemost 50:476, 1983.

57. Bick RL, Lewis M, Don Michael TA: Essential thrombocythemia presenting with intra-articular hemorrhage of the knee and thrombosis of the sino-atrial artery: A case report. Thromb Haemost 50:476, 1983.

58. Bick RL: Deep venous thrombosis: A clinical evaluation of 118 consecutive patients. Thromb Haemost 50:305, 1983.

59: Bick RL, McClain BJ: Platelet indicies as markers of acute thrombosis and response to anti-thrombotic study. Thromb Haemost 50:153, 1983.

60. Bithel TC, Parokh SJ, Strong RR: Platelet function in the Bernard-Soulier syndrome. Ann NY Acad Sci 201:145, 1972.

61. Boisvert A, MacPherson BR: The detection of platelet antibodies using a modified platelet immunofluorescence test. Am J Clin Pathol 80:839, 1983.

62. Born GVR, Bricknell J: The uptake of 5-hydroxytryptamine by blood platelets in the cold. J Physiol (Lond) 147:153, 1959.

63. Born GVR: Aggregation of blood platelets by adenosine diphosphate and its reversal. Nature 194:927, 1962.

64. Bottiger LE, Westerholm B: Thrombocytopenia. II. Drug-induced thrombocytopenia. Acta Med Scand 191:541, 1972.

65. Brady RO: Biochemical and metabolic basis of familial sphingolipidoses. Semin Hematol 9:273, 1972.

66. Brain MC, Neame PB: Thrombotic thrombocytopenia purpura and the hemolytic uremic syndrome. Semin Thromb Hemost 8:186, 1982.

67. Brown CH, Natelson EA, Bradshaw MW, Williams TW, Alfrey CP: The hemostatic defect

produced by carbenicillin. N Engl J Med 291:265, 1974.

68. Brown CN, Bradshaw MW, Natelson EA, Alfrey CP, Williams TW: Defective platelet function following the administration of penicillin compounds. Blood 47:949, 1976.

69. Brown CN, Natelson EA, Bradshaw MW: A study of the effects of ticarcillin on blood coagulation and platelet function. Antimicrob Agents Chemother 7:652, 1975.

70. Brunning RD: Morphologic alterations in nucleated blood and marrow cells in genetic disorders. Hum Pathol 1:99, 1970.

71. Buchanon GR, Handin RI: Platelet function in the Chediak-Higashi syndrome. Blood 47:941, 1976.

72. Bukowski RM, King JW, Hewlett JS: Plasmapheresis in the treatment of thrombotic thrombocytopenic purpura. Blood 50:413, 1977.

73. Burns TS, Saunders RN: Antiplatelet activity of hydralazine. Thromb Res 16:837, 1979.

74. Busch GJ, Braun WE, Carpenter CV, Carson JM, Glavanek ER, Reynolds ES, Merrill JP, Dammin GJ: Intravascular coagulation (IVC) in human renal allograft rejection. Transplant Proc 1:267, 1969.

75. Bygdeman S, Johnson I: Studies on the effect of adrenergic blocking agents on catecholamine-induced platelet aggregation and uptake of noradrenaline and 5-hydroxytryptamine. Acta Physiol Scand 75:129, 1969.

76. Byrnes JJ, Lian ECY: Recent therapeutic advances in thrombotic thrombocytopenic purpura. Semin Thromb Hemost 5:199, 1979.

77. Caen JP, Castaldi PA, Leclerc JC, Inceman S, Larrieu MJ, Probst M, Bernard J: Congenital bleeding disorders with long bleeding time and normal platelet count. I. Glanzmann's thrombasthenia (report of fifteen patients). Am J Med 41:4, 1966.

78. Caen JP: Glanzmann's thrombasthenia. Clin Haematol 1:383, 1972.

79. Camitta BM, Nathan DG, Forman EN, Parkman R, Rappeport JM, Orellana TD: Posthepatic severe aplastic anemia—an indication for early bone marrow transplantation. Blood 43:473, 1974.

80. Caranobe C, Sie P, Nouvel C, Laurent G, Pris J, Boneu B: Platelets in myeloproliferative disorders. Scand J Haematol 25:289, 1980.

81. Carpentieri U, Naggard ME: Thrombocytopenia and viral diseases. Tex Med 71:81, 1975.

82. Carroll RR, Noyes WD, Kitchens CS: High-dose intravenous immunoglobulin therapy in patients with immune thrombocytopenic purpura. JAMA 249:1748, 1983.

83. Carter AE, Eban R, Perrett RD: Prevention of postoperative deep venous thrombosis and pulmonary embolism. Br Med J 1:312, 1971.

84. Carter RL: Platelet levels in infectious mononucleosis. Blood 25:817, 1965.

85. Cavese PG, Gallucci V, Morea M, Dalla Volta S, Fasoli G, Casarotto D: Heart valve replacement with the Hancock bioprosthesis. Circulation 56 (Suppl 2):111, 1976.

86. Cazenave JP, Guccione MA, Packham MA, Mustard JF: Effects of cephalathin and penicillin G on platelet function in vitro. Br J Haematol 35:135, 1977.

87. Chesney PJ, Shahidi NT: Acute viral-induced thrombocytopenia: A review of human disease, animal models, and in vitro studies. In Lusher JM, Barnhart MI (Eds): Acquired Bleeding Disorders of Children. Masson Publishers, New York, 1981, p 65.

88. Chesterman CN, Penington DG: Platelet production and turnover: Thrombocytopenia and thrombocytosis. In Hardisty RM, Weatherall DJ (Eds): Blood and Its Disorders. Blackwell Scientific Publications, Oxford, 1982, p 971.

89. Chia YC, Machin JJ: Tuberculosis and severe thrombocytopenia. Br J Clin Pract 33:5, 1979.

90. Clare NM, Montiel MM, Lifschitz MD, Bannayan GA: Alport's syndrome associated with macrothrombopathic thrombocytopenia. Am J Clin Pathol 72:111, 1979.

91. Clarkson AR, Lawrence JR, Meadowns R, Seymour AE: The hemolytic-uremic syndrome in adults. J Med 39:227, 1970.

92. Clawson CC, White JG: Platelet interaction with bacteria: Ultrastructure of congenital afibrinogenemic platelets. Am J Pathol 98:197, 1980.

93. Clawson CC, White JG, Nerzberg MC: Platelet interaction with bacteria: Contrasting the role of fibrinogen and fibronectin. Am J Hematol 9:43, 1980.

94. Cohen LS: The pharmacology of acetylsalic acid. Semin Thromb Hemost 2:146, 1976.

95. Cohen T, Cooney DP: Cyclic thrombocytopenia: Case report and review of the literature. Scand J Hematol 12:9, 1974.

96. Cohen P, Gardner FH: Thrombocytopenia as a laboratory sign and complication of gram negative bacteremic infection. Arch Intint Med 117:113, 1966.

97. Cohn LN, Koster JK, Mee RBB, Collins JJ: Long-term follow-up of the hancock bioprosthetic valve. Circulation 60 (Suppl 1):87, 1978.

98. Cohn J. Thrombocytopenia in childhood: An evaluation of 433 patients. Scand J Haematol 16:226, 1976.

99. Cole AP: Transient thrombocytopenia in a child on sodium valproate. Dev Med Child Neurol 20:487, 1978.

100. Coller BS: Disorders of platelets. In Ratnoff OD, Forbes CD (Eds): Disorders of Hemostasis. Grune & Stratton, New York, 1984, p 73.

101. Colombani J: Auto- and isoimmune thrombocytopenia. Semin Hematol 3:74, 1966.

102. Cooper MD, Chase HP, Lowman JT, Krivit W, Good RA: Wiskett-Aldrich syndrome: An immunologic deficiency disease involving the afferent limb of immunity. Am J Med 44:499, 1968.

103. Cooper LZ, Green RH, Krugman S, Giles JP, Mirick GS: Neonatal thrombocytopenic purpura and other manifestations of rubella contracted in utero. Am J Dis Child 110:416, 1965.

104. Corash L, Shafter B, Weinberg D, Steinfield MB: Platelet sizing in whole blood total platelet populations. In Day NJ, Holmsen H, Zucker MB (Eds): Platelet Function Testing. DHEW Pub (NIH) # 78–1087, 1978, p 315.

105. Cowan DH: Effect of alcoholism on hemostasis. Semin Hematol 17:137, 1980.

106. Craig CM, Gitlin D: The nature of the hyaline thrombi in thrombotic thrombocytopenic purpura. Am J Pathol 33:251, 1957.

107. Cronberg S, Nilsson IM: Investigators in a family with thrombasthenia of moderately severe type with 16 affected family members. Scand J Haematol 5:17, 1968.

108. Crosby WH, Kaufman RM: Drug-induced thrombocytopenia. Med Ann DC 33:199, 1964.

109. Davidson C, Manohitharajah SM: Drug-induced platelet antibodies. Br Med J 3:545, 1973.

110. Day HJ, Holmsen H: Platelet adenine nucleotide "storage pool deficiency" in thrombocytopenic absent radii syndrome. JAMA 221:1053, 1972.

111. de Gruchy GC: Thrombocytopenia. In Drug-Induced Blood Disorders. Blackwell Scientific Publications, Oxford, 1975, p 118.

112. Desforges JF, Bigelow FS, Chalmers TC: The effects of massive gastrointestinal hemorrhage on hemostasis. J Lab Clin Med 43:501, 1954.

113. Des Prez RM, Steckley S, Stroud RM, Hawiger J: Interaction of histoplasma capsulatum with human platelets. J Infect Dis 142:32, 1980.

114. Diamant S, Spirer Z: Chronic thrombocytopenic purpura associated with toxoplasmosis. Br Med J 280:1505, 1980.

115. Doan CA, Bouronele BA, Wiseman BK: Idiopathic and secondary thrombocytopenic purpura: Clinical study and evaluation of 381 cases over a period of 28 years. Ann Intern Med 53:861, 1960.

116. Donckerwolcke RA, Kuijsten RH, Tiddens HA, Van Gool JD: Haemolytic uremic syndrome. Pediatrician 8:378, 1979.

117. Dumoulin-Lagrange M, Capelle C: Evaluation of automated platelet counters for the enumeration and sizing of platelets in the diagnosis and management of hemostatic problems. Semin Thromb Hemost 9:235, 1983.

118. Edelberg SB, Cohen J, Brandt NJ: Congenital hypomegakaryocytic thrombocytopenia associated with bilateral absence of the radii: Variation of the clinical picture. Hum Hered 27:147, 1977.

119. Engstrom E, Lundquist A, Soderstrom N: Periodic thrombocytopenia or tidal platelet dysgenesis in a man. Scand J Haematol 3:290, 1966.

120. Enriquez P, Neiman RS: The Pathology of the Spleen: A Functional Approach. American Society of Clinical Pathology Press, Chicago, 1976, p 1.

121. Epstein CJ, Sahud MA, Piel CF, Goodman JR, Bernfield MR, Kushner JH, Ablin AR: Hereditary macrothrombocytopathia, nephritis, and deafness. Am J Med 52:299, 1972.

122. Epstein RD, Lozner EL, Cobbey TS, Davidson CS: Congenital thrombocytopenic purpura. Purpura hemorrhagica in pregnancy and in the newborn. Am J Med 9:44, 1950.

123. Erb BD: Thrombocytopenic purpura accompanying brucellosis: A case report with demonstration of a granuloma in the bone marrow. J Tenn Med Assoc 59:876, 1966.

124. Espinoza C, Kuhn C: Viral infection of megakaryocytes in varicella with purpura. Am J Clin Pathol 61:203, 1974.

125. Evans EP, Jones GR, Bloom AL: Abnormal breakdown of adenosine diphosphate in uraemic plasma and its possible relationship to defective platelet aggregation. Thromb Res 1:323, 1972.

126. Ewald RA, Eichelberger JW, Young AA, Weiss JR, Crosby WH: The effect of dextran on platelet factor 3. Transfusion 5:109, 1965.

127. Fajardo LF: Hemtopoietic tissue. In Pathology of Radiation Injury. Masson Publishing USA, New York, 1982, p 166.

128. Fareed J, Walenga JM, Bick RL, Bermes EJ, Messmore HL: Impact of automation on the quantitation of low molecular weight markers of hemostatic defects. Semin Thromb Hemost 9:355, 1983.

129. Fareed J, Walenga JM: Current trends in hemostatic testing. Semin Thromb Hemost 9:380, 1983.

130. Feinman RD, Zabinski MP, Lubowsky J: Simultaneous measurement of aggregation and secretion. In Day HJ, Holmsen H, Zucker MB (Eds): Platelet Function Testing. DHEW Publication (NIH) # 78–1087, 1978, p 133.

131. Feinman RD, Lubowsky J, Charo I, Zabinski MP: The lumi-aggregometer: A new instrument for simultaneous measurement of secretion and aggregation. J Lab Clin Med 90:125, 1977.

132. Feldman JD, Mardiney MR, Unanue ER, Cutting H: The vascular pathology of thrombotic thrombocytopenic purpura. An immunohistochemical and ultrastructural study. Lab Invest 15:927, 1966.

133. Fialkow PJ, Faguet GB, Jacobson RV, Vardya

K, Murphy S: Evidence that essential thrombocytopenia is a clonal disorder with origin in a multipotent stem cell. Blood 58:916, 1981.

134. Folman R, Arbus GS, Churchill B, Gaum L, Huber J: Recurrence of the hemolytic-uremic syndrome in a 3½ year old child 4 months after second renal transplantation. Clin Nephrol 10:121, 1978.

135. Fonio A, Schwendener J: Die Thrombocyten des menschlichen Clutes. Huber, Bern, 1942.

136. Frick PG: Primary thrombocytopenia: Clinical, hematological, and chromosomal studies of 13 patients. Helv Med Acta 35:20, 1969.

137. Furey NL, Schmid FR, Kwaan HC, Friederici HHR: Arterial thrombosis in scleroderma. Br J Dermatol 93:683, 1975.

138. Gale RP, Champlin RE, Feig S, Fitchen JH: Aplastic anemia: Biology and treatment. Ann Intern Med 95:477, 1981.

139. Gandolfo GM, Afeltra A, Ferri GM: Plasmapheresis for thrombocytopenia. Lancet 1:1095, 1978.

140. Gangarosa EJ, Johnson TR, Ramos HS: Ristocetin-induced thrombocytopenia: Site and mechanism of action. Arch Intern Med 105:83, 1960.

141. Gardner F, Bessman JD: Thrombocytopenia due to defective platelet production. Clin Haematol 12:23, 1983.

142. Gerrard JM, Phillips DR, Rao GHR, Plow EF, Walz DA, Ross R, Karker LA, White JG: Biochemical studies of two patients with the gray platelet syndrome. J Clin Invest 66:102, 1980.

143. Gibson B, Hunter D, Naeme PB, Kelton JG: Thrombocytopenia in preeclampsia and eclampsia. Semin Thromb Hemost 8:234, 1982.

144. Glanzmann E: Hereditare hamorrhagische Thrombasthenic. Ein Beitrag zur pathhologie der Blutplattchen. Jahrb Kinderheilk 88:1, 1918.

145. Glass F, Lippon H, Kadowitz PJ: Effects of methylprednisolone and hydrocortisone on aggregation of rabbit platelets induced by arachidonic acid and other aggregating substances. Thromb Haemost 46:676, 1981.

146. Godwin NA, Ginsburg AD: May-Hegglin anomaly: A defect in megakaryocyte fragmentation. Br J Haematol 26:117, 1974.

147. Goldstein HN, Churg J, Strauss L, Gribetz D: Hemolytic-uremic syndrome. Nephron 23:263, 1979.

148. Gollub S, Shafer C, Squitieri A: The bleeding tendency associated with plasma expanders. Surg Gynecol Obstet 124:1203, 1967.

149. Gore I: Disseminated arteriolar and capillary platelet thrombosis: A morphological study of its histogenesis. Am J Pathol 26:155, 1950.

150. Gould L, Greisberg A, Lewnew GC, Roddy R, Werthamer S: Right atrial myxoma associated with thrombocytopenia and bacterial endocarditis. NY State J Med 78:2081, 1978.

151. Groover RV, Burke EC, Gordon N, Berdon WE: The genetic mucopolysaccharidoses. Semin Hematol 9:371, 1972.

152. Grottum KA, Hovig T, Holmsen H, Foss Abrahamsen A, Jeremic M, Seip M: Wiskott-Aldrich syndrome: Qualitative platelet defects and short platelet survival. Br J Haematol 17:373, 1969.

153. Gunz FW: Hemorrhagic thrombocytopenia: A critical review. Blood 15:706, 1960.

154. Gutenberger J, Trygstad CW, Stiehm ER, Opitz JM, Thatcher LG, Bloodworth JMB, Setzkorn J: Familial thrombocytopenia, elevated serum IgA levels and renal disease. Am J Med 49:729, 1970.

155. Gynn TN, Messmore HI, Friedman IA: Drug-induced thrombocytopenia. Med Clin North Am 56:65, 1972.

156. Hackett T, Kelton JG, Powers P: Drug-induced platelet destruction. Semin Thromb Hemost 8:116, 1982.

157. Hall JG, Levin J, Kuhn JP, Jottenberg E, Van Berkum KAP, McKusic V: Thrombocytopenia with absent radius (TAR). Medicine (Baltimore) 48:411, 1969.

158. Hanshaw HB: Congenital and acquired cytomegalovirus infection. Pediatr Clin North Am 13:279, 1966.

159. Hardisty RM, Wolfe NH: Haemorrhagic thrombocytopenia: A clinical and laboratory study. Br J Haematol 1:390, 1955.

160. Harker LA. Thrombokinetics in idiopathic thrombocytopenic purpura. Br J Haematol 19:95, 1970.

161. Harker LA, Finch CA: Thrombokinetics in man. J Clin Invest 48:963, 1969.

162. Harker LA: Platelet survival time: Its measurement and use. Prog Hemost Thromb 4:321, 1978.

163. Harlan JM: Thrombocytopenia due to non-immune platelet destruction. Clin Haematol 12:39, 1983.

164. Harms C: Laboratory evaluation of platelet function. In Triplett DA (Ed): Platelet Function. ASCP Press, Chicago, 1978, p 35.

165. Hartmann RC, Jonkins DE: Paroxysmal nocturnal hemoglobinuria: Current concepts of certain pathophysiological features. Blood 25:850, 1965.

166. Haskell CM: Principles of cancer chemotherapy. In Haskell CM (Ed): Cancer Treatment. W.B. Saunders, Philadelphia, 1980, p 27.

167. Hathaway WE, Bonnar J: Bleeding disorders in the newborn infant. In Perinatal Coagulation. Grune & Stratton, New York, 1978, p 115.

168. Hathaway WE: The bleeding newborn. Semin Hematol 12:175, 1975.

169. Hauglustaine D, Van Damme B, Venrenteghem Y, Michielsen P: Recurrent hemolytic uremic syndrome during oral contraception. Clin Nephrol 15:148, 1981.

170. Hawiger J, Hawiger A, Steckley S, Timmons S, Cheng C: Membrane changes in human platelets induced by lipopolysaccharide endotoxin. Br J Haematol 35:285, 1977.

171. Henry RL: Platelet function. Semin Thromb Hemost 4:93, 1977.

172. Heyns A, Lotter MG, Badenhorst PN, Kotze H, Killian FC, Herbst C, van Reenen OR, Minnaar PC: Kinetics and in vivo redistribution of "indium-labelled" platelets after intravenous protamine sulfate. Thromb Haemost 44:65, 1980.

173. Hilgard H. Hossfeld DK: Transient bleomycin-induced thrombocytopenia: A clinical study. Eur J Cancer 14:1261, 1978.

174. Hirsh J: Laboratory diagnosis of thrombosis. In Colman RW, Hirsh J, Marder VJ, Salzman E (Eds): Hemostasis and Thrombosis: Basic Principles and Clinical Practice. J.B. Lippincott, Philadelphia, 1982, p 789.

175. Hirsh J, Dacie JV: Persistent post-splenectomy thrombocytosis and thrombo-embolism: A consequence of continuing anaemia. Br J Haematol 12:14, 1966.

176. Holmsen H, Weiss HJ: Further evidence for a deficient storage pool of adenine nucleotides in platelets from some patients with thrombocytopathia—"storage pool disease." Blood 39:197, 1972.

177. Horellou MH, LeCompte T, LeCruber C, Fouque F, Chignard M, Conard J, Vargaftig BB, Drey F, Samama M: Familial and constitutional bleeding due to platelet cyclo-oxygenase deficiency. Am J Hematol 14:1, 1983.

178. Horowitz HI, Cohen DB, Martinez P, Papayoanov M: Defective ADP-induced platelet factor 3 activation in uremia. Blood 30:331, 1967.

179. Horowitz HI, Stein IM, Cohen BD, White JG: Further studies on the platelet-inhibiting effect of guanidino succinic acid and its role in uremic bleeding. Am J Med 49:339, 1970.

180. Horowitz HI, Nachman RL: Drug purpura. Semin Hematol 2:287, 1965.

181. Howard MA, Hutton RA, Hardisty RM: Hereditary giant platelet syndrome: A new disorder of platelet function. Br Med J 2:586, 1973.

182. Hoyer L: von Willebrand's disease. Prog Hemost Thromb 3:231, 1976.

183. Huguley CM, Lea JW, Butts JA: Adverse hematological reactions to drugs. Prog Haematol 5:105, 1966.

184. Imbach P, d'Apuzzo V, Hirt A, Rossi E, Vest M, Barandun S, Baumgartner C, Morell A, Schoni M, Wagner HP: High-dose intravenous gammaglobulin for idiopathic thrombocytopenic purpura in childhood. Lancet 1:1228, 1981.

185. Inceman S, Tangun V: Essential athrombia. Thromb Diath Haemorrh 33:278, 1975.

186. Ingeberg S, Stofferson E: Platelet dysfunction in patients with vitamin B_{12} deficiency. Acta Haematol 61:75, 1979.

187. Jacobson RJ, Rath CE, Perloff JK: Intravascular hemolysis and thrombocytopenia in left ventricular outflow obstruction. Br Heart J 35:849, 1973.

188. Jellett LB, Bonnin JA: Platelet thromboplastic function in polycythaemia and thrombocythaemia. Austral Ann Med 15:15, 1966.

189. Jemsbu CN, Lewis PJ, Hilgard P, Mufti GJ, Hows J, Webster J: Prostacyclin deficiency in thrombotic thrombocytopenia purpura. Lancet 2: 748, 1979.

190. Johnson GL, Leis LA, Rao GHR, White JG: Arachidonate-induced platelet aggregation in the dog. Thromb Res 14:147, 1979.

191. Jurgensen KA, Pedersen RS: Familial deficiency of prostacyclin production stimulating factor in the hemolytic-uremic syndrome of childhood. Thromb Res 21:311, 1981.

192. Kamoun P, Kleinknecht D, Duerot H, Jerome H: Platelet-serotonin in uraemia. Lancet 1:782, 1970.

193. Kaplan BS, Esseltine D: Thrombocytopenia in patients with acute post-streptococcal glomerulonephritis. J Pediatr 93:974, 1978.

194. Karpatkin S: Drug-induced thrombocytopenia. Am J Med Sci 262:69, 1971.

195. Karpatkin S, Khan O, Freedman M: Heterogeneity of platelet function. Correlation with platelet volume. Am J Med 64:542, 1978.

196. Karpatkin S, Charmatz A: Heterogeneity of human platelets. I. Metabolic and kinetic evidence suggestive of young and old platelets. J Clin Invest 48:1073, 1969.

197. Karpatkin S: Platelet volume distribution. In Day HJ, Holmsen H, Zucker MB (Eds): Platelet Function Testing. DHEW Publication (NIH) # 78–1087, 1978, p 334.

198. Kass L: Bone Marrow Interpretation. J.B. Lippincott, Philadelphia, 1979, p 1.

199. Kass L: Bone Marrow Interpretation. J.B. Lippincott, Philadelphia, 1979, p 267.

200. Kay AGL: Myelotoxicity of gold. Br Med J 1:1266, 1976.

201. Kelton JG, Neame PB, Gouldie J, Hirsh J: Elevated platelet-associated IgG in the thrombocytopenia of septicemia. N Engl J Med 300: 760, 1979.

202. Kelton JG, Blanchette VS, Wilson WE, Powers P, Pai KRM, Effer SB, Barr RD: Neonatal thrombocytopenia due to passive immunization. Prenatal diagnosis and distinction between maternal platelet allonantibodies and autoantibodies. N Engl J Med 302:1401, 1980.

203. Kelton JG, Gibbons S: Autoimmune platelet destruction: Idiopathic thrombocytopenic purpura. Semin Thromb Hemost 8:83, 1982.

204. Kjeldsberg CR, Swanson J: Platelet satellitism. Blood 43:831, 1974.

205. Klein CA, Blajchman MA: Alloantibodies and platelet destruction. Semin Thromb Hemost 8:105, 1982.

206. Knizley H, Noyes WD: Iron deficiency anemia, papilledema, thrombocytosis and transient hemiparesis. Arch Intern Med 129:483, 1972.

207. Kocsis JJ, Hernadovich J, Silver MJ, Smith JB, Ingerman C: Duration of inhibition of platelet prostaglandin formation and aggregation by ingested aspirin or indomethacin. Prostaglandins 3:141, 1973.

208. Kowalski E: Fibrinogen derivatives and their biological activities. Semin Hematol 5:45, 1968.

209. Krause JR, Lee RE: Histiocytic infiltrates. In Krause JR (Ed): Bone Marrow Biopsy. Churchill Livingstone, New York, 1981, p 171.

210. Kraytman M: Platelet size in thrombocytopenias and thrombocytosis of various origin. Blood 41:587, 1973.

211. Kurstjens R, Bolt C, Vossen M, Naanen C: Familial thrombopathic thrombocytopenia. Br J Haematol 15:305, 1968.

212. Kutti J, Weinfeld A: The frequency of thrombocytopenia in patients with heart disease treated with oral diuretics. Acta Med Scand 183:245, 1968.

213. Kwaan HC, Pierre RV, Potter EV, Gallo GE: The nature of vascular lesion in thrombotic thrombocytopenia purpura. Blood 28:986, 1966.

214. Lacey JV, Penner JA: Management of idiopathic thrombocytopenic purpura in the adult. Semin Thromb Hemost 3:160, 1977.

215. Lachner H: Hemostatic abnormalities associated with dysproteinemias. Semin Hematol 10:125, 1973.

216. Lagard M, Byron PA, Vargaftig BB, Dechavanne M: Impairment of platelet thromboxane A_2 generation and of the platelet release reaction in two patients with congenital deficiency of platelet cyclo-oxygenase. Br J Haematol 38:251, 1978.

217. Leist ER, Banwell JG: Products containing aspirin. N Engl J Med 291:710, 1974.

218. Levin J: Pathophysiology of drug-induced thrombocytopenia. In Dimitrov NV, Nodine JH (Eds): Drugs and Hematologic Reactions. Grune & Stratton, New York, 1974, p 87.

219. Levine PH: A qualitative platelet defect in severe vitamin B_{12} deficiency: Response, hyperresponse, and thrombosis after vitamin B_{12} therapy. Ann Intern Med 78:533, 1973.

220. Levine SJ, Brubaker DB: Detection of platelet antibodies using the platelet migration inhibition assay. Am J Clin Pathol 80:43, 1983.

221. Lewis JH, Zucker MB, Ferguson JH: Bleeding tendency in uremia. Blood 11:1073, 1956.

222. Lewis ML: Cyclic thrombocytopenia: A thrombopoietin deficiency? J Clin Pathol 27:242, 1974.

223. Lewis SM, Gordon-Smith EC: Aplastic and dysplastic anaemias. In Hardisty RM, Weatherall DJ (Eds): Blood and Its Disorders. Blackwell Scientific Publications, Oxford, 1982, p 1229.

224. Libre EP, Cowan DN, Watkins SP, Schulman NR: Relationships between spleen, platelets, and Factor VIII levels. Blood 31:358, 1968.

225. Ligorsky RD: TTP: True or false. Am J Med 64:913, 1978.

226. Lindsay RM, Clark WF: Platelet destruction in renal disease. Semin Thromb Hemost 8:138, 1982.

227. Lipson RL, Bayrd ED, Watkins CH: The postsplenectomy blood picture. Am J Clin Pathol 32:526, 1959.

228. Lisiewicz J: Plasma cell myeloma. In Hemorrhage in Leukemias. Polish Medical Publishers, Warsaw, 1976, p 153.

229. Lowe GDO, Reavy MM, Johnston RV, Forbes CD, Prentice CRM: Increased platelet aggregates in vascular and nonvascular illness. Correlation with plasma fibrinogen and effect of ancrod. Thromb Res 14:377, 1979.

230. Lum LG, Tubergen DG, Corash L, Blaese RM: Platelet-bound IgG in patients with the Wiskott-Aldrich syndrome. Personal observation cited by Hathaway.[168]

231. Lum LG, Tubergen DG, Corash L, Blaese RM: Splenectomy in the management of the thrombocytopenia of the Wiskott-Aldrich syndrome. N Engl J Med 302:892, 1980.

232. Lusher JM, Barnhart MI: Congenital disorders affecting platelets. Semin Thromb Hemost 4:123, 1977.

233. Lusher JM, Iyer R: Idiopathic thrombocytopenic purpura in children. Semin Thromb Hemost 3:175, 1977.

234. Malinovsky NN, Kozlov VA: Thrombosis and embolisms in heart value prosthetics. In Anticoagulant and Thrombolytic Therapy in Surgery. C.V. Mosby, St Louis, 1979, p 149.

235. Malinovsky NN, Kozlov VA: Acute arterial obstruction of aortic bifurcation and limb arteries. In Anticoagulant and Thrombolytic Therapy in Surgery. C.V. Mosby, St Louis, 1979, p 79.

236. Malmsten C, Hamberg M, Svensson J, Samuelsson B: Physiological role of an endoperoxide in human platelets: Hemostatic defect due to platelet cyclo-oxygenase deficiency. Proc Natl Acad Sci USA 72:1446, 1975.

237. Mammen EF: The endothelial cell in health and disease from the coagulationists point of view. Semin Thromb Hemost 5:165, 1979.

238. Mammen EF: Thrombotic thrombocytopenic purpura, Part 1. Semin Thromb Hemost 6:325,

1980.
239. Mammen EF: Thrombotic thrombocytopenic purpura, Part 2. Semin Thromb Hemost 7:1, 1981.
240. Marchasin S, Wallerstein RO, Aggeler PM: Variation of the platelet count in disease. Calif Med 101:95, 1964.
241. Mauer AM, de Vaux W, Lahey ME: Neonatal and maternal thrombocytopenic purpura due to quinine. Pediatrics 19:84, 1957.
242. McClure J: Idiopathic thrombocytopenic purpura in children: Diagnosis and management. Pediatrics 55:68, 1975.
243. McMillan R, Longmire RL, Xelenosky R, Donnel RL, Armstrong S: Quantitation of platelet-binding IgG produced in vitro by spleens from patients with idiopathic thrombocytopenic purpura. N Engl J Med 291:812, 1974.
244. McMillan R: Chronic idiopathic thrombocytopenic purpura. N Engl J Med 304:1135, 1981.
245. McMillin R: Immune thrombocytopenia. Clin Haematol 12:69, 1983.
246. McWilliams NB, Mauer HM: Acute idiopathic thrombocytopenic purpura in children. Am J Hematol 7:87, 1979.
247. Mennuti M, Schwarz RH, Gill F: Obstetric management of isoimmune thrombocytopenia. Am J Obstet Gynecol 118:565, 1974.
248. Meyer D, Zimmerman TS: von Willebrand's disease. In Coleman RW, Hirsh J, Marder VJ, Salzman E (Eds): Hemostasis and Thrombosis: Basic Principles and Clinical Practice. J.B. Lippincott, Philadelphia, 1982, p 64.
249. Michel H, Caen JP, Born GVR: Relation between the inhibition of aggregation and the concentration of cAMP in human and rat platelets. Br J Haematol 33:27, 1976.
250. Mielke CH, Kaneshiro MM, Maer LA, Rappaport SI: The standardized normal Ivy bleeding time and its prolongation by aspirin. Blood 34:204, 1969.
251. Mieschner PA, Graf J: Drug-induced thrombocytopenia. Clin Haematol 9:505, 1980.
252. Mieschner PA: Drug-induced thrombocytopenia. Semin Hematol 10:311, 1973.
253. Mieschner PA, Mieschner A: Immunologic drug-induced blood dyscrasias. Klin Wochenschr 56:1, 1978.
254. Miller JL: Platelet function testing: An improved approach utilizing lumi-aggregation and an interactive computer. Am J Clin Pathol 81:471, 1984.
255. Mills DCB, Robb IA, Roberts GCK: The release of nucleotides, 5-hydroxytryptamine and enzymes from blood platelets during aggregation. J Physiol (Lond) 195:715, 1968.
256. Mills DCB, Roberts GCK: Membrane active drugs and the aggregation of human blood platelets. Nature 213:35, 1967.
257. Mills DCB, Roberts GCK: Effects of adrenaline on human blood platelets. J Physiol (Lond) 193:443, 1967.
258. Minkes MS, Joist JN, Needleham P: Arachidonic acid-induced platelet aggregation independent of ADP-release in a patient with a bleeding disorder due to platelet storage pool disease. Thromb Res 15:169, 1979.
259. Mosgrave JE, Talwaker YB, Puri NC, Campbell RA, Loggan B: The hemolytic-uremic syndrome. Clin Pediatr 17:218, 1978.
260. Mueller-Eckhardt C: Idiopathic thrombocytopenic purpura (ITP): Clinical and immunologic considerations. Semin Thromb Hemost 3:125, 1977.
261. Murer EH, Siojo E: Inhibition of thrombin-induced secretion from platelets by chlortetracycline and its analogs. Thromb Haemost 47:62, 1982.
262. Murphy S: Hereditary thrombocytopenia. Clin Haematol 1:359, 1972.
263. Murphy S, Oski F, Naiman L, Lusch CJ, Goldberg S, Gardner FH: Platelet size and kinetics in hereditary and acquired thrombocytopenia. N Engl J Med 286:499, 1972.
264. Murphy S: Thrombocytosis and thrombocythaemia. Clin Haematol 12:89, 1983.
265. Murphy S: In search of a platelet coombs test. N Engl J Med 309:490, 1983.
266. Murphy S, Rosenthal DS, Weinfeld A: Essential thrombocythemia: Response during first year of therapy with melphalan and radioactive phosphorus: A polycythemia vera study group report. Cancer Treat Rep 66:35, 1982.
267. Myllyla G, Pelkonen R, Ikkala E, Apajalahti J: Hereditary thrombocytopenia: Report of three families. Scand J Haematol 4:441, 1967.
268. Nalbandian RM, Henry RL, Bick RL: Thrombotic thrombocytopenic purpura. Semin Thromb Hemost 5:216, 1979.
269. Natelson EA, Brown CH, Bradshaw MW: Influence of cephalosporin antibiotics on blood coagulation and platelet function. Antimicrob Agents Chemother 9:91, 1976.
270. Neame PB, Hirsh J, Browman G, Denburg J, D'Souza TJ, Gallus A, Brain MC: Thrombotic thrombocytopenic purpura: A Syndrome of intravascular platelet consumption. Can Med Assoc J 114:1108, 1976.
271. Neame PB, Kelton JG, Walker IR, Stewart IU, Nossel HL, Hirsh J: Thrombocytopenia in septicemia: The role of disseminated intravascular coagulation. Blood 56:88, 1980.
272. Neild GH, Rocchi G, Imberti L, Fumagalli F, Brown Z, Remuzzi G, Williams DG: Effect of cyclosporin A on prostacyclin synthesis by vascular tree. Thromb Res 32:373, 1983.
273. Nilsson LR: Chronic pancytopenia with multiple congenital abnormalities. Acta Paediatr 49:518, 1960.

274. Nishizawa EE, Wynalda DJ: Inhibitory effect of ibuprofen (Motrin) on platelet function. Thromb Res 21:347, 1981.

275. Novak R, Wilimas J: Plasmapheresis in catastrophic complications of idiopathic thrombocytopenic purpura. J Pediatr 92:434, 1978.

276. Nussbaum H, Allen B, Kagam AR, Gilbert HA, Rao A, Chan P: Management of bone metastases—multidisciplinary approach. Semin Oncol 4:93, 1977.

277. O'Brien JR: Platelet aggregation. Part I. Some effects of the adenosine phosphates, thrombin and cocaine upon platelet adhesiveness. J Clin Pathol 15:446, 1962.

278. O'Brien JR: Some effects of adrenaline and anti-adrenaline compounds on platelets in vitro and in vivo. Nature 200:763, 1973.

279. O'Brien JRL: The adhesiveness of native platelets and its prevention. J Clin Pathol 14:140, 1961.

280. O'Brien JR: Effect of anti-inflammatory agents on platelets. Lancet 1:894, 1968.

281. O'Brien JR, Shoobridge SM, Finch WJ: Comparison of the effect of heparin and citrate on platelet aggregation. J Clin Pathol 22:28, 1969.

282. Ochs ND, Slichter SJ, Harker LA, Von Behrens WE, Clark RA, Wedgwood RJ: The Wiskot-Aldrich syndrome: Studies of lymphocytes, granulocytes, and platelets. Blood 55:243, 1980.

283. Onder O, Weinstein A, Hoyer CW: Pseudothrombocytopenia caused by platelet agglutinins that are reactive in blood anticoagulated by chelating agents. Blood 56:177, 1980.

284. O'Neill EM, Varadi S: Neonatal aplastic anaemia and Fanconi's anaemia. Arch Dis Child 38:92, 1963.

285. Osborn JE, Shahadi NT: Thrombocytopenia in murine cytomegalovirus infection. J Lab Clin Med 81:53, 1973.

286. Ozer FL, Traux WE, Miesch DC, Levin WC: Primary hemorrhagic thrombocythemia. Am J Med 28:807, 1960.

287. Packham MA, Kinlough-Rathbone RL, Mustard JF: Aggregation and agglutination. In Day HJ, Holmsen H, Zucker MB (Eds): Platelet Function Testing. DHEW Publication (NIH)# 78–1087, 1978, p 66.

288. Pareti FI, Mannucci L, Capitanio A, Mills DCB: Heterogeneity of storage pool deficiency. Thromb Haemost 38:3, 1977.

289. Payne BA, Pierre RV: Pseudothrombocytopenia: A laboratory artifact with potentially serious consequences. Mayo Clin Proc 59:123, 1984.

290. Pearson HA, McIntosh S: Neonatal thrombocytopenia. Clin Haematol 7:111, 1978.

291. Pearson HA, Shulman HR, Marder VJ, Cone TE: Isoimmune neonatal thrombocytopenic purpura. Blood 23:154, 1964.

292. Pegels JG, Bruynes ECE, Engelfriet CP, Von dem Borne AEGR: Pseudothrombocytopenia: An immunologic study on platelet antibodies dependent on ethylene diamine tetra-acetate. Blood 59:157, 1982.

293. Pegels JG, Helmerhorst FM, van Leeuwen EF, van dePlas-vanDalen C, Engelfriet CP, von dem Borne AEGK: The Evans syndrome: Characterization of the responsible autoantibodies. Br J Haematol 51:445, 1982.

294. Penington DG, Lee NLY, Roxburgh AE, McGready JR: Platelet density and size: The interpretation of heterogeneity. Br J Haematol 34:365, 1976.

295. Penny R, Rozenberg MC, Firkin BG: The splenic platelet pool. Blood 27:1, 1966.

296. Perry GS, Spector BD, Schuman LM, Mandel JS, Anderson VE, McHugh RB, Hanson MR, Fahlstrom SM, Krivit W, Kersey JH: The Wiskott-Aldrich syndrome in the United States and Canada (1892–1979). J Pediatr 97:72, 1980.

297. Pfueller SL, Cosgrove LJ: Activation of human platelets in PRP via their Fc-receptor by antigen-antibody complexes or immunoglobulin G: Requirement for particle bound fibrinogen. Thromb Res 20:97, 1980.

298. Phadke KP, Isbister JP: Post-transfusion purpura. Med J Aust 1:430, 1980.

299. Pierce CH, Oshiro G, Nickerson M: Effect of methylpredisone sodium succinate (MP) on platelet aggregation. Circulation 49 (Suppl III):289, 1974.

300. Pillay VKG, Kurtzman NA, Manaligod JR, Jonasson O: Selective thrombocytopenia due to localized microangiopathy of renal allografts. Lancet 2:988, 1973.

301. Pisciotta AV, Gottschall JI: Clinical features of thrombotic thrombocytopenic purpura. Semin Thromb Hemost 6:330, 1980.

302. Plante J, Boneu B, Vaysse C, Barret A, Couzi M, Bierme R: Dipyridamole-aspirin versus low doses of heparin in the prophylaxis of deep venous thrombosis in abdominal surgery. Thromb Res 14:399, 1979.

303. Polasek T, Duckert F: Quantitative determination of platelet factor 3 activity. Thromb Diath Haemorrh 25:532, 1971.

304. Ponticelli C, Rivolta E, Imbasciati E, Rossi E, Mannucci PM: Hemolytic uremic syndrome in adults. Arch Intern Med 140:353, 1980.

305. Prankerd TAJ: Idiopathic thrombocytopenic purpura. Clin Haematol 1:327, 1972.

306. Pui CN, Wilimas J, Wang W: Evan's syndrome in childhood. J Pediatr 97:754, 1980.

307. Pullen J: Drug-induced thrombcytopenias. In Lusher JM, Barnhart MI (Eds): Acquired Bleeding Disorders in Children: Platelet Abnormalities and Laboratory Methods. Masson Publishing, USA, New York, 1981, p 49.

308. Rabiner SF: Uremic bleeding. Prog Hemost

Thromb 1:233, 1972.

309. Rabiner SF, Molinas F: The role of phenol and phenolic acids on the thrombocytopathy and defective platelet aggregation of patients with renal failure. Am J Med 49:346, 1970.

310. Raccuglia G: Gray platelet syndrome. A variety of qualitative platelet disorders. Am J Med 51:818, 1971.

311. Rajah SM, Crow MJ, Perry AF, Ahmad R, Watson DA: The effects of dipyridamole on platelet function: Correlation with blood levels in man. Br J Clin Pharmacol 4:129, 1979.

312. Rao AK, Walsh PN: Acquired qualitative platelet disorders. Clin Haematol 12:201, 1983.

313. Rattazzi L, Haimov MN: Role of the platelet in the obliterative vascular transplant rejection phenomenon. Surg Forum 21:243, 1970.

314. Remuzzi G, Livio M, Cavenaghi AE, Marchesi D, Mecca G, Donati MB, de Gaetano G: Unbalanced prostaglandin synthesis and plasma factors in uraemic bleeding. A hypothesis. Thromb Res 13:531, 1978.

315. Remuzzi G, Cavenaghe AE, Mecca G, Donati MB, de Gaetano G: Prostacyclin (PGI$_2$) and bleeding time in uremic patients. Thromb Res 11:919, 1977.

316. Remuzzi G: Treatment of the hemolytic-uremic syndrome with plasma. Clin Nephrol 12:279, 1979.

317. Remuzzi G, Rossi EC, Misiani R, Marchesi D, Mecca G, de Gaetano G, Donati MB: Prostacyclin and thrombotic microangiopathy. Semin Thromb Hemost 6:301, 1980.

318. Rendu F, Breton-Gorius J, Trugnan G, Castro-Malispina H, Andriev JM, Bereziat G, Lebret M, Caen JP: Studies on a new variant of the Hermansky-Pudlak syndrome: Qualitative ultrastructural bodies associated with a phospholipase A defect. Am J Hematol 4:387, 1978.

319. Renney JTG, O'Sullivan EF, Burke PF: Prevention of postoperative deep vein thrombosis with dipyridamole and aspirin. Br Med J 2:992, 1976.

320. Riella MC, George CRP, Hickman RO, Striker GE, Slichter SJ, Harker L, Quadracci LJ: Renal micro angiopathy of the hemolytic-uremic syndrome. Nephron 17:188, 1976.

321. Roberts WC, Bulkley BH, Morrow AG: Pathologic anatomy of cardiac valve replacement. A study of 224 necropsy patients. Prog Cardiovasc Dis 15:539, 1973.

322. Rodriquez S, Leikin S, Hiller MC: Neonatal thrombocytopenia associated with antepartum administration of thiazide drugs. N Engl J Med 207:881, 1964.

323. Roper-Drewinko P, Drewinko B, Corrigan G, Johnston D, McCredie KB, Freireich EJ: Standardization of platelet function tests. Am J Hematol 11:183, 1981.

324. Rossie EC, Levin NW: Inhibition of primary ADP-induced platelet aggregation in normal subjects after administration of nitrofurantoin (Furadantin). Clin Invest 52:2457, 1973.

325. Rossie EC, Levin NW: Inhibition of ADP-induced platelet aggregation by furosemide. J Lab Clin Med 81:140, 1973.

326. Rowan RM, Fraser C, Gray JH: Comparison of channelyser and model S plus determined platelet size measurements. Clin Lab Haematol 3:165, 1981.

327. Rysanek R, Suehla C, Spankova H, Mlejnkova M: The effect of tricyclic antidepressive drugs on adrenaline and adenosine diphosphate induced platelet aggregation. J Pharm Pharmacol 18:616, 1966.

328. Rywlin AM: Foreign cells. In Histopathology of the Bone Marrow. Little, Brown & Company, Boston, 1976, p 133.

329. Salem NH, Kouts J, Firkin BG: Circulating platelet aggregates in ischaemic heart disease and their correlation to platelet life scan. Thromb Res 17:707, 1980.

330. Salzman EW, Rosenberg RD, Smith HJ, Lindon JN, Favreau L: Effect of heparin and heparin fractions on platelet aggregation. J Clin Invest 65:621, 1980.

331. Saxon A, Kattlove H: Platelet inhibition by sodium nitroprusside, a smooth muscle inhibitor. Blood 47:957, 1976.

332. Schafer AJ, Alexander RW, Handin RT: Inhibition of platelet function by organic nitrate vasodilators. Blood 55:649, 1980.

333. Scheck R, Rasche H, Queiber W, Burkhardt H, Calvo W: Platelet dysfunction as a result of inhibition of a release (aspirin-like) defect in two identical twins. Dtsch Med Wochenschr 100:1842, 1975.

334. Schiff D, Aranda JV, Stern L: Neonatal thrombocytopenia and congenital malformations associated with administration of tolbutamide to the mother. J Pediatr 77:457, 1970.

335. Schiffer CA, Young V: Detection of platelet antibodies using a micro-enzyme-linked immunosorbent assay (ELISA). Blood 61:311, 1983.

336. Schlosser LL, Kipp MA, Wenzel FJ: Thrombocytosis in iron-deficiency anemia. J Lab Clin Med 66:107, 1965.

337. Schondorf TH, Hey D: Platelet function tests in uraemia and under acetylsalicylic acid administration. Haemostasis 3:129, 1974.

338. Schoolwerth AC, Sandler RS, Klahr S, Kissane JM: Nephrosclerosis postpartum and in women taking oral contraceptives: A report of two cases. Arch Intern Med 136:178, 1976.

339. Schulman I, Pierce M, Lukens A, Cummimbhoy Z: Studies on thrombopoiesis. I. A factor in normal plasma required for platelet production; chronic thrombocytopenia due to its deficiency. Blood 16:943, 1960.

340. Seeman PM: Membrane stabilization of drugs: Tranquilizers, steroids, and anesthetics. Int Rev Neurobiol 9:145, 1966.

341. Seidenfeld AM, Owen J, Glynn MFX: Post-transfusion purpura cured by steroid therapy in a man. Can Med Assoc J 118:1285, 1978.

342. Seip M: Hereditary hypoplastic thrombocytopenia. Acta Paediatr Scand 52:370, 1963.

343. Selner JC: More aspirin-containing drugs. N Engl J Med 292:372, 1975.

344. Sheth NK, Prankerd TAJ: Inherited thrombocytopenia with thrombasthenia. J Clin Pathol 21:154, 1968.

345. Shulman NR, Marder VJ, Hiller MC, Collier EM: Platelet and leukocyte isoantigens and their antibodies: Serologic, physiologic and clinical studies. Prog Hematol 4:222, 1964.

346. Shulman NR: A mechanism of cell destruction in individuals sensitized to foreign antigens and the implications in autoimmunity. Ann Intern Med 60:506, 1964.

347. Shulman NR: Immunoreactions involving platelets. I. A steric and kinetic model for formation of a complex from a human antibody, quinidine as a heptene, and platelets; and for fixation of complement by the complex. J Exp Med 107:665, 1958.

348. Shulman NR: Immunoreactions involving platelets. III. Quantitative aspects of platelet agglutination, inhibition of clot retraction and other reactions caused by the antibody of quinidine purpura. J Exp Med 107:697, 1958.

349. Shulman NR: Immunoreactions involving platelets. IV. Studies on the pathogenesis of thrombocytopenia in drug purpura using test doses of quinidine in sensitized individuals; their implications in idiopathic thrombocytopenic purpura. J Exp Med 107:711, 1958.

350. Siemco: The petechiometer. Package insert, Sienco Inc., Morrison CO., 1980, p. 1.

351. Silverman JL, Wurzel HA: The effect of glyceryl guiacolate on platelet function and other coagulation factors in vivo. Am J Clin Pathol 51:35, 1969.

352. Silverstein MN: Primary or hemorrhagic thrombocytopenia. Arch Intern Med 122:18, 1968.

353. Skoog WA, Lawrence JS, Adams WS: A metabolic study of a patient with idiopathic cyclical thrombocytopenic purpura. Blood 12:844, 1957.

354. Skudowitz RB, Katz J, Lurie A, Levin J, Metz J: Mechanisms of thrombocytopenia in malignant tertian malaria. Br Med J 2:515, 1973.

355. Smith CH: The purpuras. In Blood Diseases of Infancy and Childhood. C.V. Mosby Co, Saint Louis, 1972, p 760.

356. Smith MD, Smith DA, Fletcher M: Hemorrhage associated with thrombocytopenia in megaloblastic anemia. Br Med J 1:982, 1962.

357. Soppitt GD, Mitchell JRA: The effect of colchicine on human platelet behavior. J Atheroscler Res 10:247, 1969.

358. Spooner M, Meyers OO: The effect of dicumerol (3.3-methylenebis) (4-hydroxy-coumarin) on platelet adhesiveness. Am J Physiol 142:279, 1944.

359. Stacy RS: Uptake of 5-hydroxytryptamine by platelets. Br J Pharmacol 16:284, 1961.

360. Stafford BT, Crosby WH: Late onset of gold-induced thrombocytopenia. With a practical note on the injections of dimercaprol. JAMA 239:50, 1978.

361. Steiner M, Anastasi J: Vitamin E. An inhibitor of the platelet release reaction. J Clin Invest 57:732, 1976.

362. Stoll DB, Blum S, Pasquale D, Murphy S: Thrombocytopenia with decreased megakaryocytes: Evaluation and prognosis. Ann Intern Med 198:170, 1981.

363. Stuart MJ: Inherited defects of platelet function. Semin Hematol 12:233, 1975.

364. Szekely P: Systemic embolization and anticoagulant prophylaxis in rheumatic heart disease. Br Med J 1:1209, 1964.

365. Takahashi N, Nagayama R, Hattori A, Ihzumi T, Tsukada T, Shibata A: von Willebrand disease associated with familial thrombocytopenia and increased ristocetin-induced platelet aggregation. Am J Hematol 10:89, 1981.

366. Takahashi A, Ohara S, Imaoka S, Kambayashi J, Kosaki G: A simple and rapid method to detect platelet associated IgG. Thromb Res 28:11, 1982.

367. Tangun Y: Platelet aggregation and platelet factor 3 activity in myeloproliferative syndromes. Thromb Diath Haemorrh 25:241, 1971.

368. Taub RN, Rodriquez-Erdmann F, Dameshek W: Intravascular coagulation, the Shwartzman reaction and the pathogenesis of T.T.P. Blood 24:775, 1964.

369. Terada N, Baldini M, Ebbe S, Madoff MA: Interaction of influenza virus with blood platelets. Blood 28:231, 1966.

370. Tranum BL, Haut A: Thrombocytosis: Platelet kinetics in neoplasia. J Lab Clin Med 84:615, 1974.

371. Trent R, Adams E, Erhardt C, Basten A: Alterations in T-gamma-cells in patients with chronic idiopathic thrombocytopenic purpura. J Immunol 127:621, 1981.

372. Triplett DA: Platelet disorders. In Murano G, Bick RL (Eds): Basic Concepts of Hemostasis and Thrombosis. CRC Press, Boca Raton, FL, 1980, p 95.

373. Triplett DA: Qualitative or functional defects of platelets. In Triplett DA (Ed): Platelet Function: Laboratory Evaluation and Clinical Application. ASCP Press, Chicago, 1978, p 123.

374. Triplett DA: Miscellaneous lists and forms. In

Triplett DA (Ed): Platelet Function Evaluation: Laboratory Evaluation and Clinical Application. ASCP Press, Chicago, 1978, p 291.

375. Turpie AGG, de Boer AC, Genton E: Platelet consumption in cardiovascular disease. Semin Thromb Hemost 8:161, 1982.

376. Vaughn-Neil EF, Ardeman S, Bevan G, Blakeman AC, Jenkins WJ: Post-transfusion purpura associated with unusual platelet antibody (Anti-PL[B1]). Br Med J 1:436, 1975.

377. Veenhoven WA, Van Der Schans GS, Huiges W, Metting-Scherphuis HE, Halie MR, Nieweg NO: Pseudothrombocytopenia due to agglutinins. Am J Clin Pathol 72:1005, 1979.

378. Vipan WH: Quinine as a cause of purpura. Lancet 2:37, 1865.

379. Vizcaino GJ, Diez-Ewald M: Autoimmune thrombocytopenic purpura. Comparison of three different methods for the detection of platelet antibodies. Am J Hematol 14:279, 1983.

380. Volk BW, Adachi M, Schneck L: The pathology of the spingolipidoses. Semin Hematol 9:317, 1972.

381. Von Behrens WE: Mediterranean macrothrombocytopenia. Blood 46:199, 1975.

382. von dem Borne AEG, van Leeurwen EF, von Riesz LE, van Boxtel CJ, Engelfriet CP: Neonatal alloimmune thrombocytopenia: Detection and characterization of the responsible antibodies by the platelet immunofluorescence test. Blood 57:649, 1981.

383. von dem Borne AEGK, von Reisz E, Verheugt FWA, ten Cate JW, Kope JG, Engelfrict CP, Nijenhuis LE: Bak-a, a new platelet-specific antigen involved in neonatal alloimmune thrombocytopenia. Vox Sang 39:113, 1980.

384. Von Gasset C, Gautier E, Steck A, Siebenmann RE, Oechslin R: Hamolytisch-Uraemische syndrome: Bilaterale Nierenrindennekrosen bie akuten erworbenen hamolytischen Anamien. Schweiz Med Wochenschr 85:905, 1955.

385. Vossaugh P, Leikin J, Avery G, Monif G, Sever T: Neonatal thrombocytopenia in association with rubella. Acta Haematol 35:158, 1966.

386. Wang W, Herrod H, Pui CH, Presbury G, Wilimas J: Immunoregulatory abnormalities in Evans syndrome. Am J Hematol 15:381, 1983.

387. Weinfeld A, Branehog I, Kutti J: Platelets in the myeloproliferative syndrome. Clin Haematol 4:373, 1975.

388. Weintraub RM, Pechet L, Alexander B: Rapid diagnosis of drug-induced thrombocytopenic purpura. JAMA 180, 1962.

389. Weiss HJ: Pathophysiology and detection of clinically significant platelet dysfunction. In Baldini MG, Ebbe S (Eds): Platelets. Production, Function, Transfusion, and Storage. Grune & Stratton, New York, 1974, p 253.

390. Weiss HJ, Lages BA, Witte LD, Kaplan KL, Goodman DS, Nossel HL, Baumgartner HR: Storage pool disease: Evidence for clinical and biochemical heterogeneity. Thromb Haemost 38:3, 1977.

391. Weiss HJ: Platelet aggregation, adhesion, and adenosine diphosphate release in thrombopathia (platelet factor-3 deficiency): A comparison with Glanzmann's thrombasthenia and von Willebrand's disease. Am J Med 43:570, 1967.

392. Weiss HJ, Ames RP: Ultrastructural findings in storage pool disease and aspirin-like defects of platelets. Am J Pathol 71:447, 1973.

393. Weiss HJ, Rogers J: Thrombocytopathia due to abnormalities in platelet release reaction: Studies on six unrelated patients. Blood 39:187, 1972.

394. Weiss HJ: Antiplatelet drugs: pharmacological aspects. In Platelets: Pathophysiology and Antiplatelet Drug Therapy. Alan R Liss, New York, 1982, p 45.

395. Weiss HJ: Pharmacology of platelet inhibition. Prog Hemost Thromb 1:199, 1972.

396. Weiss HJ, Eichelberger JW: The detection of platelet defects in patients with mild bleeding disorders: Use of quantitative assay for platelet factor 3. Am J Med 32:872, 1962.

397. Weiss HJ: Antiplatelet drugs in clinical medicine. In: Platelets: Pathophysiology and Antiplatelet Drug Therapy. Alan R Liss, New York, 1982, p 75.

398. Weksler BB, Gillik M, Pink J: Effect of propanolol on platelet function. Blood 49:185, 1977.

399. Weksler BB: Prostacyclin. Prog Hemost Thromb 6:113, 1982.

400. Wessler S, Gitel SN: Heparin: New concepts relevant to clinical use. Blood 53:525, 1979.

401. Whitaker JA, Sartain P, Shahedy M: Hematological aspects of congenital syphilis. J Pediatr 66:629, 1965.

402. White JG, Raynor ST: The effects of trifluoroperazine, an inhibitor of calmodulin on platelet function. Thromb Res 18:279, 1980.

403. White JG: Effects of colchicine and vinca alkaloids on human platelets. I. Influence on platelet microtubules and contractile function. Am J Pathol 53:281, 1968.

404. White JG: Ultrastructural studies of the gray platelet syndrome. Am J Pathol 95:445, 1979.

405. Widerlov E, Karlman I, Storsater J: Hydralazine-induced neonatal thrombocytopenia. N Engl J Med 303:1235, 1980.

406. Wiley JS, Chesterman CN, Morgan FJ, Castaldi PA: The effect of sulfinpyrazone on the aggregation and release reactions of human platelets. Thromb Res 14:23, 1979.

407. Williams DM, Lynch RE, Cartwright GE: Drug-induced aplastic anemia. Semin Hematol 10:195, 1973.

408. Wilson JJ, Neame PB, Kelton JG: Infection-in-

duced thrombocytopenia. Semin Thromb Hemost 8:217, 1982.

409. Winocour PD, Kinlough-Rathbone RL, Mustard JF: The effect of the phospholipase inhibitor mepacrine on platelet release reaction, and fibrinogen binding to the platelet surface. Thromb Haemost 45:257, 1981.

410. Wolf SM, Shulman NR: Inhibition of platelet energy production and release reaction by PGE$_1$, theophylline and cAMP. Biochem Biophys Res Commun 41:128, 1970.

411. Wolff JA: Wiskott-Aldrich syndrome: Clinical, immunologic, and pathologic observations. J Pediatr 70:221, 1967.

412. Wu KK, Hoak JC: A new method for the quantitative detection of platelet aggregates in patients with arterial insufficiency. Lancet 2:924, 1974.

413. Yam LT, McMillan R, Tauassoli M, Crosby WH: Splenic hemopoiesis in idiopathic thrombocytopenic purpura. Am J Clin Pathol 62:830, 1974.

414. Zahavi J: Acquired "storage pool disease" of platelets. Thromb Haemost 35:501, 1976.

415. Zeigler Z: In vitro granulocyte-platelet rosette formation mediated by an IgG immunoglobulin. Haemostasis 3:282, 1974.

416. Zeigler Z, Murphy S, Gardner FH: Post-transfusion pupura: A heterogeneous syndrome. Blood 45:529, 1975.

417. Zieve PD, Solomon HM: Effects of diuretics on the human platelet. Am J Physiol 215:650, 1968.

418. Zucker S, Meilke H, Durocher JR, Crosby WH: Oozing and bruising due to abnormal platelet function. Ann Intern Med 76:725, 1971.

419. Zucker MB, Peterson J: Effect of acetylsalicylic acid, other nonsteroidal anti-inflammatory agents, and dipyridamole on human blood platelets. J Lab Clin Med 76:66, 1970.

420. Zucker MB: Effect of heparin on platelet function. Thromb Diath Haemorrh 33:63, 1975.

5

Congenital Coagulation Factor Defects and von Willebrand's Disease

Hereditary defects of the blood proteins leading to hemorrhagic and associated disease states are the topic of this chapter, and specific acquired inhibitors of isolated coagulation proteins leading to hemorrhage, thrombosis, and thromboembolus are discussed in Chapter 12. The clinical manifestations of coagulation factor disorders are different from those previously discussed for vascular or platelet defects (Chapters 3 and 4). Coagulation factor disorders are characterized by deep tissue bleeding, including intraarticular bleeding with resultant crippling hemarthrosis, deep intramuscular bleeding, and, at times, intracranial bleeding, which can be life-threatening.[16] In addition, patients with single or multiple coagulation factor defects have moderate to severe mucosal membrane hemorrhage, whereas patients with vascular and platelet defects more commonly experience mild to moderate mucosal membrane hemorrhage.[17] Thus, mucosal membrane bleeding tends to be much more severe with single or multiple coagulation factor deficiencies. Mucosal membrane hemorrhage may be gastrointestinal, genitourinary, intrapulmonary, from paranasal sinuses, or may be manifested as diffuse, bilateral epistaxis.

Patients tend to develop large ecchymoses but do not develop petechiae and purpura except in von Willebrand's disease.[18] Petechiae and purpura are hallmark findings of vascular and platelet defects and are not generally found in coagulation protein defects, with the exception of von Willebrand's disease, which is a blood protein defect manifested clinically as an endothelial-platelet interaction problem.[12] However, patients with coagulation protein defects may develop petechiae and purpura in conjunction with other hemostasis compartment defects; this may occur, for example, in disseminated intravascular coagulation (DIC)-type syndromes in which a patient may have a blood protein problem plus a platelet problem plus (potentially) a vascular problem, or it may occur if the patient with a blood protein defect has an isolated platelet or vascular defect; such an associated defect may be hereditary, acquired, or drug-induced.[18,19] Clinical and laboratory findings of coagulation factor disorders are summarized in Table 5–1.

The vast majority of clinically significant coagulation protein disorders will be detected by noting prolongation of global tests of coagulation, those tests that depend on the conversion of fibrinogen to fibrin for an end-point determination.[16–18] These include such tests as the prothrombin time, the activated partial thromboplastin time (PTT), the thrombin time, the Lee-White clotting time, the activated clotting time, and the whole blood clotting time. One or a combination of these global tests will usually be prolonged in clinically significant coagulation protein defects. The other screening tests of hemostasis are normal in patients with isolated coagulation protein problems. The template bleeding time is normal in hemophilia patients. A definitive diagnosis of the particular coagulation factor defects present usually requires a specific quantitative factor assay after demonstrating prolongation of one or several of the aforementioned global tests of coagulation. The coagulation factor disorders are summarized in Table 5–2. The hereditary defects are almost always a single factor deficiency or dysfunction as opposed to the acquired defects, which usually involve multi-factor deficiencies, such as those seen in patients with acute or

Table 5-1 Clinical and Laboratory Findings of Coagulation Factor Disorders

Clinical
  Deep tissue hemorrhage
    Intramuscular bleeding
    Intra-articular bleeding
    Intracranial bleeding
  Moderate to severe mucosal membrane hemorrhage
    Gastrointestinal
    Genitourinary
    Intrapulmonary
  Large subcutaneous hematomas
  Petechiae and purpura not present
    (except von Willebrand's)
Laboratory
  Prolongation of global tests dependent on the conversion of fibrinogen to fibrin
    Prothrombin time
    PTT
    Thrombin time
    Lee-White clotting time
    Whole blood clotting time
    Activated clotting time
  Other screening tests normal
    Platelet count
    Template bleeding time*
    Peripheral blood smear
  Definitive diagnosis usually requires a specific quantitative factor assay

* Except von Willebrand's disease.

Table 5-2 Coagulation Factor Disorders

Hereditary defects
  (usually monofactorial deficiency or dysfunction)
    Hemophilias
    von Willebrand's disease
    Deficiencies of Factors II, VII, IX, or X (rare)
    Fibrinogen defects
    Other single factor defects (Factors V, XI, XIII)
    Contact activation defects
    Kininogen defects
Acquired defects
  (usually multifactorial deficiency or dysfunction)
    Disseminated intravascular coagulation syndromes
    Primary fibrinolytic syndromes
    Liver disease
    Circulating anticoagulants
    Drug-induced

Table 5-3 Hereditary Coagulation Factor Defects

Afibrinogenemia, hypofibrinogenemia, dysfibrinogenemia
Factor II defects
Factor V defects
Factor VII defects
Factor VIII:C defects (hemophilia A)
Factor VIII:vW defects (von Willebrand's)
Factor IX defects (hemophilia B)
Factor X defects
Factor XI defects
Factor XII defects (Hageman factor)
Factor XIII defects
Passovoy defect
Prekallikrein defects (Fletcher factor)
Kininogen defects (Williams, Fitzgerald, Reid, Flaujeac, Fujiwara factors)
Fibrinolytic system defects

chronic liver disease, generalized intravascular proteolytic syndromes, such as DIC, or primary fibrinolytic syndromes.

The hereditary coagulation factor disorders are summarized in Table 5-3. The afibrinogenemias, hypofibrinogenemias, and dysfibrinogenemias are quite rare. However, the dysfibrinogenemias may be more common than previously appreciated because only during the past two decades has awareness of this disorder been appreciated, thus leading to laboratory testing for its presence. Isolated deficiencies of Factors II, V, VII, or X are extremely rare clinical oddities. Isolated Factor XII deficiency, Fletcher factor deficiency, and Fitzgerald factor deficiency are also rare; however, until more widespread screening is done, as specific assays become generally available to most clinical laboratories, the actual incidence of these disorders will remain undefined. The three hemophilias occur in approximately 1 in 8000 to 10,000 male births in the United States, although differences in the incidence of hemophilias are noted regionally and worldwide.[47]

Fibrinogen Defects

Congenital abnormalities of fibrinogen consist of afibrinogenemia, hypofibrinogenemia, or dysfibrinogenemia. A very important concept is that most of the isolated coagulation factor disorders may occur because of absence of the protein or the presence of a dysfunctional protein that has abnormal or absent biologic coagulant activity. This concept will be exemplified by a discussion of afibrinogenemia, hypofibrinogenemia, and dysfibrinogenemia. Congenital abnormalities of fibrinogen are summarized in Table 5–4. These abnormalities may be quantitative or qualitative. Both types of defects are inherited as autosomal dominant traits.[91] The quantitative defects are hypofibrinogenemia, representing the heterozygote, and afibrinogenemia, representing the homozygous patient. The hypofibrinogenemic patient will have approximately 50% normal fibrinogen levels; however, the afibrinogenemic patient has essentially no fibrinogen present. Interestingly, some patients who are severely afibrinogenemic do have very small amounts of fibrinogen detectable by immunologic techniques, usually measured as 5 to 10 mg/dL. However, this may represent cross-reactivity with a fibrinogen-like protein such as fibronectin.

The qualitative defects of fibrinogen consist of the dysfibrinogenemias; these are also manifested in the homozygous or heterozygous state. If the patient is homozygous, all fibrinogen will be dysfunctional. If, however, the patient is heterozygous, only 50% of circulating fibrinogen will be dysfunctional.

The hypofibrinogenemic patient rarely has clinical bleeding. Some, however, have a mild bleeding tendency, but most patients only bleed significantly after surgical or traumatic stress. The afibrinogenemic patient does have occasional spontaneous hemorrhage.[114] This can be manifested as gastrointestinal blood loss in the form of melena, hematochezia, or hematemesis; patients may develop large hematomas or massive hematemesis and hypermenorrhagia, and frequently they have umbilical stump bleeding, gingival bleeding with toothbrushing, and other mucosal membrane bleeding.[16,114] Intra-articular bleeding with resultant hemarthroses and occasional intracranial bleeding occurs.[140] The clinical manifestations

of congenital hypofibrinogenemia and afibrinogenemia are listed in Table 5–5, and the laboratory diagnosis is given in Table 5–6. Global tests of coagulation, such as whole blood clotting time, recalcification time, activated PTT, prothrombin time, or reptilase time will have prolonged values in the hypofibrinogenemic (heterozygous) patient.[16,114] However, the same global test values, dependent on the conversion of fibrinogen to fibrin, will be markedly prolonged or infinite in the afibrinogenemic (homozygous) patient.[16,114] When measuring fibrinogen concentration by coagulation tests, protein precipitation, or immunologic techniques, hypofibrinogenemic patients (heterozygotes) will have fibrinogen levels approximately 50% of normal. However, afibrinogenemic patients (homozygotes) will demonstrate no detectable fibrinogen.

Patients with congenital dysfibrinogenemia often display no hemorrhagic diathesis; however, some do have a mild bleeding tendency and easy and spontaneous bruising.[114,115,135,144] Patients with dysfibrinogenemia may have profuse and prolonged bleeding after trauma or surgery and females may have excessive menstrual flow. These findings are most commonly seen in homozygous patients in whom all fibrinogen is dysfunctional; heterozygous patients with 50% normal functioning fibrinogen are often asymptomatic. Several types of congenital dysfibrinogenemia have been associated

Table 5–4 Hereditary Fibrinogen Defects

Autosomal dominant traits
Quantitative fibrinogen defects
  Hypofibrinogenemia (heterozygous patient)
  Afibrinogenemia (homozygous patient)
Qualitative fibrinogen defects (dysfibrinogenemias)
  All fibrinogen defective (homozygous patient)
  Half of fibrinogen defective (heterozygous patient)

Table 5–5 Clinical Manifestations of Quantitative Fibrinogen Defects

Hypofibrinogenemia
  Spontaneous hemorrhage is rare
  Some with a mild bleeding tendency
  May have severe bleeding with surgery or trauma
Afibrinogenemia
  Spontaneous hemorrhage may occur
  Gastrointestinal bleeding
  Subcutaneous hematomas
  Prolonged and excessive menstrual bleeding
  Common types of hemorrhage
    Umbilical stump bleeding
    Gingival bleeding
    Mucosal membrane bleeding
    Intra-articular bleeding
    Intracranial bleeding

Table 5–6 Laboratory Manifestations of Quantitative Fibrinogen Defects

Global coagulation tests	Afibrinogenemia	Hypofibrinogenemia
Whole blood clotting time	Infinite	Prolonged
PTT	Infinite	Prolonged
Prothrombin time	Infinite	Prolonged
Thrombin time	Infinite	Prolonged
Reptilase time	Infinite	Prolonged
Activated clotting time	Infinite	Prolonged
Fibrinogen concentration		
Coagulation tests	0%	Reduced
Precipitation tests	0%	Reduced
Immunologic tests	0%	Reduced
Other tests		
Template bleeding time	Boarderline	Normal
Platelet function (aggregation)	Abnormal	Abnormal

with a thrombotic tendency. These are fibrinogens Baltimore,[13] Chapel Hill,[34] Charlottesville,[106] Copenhagen,[175] Marburg,[57] Naples,[155] New York,[7] Oslo I,[48] Paris II,[174] and Wiesbaden.[211] Clinical findings of congenital dysfibrinogenemia are summarized in Table 5–7. Global coagulation tests, including whole blood clotting time, recalcification time, activated PTT, prothrombin time, reptilase time, or thrombin time will have normal or moderately prolonged values in the heterozygote dysfibrinogenemic patient; in general, 100 mg% functional fibrinogen will render a normal clotting time with the aforementioned global coagulation tests.

Laboratory manifestations of congenital dysfibrinogenemia are summarized in Table 5–8. When measuring fibrinogen concentration by clot-based techniques, the heterozygote dysfibrinogenemic patient is found to have reduced levels, but the homozygote dysfibrinogenemic patient has no detectable fibrinogen by clotting technique. Protein precipitation

Table 5–7 Clinical Manifestations of Qualitative Fibrinogen Defects (Dysfibrinogenemias)

Heterozygous patients
  Seldom have hemorrhage
  May bleed with surgery or trauma
Homozygous patients
  Some are asymptomatic
  Some with spontaneous bleeding
  Easy bruising is common
  Severe bleeding with surgery or trauma
  Excessive menstrual bleeding common

Table 5–8 Laboratory Manifestations of Qualitative Fibrinogen Defects (Dysfibrinogenemias)

Global coagulation tests	Homozygote	Heterozygote
Whole blood clotting time	Infinite	Prolonged
Prothrombin time	Infinite	Prolonged
PTT	Infinite	Prolonged
Thrombin time	Infinite	Prolonged
Reptilase time	Infinite	Prolonged
Activated clotting time	Infinite	Prolonged
Fibrinogen concentration		
Coagulation tests	0%	Reduced
Precipitation tests	100%	100%
Immunologic tests	100%	100%
Other tests		
Template bleeding time	Normal	Normal
Platelet function (aggregation)	Normal	Normal

methods for fibrinogen determination will reveal both the heterozygous or homozygous dysfibrinogenemic patient to have normal fibrinogen levels. Immunologic fibrinogen determination techniques will also demonstrate normal levels of fibrinogen in heterozygous and homozygous dysfibrinogenemic patients.

In most instances of congenital dysfibrinogenemia, the exact defect accounting for defective function of the fibrinogen molecule is not known. The congenital dysfibrinogenemias are listed in Table 5–9. Most that have been characterized have crucial amino acid substitutions, defects of fibrinopeptide A or B release, or abnormal carbohydrate content.[114,115,128,135,144,145,161] Fibrinogen Detroit (Fig. 5–1) was the first congenital dysfibrinogenemia in which the mechanism for dysfunction was carefully evaluated and defined. Dysfibrinogenemia Detroit represents the second molecular defect leading to a clinically significant disease found in medicine; the first, of course, was sickle cell anemia. In Figure 5–1 is shown the A-alpha, B-beta, and gamma chains and the amino acid sequence of fibrinopeptide A. Fibrinopeptide A consists of 16 amino acids; thrombin cleaves an arginine-glycine bond, between arginine 16 and glycine 17. For this cleavage to occur, thrombin must attach to a thrombin-binding site, three amino acids removed, at position 19. In Fibrinogen Detroit the amino acid serine has been substituted for arginine at position 19; thus, thrombin binding cannot occur and there is no cleavage of the arginine-glycine bond. Thus, fibrinopeptide A cannot be removed and fibrinogen cannot be converted into fibrin monomer.[27,116] These patients have a hemorrhagic diathesis, since they are unable to make fibrin monomer and a resultant fibrin clot.[114,115]

The differential diagnostic laboratory findings of quantitative and qualitative defects of fibrinogen are summarized in Table 5–10. Patient 1 is afibrinogenemic and demonstrates absence of fibrinogen by clotting time and by protein precipitation and absent to trace amounts of fibrinogen by immunologic techniques. Patient 2 is hypofibrinogenemic and thus has approximately 50% of normal fibrinogen levels. Patient 3 is homozygous dysfibrinogenemic; all of this patient's fibrinogen is dysfunctional. Clot-based assays will reveal absence of clottable fibrinogen; however, protein precipitation assays or immunologic assays reveal normal levels of fibrinogen. Patient 4 is heterozygous dysfibrinogenemic and 50% of the fibrinogen is functional. Protein precipitation assays and immunologic assays demonstrate normal fibrinogen levels.

Table 5–9 Dysfibrinogenemias*

City	Year	City	Year
Amsterdam	1971	Matika	1976
Baltimore	1964	Metz	1972
Bern	1978	Mexico	1978
Bethesda I	1970	Montreal I	1972
Bethesda II	1972	Montreal II	1975
Bethesda III	1979	Montreal III	1976
Bondy	1980	Munich	1980
Boulogne	1975	Nagoya	1979
Buenos Aires I	1975	Naifa	1981
Buenos Aires II	1978	Nancy	1971
Caracas I	1975	Naples I	1977
Caracas II	1977	Naples II	1979
Chapel Hill I	1975	Newark	1979
Chapel Hill II	1977	New Orleans	1977
Chapel Hill III	1983	New York I	1975
Charlottesville	1977	New York II	1979
Chicago	1981	Oklahoma	1970
Clermont-Ferrand	1975	Oslo I	1967
Cleveland I	1967	Oslo II	1977
Cleveland II	1973	Paris I	1963
Copenhagen	1979	Paris II	1968
Detroit	1968	Paris III	1974
Frankfurt I	1979	Paris IV	1978
Frankfurt II	1979	Parma	1958
Freiburg	1979	Petoskey	1980
Geneva	1972	Philadelphia	1974
Giessen I	1972	Pontoise	1978
Giessen II	1975	Puerto Rico	1979
Giessen III	1977	Quebec I	1978
Hannover	1977	Quebec II	1978
Harva	1973	Saint Louis	1968
Homburg	1979	Saint Mande I	1976
Houston	1978	Saint Mande II	1976
Iowa City	1973	Seattle	1977
Istanbul	1970	Tokyo	1975
Lille	1978	Troyes	1972
Logrono	1979	Valencia	1974
London	1978	Vancouver	1963
Los Angeles	1970	Versailles	1979
Louvain	1970	Vienna	1973
Manchester	1979	Wiesbaden I	1971
Manila	1974	Wiesbaden II	1973
Marburg	1977	Zurich I	1965
Marseille	1980	Zurich II	1970

* The dysfibrinogenemias are named after the city from which the patient originated.

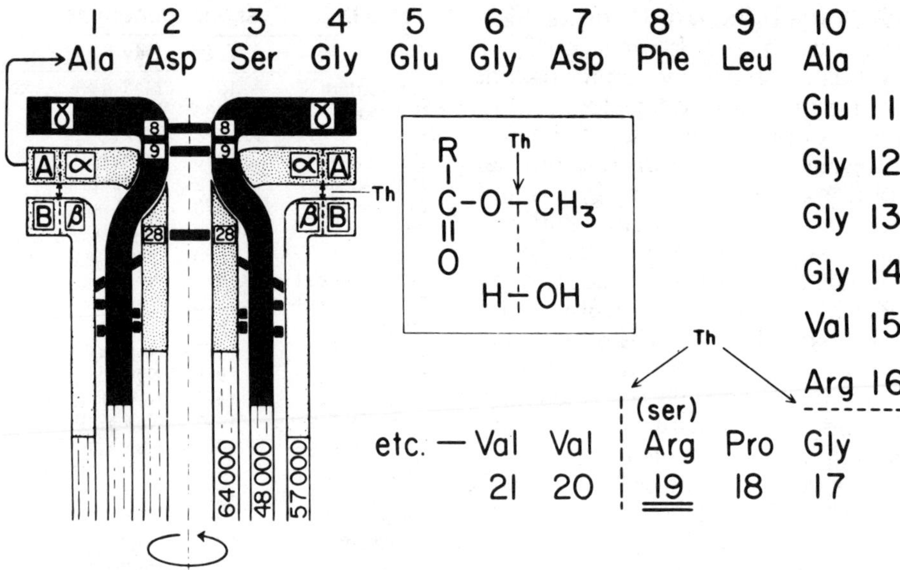

Fig. 5–1. Fibrinogen Detroit. (Courtesy of E.F. Mammen.)

Table 5–10   Differential Diagnosis of Quantitative and Qualitative Fibrinogen Defects

	Patient			
	1	2	3	4
Clotting tests	0%	50%	0%	50%
Precipitation tests	0%	50%	100%	100%
Immunologic tests	0%	50%	100%	100%
Diagnosis	Afibrinogenemia	Hypofibrinogenemia	Dysfibrinogenemia, type I	Dysfibrinogenemia, type II

The therapy of afibrinogenemia, hypofibrinogenemia, and dysfibrinogenemia is component replacement therapy when significant bleeding occurs or when extensive surgery, likely to compromise hemostasis severely, is planned. Whole blood or plasma can be used; however, the best therapeutic component for these patients is cryoprecipitate.[16,114] Bleeding is usually controlled easily by infusing enough cryoprecipitate, or other fibrinogen-containing components to render a clottable (functional) fibrinogen level of 75 to 100 mg/dL.

Factor II Defects

Congenital Factor II (prothrombin) defects are extremely rare, with less than 40 families being described.[12,60,61,141,153] Prothrombin defects are inherited as autosomal recessive and both quantitative and qualitative types have been described.[117] The quantitative defects are the hypoprothrombinemias and aprothrombinemias; patients are referred to as cross-reacting material negative (CRM−) if they have an absence of Factor II and they are referred to as cross-reacting material positive (CRM+) if they have a dysfunctional form of Factor II.

This terminology is commonly used to distinguish quantitative and qualitative (dysprothrombinemias) defects. The quantitative defects are more common than the qualitative defects.[117] Since prothrombin defects are inherited as autosomal recessive, four subtypes are noted. In the quantitative prothrombin defects, heterozygous patients will have approximately 50% of normal prothrombin levels and homozygous patients will have very low or absent prothrombin levels. Similarly, patients with qualitative defects may be heterozygous or homozygous; heterozygous patients will have both functional (50%) and dysfunctional (50%) prothrombin, whereas homozygous patients will have essentially no functionally normal prothrombin. As with fibrinogen defects, the quantitative versus qualitative prothrombin defects can be precisely characterized by doing both functional and immunologic assays.[20] In patients with quantitative defects results of functional and immunologic assays will be concordant; however, in the dysprothrombinemias, functional, clot-based, assays will show decreased or absent prothrombin levels, but immunologic assays will reveal normal levels (discordant results). In this regard, several of the dysprothrombinemias have also been associated with a moderate quantitative defect (dysprothrombinemias Habana,[170] Houston,[208] Metz,[158] Molise,[62] and Quick[156]). Precise mechanisms accounting for dysfunctional prothrombin, when known, have recently been reviewed (Table 5–11).

The clinical features of prothrombin defects are what one would expect with an isolated coagulation factor disorder;[16,117] homozygous patients can have severe spontaneous bleeding consisting of large hematomas and ecchymoses, and life-threatening mucosal membrane hemorrhage. Heterozygous patients can have

similar bleeding and may have severe bleeding with surgery or trauma. The clinical and laboratory features of congenital Factor II defects are summarized in Table 5–12. Once the diagnosis of a congenital Factor II defect is made, an immunologic assay of Factor II should be performed to differentiate between a qualitative or quantitative defect.[20]

Management of congenitally defective Factor II patients is required when clinically significant hemorrhage occurs or surgery is contemplated. Prothrombin complex concentrates are the the therapy of choice; however, plasma may also be used.[16] The level of functional Factor II should be raised to approximately 50% of normal to stop hemorrhage or to afford surgical hemostasis in presurgical patients. The half-life of Factor II is approximately 3 days; thus, infusions need not be frequent.

Factor V Defects

Factor V deficiency was first described by Owren[150] and is extremely rare, with approximately 30 cases being reported.[139,179,197] The defect is inherited as

Table 5–11 Dysprothrombinemias*

Name	Year	Reference
Barcelona	1971	93
Brussels	1974	94
Cardeza	1969	184
Denver	1980	142
Gainesville	1981	190
Habana	1983	170
Houston	1980	208
Madrid	1979	15
Metz	1979	158
Molise	1978	62
Padua	1974	63
Quick	1978	156
Salakta	1984	14
San Juan	1974	185

* Like the other qualitative coagulation protein defects, the dysprothrombinemias are named after the city from which the patient originated.

Table 5–12 Clinical and Laboratory Manifestations of Prothrombin (Factor II) Defects

Clinical
  Homozygous patients
    Severe spontaneous hemorrhage: many sites
    Severe bleeding with surgery or trauma
    Large hematomas and ecchymoses
    Severe mucosal membrane bleeding
  Heterozygous patients
    Rare spontaneous hemorrhage
    Mild mucosal membrane hemorrhage
    Potentially severe bleeding with surgery or trauma
Therapy
  Level of Factor II should be raised to 50%
  Prothrombin complex concentrates every 3 days or
    fresh frozen plasma every 3 days
Laboratory
  Prolonged prothrombin time
  Prolonged PTT
  Normal thrombin time
  Normal template bleeding time
  Normal platelet function
  Definitive diagnosis usually requires quantitative Factor II assay

an autosomal recessive trait. Factor V deficiency has also been referred to as parahemophilia.[150,179] There have been some cases of combined congenital Factor VIII and V deficiency and combined Factor V deficiency associated with von Willebrand's disease.[179,194,197] It has been suggested that combined Factor V and Factor VIII deficiency may actually represent congenital protein C inhibitor deficiency; however, this remains to be clarified.[59,129] Most patients thus far studied have been CRM− or have an absence of Factor V. Recently, however, several cases of dysfunctional Factor V have been described.[35] The clinical features include moderate to severe mucosal membrane bleeding, large hematomas, and large ecchymoses. Bleeding with surgery can be particularly severe and spontaneous intra-articular bleeding episodes have been described. Heterozygous patients rarely have spontaneous bleeding, but propensity to hemorrhage correlates very poorly with levels of circulating Factor V.[16,118]

The laboratory diagnosis is suggested by noting prolongation of the prothrombin time and the PTT. A specific diagnosis depends on a quantitative Factor V assay. There are no Factor V concentrates available and patients are managed with infusions of fresh frozen plasma at approximately 10 mL/kg total body weight or with cryoprecipitate.[16,118] The Factor V levels should be kept above 30% for hemostasis; since the half-life of Factor V is about 24 hours, infusions need only be daily. The clinical and laboratory characteristics of congenital Factor V deficiency are summarized in Table 5–13.

Factor VII Defects

Factor VII deficiency is inherited as an autosomal recessive[5] and is extremely rare, less than 150 cases having been reported.[119,159,178,195] Both the absent (CRM−) and dysfunctional (CRM+) forms of the disease exist;[43,69] the absence of Factor VII appears more common than dysfunctional Factor VII defects. The clinical features are similar to other congenital single factor defects and consist of

Table 5–13 Manifestations of Factor V Defects

Clinical characteristics
Autosomal recessive
About 30 cases reported
Severe mucosal membrane hemorrhage
Large subcutaneous hematomas
Spontaneous ecchymoses
Severe bleeding with surgery or trauma
Heterozygous patients usually asymptomatic
Laboratory characteristics
Prolonged prothrombin time
Prolonged PTT
Normal thrombin time
Normal template bleeding time
Normal platelet function
Definitive diagnosis requires a quantitative Factor V assay
Therapy
Fresh frozen plasma at 10.0 mL/kg daily (keep patient above 30% activity)

intra-articular bleeding with hemarthroses, more common in male patients, severe epistaxis, and other mucosal membrane-type bleeding, including gastrointestinal, genitourinary, and intrapulmonary hemorrhage.[16,119] Patients may have significant life-threatening hemorrhage with surgery or trauma. Umbilical stump bleeding is also common. Spontaneous bleeding rarely occurs in heterozygous patients unless trauma or surgery is experienced. The clinical and laboratory features of Factor VII deficiency are summarized in Table 5–14. The dysfunctional Factor VII defects have been reported by several investigators.[31,42,43–69]

The laboratory diagnosis depends on noting a prolonged prothrombin time and a normal PTT. When this combination of abnormalities is noted, a Factor VII assay should be performed. The Stypven time (prothrombin time with Russell's viper venom) is normal.[16,119] The management of homozygous patients, when clinically significant hemorrhage occurs, is with prothrombin complex concentrates or plasma. It should be noted that several of the commercially available prothrombin complex concentrates contain minimal or no Factor VII. Thus, if treating a patient with Factor VII deficiency, the characteristics of available concentrates must be known. The Factor VII levels should be maintained at 30% of normal; infusions

Table 5–14 Manifestations
of Factor VII Defects

Clinical manifestations
  Autosomal recessive trait
  About 150 cases reported
  Absence form (CRM⁻) and dysfunctional form (CRM⁺)
    exist
  Intra-articular bleeding
  Severe epistaxis
  Umbilical stump bleeding occasionally
  Mucosal membrane hemorrhage common
  Gastrointestinal
  Genitourinary
  Intrapulmonary
  Profuse bleeding with surgery or trauma
  Heterozygous patients rarely bleed spontaneously
  Heterozygous patients bleed with surgery or trauma
Laboratory manifestations
  Prolonged prothrombin time
  Normal PTT
  Normal Russell's vipor venom time
  Normal template bleeding time
  Normal platelet function (aggregation)
  Definitive diagnosis requires quantitative Factor VII
    assay
Therapy
  Raise Factor VII to >30%
  Fresh frozen plasma
  Some prothrombin complex concentrates

need to be frequent in bleeding or surgical patients, since the plasma half-life of Factor VII is about 4 to 6 hours.

Factor VIII:C Defects

The hemophilias are more common congenital coagulation defects than those previously discussed. The incidence of hemophilia is about 1 in 10,000 male births, although regional differences are observed.[47,56,105] Before discussing hemophilias and von Willebrand's disease, the properties and nomenclature of the Factor VIII macromolecular complex will be summarized to avoid confusion and lend uniformity to this discussion (Fig. 5–2). The Factor VIII macromolecular complex is comprised of three discrete portions and two discrete biologic activities.[77,84,85] The low molecular weight portion is responsible for procoagulant activity in the conversion of Factor X to Factor Xa (Chapter 1); this portion is commonly designated Factor VIII:C (for Factor VIII coagulant activity). It is Factor VIII:C

that is measured in the PTT test system and the traditional PTT-derived Factor VIII coagulant assay. With a great deal of difficulty, homologous nonprecipitating antibodies can be harvested against highly purified Factor VIII:C; these antibodies react with a moiety referred to as Factor VIII:CAg.[86] In general, Factor VIII:C and Factor VIII:CAg levels parallel each other in normal persons and in most, but not all, hemophilic patients.[44] A second discrete identifiable portion of the Factor VIII macromolecular complex is a high molecular weight portion, referred to as Factor VIII:R.[85,86] Heterologous precipitated antibodies, usually goat or rabbit, can easily be harvested against this portion. The moiety with which these heterologous antibodies react is referred to as Factor VIII:RAg (Factor VIII related antigen).[85,86,120] The third discrete portion of the Factor VIII macromolecular complex is an integral portion of Factor VIII:R that contains the biologic activity responsible for normal platelet function, normal vascular function, and normal template bleeding times. This biologic activity (function) is referred to as von Willebrand factor or Factor VIII:vW. Factor VIII:vW is synonymous with ristocetin cofactor activity (Factor VIII:RCo); however, the term "Factor VIII:vW" will be used throughout this discussion.

Hemophilia A, referred to as classic hemophilia, is inherited as a sex-linked recessive and is a deficiency or defect of Factor VIII:C.[16,120] Approximately 90% of patients have a deficiency of both Factor VIII:C and Factor VIII:CAg and are, thus, truly deficient CMR−, or Factor VIII:C−. The remaining patients, approximately 10%, are missing Factor VIII:C activity but have normal Factor VIII:CAg; thus, these patients have dysfunctional Factor VIII:C.[44] These patients are referred to as CRM+, or Factor VIII:C+ patients. A positive family history is elicited in 70% of hemophilic patients, and in approximately 30% of patients the gene appears to arise spontaneously, representing a high mutation rate.[16] Factor VIII:C− and Factor VIII:C+ patients have similar clinical courses. Hemophilic patients typically experience hemorrhage, primarily manifested as deep tissue bleeding.[16,120,202] The types of bleeding are usually deep intramuscular bleeding, intra-articular bleeding with resultant joint fibrosis, referred to as hemarthrosis, and potentially fatal intracranial bleeding.[16,75,120,192,202] Patients may also commonly have hematuria.[189] Particularly severe and potentially crippling bleeding can occur when hemorrhage into one of the closed muscular compartments of the extremities occur; this can result in anterior or posterior compartmental compression syndrome leading to vascular or peripheral nerve compromise or subsequent fibrotic tissue formation.[16,120,177,202]

The severity of bleeding in hemophilia A closely parallels the level of circulating Factor VIII:C. Severe bleeders are those who have 0 to 5% of circulating Factor VIII:C or who have circulating inhibitors to Factor VIII:C.[16,120,202] These patients have severe spontaneous deep tissue bleeding episodes of the type earlier described. They are usually diagnosed in early childhood, usually at circumcision, or at the initiation of crawling when patients begin to demonstrate spontaneous bleeding into the knees and elbow joints.[16] Moderate hemophilia occurs in those who have 5 to 10% circulating Factor VIII:C levels. These patients have minimal to moderate numbers of spontaneous bleeding episodes, but bleed profusely when subjected to surgery or trauma. Mild hemophilia occurs in those who have 10 to 40% circulating Factor VIII:C. Patients with mild hemophilia rarely have spontaneous bleeding, but may have severe and life-threatening bleeding with surgical or traumatic stress. It is important to realize that severe hemophilia is usually clinically obvious and, in general, these patients are identified early in life. However, mild hemophilia may not be identified until surgical or traumatic bleeding occurs. For this reason, a sensitive activated PTT and reliable associated reagents are of paramount importance when using this test as a presurgical screening procedure or when using it to evaluate a bleeding patient for potential hemophilia. Numerous recently published studies have addressed the sensitivity and reliability of the activated PTT and associated reagents; for specific information and recommendations the reader is referred to these references.[50,71–73,79]

The differential PTT was a popular test in the past, and sometimes used to aid in a diagnosis of hemophilia; however, with the general availability of good activated PTT reagents and Factor VIII:C quantitative assay reagents, the early identity of severe and moderate hemophilia, and the relative insensitivity of the differential PTT to mild deficiencies, this test is seldom, if ever, indicated.[16,18,19] The key to a rapid diagnosis of hemophilia A is to note a prolonged PTT with a normal prothrombin time in a (usually) male child who has a positive bleeding history or a positive family history; in this setting, the chances are approximately 85% the child will have Factor VIII:C deficiency and, thus, logic would dictate a quantitative Factor VIII assay to be performed. If this were negative in the aforementioned setting, a Factor IX:C and subsequently, if warranted, a Factor XI:C assay would be in order. The clinical features of hemophilia A are summarized in Table 5–15.

Approximately 10% of hemophilia A patients develop anti-VIII:C antibodies.

Table 5–15 Clinical Manifestations of Hemophilia A

Characteristic clinical findings
Sex-linked recessive
Absence of Factor VIII:C in 90% (CRM⁻)
Presence of dysfunctional Factor VIII:C (CRM⁺) in 10%
Deep tissue hemorrhage
Intra-articular hemorrhage
Intracranial hemorrhage
Intramuscular hemorrhage
Compartmental compression syndromes
Clinical course parallels Factor VIII:C level
Severe (0 to 5%): many spontaneous bleeds
Moderate (5 to 10%): occasional spontaneous bleeds
Mild (10 to 40%): rare spontaneous bleeds
Severe bleeding with surgery or trauma
Anti-VIII:C antibody in 10% (usually IgG-kappa)
Hemophilia A accounts for 85% of hemophilic patients
Most patients are male (sex-linked recessive)
Characteristic laboratory findings
Prolonged PTT
Normal prothrombin time
Normal template bleeding time
Platelet dysfunction (aggregation) may be seen in very severe patients
Differential PTT of little or no value

These are most commonly IgG_4 kappa.[16,120,152,209] The development of antibodies was initially thought to be related to the source of Factor VIII, with the commercially available Factor VIII concentrates originally being incriminated. However, a large multicenter trial suggests no correlation between the development of antibodies and the source of Factor VIII; the incidence of antibody formation in this study was equal with concentrates, cryoprecipitate, or plasma.[24] The anti-VIII:C antibody is long-acting and may require a long incubation in the PTT system for demonstration. Thus, it is wise to incubate the activated PTT system for 15, 30, 45, and 60 minutes in order to demonstrate the presence or absence of Factor VIII:C antibody. Reliable screening and assay procedures have been published and reagents are readily available.[95,148,209] Factor VIII:C antibodies are irreversible; once the antibody combines with Factor VIII:C, biologic activity is lost, unlike other types of inhibitors that will be discussed in subsequent chapters.

The therapy of hemophilia A is dependent on the site and severity of hemorrhage. Mild bleeding can often be controlled with cold compresses, topical thrombin when necessary, and other supportive measures.[16] Serious bleeding episodes, including intra-articular, should be treated with Factor VIII concentrates.[1,4,16,55,120,207] Factor VIII concentrates are more commonly used and are preferred over cryoprecipitate. Cryoprecipitate may have unreliable amounts of Factor VIII:C, and a large amount of fibrinogen, potentially leading to renal damage, is infused and, in addition, the response to Factor VIII concentrate is quite predictable. In general, the infusion of 25 U/kg will render a 50% increase in activity in a hemophilia A patient; a level of 50% normal activity should readily achieve hemostasis in most instances.[4,16,120] A more precise formula for calculating a dose of Factor VIII concentrate is given in Table 5–16. This method is prefered for nonemergent replacement, for example, preoperatively. The biologic half-life of infused Factor VIII:C is between 8 and 12 hours and infusions, especially in surgical patients, patients undergoing physical

Table 5–16 Factor VIII:C Concentrate Dose Calculation in Hemophilia A

Units needed = (desired level − initial level) = units needed

Total units needed = units needed × 0.6 × body weight (kg)

and

$$\text{Milliliters of concentrate needed} = \frac{\text{Total units needed}}{\text{Units/mL in concentrate}}$$

therapy, or any patient requiring several days or weeks of constant therapy, needs to be adjusted appropriately, based on the formula given and frequent quantitative Factor VIII:C assays.

For some orthopedic, cardiac, and neurosurgical procedures, the Factor VIII:C level should be maintained from 80 to 100% of normal.[4,16,32,55,58,120] When the patient does not demonstrate the expected postinfusion rise in Factor VIII:C activity, an inhibitor should be strongly suspected and appropriate testing done. When Factor VIII inhibitors are found, they should be quantitatively titered. Low titer inhibitors can be overcome and treated with Factor VIII concentrates.[98,183] In this instance, the inhibitor is quantitated and an appropriate amount of Factor VIII concentrate is given to exactly neutralize the inhibitor; following this, it can be assumed the patient is at 0% Factor VIII:C and then an appropriate amount of concentrate is infused using the formula in Table 5–18 to obtain the desired Factor VIII:C level. High titers of antibodies are treated with "activated" prothrombin complex concentrates; the response is generally, but not consistently, good.[55,112,152] Anti-VIII antibodies in hemophilic patients are generally not responsive to immunosuppressive therapy.[152]

Both Factor VIII and Factor IX concentrates are associated with a risk of hepatitis; the risk is greater with Factor IX concentrates. Many patients never develop clinical manifestations, but demonstrate elevated transaminases and seropositivity. In the past, patients with blood groups A, B, and AB developed allergic reactions to concentrates, due to the presence of anti-A or anti-B agglutinins; however, this problem has been almost entirely eradicated by mixing appropriate proportions of A, B, and AB donor pools.[24,55,180] An additional problem of Factor IX concentrates is that of thrombogenicity; this will be discussed in the section dealing with hemophilia B. Some hemophiliac patients are fortunate enough to be on prophylactic "home therapy." In these individuals various dosage schedules have been divised whereby the patient is infused with enough Factor VIII concentrate to maintain Factor VIII:C at a minimal or "nonbleeding" level. This type of therapy is, however, extremely expensive and may be associated with frequent complications.

Methods of detecting carriers of hemophilia A and B have recently been described and approach 90% accuracy.[101,162,163] By measuring Factor VIII:RAg in conjunction with Factor VIII:C, the carrier state can potentially be detected. The ratio of Factor VIII:RAg to Factor VIII:C in carriers should be 2:1. Thus, the sampling of fetal blood in utero can be accomplished in high-risk carriers.

Factor IX Defects

Factor IX deficiency is also known as hemophilia B, Christmas disease, or plasma thromboplastin component deficiency.[3,16,25,121] This disorder, like hemophilia A, is also inherited as a sex-linked recessive.[16,121,162] The clinical features are identical to those of hemophilia A and consist of deep tissue bleeding, including intra-articular bleeding with hemarthroses, intramuscular bleeding, intracranial bleeding, and potentially severe mucosal membrane hemorrhages.[16,55,121] The disease can be clinically divided into patients who are mild, moderate, or severe.[16,121] Correlation between Factor IX:C and severity of the disease is the same as that noted with Factor VIII deficiency. Seventy to 90% of patients are truly deficient in Factor IX:C and are CRM−. However, 10 to 30% of patients are CRM+.[45,121,146,167] As an additional variable, some CRM+ patients have prolonged ox brain thromboplastin times and others are normal; thus, three variants of hemophilia B exist.[33,51,80,96,121] Another

variant is hemophilia B Leyden, in which the Factor IX:C levels increase with age.[203] Additional named variants are Factor IX Chapel Hill and Factor IX Alabama.[36,37] The clinical features of hemophilia B are summarized in Table 5–17, and the variants are summarized in Table 5–18. Approximately 60 to 70% of patients will have a positive family history. Patients will characteristically have a prolonged activated PTT and a normal prothrombin time.[16,121] The diagnosis is usually made when these conditions are present and the Factor VIII:C assay is normal. In this circumstance the next logical assay to be performed would be a Factor IX assay. Management, like that for hemophilia A, depends on the clinical significance of hemorrhage. Mild bleeding is best controlled by local supportive measures, including cold compresses and, when appropriate, topical thrombin.[16] Severe bleeding or preparation for surgery is managed with Factor IX containing prothrombin complex concentrates.[16,23,30,121,191,199]

The hazards of these concentrates are hepatitis and thrombogenicity, including the initiation of DIC-type syndromes in recipients.[16,26,121,164,210] Potential for

Table 5–17 Clinical Manifestations of Hemophilia B (Factor IX Deficiency)

Characteristic Clinical Findings
Sex-linked recessive
Absence of Factor IX in 70 to 90% (CRM⁻)
Presence of dysfunctional Factor IX in 10 to 30% (CRM⁺)
Deep tissue hemorrhage
Intra-articular hemorrhage
Intracranial hemorrhage
Intramuscular hemorrhage
Compartmental compression syndromes
Clinical course parallels Factor IX level
Severe (0 to 5%): many spontaneous bleeds
Moderate (5 to 10%): occasional spontaneous bleeds
Mild (10 to 40%): rare spontaneous bleeds
Severe bleeding with surgery or trauma
Anti-IX antibody in 7 to 10% (usually IgG-lambda)
Hemophilia B accounts for 10 to 15% of hemophilic patients
Most patients are male (sex-linked recessive)
Characteristic laboratory findings
Prolonged PTT
Normal prothrombin time
Normal template bleeding time
Platelet dysfunction (aggregation) may be seen in very severe patients
Differential PTT of little or no value

Table 5–18 Variants of Hemophilia B*

Factor IX Protein	Ox Brain Thromboplastin Time	Term Used
CRM$^+$	Normal	Hemophilia B$^+$
CRM$^+$	Long	Hemophilia B^+_M
CRM$^-$	Normal	Hemophilia B$^-$
CRM$^-$	Long	Hemophilia B^-_M

* Others: Factor IX Chapel Hill (CRM$^+$); Factor IX Alabama (CRM$^+$); Hemophilia B Leyden (IX levels increase with age)

thrombogenicity is carefully monitored in each lot of concentrate by use of the nonactivated PTT. A lot that causes shortening of the nonactivated PTT is considered potentially thrombogenic.[210] An additional stability test to ensure against the generation of thrombin or Factor X_a is to add 0.1 mL of concentrate to 1 mL of citrated plasma drawn from the patient and observing the mixture for clot formation for a full 5 minutes before infusion of the material.[16] Approximately 5 to 7% of patients with Factor IX deficiency develop anti-IX antibodies.[16,121] The only therapy for this complication is to neutralize the antibody with prothrombin complex concentrate, followed by raising the Factor IX:C level to the desired range to achieve hemostasis. Like Factor VIII antibodies, Factor IX antibodies in hemophilia B pa-

Table 5–19 Laboratory Evaluation of Hemophilias

Older Methods (Nonautomated)	Newer Methods (Automated)
Prothrombin time	External pathway generated thrombin* (Prothrombin equivalent)
PTT	Internal pathway Generated thrombin (PTT equivalent)
PTT-derived assays	
Factor VIII:C	Factor VIII:C*†
Factor IX:C	Factor IX:C*†
Factor XI:C	Factor XI:C*†
Differential PTT	Factor VIII:RAg†
Factor VIII inhibitors	Factor VIII inhibitors*†

* Synthetic substrates.
† Immunologic or ELISA assays.

tients also respond poorly to immunosuppressive therapy.[152] New and old laboratory modalities for evaluating hemophilias are summarized in Table 5–19.

Factor X Defects

Factor X deficiency is an extremely rare disorder, with some 50 families being described.[16,81,122,143,196] The disorder is inherited as an autosomal recessive; homozygous patients have very low Factor X:C levels and heteroxygotes have about 50% of normal Factor X:C activity. Both the absent form, Factor X:C$-$ and dysfunctional form, Factor X:C$+$ are known to exist,[46,122] and the clinical features are similar for both forms.[16,122,162] Factor X Friuli was the first described dysfunctional form.[67] Factor X deficient patients are more prone to have severe mucosal membrane and skin hemorrhages and fewer deep tissue hemorrhages than those seen in the hemophilias.[122] Mucosal membrane hemorrhages can be from any site and is often quite severe in homoxzygous patients. Umbilical stump bleeding is a particularly common early manifestation of Factor X deficiency.[70]

The activated PTT and prothrombin time are markedly prolonged in homozygous patients and mildly prolonged or, at times, normal in heterozygous patients.[16,122] In addition, since Russell's viper venom will activate Factor X in vitro, this test is also prolonged.[11,16,122] The Russell's viper venom time, however, may be normal in some Factor X:C$+$ patients.[67] The aforementioned findings should prompt a quantitative Factor X:C assay for definitive diagnosis. Since hemostasis can be achieved with 15 to 20% levels of Factor X, management can often be achieved with plasma infusions.[16,122] Serious bleeding, or the achieving of higher levels for surgery, can be accomplished with prothrombin complex concentrates when the desired potential clinical benefits outweigh the potential hazards of hepatitis or thrombosis.[16,200] The clinical and laboratory findings of Factor X defects are given in Table 5-20.

Table 5–20 Manifestations
of Factor X Defects

Clinical characteristics
Autosomal recessive trait
Absence form (CRM−) and dysfunctional form
(CRM+) exist
Factor X Friuli was first dysfunctional form
Severe mucosal membrane hemorrhages are typical
Umbilical stump bleeding is common
Severe bleeding occurs with surgery or trauma
Laboratory characteristics
Prolonged PTT
Prolonged prothrombin time
Russell's vipor venom time, usually prolonged
Normal template bleeding time
Normal platelet function (aggregation)
Therapy
Raise Factor X level to 15 to 20%
Fresh frozen plasma
Prothrombin complex concentrates

Factor XI Defects

Factor XI deficiency is also referred to as plasma thromboplastin antecedent deficiency, Rosenthal's disease, or hemophilia C; this latter term should probably be abandoned.[16,123] The disorder was first described by Rosenthal and co-workers[168] in 1953.[168] Factor XI deficiency was initially thought to be inherited as an autosomal dominant; however, more recent and thorough studies have revealed it to be inherited as an incomplete autosomal recessive trait.[123,160,168] Homozygous patients have approximately 1% Factor X, whereas heteroxygotes have approximately 50% of normal Factor X levels.[16,123,160] A high incidence occurs in Jewish patients of Russian descent (Ashkenazic Jews), and in this population homozygotes comprise approximately 0.2% of the population and heterozygotes may comprise as much as 11% of this population.[16,123,181,182] Many other races are also affected. All patients thus far studied appear to have a true impaired Factor XI synthesis defect, since no dysfunctional forms have yet been described.

The clinical features are amazingly variable and quite confusing.[16,40,123] Homozygous patients have spontaneous bleeding from mucosal membranes that may be quite serious; however, deep tissue bleeding, including intra-articular bleeding, is extremely rare. Up to 50% of homozygous patients may experience serious and life-threatening bleeding with surgery or trauma.[16,40,123,169] Bleeding from the oral mucosal or the genitourinary tract is a particular problem and has been ascribed to the enhanced fibrinolytic activity that may occur in these areas.[134,187] Most heterozygous patients have no bleeding; however, a few patients may have spontaneous mucosal membrane hemorrhages, especially epistaxis, and some will have minor bleeding with surgery or trauma.[16] Homozygous patients may have no bleeding, minimal bleeding, or profuse bleeding.[16,40,123] In addition, the severity of bleeding does not correlate well with levels of circulating Factor XI.[16] Patients may have a marked change in their clinical course; a nonbleeding patient or a patient with minimal bleeding, may, in the course of the disease, become a spontaneous or severe bleeder. Alternatively, a frequently bleeding patient may become a nonbleeding patient. These changes in the clinical course often have no relationship to changes in circulating Factor XI. Clinical and laboratory manifestations of Factor XI deficiency are summarized in Table 5–21.

From the laboratory diagnostic standpoint, some patients will present with a negative bleeding history and some will present with an appropriate positive bleeding history. Patients with Factor XI deficiency will demonstrate a prolonged activated PTT and normal prothrombin time.[16,107,123] Unless the patient is a female, in which case a Factor XI level should be considered immediately, the diagnosis is usually made by noting a patient with a typical personal or family history or significant bleeding and a prolonged PTT, a normal prothrombin time, a normal Factor VIII and Factor IX level, and a subsequent decreased level of Factor XI.[16,18,19,123] Management is primarily through the use of fresh frozen plasma infused at 10 mL/kg/day for significant bleeding episodes or in preparation for surgery.[16,55,123] The Factor XI levels should be raised to 30 to 40% of normal to achieve hemostasis. Factor IX concen-

Table 5–21 Clinical and Laboratory Manifestations of Factor XI Defects

Clinical
  Incomplete autosomal recessive trait
  Highly variable clinical course
  Most common in Ashkenazic Jews
  Many other races also affected
  Spontaneous mucosal membrane hemorrhage common
  Spontaneous deep tissue hemorrhage rare
  Severe bleeding may occur with surgery or trauma
  Little correlation between bleeding and Factor XI level
  An individual clinical course may change dramatically
  Heterozygous patients rarely bleed
  Oral mucosal bleeding unusually common
  Genitourinary bleeding unusually common
Laboratory
  Bleeding history may be positive or negative
  Prolonged PTT
  Normal prothrombin time
  Normal template bleeding time
  Normal platelet function (aggregation)
  Definitive diagnosis requires Factor XI assay
  Factor XI assay should be first assay done in a female child with prolonged partial thromboplastin time and normal prothrombin time

trates have been used to control clinically significant hemorrhage in rare instances; some preparations of prothrombin complex concentrates contain large amounts of Factor XI.[21] However, this is not true for all commercially available concentrates, and if a patient does not respond to infusions of fresh frozen plasma and the use of prothrombin complex concentrates is considered, the concentrate must be assayed to know if Factor XI is present in significant amounts.[16,21]

Factor XII Defects

Congenital Factor XII deficiency was first described by Ratnoff and Colopy[165] in 1955; since then several hundred cases have been reported.[16,55,162] The name of the first patient studied by Ratnoff and Colopy was John Hageman, and the disorder is thus also commonly referred to as Hageman trait.[165] In most instances, the disorder is inherited as an autosomal recessive, but instances of autosomal dominant inheritance have also been described.[162] Homozygous patients of the autosomal

recessive variety have very low levels of Factor XII; heterozygotes can be quite variable, but tend to have around 50% of normal Factor XII activity. The disorder is known to exist in the absence form, Factor XII:C− and the dysfunctional form, Factor XII:C+ (CRM+).[171] However, the absent form appears much more common than the dysfunctional variety.

In many instances, Factor XII deficiency is found by chance when a screening PTT is performed and noted to be markedly prolonged, often in a routine presurgical patient.[16,18,19] Since this is the manner in which many patients present, it is assumed and classically incorrectly taught that patients with Factor XII deficiency have no bleeding diathesis. In fact, some patients do have a mild bleeding tendency and life-threatening bleeding can occur, although rarely.[49,165] Of particular interest, patients with Factor XII deficiency have defective surface-mediated activation of fibrinolysis and many patients with Factor XII deficiency have died of thrombosis or thromboembolism.[10,68,78,133] John Hageman, a railroad worker, died from a pulmonary embolus following hip fracture.[166] Thus, it appears that an inordinantly large number of patients with Factor XII deficiency have died of a myocardial infarction (thrombus?) or pulmonary embolus. In addition, patients may have defects in neutrophil or macrophage chemotaxis.[38]

As previously mentioned, the diagnosis is most commonly made by noting a markedly prolonged PTT and normal prothrombin time and thrombin time in an asymptomatic patient or a patient with a mild hemorrhagic diathesis.[16,165] A definitive diagnosis requires specific quantitative Factor XII assay by clot-based or synthetic substrate techniques; both assays are readily available.[20] An additional laboratory finding is prolongation of the euglobulin clot lysis time, although fibrinolytic system components are normal.[124] Since hemorrhage is rare, replacement therapy is generally not required. In those exceptionally rare patients with significant hemorrhage, replacement should be with fresh frozen plasma. It is not known if prophylactic fibrinolytic enhancement therapy is indicated in Factor XII deficient patients; perhaps more experience will eventually dictate some type of prophylaxis for thrombosis, such as stanozolol enhancement of fibrinolysis. Certainly, when thrombosis or thromboembolism occurs, it should be treated appropriately. Findings of Factor XII defects are given in Table 5–22.

Prekallikrein Defects

Prekallikrein deficiency was first noted by Hathaway in 1965, when children from a consanguineous marriage were involved in a fire. After recuperation from burns, tonsillectomies were contemplated and the preoperative PTT was markedly prolonged in 4 of 14 children. The defect was noted to correct with Factor XII deficient plasma and the new disorder was referred to as Fletcher trait, after the surname of the family.[74] The mode of inheritance is unclear or variable; some have described autosomal recessive characteristics, whereas others have noted autosomal dominance.[124] Although the majority of patients thus far studied have a true deficiency (CRM−), several instances of a dysfunctional form (CRM+) have also been described.[172] Patients with prekallikrein

deficiency have no bleeding tendency, although these patients, like those with Factor XII deficiency, also have defective activation of the fibrinolytic system.[53,124] The diagnosis is suggested when noting a markedly prolonged PTT and a normal prothrombin time and thrombin time in an asymptomatic individual, usually during presurgical screening procedures.[16,18,19,124] The diagnosis is made by performing a specific prekallikrein assay by clot-based or synthetic substrate-based techniques; both types of assays are readily available. A characteristic of prekallikrein deficiency is the noting of correction of the PTT when incubating the PTT system for 10 minutes with kaolin, Celite, silica, or ellagic acid.[52,74] This test should not be used for a diagnosis, since the same phenomena can be noted with Passovoy deficiency; an erroneous interpretation could lead to a missed diagnosis of Passovoy defect and a potential bleeding problem. The features of prekallikrein deficiency are summarized in Table 5–23.

Kininogen Defects

High molecular weight kininogen deficiency is known by a variety of surnames, including the most common, Fitzgerald trait.[173] However, the defect is also known as Williams trait,[39] Flaujeac trait,[103] Fujiwara trait,[149] and Reid trait.[113] The disorder is inherited as an autosomal recessive. Pa-

---

Table 5–22 Manifestations of Factor XII Defects (Hageman Factor)

Clinical characteristics
  Autosomal recessive trait: most patients
  Autosomal dominance: few patients
  Absence form (CRM−) and dysfunctional form
    (CRM+) exist
  Defect is often found by chance via prolonged PTT
  Many have a mild bleeding tendency
  Fatal bleeding has occurred
  Most have defective surface-mediated fibrinolytic
    activation
  High incidence of fatal thrombosis or
    thromboembolism
Laboratory characteristics
  Markedly prolonged PTT
  Normal prothrombin time
  Normal template bleeding time
  Normal platelet function (aggregation)
  Definitive diagnosis requires Factor XII assay
Therapy
  Plasma replacement for hemorrhage
  Anticoagulants for thrombosis or thromboembolus

Table 5–23 Manifestations of Prekallikrein Deficiency (Fletcher Factor)

Clinical characteristics
  Autosomal recessive and dominant cases described
  Majority have absence of protein (CRM−)
  Some have dysfunctional protein (CRM+)
  No hemorrhagic tendency yet described
  Defective surface-mediated activation of fibrinolysis
Laboratory characteristics
  Prolonged PTT*
  Normal prothrombin time
  Normal template bleeding time
  Normal platelet function (aggregation)
  Definitive diagnosis requires prekallikrein assay

---

* Correction of PTT with long incubation (10 minutes) is characteristic, but should not be used as a diagnostic tool; the same findings may be seen in Passovoy defect.

tients do not have a hemorrhagic tendency, but do have abnormal surface-mediated activation of fibrinolysis, as noted by a long euglobulin clot lysis time.[124] All patients thus far studied have a true deficiency of high molecular weight kininogen. Fitzgerald and Rein traits represent a deficiency of high molecular weight kininogen; however, Williams, Fleaujac, and Fujiwara traits represent a deficiency of both high and low molecular weight kininogen. These last three forms of deficiency are also deficient in prekallikrein.

The diagnosis is suspected by noting a prolonged PTT and a normal prothrombin time and thrombin time, noncorrecting of the PTT with prolonged incubation in an asymptomatic individual usually during a routine preoperative screening work-up.[16,18,19,124] A definitive diagnosis is made by immunologic assay for high molecular weight kininogen.[82,97,124] Individuals are asymptomatic but have abnormal surface-activated fibrinolysis as well as defective neutrophil or macrophage chemotaxis. In one individual abnormal inflammatory responses were noted.[173] The features of high molecular weight kininogen deficiency are summarized in Table 5–24.

Passovoy Defect

Passovoy deficiency was first described by Hougie and associates[82] in 1975. The disorder appears to be inherited as an autosomal dominant. The molecular characteristics are thus far unknown. Patients typically have a moderate bleeding tendency characterized by mucosal membrane bleeding, including epistaxis, easy and spontaneous bruising, and excessive menstrual flow.[82,83,92] Intra-articular bleeds are uncommon. Severe bleeding may occur with trauma or surgery. The PTT is moderately prolonged and the prothrombin time and thrombin time are normal.[82,83,92] The PTT will shorten with incubation, and thus the disorder can be erroneously confused with prekallikrein deficiency.[83] Plasma infusions are used for traumatic or surgical hemorrhage. The features of Passovoy defect are noted in Table 5–25.

Antiplasmin Defects

Alpha-2-antiplasmin deficiency is inherited as an autosomal recessive; alpha-2-antiplasmin levels are less than 10% in homozygous patients and about 50% in heterozygous individuals.[125] Thus far no dysfunctional forms have been noted and

Table 5–24 Manifestations of High Molecular Weight Kininogen Deficiency

Clinical characteristics
Autosomal recessive trait
No hemorrhagic tendency
Abnormal surface-mediated activation of fibrinolysis
Variety of synonyms
Fitzgerald trait: HMW* kininogen only
Reid trait: HMW kininogen only
Williams trait: HMW plus LMW* kininogen
Flaujeac trait: HMW plus LMW kininogen
Fujiwara trait: HMW plus LMW kininogen
Laboratory characteristics
Prolonged PTT
Normal prothrombin time
Normal template bleeding time
Normal platelet function (aggregation)
Definitive diagnosis requires immunologic assay for high molecular weight kininogen

* HMW: high molecular weight; LMW: low molecular weight.

Table 5–25 Manifestations of Passovoy Defect

Clinical characteristics
Autosomal dominant trait
Moderate hemorrhagic tendency
Mucosal membrane bleeding is typical
Easy and spontaneous bruising is typical
Severe hemorrhage occurs with surgery or trauma
Laboratory characteristics
Prolonged PTT
Normal prothrombin time
Normal thrombin time
Normal template bleeding time
Normal platelet function (aggregation)
PTT will shorten with long incubation times (10 minutes) and this disorder can be mistaken for prekallikrein deficiency
Therapy
Fresh frozen plasma for hemorrhage or preparation for surgery

all patients studied to date have parallel levels of biologic and immunologic alpha-2-antiplasmin.[8,9,102,138,212] Bleeding can be severe in homozygous patients and typically consists of mucosal membrane bleeding, with hematuria predominating, large subcutaneous hematomas, spontaneous bruising, and severe bleeding with trauma.[8,9,102,130,138,212] Intra-articular bleeding may also occur. Laboratory tests are generally normal except for a short euglobulin lysis time and low to nonexistent levels of alpha-2-antiplasmin by biologic or synthetic substrate assay.[8,102,125,212] Occasionally, elevated fibrin(ogen) degradation products may be seen. The therapy of choice is epsilon-aminocaproic acid given as 10 mg/kg three times daily, orally or intravenously.[9,125] The findings of antiplasmin deficiency are given in Table 5–26.

Factor XIII Defects

Congenital Factor XIII deficiency has been described in more than 100 families and is inherited as an autosomal recessive, although originally thought to be sex-linked.[100,109,126] A high incidence of consanguinity has been noted.[100,109] Factor XIII is a dimeric protein consisting of an alpha and beta chain.[109] Homozygous patients are missing the alpha chain, which contains the site at which thrombin activates Factor XIII. Homozygotes may also have decreased levels of the beta chain, but patients have been described who have absent or normal beta chains. Heterozygotes generally have decreased alpha and beta chains. Thus, if immunologic techniques are used to assay Factor XIII, anti-alpha chain and anti-beta chain antibodies must be used; the techniques are available.[88,90,109,126]

The clinical manifestations of Factor XIII deficiency are characteristic and the bleeding diathesis only occurs in homozygotes because only 10% of normal Factor XIII levels are necessary for normal fibrin monomer cross-linking to occur.[100,109,126] Ninety percent of patients demonstrate delayed umbilical stump bleeding at childbirth, and this finding should immediately prompt a strong suspicion of Factor XIII deficiency, or less likely, afibrinogenemia or homozygous dysfibrinogenemia, since only in these disorders is umbilical stump bleeding characteristic.[16,100,109,126] Patients with homozygous Factor XIII deficiency also characteristically have significant deep tissue hemorrhages, especially into muscle and muscle compartments; these most commonly develop several days after minor trauma but may occur spontaneously.[100] Many patients develop subsequent destruction of bone and pseudotumors; these are especially prominant in the thigh and gluteal areas.[100] The most common cause of death is that of intracranial hemorrhage, which occurs in Factor XIII deficiency more commonly than in any of the other congenital coagulation protein defects. Bleeding is also commonly preceded by minor trauma occurring several days previously.[100,126] Although deep tissue bleeding is common, intra-articular bleeds are rare. In addition, although patients have delayed post-traumatic bleeding, postsurgical bleeding is less commonly a problem. Most homozygous males are sterile and a high incidence of spontaneous abortion is seen in homozygous females.[100] It has been suggested that Factor XIII is not only involved in adequate wound healing, by possibly cross-linking collagen as well

Table 5–26 Manifestations of Antiplasmin Deficiency

Clinical characteristics
  Autosomal recessive
  All described are CRM−
  Severe mucosal membrane hemorrhage
  Genitourinary bleeding is characteristic
  Large subcutaneous hematomas
  Easy and spontaneous bruising
  Severe bleeding with surgery or trauma
  Intra-articular bleeding has occurred
Laboratory characteristics
  Normal prothrombin time
  Normal PTT
  Normal template bleeding time
  Normal platelet function (aggregation)
  Definitive diagnosis requires assay for alpha-2-antiplasmin
Therapy
  Epsilon-aminocaproic acid: 10 mg/kg. three times daily

as fibrin, but may also be necessary for normal implantation of a fertilized ova into the uterine decidua.[100]

A screening test for the presence or absence of Factor XIII consists of observing for clot solubility or insolubility in 5 M urea or 1% monochloroacetic acid, two agents that will disrupt hydrophobic bonds, but not the gamma glutamyl-lysine bonds created by Factor XIII$_a$.[16,18,19,126] These solubility tests are, however, poor screening techniques because they are insensitive to levels slightly more than 1% normal activity and thus potential deficient bleeders can be missed.[126] More specific techniques are available, including assays for gamma-gamma dimer (cross-linked by Factor XIII), radioactive amine incorporation tests, latex agglutination inhibition tests, or radioimmunoassay.[88,90,109]

Therapy for Factor XIII deficiency consists of infusion of fresh frozen plasma at 10 mL/kg every 7 to 10 days. Alternatively, cryoprecipitate can be used. Adequate levels of Factor XIII are also given to the surgical patient who may have received several units of whole blood. Characteristic findings of Factor XIII defects are noted in Table 5–27.

Table 5–27 Manifestations of Factor XIII Defects

Clinical characteristics
Autosomal recessive trait
Most patients have absence of alpha chain (CRM−)
Umbilical stump bleeding in 90%
Delayed deep tissue hemorrhage is typical
Intramuscular
Intracranial
Pseudotumors often develop
Most common cause of death is intracranial bleed
Most homozygous males are sterile
Most homozygous females have miscarriages
Heterozygous patients usually asymptomatic
Laboratory characteristics
Clot solubility in urea or monochloroacetic acid
Clot solubility is a poor diagnostic tool
Therapy
Fresh frozen plasma or cryoprecipitate every 7 to 10 days

von Willebrand's Disease

von Willebrand's disease, first reported in 1926,[204] was initially noted in families living on the Aland islands off the coast of Sweden in the Gulf of Bothnia. The islands have since been renamed Ahvenanmaa. The original patients described had a severe bleeding disorder that was autosomally inherited. A prolonged bleeding time, normal clot retraction, normal platelet counts, and a normal coagulation time were characteristic. This original group, who were initially labeled as "pseudohemophiliacs," were restudied by the use of a capillary "thrombometer" several years later by von Willebrand and Jurgens; this closer evaluation revealed prolonged thrombometer times and patients were then labeled as having "constitutional thrombopathy."[205] The criteria for a diagnosis became (1) a bleeding tendency, (2) autosomal inheritance, (3) a normal platelet count, (4) a long bleeding time, and (5) a normal whole blood clotting time.

In 1953, Alexander, Quick, and Larrieu simultaneously discovered a new characteristic of von Willebrand's syndrome, that of low Factor VIII levels.[6,104,157] This important discovery acted as a catalyst to launch investigations that have subsequently led to a more complete understanding of the biology of the Factor VIII macromolecular complex, classic hemophilia, and von Willebrand's disease. In 1971 Zimmerman and associates[213] developed an antibody to Factor VIII and were able to demonstrate the presence of an antigen (Factor VIII:RAg) in normal and hemophiliac plasma, but not in von Willebrand's plasma. This discovery initiated the era of molecular biology of hemophilia, von Willebrand's disease, and Factor VIII moieties, and provided a tool for the discovery and defining of von Willebrand types as well as the separately recognized portions or activities of the Factor VIII macromolecular complex. A concept of the complex is depicted in Figure 5–2.[77,84,85,89,214] Factor VIII:C is a low molecular weight portion that is attached to a high molecular weight portion referred to as Factor VIII:R. Factor VIII:C is re-

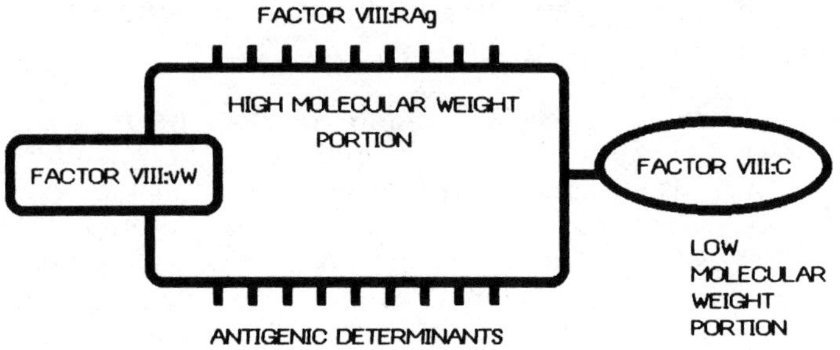

Fig. 5–2. Factor VIII macromolecular complex.

sponsible for procoagulant activity; it is the biologic activity responsible for serving as a cofactor or determiner in the conversion of Factor X to Factor X_a and is the factor that is defective in classic hemophilia.[77] This factor is probably synthesized in many cellular sites, but not the endothelium. Factor VIII:C has no other known biologic activity. Factor VIII:R is comprised of Factor VIII:RAg (to heterologous antibody) and Factor VIII:vW. Factor VIII:vW is an integral part of the high molecular weight portion and is that biologic activity that is necessary for normal bleeding times, normal platelet aggregation to ristocetin, normal platelet adhesion to subendothelial surfaces, and a normal platelet-endothelial interaction.[77,84,85,89,206,214] Factor VIII:R is a polymerized multimeric moiety and is

synthesized in the endothelium of arteries and veins and in platelets and megakaryocytes.[77,84,85,87,89,154,193,206,214] It is thought that Factor VIII:R may induce the synthesis or release of Factor VIII:C, thus accounting for a well-known phenomena; when the von Willebrand patient is transfused with normal plasma, hemophilic plasma, or cryoprecipitate, there is a marked and sustained rise in Factor VIII:C.[28,41,84,85,214] The Factor VIII:C response to transfusions in hemophilia and von Willebrand's disease are compared and contrasted in Figure 5–3.

The bleeding in von Willebrand's disease is reminiscent of a platelet-vascular problem and consists of purpura, easy and spontaneous bruising, hypermenorrhagia, mucosal membrane bleeding, including gastrointestinal and genitourinary

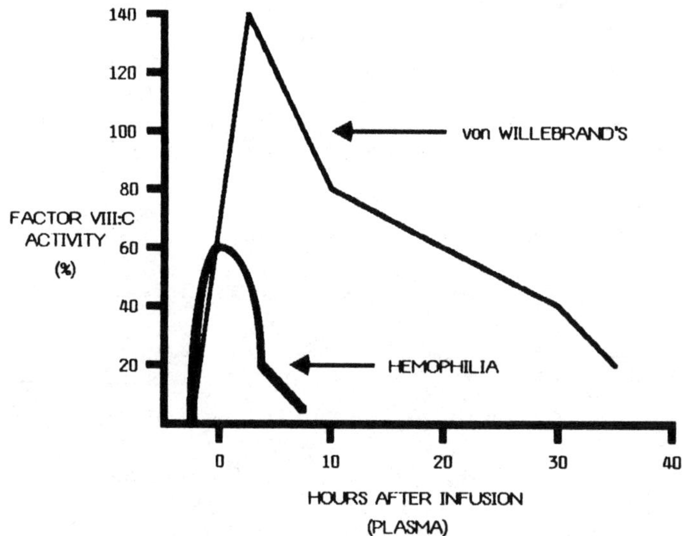

Fig. 5–3. Transfusion response in hemophilia and von Willebrand's disease.

hemorrhage, and bilateral epistaxis.[16,120] Bleeding often in the form of bilateral epistaxis and easy and spontaneous bruising can typically begin in early childhood, and this constellation of findings should prompt an early suspicion of von Willebrand's disease. Deep tissue bleeding and intra-articular bleeding are far less common than mucosal membrane bleeding. Hemorrhage, however, can be profuse with surgery or trauma. Clinical features of von Willebrand's syndrome are summarized in Table 5–28. There are four recognized subtypes of von Willebrand's syndrome.[29,54,87,127,132,151,186,188] However, a recent study showing a high degree of variability in the laboratory features in any individual patient over a given period of time suggests that these subtypes may be in error or alternatively that many patients put into one type, based on study at a single time, may, in fact, not be correctly classified.[2] The results of this study would also suggest that if a patient has a history suggestive of von Willebrand's disease, but fails to meet the diagnostic laboratory criteria, the patient should be restudied at another time. The currently generally accepted types of von Willebrand's disease are as follows.

1. Homozygous von Willebrand's disease is characterized by severe bleeding at the sites previously mentioned and a high incidence of consanguinity. The bleeding time is usually markedly prolonged. Ristocetin cofactor activity is markedly abnormal or absent and Factor VIII:RAg and Factor VIII:vW are markedly reduced or absent. Factor VIII:C and Factor VIII:CAg are reduced but not as profoundly as Factor VIII:vW and Factor VIII:RAg.

2. Heterozygous von Willebrand's type I is inherited as an autosomal dominant and is characterized by concordant decreases in Factor VIII:C, Factor VIII:CAg, Factor VIII:vW, and Factor VIII:RAg. This type, thus, is a quantitative defect in the entire Factor VIII macromolecular complex.

3. Heterozygous von Willebrand's type II is subdivided into two forms. Type IIA is inherited as an autosomal dominant and appears to represent a dysfunction of Factor VIII:vW. There is absent or almost nonexistent Factor VIII:vW activity and discordance with levels of Factor VIII:C, Factor VIII:CAg, and Factor VIII:RAg, all of which are usually much higher than levels of Factor VIII:vW. This suggests a dysfunction of the complex rather than a quantitative defect. In this form of the disease it appears that there is depolymerization of the macromolecular complex, with many monomeric forms circulating. This type may therefore represent an abnormality of polymerization ability of the complex. Type IIB is also inherited as an autosomal dominant and has the same discordant findings as seen in type IIA. There are normal or near normal Factor VIII:C, Factor VIII:CAg, and moderately reduced levels of Factor VIII:RAg. The two major differences from type IIA are that there is enhanced platelet aggregability to ristocetin (enhanced Factor VIII:RCo activity) and although this form also appears to be associated with a defect in polymerization, there are fewer of the monomeric forms and more of the polymerized forms circulating that are typically seen in type IIA. The types of von Willebrand's syndrome are characterized in Table. 5–29.

The laboratory diagnosis of von Willebrand's disease can be complex and complicated.[2,16,28,85,120,214] This complexity is

Table 5–28 Clinical Manifestations of von Willebrand's Disease

Clinical characteristics
Variable inheritance
Easy and spontaneous bruising
Petechiae and purpura
Mucosal membrane hemorrhage
Genitourinary
Gastrointestinal
Intrapulmonary
Gingival bleeding
Bilateral epistaxis in early childhood
Deep tissue bleeding rare
Hemorrhage may be severe with surgery or trauma
Therapy
Cryoprecipitate: 1 to 3 bags per 10 kg. body weight
Fresh frozen plasma to Factor VIII:C>75%
Monitor template bleeding time (variable)
Desmopression may be of benefit in selected types

Table 5-29 Clinical Variants of von Willebrand's Disease

Homozygous von Willebrand's disease
  Severe hemorrhage of many sites
  High incidence of consanguinity
  Very prolonged template bleeding time
  Very decreased (or absent) Factor VIII:vW
    (ristocetin cofactor)
  Reduced Factor VIII:C
  Reduced Factor VIII:RAg
Heterozygous von Willebrand's disease, type I
  Autosomal dominant trait
  Concordant decreases in
    Factor VIII:C
    Factor VIII:CAg
    Factor VIII:vW
    Factor VIII:RAg
  A quantitative defect in entire
  Factor VIII complex
Heterozygous von Willebrand's disease type IIA
  Autosomal dominant trait
  Discordant decreases in
    Factor VIII:C (reduced)
    Factor VIII:CAg (reduced)
    Factor VIII:RAg (reduced)
    Factor VIII:vW (absent)
Heterozygous von Willebrand's disease, type IIB
  Autosomal dominant trait
  Discordant findings, as in type IIA
  Factor VIII:C near normal
  Factor VIII:RAg moderately reduced
  Enhanced platelet agglutination to ristocetin
  Defective Factor VIII complex polymerization
  A qualitative defect in the Factor VIII complex with
    depolymerization of the complex

Table 5-30 Methods for the Evaluation of von Willebrand's Disease

Old Methods	New Methods
Manual	Manual
PTT	Factor VIII:RAg
Factor VIII:C	Ristocetin aggregation
Duke bleeding time	Ristocetin cofactor
Ivy bleeding time	Template bleeding time
Lee-White clotting time	Aspirin tolerance test
	Petechiometer test
	Automated*
	Intrinsic pathway
	Generated thrombin
	(automated PTT)
	Factor VIII:C
	Factor VIII:CAg
	Factor VIII:RAg

* Synthetic substrates, immunoassays, ELISA assays.

further enhanced by the noting of variability and changing of laboratory parameters in a given patient, as well as the past popularity of tests that are notoriously unreliable in von Willebrand's disease and are no longer recommended for use: ristocetin-induced platelet aggregation and the platelet adhesion techniques using glass bead columns.[76,110,137,201,215] The ristocetin cofactor assay has replaced ristocetin-induced aggregation and is a reasonably sensitive test. However, the primary laboratory tests are the Factor VIII:C and Factor VIII:RAg and template bleeding time used in conjunction with Factor VIII:RCo assay.[2,16,85,120,137,214,215] Older and newer laboratory tests for the diagnosis of von Willebrand's disease are given in Table 5-30.

The therapy of choice for patients with von Willebrand's disease is cryoprecipitate, which contains abundant levels of Factor VIII:R.[16,85,120,137,215] The amount of cryoprecipitate currently used is variable because the amount of Factor VIII:R is variable and the response, by monitoring correction of the bleeding time, is also quite variable. However, a rough guideline is to give one to three bags of cryoprecipitate per day per 10 kg total body weight. The presurgical patient should receive three bags per 10 kg the morning of the day of surgery. If cryoprecipitate is not available, infusions of fresh frozen plasma to raise the Factor VIII:C level to 80 to 100% of normal or to normalize the bleeding time can be used; this dose requirement is about 10 to 15 mL/kg/day. The use of desmopressin has also been of benefit in maintaining hemostasis in patients with von Willebrand's disease, although the response may depend on the type.[111,176,198] The usual dose is 0.2 to 0.5 μg/kg diluted in 30 mL of normal saline, with infusions over 15 minutes every 24 to 48 hours. Factor VIII concentrates should not be used for von Willebrand's disease because they appear to contain very little of the Factor VIII:R or Factor VIII:vW activity. Table 5-31 compares and contrasts findings of hemophilia A and von Willebrand's disease.

Other Rare Defects

Other rare hereditary protein defects leading to a hemorrhagic disorder have

Table 5–31 von Willebrand's Disease and Hemophilia A

	von Willebrand's	Hemophilia A
Inheritance	Autosomal dominant	Sex-linked recessive
Bleeding time	Long	Normal
Factor VIII:C	Moderate decrease	Marked decrease
Factor VIII:RAg	Decreased	Normal
Factor VIII:vW	Decreased	Normal
Platelet adhesion	Abnormal	Normal
Clinical Features	Mucosal bleeds, petechiae, purpura	Deep tissue bleeding

also been described. An alpha-1-antitrypsin variant causing a severe life-long bleeding diathesis in a 10-year-old boy was described in 1978 by Lewis and co-workers.[108] The inhibitory action was similar to that of heparin, but was not bound to barium citrate or inhibited by protamine; evaluation of the inhibitor revealed it to be a double-banded alpha-1-antitrypsin. The defect is referred to as "antithrombin Pittsburg." A similar case has been reported by Messmore and co-workers.[136] A similar family was recently seen by this author in Bakersfield; in this instance, however, the defect in the patient and the four children was found to be a biologically hyperactive antithrombin III variant.[22] A 32-year-old female presented with a life-long history of easy and spontaneous bruising and severe bleeding requiring transfusions after dental extraction and appendectomy. Her four children had never been stressed by surgery or trauma, but had life-long histories of easy and spontaneous bruising. The diagnosis was suspected by noting that it required four thrombin-clot tubes to remove fibrinogen to perform fibrin(ogen) degradation product titers. Following this, an evaluation revealed this family to have normal immunologic antithrombin III levels, but twice normal biologic activity by several different methods.

Congenital protein C inhibitor deficiency has been reported by both Marler and Griffin[129] and Giddings and associates,[59] and the patients were deficient in Factor V and Factor VIII:C. Four unrelated patients were studied by Marler and Griffin, although the clinical manifestations were not discussed. Giddings and associates[59] reported an additional two cases of protein C inhibitor deficiency,

both were also associated with combined Factor V and Factor VIII:C deficiency. In this report all patients studied who had only an isolated singular Factor V or isolated Factor VIII:C deficiency had normal protein C inhibitor activity. Because of these findings, it has been suggested that many previously reported cases of combined Factor V and Factor VIII:C deficiency may, upon reevaluation, be found to represent congenital protein C inhibitor deficiency.

Newer and older methods for diagnosing hereditary coagulation protein defects are summarized in Table 5–32. Both older

Table 5–32 Methods for the Evaluation of Congenital Coagulation Defects

Old Methods (Manual)	New Methods (Automated)
Prothrombin time	External pathway generated thrombin (prothrombin time equivalent)*
Activated PTT	Internal pathway generated thrombin (PTT equivalent)*
Factor assays	Factor assays
Fibrinogen	Fibrinogen[†]
Factor II	Factor II*[†]
Factor V	Factor V*[†]
Factor VII	Factor VII*[†]
Factor VIII:C	Factor VIII:C*[†]
Factor VIII:RAg	Factor VIII:CAg*[†]
Factor IX	Factor VIII:RAg*[†]
Factor X	Factor IX*[†]
Factor XI	Factor X*[†]
Factor XII	Factor XI*[†]
Prekallikrein	Factor XII*[†]
Clot Solubility	Prekallikrein*[†]
Bleeding times	High molecular weight kininogen[†]
	Factor XIII*[†]
	Antiplasmin*[†]

* Synthetic substrates.
[†] Immunoassays, ELISA, laser nephelomety.

manual techniques as well as newer automated techniques are depicted. Acquired coagulation factor defects, both single and multiple, leading to hemorrhage and congenital protein defects leading to thrombotic problems will be discussed in appropriate subsequent chapters.

References

1. Abildgaard CF, Simone JV, Corrigan JJ, Seeler RA, Edelstein G, Vanderheiden J, Schulman I: Treatment of hemophilia with glycine-precipitated Factor VIII. N Engl J Med 275:471, 1966.
2. Abildgaard U, Suzuki Z, Harrison J, Jefcoat K, Zimmerman TS: Serial studies in von Willebrand's disease: Variability versus "variants". Blood 56:712, 1980.
3. Aggeler PM, White SG, Glendening MB, Page EW, Leake TB, Bates G: Plasma thromboplastin component (PTC) deficiency: A new disease resembling hemophilia. Proc Soc Exp Biol Med 79:692, 1952.
4. Aledort LM: The management of hemophilia: A perspective. Drug Therapy 1:1, 1971.
5. Alexander B, Goldstein R, Landwehr G, Cook CD, Addelson E, Wilson C: Congenital SPCA deficiency. A hitherto unrecognized coagulation defect with hemorrhage rectified by serum and serum fractions. J Clin Invest 30:596, 1952.
6. Alexander B, Goldstein R: Dual hemostatic defect in pseudohemophilia. J Clin Invest 32:551, 1953.
7. Al-Mondhiry HAB, Bilezikian SB, Nossel HL: Fibrinogen "New York"—an abnormal fibrinogen associated with thromboembolism: functional evaluation. Blood 45:607, 1975.
8. Aoki N, Saito H, Kamiya T, Koie K, Sakata Y, Kabakura M: Congenital deficiency of alpha-2-plasmin inhibitor associated with severe hemorrhagic tendency. J Clin Invest 63:877, 1979.
9. Aoki N, Sakata Y, Matsuda M, Tateno K: Fibrinolytic states in a patient with congenital deficiency of alpha-2-plasmin inhibitor. Blood 55:483, 1980.
10. Azner J, Pavnon A Fernandez: Thromboembolic accidents in patients with congenital deficiency of Factor XII. Thromb Diath Haemorrh 31:525, 1974.
11. Bachmann F, Duckert F, Koller F: The Stuart-Prower factor assay and its clinical significance. Thromb Diath Haemorrh 2:24, 1958.
12. Baudo F, De Caltado F, Josso F, Silvello L: Hereditary hypoprothrombinemia. True deficiency of Factor II. Acta Haematol 47:243, 1972.
13. Beck EA, Shainoff JR, Vogel A, Jackson DP: Functional evaluation of an inherited abnormal fibrinogen: Fibrinogen "Baltimore". J Clin Invest 50:1874, 1971.
14. Bezeaud A, Drouet L, Soria C, Guillin MC: Prothrombin Salakta: An abnormal prothrombin characterized by a defect in the active site of thrombin. Thromb Res 34:507, 1984.
15. Bezeaud A, Guillin MC, Olmeda F, Quintana M, Gomez N: Prothrombin Madrid: A new familial abnormality of prothrombin. Thromb Res 16:47, 1979.
16. Bick RL: Hereditary plasma protein disorders. In Murano G, Bick RL (Eds): Basic Concepts of Hemostasis and Thrombosis. CRC Press, Boca Raton, FL, 1980, p 149.
17. Bick RL: Vascular disorders associated with thrombohemorrhagic phenomena. Semin Thromb Hemost 5:167, 1979.
18. Bick RL: A systematic approach to the diagnosis of bleeding disorders. In Murano G, Bick RL (Eds): Basic Concepts of Hemostasis and Thrombosis. CRC Press, Boca Raton, FL, 1980, p 81.
19. Bick RL, Shanbrom E: A systematic approach to the diagnosis of bleeding disorders. Med Counterpoint 6:27, 1972.
20. Bick RL: Clinical hemostasis practice: The major impact of laboratory automation. Semin Thromb Hemost 9:139, 1983.
21. Bick RL, Adams T, Radack K: Surgical hemostasis with a Factor XI-containing concentrate. JAMA 229:163, 1974.
22. Bick RL: Personal observations, 1980.
23. Bidwell E, Booth JM, Dike GWR, Denson KWE: The preparation for therapeutic use of a concentrate of Factors IX containing also Factors II, VII, and X. Br J Haematol 13:568, 1967.
24. Biggs R: Jaundice and antibodies directed against Factors VIII and IX in patients treated for haemophilia or Christmas disease in the United Kingdom. Br J Haemaol 26:313, 1974.
25. Biggs R, Douglas AM, Macfarlane RA, Dacie JV, Pitney WR, Merskey C, O'Brien JR: Christmas disease: A condition previously mistaken for haemophilia. Br Med J 2:1378, 1952.
26. Blatt PM, Lundblad RL, Kingdon HS, McLean G, Roberts HR: Thrombogenic materials in prothrombin complex concentrates. Ann Intern Med 81:766, 1974.
27. Blomback M, Blomback B, Mammen EF, Prasad AS: Fibrinogen Detroit—a molecular defect in the N-terminal disulfide knot of human fibrinogen? Nature 218:134, 1968.
28. Blomback M, Jorpes JE, Nilsson IM: von Willebrand's disease. Am J Med 34:236, 1963.
29. Bowie EJW, Didisheim P, Thompson JH, Owen CA: The spectrum of von Willebrand's disease. Thromb Diath Haemorrh 18:40, 1970.
30. Breen FA, Tullis JL: Prothrombin concentrates

in treatment of Christmas disease and allied disorders. JAMA 208:1848, 1969.

31. Briet E, Loeliger A, Van Tilburg NH, Veltkamp JJ: Molecular variant of Factor VII. Thromb Haemost 35:289, 1976.

32. Brockman SK, Aprill SN, Rabiner FS: Aortic valve replacement in hemophilia: Report of a case. JAMA 222:660, 1972.

33. Brown PE, Hougie C, Roberts HR: The genetic heterogeneity of hemophilia B. N Engl J Med 283:61, 1970.

34. Carrell N, Gabriel DA, Blatt PM, Carr ME, McDonagh J: Hereditary dysfibrinogenemia in a patient with thrombotic disease. Blood 62:439, 1983.

35. Chiu HC, Whitaker E, Coleman R: Heterogeneity of human Factor V deficiency: Evidence for the existance of antigen-positive variants. J Clin Invest 72:493, 1983.

36. Chung KS, Madar DA, Goldsmith JC, Kingdon HS, Roberts HR: Purification and characterization of an abnormal Factor IX (Christmas factor) molecule. Factor IX Chapel Hill. J Clin Invest 62:1078, 1978.

37. Chung KS, Goldsmith JC, Roberts HR: Purification and characterization of an abnormal Factor IX Alabama (IX$_{Ala}$). XVII Congress of the International Society of Haematology, Paris. (Abstr.) 1978, p 859.

38. Colman RW, Wong PY: Participation of Hageman factor dependent pathways in human disease states. Thromb Haemost 38:751, 1977.

39. Colman RW, Bagdasarian A, Talamo RC, Scott CF, Seavey M, Guimaraes JA, Pierce JV, Kaplan AP: Williams trait. Human kininogen deficiency with diminished levels of plasminogen proactivator and prekallikrein associated with abnormalities of the Hageman factor-dependent pathways. J Clin Invest 56:1650, 1975.

40. Conrad FG, Breneman WL, Grisham DB: A clinical evaluation of plasma thromboplastin antecedent (PTA) deficiency. Ann Intern Med 62:885, 1965.

41. Cornu P, Larrieu MJ, Caen J, Bernard J: Transfusion studies in von Willebrand's disease: Effect on bleeding time and Factor VIII. Br J Haematol 9:189, 1963.

42. Croze M, Brizard CP: Factor VII Padua I, another case. Haemostasis 11:185, 1982.

43. Denson KWE, Conrad J, Samama M: Genetic variants of Factor VII. Lancet 1:1234, 1972.

44. Denson KWE, Biggs R, Haddon ME, Borrett R, Cobb K: Two types of hemophilia (A$^+$ and A$^-$): A study of 48 cases. Br J Haematol 17:163, 1969.

45. Denson KWE, Biggs R, Mannucci PM: An investigation of three patients with Christmas disease due to an abnormal type of Factor IX. J Clin Pathol 21:160, 1968.

46. Denson KWE, Lurie A, De Cataldo F, Mannucci PM: The Factor X defect: Recognition of abnormal forms of Factor X. Br J Haematol 18:317, 1970.

47. Department of Health, Education and Welfare: National Heart and Lung Institute Blood Resource Studies, Vol 3, Pilot Study of Hemophilia Treatment in the United States. U.S. Government Printing Office, Washington, D.C., 1972.

48. Egeberg O: Inherited fibrinogen abnormality causing thrombophilia. Thromb Diath Haemorrh 17:176, 1967.

49. Egeberg O: Factor XII defect and hemorrhage. Evidence for a new type of hereditary hemostatic disorder. Thromb Diath Haemorrh 23:432, 1970.

50. Elodi S, Varadi K, Hollan SR: Some sources of error in the one-stage assay of Factor VIII. Haemostasis 7:1, 1978.

51. Elodi S, Puskas E: Variants of haemophilia B. Thromb Diath Haemorrh 28:489, 1972.

52. Entes K, LaDuca FM, Tourbaf KD: Fletcher factor deficiency, source of variations of the activated partial thromboplastin time. Am J Clin Pathol 75:626, 1981.

53. Estelles A, Aznar J, Espana F: The absence of release of the plasminogen activator after venous occlusion in a Fletcher trait patient. Throm Haemost 49:66, 1983.

54. Firkin B, Firkin F, Scott L: von Willebrand's disease type B: A newly defined bleeding diathesis. Aust N.Z. J Med 3:225, 1973.

55. Forbes CD: Clinical aspects of the hemophilias and their management. In Ratnoff OD, Forbes CD (Eds): Disorders of Hemostasis. Grune & Stratton, New York, 1984, p 177.

56. Francis RB, Kasper CK: Reproduction in hemophilia. JAMA 250:3192, 1983.

57. Fuchs G, Egbring R, Havemann K: Fibrinogen Marburg. A new genetic variant of fibrinogen. Blut 34:107, 1977.

58. George JN, Breckenridge RT: The use of Factor VIII and Factor IX concentrates during surgery. JAMA 214:1673, 1970.

59. Giddings JC, Sugrue A, Bloom AL: Quantitation of coagulant actigens and inhibition of activated Protein C in combined Factor V and VIII deficiency. Br J Haematol 52:495, 1982.

60. Gill F, Shapiro SS, Schwartz E: Severe congenital hypoprothrombinemia. J Pediatr 94:264, 1978.

61. Girolami A: The hereditary transmission of "true" hypoprothrombinemia. Br J Haematol 21:695, 1971.

62. Girolami A, Cocceri S, Palareti G, Poggi M, Burul A, Capellato G: Prothrombin Molise: A "new" congenital dysprothrombinemia, double heterozygosis with an abnormal prothrombin and "true" prothrombin deficiency. Blood 52:115, 1978.

63. Girolami A, Bareggi G, Burnetti A, Sticchi A: Prothrombin Padua: A "new" congenital dysprothrombinemia. J Lab Clin Med 84:654, 1974.

64. Girolami A, Falezza G, Patrassi G, Stenico M, Vittore L: Factor VII Verona coagulation disorder: Double heterozygosis with an abnormal Factor VII and heterozygous Factor VII deficiency. Blood 50:603, 1977.

65. Girolami A, Fabris F, Zanon R Dal Bo, Chiotto G, Burul A: Factor VII Padua: A congenital coagulation disorder due to an abnormal Factor VII with a peculiar activation pattern. J Lab Clin Med 91:387, 1978.

66. Girolami A, Cattarozzi G, Dal Bo Zanon R, Cella G, Toffanin F: Factor VII Padua 2: Another Factor VII abnormality with defective ox brain thromboplastin activation and a complex hereditary pattern. Blood 54:46, 1979.

67. Girolami A, Molaro G, Lazzarin M, Scarpa R, Brunetti A: A "new" congenital haemorrhagic condition due to the presence of an abnormal Factor X (Factor X Friuli): Study of large kindred. Br J Haematol 19:179, 1970.

68. Glueck HI, Roehll W: Myocardial infarction in a patient with a Hageman (Factor XII) defect. Ann Intern Med 64:390, 1966.

69. Goodnight SH, Feinstein DI, Osterud B, Rapaport SI: Factor VII antibody-neutralizing material in hereditary and acquired Factor VII deficiency. Blood 38:1, 1971.

70. Grosse KP, Seiler G, Niedhardt B, Schricker TH, Kroehling M: Kongenitaler faktor X-Mangel. Fallbericht und literaturubersicht. Monatsschr Kinderheilkd 127:285, 1979.

71. Harms CA, Triplett DA, Koepke JA: Factor VIII (antihemophilic factor) assay results in the 1976 College of American Pathologists survey program. Am J Clin Pathol 70:560, 1978.

72. Harper TA, Chauhan K: A collaborative study on the suitability of commercial, assayed plasmas for one-stage Factor VIII assays. Am J Clin Pathol 77:614, 1982.

73. Harker TA, Bailey EL, Chauhan K: Reliability of "standard" plasmas used by clinical laboratories for one-stage Factor VIII assays. Am Clin Pathol 75:197, 1981.

74. Hathaway WE, Belhasen LP, Hathaway HS: Evidence for a new plasma thromboplastin factor. I. Case report, coagulation studies, and physicochemical properties. Blood 26:521, 1965.

75. Helske T, Ikkala E, Myllyla G, Nevanlinna HR, Rasi V: Joint involvement in patients with severe haemophilia A in 1957-59 and 1978-79. Br J Haematol 51:643, 1982.

76. Hirsh J: Laboratory diagnosis of thrombosis. In Coleman RW, Hirsh J, Marder VJ, Salzman EW, (Eds): Hemostasis and Thrombosis: Basic Principles and Clinical Practice. JB, Lippincott,

Philadelphia, 1982, p 789.

77. Hirshgold EJ: Properties of Factor VIII (antihemophilic factor). Prog Hemost Thromb 2:99, 1974.

78. Hoak JC, Swanson LW, Warner ED, Connor WE: Myocardial infarction associated with severe Factor XII deficiency. Lancet 2:884, 1966.

79. Hoffman JJML, Meulendijk PN: Comparison of reagents for determining the activated partial thromboplastin time. Thromb Haemost 39: 640, 1978.

80. Hougie C, Twomey JJ: Hemophilia Bm: A new type of Factor IX deficiency. Lancet 1:698, 1967.

81. Hougie C, Barrow EM, Graham JB: Stuart clotting defect. I. Segregation of an hereditary haemorrhagic state from the heterogeneous group heretofore called stable factor (SPCA) deficiency. J Clin Invest 36:485, 1957.

82. Hougie C, McPherson RA, Aronson L: Passovoy factor: A hitherto unrecognized factor necessary for haemostasis. Lancet 290, 1975.

83. Hougie C, McPherson RA, Brown JE, Lakin-Thomas PL, Melaragno A, Aronson L, Baugh RF: The Passovoy defect. Further characterization of a hereditary hemorrhagic diathesis. N Engl J Med 298:1045, 1978.

84. Hoyer LW: Immunologic properties of antihemophilic factor. Prog Hematol 8:191, 1973.

85. Hoyer LW: von Willebrand's disease. Prog Hemost Thromb 3:231, 1976.

86. Hoyer LW, Breckenridge RT: Immunologic properties of antihemophilic factor (AHF Factor VIII). II. Properties of cross-reacting material. Blood 35:809, 1970.

87. Hoyer LW, Rizza CR, Tuddenham EGD, Carta CA, Armitage H, Rotblat F: von Willebrand factor multimer patterns in von Willebrand's disease. Br J Haematol 55:493, 1983.

88. Ikematsu S, McDonagh RP, Reisner HM, Skrzynia C, McDonagh J: Immunochemical studies of human Factor XIII. Radioimmunoassay for the carrier subunit of the zymogen. J Lab Clin Med 97:662, 1981.

89. Irwin JF: Factor VIII in von Willebrand's disease. Semin Thromb Hemost 2:85, 1985.

90. Isreals ED, Paraskevus F, Isreals LG: Immunological studies of coagulation Factor XIII. J Clin Invest 52:2398, 1973.

91. Jackson DP, Beck EA, Charache P: Congenital disorders of fibrinogen. Fed Proc 24:816, 1965.

92. Jackson JM, Marshall LR, Herrmann RP: Passovoy factor deficiency in five western Australian kindreds. Pathology 13:517, 1981.

93. Josso F, De Sanchez JM, Lavergne JM, Menache D, Soulier JP: Congenital abnormality of the prothrombin molecule (Factor II) in four siblings: Prothrombin Barcelona. Blood 38:9, 1971.

94. Kahn MJP, Govaerts A: Prothrombin Brussels,

a new congenital defective protein. Thromb Res 5:141, 1974.

95. Kasper CK, Aledort LM, Counts RB, Edson JR, Fratantoni J, Green D, Hampton JW, Hilgartner MW, Lazerson J, Levine PH, McMillan CW, Pool JG, Shapiro SS, Shulman NR, van Eys J: A more uniform measurement of Factor VIII inhibitors. Thromb Diath Haemorrh 34:869, 1975.

96. Kasper CK, Osterud B, Minami JY, Shonick W, Rapaport SI: Hemophilia B: Characterization of genetic variants and detection of carriers. Blood 50:351, 1977.

97. Kerbiriou-Nabius DM, Garcia FO, Larrieu MJ: Radioimmunoassays of human high and low molecular weight kininogens—in plasmas and platelets. Br J Haematol 56:273, 1984.

98. Kernoff PBA, Thomas ND, Lilley PA, Matthews KB, Goldman E, Tuddenham EGD: Clinical experience with polyelectrolyte-fractionated porcine Factor VIII hemophiliacs with antibodies to Factor VIII. Blood 63:31, 1984.

99. Kernoff LM, Hughes J, Denson K: Clinical and laboratory observations in congenital Factor VIII deficiency. Thromb Haemost 46:1088, 1981.

100. Kitchens CS, Newcomb TF: Factor XIII. Medicine Baltimore 58:413, 1979.

101. Klein HG, Aledort LM, Bouma BH, Hoyer LW, Zimmerman TS, de Mets DL: A cooperative study for the detection of the carrier state of classic hemophilia. N Engl J Med 296:959, 1977.

102. Kluft C, Vallenga E, Brommer EJP, Wijngaards G: A familial hemorrhagic diathesis in a Dutch family: An inherited deficiency of alpha-2-antiplasmin. Blood 59:1169, 1982.

103. Lacombe MJ, Varet B, Levy JP: A hitherto undescribed plasma factor acting at the contact phase of blood coagulation (Flaujeac factor): Case report and coagulation studies. Blood 46:761, 1975.

104. Larrieu MJ, Soulier JP: Deficit en facteur antihemophilique A chez un fille associé a un trouble du saignement. Rev Haematol 8:361, 1953.

105. Larsson SA, Nilsson IM, Blomback M: Current status of Swedish hemophiliacs. Acta Med Scand 212:195, 1982.

106. Laugen RH, Bithell: Fibrinogen Charlottesville: Hereditary dysfibrinogenemia characterized by slow fibrinopeptide release and competitive inhibition of thrombin. Blood 50:273, 1977.

107. Leiba H, Ramot B, Many M: Hereditary and coagulation studies in ten families with Factor XI (plasma thromboplastin antecedent) deficiency. Br J Haematol 11:654, 1965.

108. Lewis JH, Iammarino RM, Spero JA, Hasiba U: Antithrombin Pittsburgh: An alpha-1-antitrypsin variant causing hemmorrhagic disease

Blood 51:129, 1978.

109. Lorand L, Losowsky MS, Miloszewski K: Human Factor XIII: Fibrin-stabilizing factor. Prog Hemost Thromb 5:245, 1980.

110. Lowe GDO: Laboratory evaluation of hypercoagulability. Clin Haematol 10:407, 1981.

111. Lundlam CA, Peake IR, Allen N, Davies BL, Furlong RA, Bloom AL: Factor VIII and fibrinolytic response to deamino-8-D-arginine vasopressin in normal subjects and dissociate response in some patients with haemophilia and von Willebrand's disease. BR J Haematol 45:499, 1980.

112. Lusher JM, Blatt PM, Penner JA, Aledort LM, Levine PH, White GC, Warrier AI, Whtiehurst DA: Autoplex versus proplex: A controlled, double-blind study of effectiveness in acute hemarthroses in hemophiliacs with inhibitors to Factor VIII. Blood 62:1135, 1983.

113. Lutcher CL: Reid trait: A new expression of high molecular weight kininogen (HMW kininogen) deficiency. Clin Res 24:47, 1976.

114. Mammen EF: Fibrinogen abnormalities. Semin Thromb Hemost 9:1, 1983.

115. Mammen EF: Congenital abnormalities of the fibrinogen molecule. Semin Thromb Hemost 1:184, 1974.

116. Mammen EF, Prasad AS, Barnhart MI, Hu CC: Congenital dysfibrinogenemia: Fibrinogen Detroit. J Clin Invest 48:235, 1969.

117. Mammen EF: Factor II abnormalities. Semin Thromb Hemost 9:13, 1983.

118. Mammen EF: Factor V deficiency. Semin Thromb Hemost 9:19, 1983.

119. Mammen EF: Factor VII abnormalities. Semin Thromb Hemost 9:19, 1983.

120. Mammen EF: Factor VIII abnormalities. Semin Thromb Hemost 9:22, 1983.

121. Mammen EF: Factor IX abnormalities. Semin Thromb Hemost 9:28, 1983.

122. Mammen EF: Factor X abnormalities. Semin Thromb Hemost 9:31, 1983.

123. Mammen EF: Factor XI deficiency. Semin Thromb Hemost 9:34, 1983.

124. Mammen EF: Contact factor abnormalities. Semi Thromb Hemost 9:36, 1983.

125. Mammen EF: α-2-Antiplasmin deficiency. Semin Thromb Hemost 9:52, 1983.

126. Mammen EF: Factor XIII deficiency. Semin Thromb Hemost 9:10, 1983.

127. Mannucci PM: Spectrum of von Willebrand's disease: A study of 100 cases. (Italian working group report). Br J Haematol 35:101, 1977.

128. Marder VJ: The functional defects of hereditary dysfibrinogens. Thromb Haemost 36:1, 1976.

129. Marler RA, Griffin JH: Deficiency of protein C inhibitor in combined Factor V/VIII deficiency disease. J Clin Invest 66:1186, 1980.

130. Marsh N: Fibrinolysis and disease. In Fibrinolysis. John Wiley & Sons, New York, 1981, p 125.

131. Mazzucconi MG, Mandelli F, Mariani G, Briet E, Veltkamp JJ, Mariana G, Briet E, Veltkamp JJ: A CRM-positive variant of Factor VII deficiency and the detection of heterozygotes with the assay of Factor-like antigen. Br J Haematol 36:127, 1977.

132. McCarroll DR, Ruggeri ZM, Montgomery RR: Correlation between circulating levels of von Willebrand's antigen II and von Willebrand factor: Discrimination between type I and type II von Willebrand's disease. J Lab Clin Med 103:704, 1984.

133. McPherson RA: Thromboembolism in Hageman trait. Am J Clin Pathol 68:420, 1977.

134. Megguier RJ: Fibrinolytic activity in human dental sockets after extractions. J Oral Surg 29:321, 1971.

135. Menache' D: Abnormal fibrinogens: A review. Thromb Diath Haemorrh 29:525, 1973.

136. Messmore HL, Parvez Z, Fareed J: Isolation and partial characterization of a novel circulating antithrombin. Thromb Haemost 42:123, 1979.

137. Meyer D, Zimmerman TS: von Willebrand's disease. In Coleman RW, Hirsh J, Marder VJ, Salzman EW (Eds): Hemostasis and Thrombosis: Basic Principles and Clinical Practice. J.B. Lippincott, Philadelphia, 1982, p 64.

138. Miles LA, Plow EF, Donnelly KJ, Hougie C, Griffin JH: A bleeding disorder due to deficiency of alpha-2-antiplasmin. Blood 59:1246, 1982.

139. Mitterstieler G, Muller W, Geir W: Congenital Factor V deficiency. A family study. Scand J Haematol 21:9, 1978.

140. Montgomery R, Natelson SE: Afibrinogenemia with cerebral hematoma. Am J Dis Child 131:555, 1977.

141. Montgomery RR, Otsuka A, Hathaway WE: Hypoprothrombinemia: Case report. Blood 51:299, 1978.

142. Montgomery RR, Corrigan JJ, Clarke S, Johnson J: Prothrombin Denver—a new dysprothrombinemia. Circulation 62 (Suppl. III):279, 1980.

143. Mori K, Sakai H, Nakano N, Suzuki S, Sugai K, Hisa S, Goto Y: Congenital Factor X deficiency in Japan. Tohoku J Exp Med 133:1, 1981.

144. Morse EE: Fibrinogen and dysfibrinogenemia. Ann Clin Lab Sci 10:351, 1980.

145. Morse EE: The fibrinogenopathies. Ann Clin Lab Sci 8:234, 1978.

146. Neal WR, Tayloe DT, Cederbaum AI, Roberts HR: Detection of genetic variants of hemophilia B with an immunosorbent technique. Br J Haematol 25:63, 1973.

147. Nilsson IM: Report of the working party on Factor VIII-related antigens. Thromb Haemost 39:511, 1978.

148. Noren I: Clinical application of a new assay of Factor VIII and Factor VIII inhibitors. Thromb Res 1:19, 1972.

149. Oh-Ishi S, Ueno A, Uchida Y, Katori M, Hayashi H, Hoya H, Kitajima K, Kimura I: Abnormalities in the contact activation through Factor XII in Fujiwara trait: A deficiency in both high and low molecular weight kininogens with low level of prekallikrein. Tohoku J Exp Med 133:67, 1981.

150. Owren PA: Parahemophilia, haemorrhagic diathesis due to absence of a previously unknown clotting factor. Lancet 1:446, 1947.

151. Peake IR, Bloom AL, Giddings JL: Inherited variants of Factor VIII-related protein in von Willebrand's disease. N Engl J Med 291:113, 1974.

152. Penner JA, Kelly PE: Management of patients with Factor VIII or IX inhibitors. Semin Thromb Hemos 1:386, 1975.

153. Pina-Cabral JM, Justica B: Congenital hypoprothrombinemia in a Portuguese family. Thromb Diath Haemorrh 30:451, 1973.

154. Piovella F, Nalli G, Malamani GD, Majolino I, Frassoni F, Sitar GM, Ruggeri A, Dell-Orbo C, Ascari E: The ultrastructural localization of Factor VIII-antigen in human platelets, megakaryocytes and endothelial cells utilizing a ferritin-labelled antibody. Br J Haematol 39:209, 1978.

155. Quattrone A, Colucci M, Donati MB, Mussoni L, Roncaglioni MC, Semeraro N, Carlomango S, Bonavita S: Cerebral thrombosis in two young siblings with dysfibrinogenemia. Neurosci Lett 3:54, 1979.

156. Quick AJ, Pisciotta AV, Hussey CV: Congenital hypoprothrombinemic states. Arch Intern Med 95:2, 1955.

157. Quick AJ, Hussey CV: Hemophilic condition in the female. J Lab Clin Med 42:929, 1953.

158. Rabiet MJ, Elion J, Labie D, Josso J: Prothrombin Metz: Purification and characterization of a variant of human prothrombin. Thromb Haemost 42:57, 1979.

159. Ragni MV, Lewis JH, Spero JA, Hasiba: Factor VII deficiency. Am J Hematol 10:79, 1981.

160. Rapaport SI, Proctor RR, Patch MJ, Yettra: The mode of inheritance of PTA deficiency: Evidence for the existence of major PTA deficiency and minor PTA deficiency. Blood 18:149, 1961.

161. Ratnoff OD, Forman WB: Criteria for the differentiation of dysfibrinogenemic states. Semin Hematol 13:141, 1976.

162. Ratnoff OD: The molecular basis of hereditary clotting disorders. Prog Hemost Thromb 1:39, 1972.

163. Ratnoff OD, Jones PK: The laboratory diagnosis of the carrier state for classic hemophilia. Ann Intern Med 86:521, 1977.

164. Ratnoff OD, Prothrombin complex concentrates: A cautionary note. Ann Intern Med

81:852, 1974.

165. Ratnoff OD, Colopy JE: A familial hemorrhagic trait associated with a deficiency of clot-promoting fraction of plasma. J Clin Invest 34:602, 1955.

166. Ratnoff OD, Busse RJ, Sheon RP: The demise of John Hageman. N Engl J Med 279:760, 1968.

167. Roberts HR, Grizzle JE, McLester WD, Penick: Genetic variants of hemophilia B: Detection by means of a specific inhibitor. J Clin Invest 47:360, 1968.

168. Rosenthal RL, Dreskin OH, Rosenthal N: New hemophilial-like disease caused by deficiency of a third plasma thromboplastin factor. Proc Soc Exp Biol Med 82:171, 1953.

169. Rosenthal RL: Factor XI: General review. Bibl Haematol 23:1350, 1965.

170. Rubio R, Almagro D, Cruz A, Corral JF: Prothrombin Habana: A new dysfunctional molecule of human prothrombin associated with a true prothrombin deficiency. Br J Haematol 54:553, 1983.

171. Saito H, Scott JG, Movat HZ, Scialla SJ: Molecular heterogeneity of Hageman trait (Factor XII deficiency). Evidence that two of 49 subjects are cross-reacting material positive (CRM+). J Lab Clin Med 94:256, 1979.

172. Saito H, Goodnough LT, Soria J, Soria C, Aznar J, Espana F: Heterogeneity of human prekallikrein deficiency (Fletcher trait). Evidence that five of 18 cases are positive for cross-reacting material. N Engl J Med 305:910, 1981.

173. Saito H, Ratnoff OD, Waldmann R, Abraham JP: Fitzgerald trait: Deficiency of a hitherto unrecognized agent, Fitzgerald factor, participating in surface-mediated reactions of clotting, fibrinolysis, generation of kinins, and the property of diluted plasma enhancing vascular permeability (PF/DIL). J Clin Invest 55:1082, 1975.

174. Samama M, Soria J, Soria C: Congenital and acquired dysfibrinogenemia. in Poller L (Ed): Recent Advances in Blood Coagulation. Churchill Livingstone, London, 1977, p 313.

175. Sandjerg-Hamsen M, Clemmensen I,: An abnormal fibrinogen (Copenhagen) associated with severe thromboembolic disease, but with normal absorption of plasminogen. Thromb Haemost 42:137, 1979.

176. Schmitz-Huebner U, Balleisen L, Arends P, Pollmann H, Sutor AH: DDAVP-induced changes of Factor VIII-related activities and bleeding time in patients with von willebrand's syndrome. Haemostasis 9:204, 1980.

177. Schreiber RR: Musculo-skeletal system—radiologic findings. In Brinkhous KM, Hemker HC (eds): Handbook of Hemophilia. Elsevier Publishing, New York, 1975, p 333.

178. Schricker KT: Congenital Factor VII deficiency. Med Klin 76:24, 1981.

179. Seeler RA: Parahemophilia. Factor V deficiency. Med Clin North 56:119, 1972.

180. Seeler RA: Hemolysis due to anti-A and anti-B in Factor VIII preparations. Arch Intern Med 130:101, 1972.

181. Seligsohn U: High gene frequency of Factor XI (PTA) deficiency in Ashkenazi Jews. Blood 51:1223, 1978.

182. Seligsohn U, Modan M: Definition of the population at risk of bleeding due to Factor XI deficiency in Ashkenazi Jews and the value of the activated partial thromboplastin time in its detection. Isr J Med Sci 17:413, 1981.

183. Shanbrom E: Rapid correction of AHF deficiency by antihemophilic factor—method four, with special reference to inhibitors. Bibl Haematol 34:52, 1970.

184. Shapiro SS, Martinez J, Holburn RR: Congenital dysprothrombinemia: An inherited structural disorder of human prothrombin. J Clin Invest 48:2251, 1969.

185. Shapiro SS, Maldonado NI, Fradera J, McCord S: Prothrombin San Juan: A complex new dysprothrombinemia. J Clin Invest 53:73, 1974.

186. Shoa'i I, Lavergne JM, Ardaillou N, Obert B, Ala F, Meyer D: Heterogeneity of von Willebrand's disease: Study of 40 Iranian cases. Br J Haematol 37:67, 1977.

187. Sidi A, Seligsohn U, Jonas P, Many M: Factor XI deficiency: Detection and management during urological surgery. J Urol 119:528, 1978.

188. Silwer J, Nilsson IM: On a Swedish family with 51 members affected by von Willebrand's disease. Acta Med Scand 175:627, 1964.

189. Singher LJ: Renal and urological complications of hemophilia. In Brinkhous KM, Hemker HC (Eds): Handbook of Hemophilia. Elsevier Publishing, New York, 1975, p 377.

190. Smith LG, Coone LAN, Kitchen CS: Prothrombin Gainesville. A dysprothrombinemia in a pair of identical twins. Am J Hematol 11:223, 1981.

191. Soulier JP, Josso F, Steinbuch M, Cosson A: The therapeutic use of fraction P.P.S.B. Bibl Haematol 29:1127, 1968.

192. Spiyack AR, Avioli LV: Orthopedic and medical treatment of patients with hemophilia. Arch Intern Med 143:1431, 1983.

193. Sultan Y, Bouma BN, de Graaf S, Simeon J, Caen JP, Sixma JJ: Factor VIII related antigen in platelets of patients with von Willebrand's disease. Thromb Res 11:23, 1977.

194. Suzuki K, Nishioka J, Hashimoto S, Kamiya T, Saito H: Normal titer of functional and immunoreactive protein-C inhibitor in plasma of patients with congenital combined deficiency of Factor V and Factor VIII. Blood 62:1266, 1983.

195. Takamatsu J, Hayashi K, Ogata K, Kamiya T,

Koie K: A family of congenital Factor VII deficiency. Rinsho Ketsueki 21:834, 1980.

196. Telfer TP, Denson KWE, Wright DR: A "new" coagulation defect. Br J Haematol 2:308, 1956.

197. Terheggen HG: Faktor V—Mangel bei einem 8 monate alten Madchen. Monatsschr Kinderheilkd 119:627, 1971.

198. Theiss W, Schmidt G: DDAVP in von Willebrand's disease: Repeated administration and the behavior of the bleeding time. Thromb Res 13:1119, 1978.

199. Tullis JL, Melin M, Jurigian P: Clinical use of human prothrombin complex concentrates. N Engl J Med 273:667, 1965.

200. Tullis JL, Melin M: Management of Christmas disease and Stuart-Prower deficiency with a prothrombin-complex concentrate (Factors II, VII, IX, X). Bibl Haematol 29:1134, 1968.

201. Turrito VT, Baumgartner HR: Platelet-surface interactions. In Coleman RW, Hirsh J, Marder VJ, Salzman EW (Eds): Hemostasis and Thrombosis: Basic Principles and Clinical Practice. J.B. Lippincott, Philadelphia, 1982, p 64.

202. Veltkamp JJ: Clinical features of hemophilia. In Brinkhouse KM, Hemker HC (Eds): Handbook of Hemophilia. Elsevier Publishing, New York, 1975, p 371.

203. Veltkamp JJ: Meilof J, Remmelts HG, Vander Vlerg D, Loeliger EA: Another genetic variant of haemophilia B: Haemophilia B-Leyden. Scand J Haematol 7:82, 1970.

204. von Willebrand EA: Hereditar pseudohamofili. Finska Laeksaellsk Handl 68:87, 1926.

205. Von Willebrand EA, Juergens R: Veber ein neues vererbbares Blutungsuebel: Konstitutionelle. Dtsch Arch Klin Med 175:453, 1933.

206. Walsh RT: The platelet in von Willebrand's disease: Interactions with ristocetin and Factor VIII. Semin Thromb Hemost 2:105, 1975.

207. Webster WP, Roberts HR, Thelin GM, Wagner RH, Brinkhous KM: Clinical use of a new glycine-precipitated antihemophilic fraction. Am J Med Sci 250:643, 1965.

208. Weinger RS, Rudy C, Moake JL, Olson JD, Cimo PL: Prothrombin Houston: A dysprothrombin identifiable by crossed immunoelectrofocusing and abnormal Echis carcinatus venom activation. Blood 55:811, 1980.

209. Weiss AE: Circulating inhibitors in hemophilia A and B: Epidemiology and methods of detection. In Brinkhous KM, Hemker HC (Eds): Handbook of Hemophilia. Elsevier Publishing, 1975, p 629.

210. White GC, Roberts HR, Kingdon HS, Lundblad RL: Prothrombin complex concentrates: Potentially thrombogenic materials and clues to the mechanism of thrombosis in vivo. Blood 49:159, 1977.

211. Winckelmann G: Kongenitale Dysfibrinogenamie bericht uber eine neue Familie (Fibrinogen "Wiesbaden"). Thromb Diath Haemorrh 55:345, 1973.

212. Yoshioka A, Kamitsuji H, Takase T, Iida Y, Tsukada S, Mikama S, Fukui H: Congenital deficiency of alpha-2-plasmin inhibitor in three sisters. Haemostasis 11:176, 1982.

213. Zimmerman TS, Ratnoff OD, Powell AE: Immunologic differentiation of classic hemophilia (Factor VIII deficiency) and von Willebrand's disease. J Clin Invest 50:244, 1971.

214. Zimmerman TS, Ruggeri ZM: von Willebrand's disease. Prog Hemost Thromb 6:203, 1982.

215. Zimmerman TS, Ruggeri ZM: von Willebrand's disease. Clin Haematol 12:175, 1983.

6
Disseminated Intravascular Coagulation and Related Syndromes

Disseminated intravascular coagulation (DIC) is not an independent disease entity, but rather an intermediary mechanism of disease, and in that capacity it is usually seen in association with well-defined clinical entities.[20,21] In addition, the pathophysiology of DIC serves as an intermediary mechanism of disease in several localized processes that, in many instances, remain organ specific. This catastrophic syndrome spans all areas of medicine and presents a wide clinical spectrum that remains confusing to many. The syndrome of DIC was referred to in early literature as "consumptive coagulopathy."[190,287] This is not an appropriate term, since very little is consumed in DIC; most factors and plasma constituents are plasmin biodegraded. Terminology that followed this initial descriptive phrase was that of defibrination syndrome.[101,226] However, a more appropriate term would be defibrinogenation syndrome. DIC is the most common term used for this disease entity and is a good descriptive pathophysiologic term if one accepts coagulation as representing hemorrhage plus thrombosis.[22]

Most consider DIC to be a systemic hemorrhagic syndrome; however, this is only because hemorrhage is obvious and often is impressive. What is less commonly appreciated is the significant amount of microvascular thrombosis and, in some instances, large vessel thrombosis that is also occurring. In fact, the hemorrhage is often easy to contend with in patients with fulminant DIC, and it is the small vessel and large vessel thrombosis with impairment of blood flow, ischemia, and associated end organ damage that usually leads to irreversible morbidity and mortality of the patient. Thus, DIC is a syndrome associated with hemorrhage that

is often clinically obvious, but also associated with diffuse thromboses that may lead to irreversible end organ damage and death; it is this latter complication that is difficult to stop or reverse. Acute versus chronic DIC and the attendant differences in clinical manifestations, laboratory findings, and treatment will be discussed. However, it should be realized that these are often pure and often theoretical clinical spectrums of a disease continuum, and patients may present anywhere in this continuum and, in fact, may lapse from one end of the spectrum to the other.

Historical Perspectives

The first description of DIC was given in a lecture delivered by Walter H. Seegers, then Professor and Chairman of the Department of Physiology at Wayne State University, to the Cincinnati Academy of Medicine on April 18, 1950, and subsequently published.[297] In this lecture Seegers gave special reference to Factor V, which had recently been discovered, and he postulated that "thromboplastin" may gain access to the maternal circulation and cause hemorrhagic problems. Several essential steps in developing this concept were discussed, thus serving as the first logical thinking with respect to the pathologic description of DIC. Seegers recognized that thromboplastin was present in many tissues and that it could initiate the blood clotting mechanism directly by activating prothrombin. In addition, when thromboplastin was deliberately placed in the circulation of animals, a variety of pathologic responses were obtained. Seegers also recognized that in experimental animal models mechanical trauma of the placenta released material that was likely to be thromboplastin and induced a variety of pathologic changes in the animal. Also, a study of human cases revealed that many of the pathologic lesions corresponded to those produced by thromboplastin in animal models. Shortly before delivering this lecture, Seegers and his colleague Charles L. Schneider had been able to demonstrate that amniotic fluid and placenta contained a large amount of thromboplastin. Seegers also noted that during observations in animal models the injection of thromboplastin caused cessation of blood flow in small vessels altogether, and if the animals were carefully examined it was noted that death was due to characteristic intravascular thrombotic lesions and that thromboembolism was disseminated throughout the pulmonary vascular tree. It was additionally noted that the central nervous system was damaged by perivascular hemorrhage and liver necrosis was present. Thus, Seegers not only delivered the first description of DIC and offered a pathophysiologic mechanism, but also recognized that hemorrhage plus thrombosis is the usual clinical result. These observations were extended to several patients who were also discussed in this early lecture. Three of these patients had eclampsia. Seegers described a case of complete placental abruptio with nearly complete "defibrination" in the patient; this was demonstrated by repeated laboratory assays for circulating fibrinogen.

These studies were expanded on and again reported on at the Fourth American Congress on Obstetrics and Gynecology in 1951 by Seegers and Schneider.[298] During this presentation the investigators focused attention on thromboplastin and reviewed reasons why thromboplastin might be responsible for a group of "perplexing disorders" of late pregnancy, including intracranial hemorrhage, shock associated with obstetric accidents, the hemorrhagic diathesis of pregnancy, and toxemia of pregnancy. They also recognized that thromboplastin led to an underlying disease process of intravascular coagulation, with thromboplastin presumably entering the bloodstream. Although this material initiates the blood clotting

mechanism or procoagulant system, it may be carried some distance and mixed with a variable volume of blood before fibrin starts to form in the microcirculation. This process of coagulation then results in a depletion of fibrinogen and a resultant extensive defibrination. Following this, blood was noted to be refractory to further injections of thromboplastin because of inadequate fibrinogen. They stated "by the same token however, animals are subject to grave danger due to uncontrolled hemorrhage, for an important portion of the hemostatic mechanism has been depleted." They concluded by pointing out that the mechanism of thromboplastin introduction to the systemic maternal circulation needed to be considered a factor in several complications of late pregnancy and not simply as one type of complication because the resultant foci of tissue destruction in different organs will cause different clinical dysfunctional manifestations. Also during this same presentation, Seegers and Schneider documented and quantitated the amount of thromboplastin or procoagulant material that could be obtained from the placental, decidua, and amniotic fluid. In addition, they presented a hypothetical mechanism by which intravascular coagulation might occur due to this thromboplastin material. It was proposed that maternal blood within a retroplacental hematoma became admixed with material fragmented from or leached out of the torn uterine decidua within which the hematoma was enclosed. This mixture, rich in thromboplastin material from the decidua, could then enter the circulation by one path or another, with the most likely path being into the maternal lake within the placenta. Once within the maternal lake, this admixture would be likely to be distributed throughout the maternal circulation. Thus, these are the first descriptions of clinical DIC.

In the same year in the Harvey Lectures Seegers further reported on decreases in Factor V as well as fibrinogen during the hemorrhagic complications of pregnancy.[299] In 1952 this important work was further expanded and reported, in which the role of the accelerated conversion of prothrombin to thrombin, thus leading to subsequent defibrinogenation and complications of pregnancy, was described.[165] In 1953, this original work was again extended to the clinical field and Seegers and co-workers[322] gave guidelines for early ceserean section to abort the hemorrhagic syndrome, which they called "defibrination." Major clinical extensions of this initial observation were shortly thereafter reported by Ratnoff and colleagues.[280,281] Many profound observations were imparted, including the recognition that the hemorrhagic syndromes of pregnancy included premature separation of the placenta, amniotic fluid embolism, the presence of a dead fetus in utero, and severe preeclampsia, or frank toxemia of pregnancy. In addition, they recognized that a generalized bleeding tendency may occur as a sequel to "criminal abortion." In addition, it was noted that the treatment of a patient with a hemorrhagic diathesis associated with premature separation of the placenta consisted most importantly of early evacuation of the uterus, and it was pointed out that if labor did not occur promptly, it was thus difficult to keep a patient out of shock, or if laboratory tests revealed progressive hypofibrinogenemia, it was probably in the best interest of the patient to empty the uterus promptly by ceserean section. The reader will appreciate that this was profound thinking for 1955. In addition, in the conclusion of this article it was recognized that more than simple hypofibrinogenemia accounted for the hemorrhagic syndromes associated with pregnancy, and it was also noted that an "unexplained prolongation of the clotting time and associated severe thrombocytopenia" were present. Thus, it was again recognized that multiple hemostatic defects were present. In addition, Dr. Ratnoff and co-workers were the first to note that in individuals with amniotic fluid embolism, hemorrhagic symptoms appeared even though the concentration of fibrinogen in the plasma did not seem to be sufficiently low to account adequately for ineffective hemostasis. This then, rendered the first description of a multifaceted defect that accounted for the hemorrhage of DIC.

Additional observations were that "fibrinolysin was thought to be present," thus also rendering the first description of secondary activation of the fibrinolytic system and probably the most important cause of hemorrhage in these patients. In addition, in this report by Ratnoff and co-workers is to be found the first report of septicemia associated with DIC, two patients being described who had undergone attempts at self-induced abortion and subsequently developed bacteremia with gram-negative coliform bacilli (this represents the first description of septicemia and disseminated intravascular coagulation).

In 1962, Ratnoff and Nebehay[282] carefully described the severe alterations in blood coagulation that may sometimes contribute to the bleeding tendency and shock in the Waterhouse-Friderichsen syndrome. Also described was a case of DIC associated with incoagulable blood with prolonged clotting and bleeding times, thrombocytopenia, and low levels of fibrinogen, Factor V, and Factor VII in a patient with the Waterhouse-Friderichsen syndrome induced by infection with pneumococcus. Following this, additional reports of DIC began to appear in the literature and finally in the mid-1960s it became a clinically accepted and readily recognized syndrome. However, we owe our basic understanding and appreciation of this syndrome to the astute clinical and laboratory observations of Seegers and Ratnoff and their co-workers. The reader is encouraged to peruse these early descriptions of DIC for a complete appreciation of the discoveries that may be made by careful and astute observation, both biochemically and clinically.

Etiology of Disseminated Intravascular Coagulation

Acute

DIC is usually seen in association with well-defined clinical entities (Table 6–1). Obstetrical accidents are common events leading to DIC, such as amniotic fluid embolism. Amniotic fluid has thromboplastin-like (platelet factor 3-like or phospholipoprotein-like) activity.[80,206,321] Amniotic fluid may be released into the uterine and then subsequently the sys-

Table 6–1 Conditions Associated with Acute Disseminated Intravascular Coagulation

Obstetric accidents
  Amniotic fluid embolism
  Placental abruption
  Retained fetus syndrome
  Eclampsia
Intravascular hemolysis
  Hemolytic transfusion reactions
  Minor hemolysis
  Massive transfusions
Bacteremia
  Gram-negative (endotoxin)
  Gram-positive (bacterial mucopolysaccharides)
Viremias
  Cytomegalovirus
  Hepatitis
  Varicella
Disseminated malignancy
Leukemia
  Acute promyelocytic
  Acute myelomonocytic
  Many others
Burns
Crush injuries and tissue necrosis
Liver disease
  Obstructive jaundice
  Acute hepatic failure
Prosthetic devices
  (LeVeen shunting, aortic assist)
Vascular disorders

temic maternal circulation and thus activate the coagulation sequence at points where platelet factor 3 would normally activate the system, including the conversion of Factor X to Xa and prothrombin to thrombin. In instances of placental abruption, placental enzymes and/or tissues, including thromboplastin-like material, may be released into the uterine and subsequently the systemic maternal circulation and likewise lead to activation of the coagulation system. In DIC associated with the retained fetus syndrome the incidence of DIC approaches 50% if the woman retains a dead fetus in utero for greater than 5 weeks. The first findings are usually those of a chronic compensated DIC, which then amplify into a more fulminant hemorrhagic-thrombotic DIC. In this instance necrotic fetal tissue as well as enzymes derived from necrotic fetal tissue are released into the uterine and then the systemic maternal circulation and act at various points to activate the procoagulant system and trigger an episode of acute DIC.[138,320]

Intravascular hemolysis of any etiology, even of minimal degree, is a common triggering event for DIC, and a frank hemolytic transfusion reaction is certainly a triggering event. During hemolysis, the release of red cell adenosine diphosphate (ADP) or red cell membrane phospholipoprotein may activate the procoagulant system and in clinical practice either, or a combination, of these may account for episodes of DIC associated with major or minor hemolysis.[105,184,189,277,326] An example of this is the use of multiple transfusions with banked whole blood over a short period of time, such as 5 to 10 U within a 24-hour period, which will provide a significant trigger for DIC via the aforementioned mechanisms. Thus, hemolysis due to a frank hemolytic transfusion reaction or even to a minor hemolytic reaction with release of red cell ADP or red cell membrane phospholipoprotein is capable of providing a trigger for activation of the procoagulant system and a subsequent episode of acute DIC.

Septicemia is often associated with DIC. An early organism to be associated with DIC was the meningococcus.[1,213,340] Later, other gram-negative organisms were also noted to provide a triggering event for DIC.[87,149,342] The triggering mechanisms have been well described and consist of the initiation of coagulation by endotoxin: bacterial coat lipopolysaccharide.[79,214] Endotoxin has the ability to activate Factor XII to XIIa, to induce a platelet release reaction, to cause endothelial sloughing with subsequent activation of Factor XII to XIIa or Factor XI to XIa, or to initiate a release of granulocyte procoagulant materials; any one of these might independently trigger DIC. However, what is most likely commonly seen is a clinical summation of several or all of these activation sequences. Following this, numerous gram-positive organisms were also noted to be associated with DIC; the mechanisms have been aptly described.[89,289] Bacterial coat mucopolysaccharides may demonstrate exactly the same activity as endotoxin, namely, the activation of Factor XII to Factor XIIa, a platelet release reaction, endothelial sloughing, or the release of granulocyte procoagulant materials, any one of which may initiate DIC. However, as with gram-negative endotoxemia, what is most likely commonly seen is a clinical summation of several or all of these activation mechanisms.

Numerous viremias have been reported to be associated with DIC, and the most common are varicella, hepatitis, or cytomegalovirus infections.[125,215] However, many other acute viremias may also induce DIC.[21] The exact triggering mechanisms are poorly documented, although the most likely is that of circulating antigen-antibody complex-induced activation of Factor XII, a platelet release reaction, or endothelial sloughing with subsequent exposure of subendothelial collagen and basement membrane.[251,284,293] Severe viral hepatitis and hepatic failure can lead to DIC. In addition, intrahepatic or extrahepatic cholestasis may be accompanied by acute DIC; the mechanisms will be discussed in Chapter 7.

Malignancy is often associated with DIC and most individuals with disseminated solid malignancy will have at least laboratory evidence of DIC that may or may not become clinically manifest. If one therefore looks for laboratory evidence of DIC in patients with disseminated solid malignancy, it is almost always found.[23,24,227,325] There are many mechanisms by which malignancy may provide a trigger for initiation of DIC. One such mechanism is simply neovascularization of tumor; the "new vasculature" is comprised of abnormal endothelial lining that may activate the procoagulant system by several mechanisms.[122,123] In addition, solid tumors may release necrotic tumor tissue or tumor cell enzymes into the systemic circulation and activate the coagulation sequence.[303,339] Other mechanisms may also be operative in malignancy; for example, the sialic acid moiety of mucin in mucinous adenocarcinoma tissue is capable of the nonenzymatic activation of Factor X to Factor Xa which may then lead to an acute or chronic compensated DIC that may manifest itself in the usual manner or may be manifested as multiple or single thrombosis.[271,272] It has long been debated whether prostatic carcinoma is

associated with a primary hyperfibrinogenolytic syndrome or DIC.

Rapaport and Chapman[279] have clearly shown that malignant prostatic tissue secretes enzyme-type materials that are capable of activating the coagulation system and are associated with the usual secondary fibrinolytic response, which represents a typical DIC syndrome.[98,267] In addition, these investigations have also demonstrated that malignant prostatic tissue may secrete materials that independently activate the fibrinolytic system, converting plasminogen to plasmin. Thus, in prostatic carcinoma, patients develop a typical DIC syndrome with secondary fibrinolysis and develop primary activation of the fibrinolytic system; thus, an overwhelming fibrinolytic response is seen in these patients. This accounts for the clinical observation that these patients far more commonly present with hemorrhage rather than thrombosis.

Studies done at the Mayo Clinic have revealed that there is a direct correlation between laboratory findings of DIC before transurethral prostatectomy and degree of blood loss after prostatectomy, suggesting that it is prudent to look for evidence of DIC, as defined by elevated fibrin(ogen) degradation products (FDP) and circulating soluble fibrin monomer, since this may well predict those patients who will bleed after surgery and may predict the need for postoperative blood replacement.[229] Pancreatic carcinoma has been classically associated with migratory thrombophlebitis and the mechanisms have been carefully studied and described.[129,161] In this instance, the migratory thrombophlebitis is nothing more than a clinical manifestation of DIC. The incidence of thrombophlebitis in carcinoma of the pancreas is much higher in patients with carcinoma of the body or tail as opposed to those of the head of the pancreas. When a carcinoma is present in the body or tail of the pancreas there is minimal ductal obstruction, and thus a large amount of trypsin is released into the systemic circulation. Trypsin, a serine protease, possesses activity much like thrombin or Factor Xa and thus may activate the coagulation system and a typical DIC-type syndrome results.

The clinical manifestation is more commonly thrombosis than hemorrhage, as opposed to that seen in prostatic carcinoma. Alternatively, if the carcinoma is located in the head of the pancreas, ductal obstruction is pronounced and only minimal trypsin release occurs and disseminated thromboses are much less commonly seen. In summary, many patients with disseminated solid malignancy demonstrate laboratory evidence of DIC. However, many patients never develop overt clinical manifestations of acute DIC even though a significant number may have clinical manifestations of a chronic compensated DIC if it is suspected and subsequently looked for and documented.

Patients with acute or chronic leukemia are also common candidates for DIC. The most common acute leukemia associated with DIC is hypergranuler promyelocytic. The mechanisms for this have been carefully investigated and described by Gralnick[132] and Gralnick and Tan[130] as well as others,[199,200,278] and consistent of the release of procoagulant material from granules of the progranulocyte. Furthermore, Gralnick and associates[131] and Bennett[18] have demonstrated that the use of heparin or miniheparin before the initiation of cytotoxic chemotherapy may ward off the development of DIC and may significantly prolong survival.

It has certainly been my experience that if a patient with acute promyelocytic leukemia does not actually present with findings of DIC, the patient will almost always develop acute DIC when cytotoxic chemotherapy is initiated; chemotherapy results in a large population cell "kill" and resultant release of granule procoagulant material into the systemic circulation and subsequent DIC.[21]

The next most common leukemia to be associated with DIC is acute myelomonocytic.[268] However, any acute leukemia may be associated with DIC and may significantly alter the prognosis of patients.[21,199,200,268]

Any of the chronic leukemias can be associated with DIC, although much less commonly than the acute leukemias. Malignancies commonly associated with DIC are listed in Table 6–2. Acidosis, and less commonly alkalosis, may also provide triggers for DIC.[16,21,216,228] In acidosis the

Table 6–2 Malignancies Most Commonly Associated with Disseminated Intravascular Coagulation

Gastrointestinal
Pancreas
Prostate
Lung
Breast
Ovary
Malignant melanoma
Myeloma
Acute promyelocytic leukemia
Acute myelomonocytic leukemia
Acute myeloblastic leukemia
Lymphomas (immunoblastic)
Hodgkin's disease
Biliary cancer

triggering event is most likely due to endothelial sloughing with the attendant activation of Factor XII to XIIa or XI to XIa or platelet release with a subsequent activation of the procoagulant system. However, the mechanisms that are potentially operative in cases of alkalosis remain unclear.

Patients with extensive burns are also ideal candidates for DIC and several mechanisms may be operative.[158,292] Microhemolysis with the attendant release of red cell membrane phospholipid or red cell ADP may provide the trigger. In addition, necrotic burn tissue may be associated with the release of tissue materials and/or cellular enzymes into the systemic circulation to initiate a DIC-type process. Any patient with a large degree of crush injury and attendant tissue necrosis may also develop DIC by the release of tissue enzymes and/or phospholipoprotein-like material into the systemic circulation.[21,216]

Selected vascular disorders and other miscellaneous disorders may also be associated with acute DIC. However, these are more commonly associated with a chronic DIC syndrome.[21,25,26] In particular, all are familiar with the Kasabach-Merritt syndrome, the association of giant cavernous hemangiomas and DIC.[160,173] Up to 25% of patients with giant cavernous hemangiomas will develop a chronic low-grade "compensated" DIC that may or may not progress into an acute DIC. The progression into an acute DIC from a chronic compensated DIC may occur with or without any particular identifiable reason. Approximately 50% of patients with hereditary hemorrhagic telangiectasia will also have a chronic DIC syndrome and many of these individuals may develop an acute DIC process for unexplained reasons.[27,28] Patients with small vessel disease, such as vasospastic phenomena, including Raynaud's syndrome, or severe diabetic angiopathy or angiopathy associated with autoimmune disorders may also develop chronic DIC, which may or may not become an acute process.[175] Vascular disorders associated with DIC are given in Table 6–3.

Many chronic inflammatory disorders, including sarcoidosis, Crohn's disease, and ulcerative colitis, may also be associated with compensated DIC. Selected prosthetic devices may also provide a triggering event for DIC. Exposure of the blood to foreign surfaces is often linked with activation of the procoagulant system, and this may provide a major obstacle in the use of certain prosthetic devices. The use of prosthetic devices has become extremely commonplace in the management of patients with vascular disease, cardiac disease, renal disease, and ascites. The hemostatic complications that accompany the insertion of prosthetic devices include activation of coagulation factors, "consumption" of coagulation factors as well as other plasma proteins and platelets, and the generation of microthrombi, which may be of no clinical consequence. In addition, thrombosis or thromboembolism may also give rise to serious life-threatening problems with prosthetic devices.[29] Intra-aortic balloon assist is a widely utilized clinical maneuver to control postmyocardial infarction, cardiogenic shock, and to stabilize selected patients after bypass surgery. Activation of the coagulation system with an attendant low-grade DIC that may become fulminant and acute may accompany the use of these devices.[29] LeVeen valve shunting for peritoneovenous shunting has become a common palliative procedure for the treatment of intractable ascites associated with severe liver disease or malignant ascites. A generalized DIC-type syndrome is often seen with the use of the LeVeen shunt.[29] It has been noted that the removal of ascitic fluid at the time of valve implantation, as well as the use of selected anticoagulants, may abort DIC in these patients.[79]

Chronic

Chronic DIC is a compensated event and again represents the pure end of a clinical spectrum that may not always represent reality.[258] Those conditions that are most commonly associated with a chronic DIC-type process are depicted in Table 6–4. Obstetrical accidents are common causes of chronic DIC, and the retained fetus syndrome usually presents as an acute DIC process. However, many individuals with retained dead fetus may develop a chronic-type DIC syndrome that then slowly amplifies into a more fulminant acute process.[276] Likewise, eclampsia represents the straightforward pathophysiology of DIC that sometimes remains chronic and often remains organ specific with respect to remaining localized to the renal and placental microcirculation; however, in approximately 10% of women the process may become a systemic process and may become acute and fulminant.[64,286]

Many patients undergoing hypertonic saline-induced abortion develop a chronic DIC-type process that in some instances becomes acute and in some remains chronic and compensated until the abortion is completed.[318] Cardiovascular diseases may likewise be associated with chronic DIC and on rare occasions patients with acute myocardial infarction

Table 6–3 Disseminated Intravascular Coagulation and Vascular Disorders or Defects

Kasabach-Merritt Syndrome
Hereditary hemorrhagic telangiectasia
Raynaud's disease
Leriche's syndrome
Vascular prostheses
Autoimmune disorders with vasculitis
Microangiopathic hemolytic anemias
Hemolytic-uremic syndrome
Thrombotic thrombocytopenic purpura (rarely)
Malignant hypertension
Glomerulonephritis
Hemangio(endothelio)sarcoma
Arterio-venous fistulae

Table 6–4 Conditions Associated with Chronic Disseminated Intravascular Coagulation

Obstetrical accidents
  Eclampsia
  Retained fetus syndrome
  Saline-induced abortion
Cardiovascular diseases
  Acute myocardial infarction
  Peripheral vascular diseases
  Leriche's syndrome
Metastatic malignancy
Hematologic diseases
  Paroxysmal nocturnal hemoglobinuria
  Polycythemia vera
  Agnogenic myeloid metaplasia
Collagen vascular disorders
  (especially if a microvascular component)
Renal disorders
  Glomerulonephritis
  Renal Angiopathies
  Hemolytic-uremic syndrome
Miscellaneous
  Allergic vasculitis
  Sarcoidosis
  Amyloidosis
  Chronic inflammatory disorders
  Diabetes mellitus
  Hyperlipoproteinemias

may develop a chronic compensated or, alternatively, acute fulminant DIC-type process.[259] The mechanisms remain unclear but may simply be due to shock, hypoxia, and acidosis, with resultant endothelial sloughing or activation of the contact activation system via stasis. Peripheral vascular diseases, such as giant cavernous hemangiomas, hereditary hemorrhagic telangiectasia, Leriche's syndrome, and selected small vessel diseases may lead to a chronic compensated DIC process that may remain chronic or may progress to a more acute phase.[85,295]

The vast majority of patients with disseminated malignancy have laboratory findings of a chronic DIC-type process, although many of these individuals never develop specific clinical signs and symptoms of DIC. Pulmonary hemorrhage appears to be a very early and prominent sign of chronic DIC in the patient with malignancy.[24,288] Approximately 75% of patients with malignancy and chronic DIC will eventually develop clinical evidence of this syndrome, and 25% will develop some type of significant thrombotic event.[20,21] As will be discussed under Therapy, many individuals with chronic DIC and malignancy may show marked correction of both their clinical hemorrhage and thrombosis as well as laboratory findings of DIC when aggressive antineoplastic therapy is instituted.[9,21,24,92,313] Many hematologic disorders have also been associated with DIC, such as agnogenic myeloid metaplasia, and a significant number of patients with polycythemia rubra vera have clinical and laboratory findings of an underlying chronic compensated DIC-type process.[23,24,96,308] There is an increased tendency for thrombosis or thromboembolus in patients with paroxysmal nocturnal hemoglobinuria, and this represents a DIC-type process that is clinically manifested primarily as thrombosis.[147,217]

Collagen vascular diseases may also be associated with DIC, and any patient with a collagen vascular disorder, especially when associated with significant small vessel involvement, may develop DIC. This DIC, usually in a chronic compensated form, may be seen in patients with severe rheumatoid arthritis, systemic lupus erythematosus. Sjögren's syndrome, dermatomyositis, and scleroderma. Again, this is most commonly seen when these disorders are associated with a severe microvascular component.[20,21,291]

Hemolytic-uremic syndrome (HUS), like eclampsia, shares similar pathophysiology to DIC. However, HUS often remains organ specific and localized to the renal microcirculation.[174,178] In approximately 10% of patients with HUS the condition becomes systemic.[21] It should be appreciated that when patients with HUS are seen, it is often clinically impossible to know whether the disease started as a primary insult to the renal vasculature and subsequent activation of the coagulation system or whether there was a primary activation of the coagulation system that initiated a localized or systemic DIC process that then subsequently induced local damage to the renal microcirculation secondary to fibrin deposition. No matter where the process started, the clinical manifestations may be quite similar; more importantly, when a patient with HUS is seen, it is often impossible to know where the cycle was initiated.

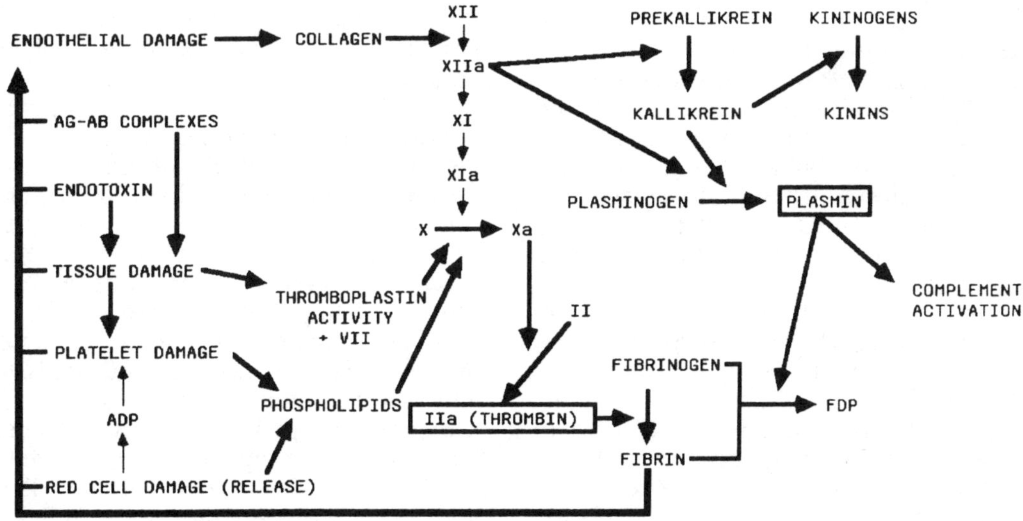

Fig. 6–1. Triggering mechanisms in DIC.

Numerous miscellaneous disorders have been reported to be associated with DIC, including allergic vasculitis, including Henoch-Schönlein purpura and the allergic purpuras, sarcoidosis, amyloidosis, chronic ulcerative/inflammatory conditions including Crohn's disease, ulcerative colitis, and severe diabetes mellitus, especially when associated with a significant microvascular component.[117, 162,166] In addition, a chronic compensated DIC-type syndrome may occur in patients who have hyperlipoproteinemias types II and IV.[76] On rare occasions, patients may develop a chronic DIC-type process for which no etiology can be found.[20,21]

Figure 6–1 serves to exemplify how a wide variety of seemingly unrelated pathophysiologic insults can give rise to the same common final pathway, the syndrome referred to as DIC. There are many disorders that can give rise to endothelial damage, circulating antigen-antibody complex, endotoxemia, tissue damage of any type (with resultant release of tissue procoagulant materials or tissue procoagulant enzymes), platelet damage and subsequent release, or red cell damage.[12,97,107] When one of these types of insults occurs, there is a wide range of potential activation pathways that may eventually give rise to systemically circulating plasmin plus systemically cir-

culating thrombin. When these two enzymes are circulating systemically, DIC is the result.[20,21,121,139,155] In many instances, the pathway leading from the initial pathophysiologic insult to the generation of systemic thrombin and plasmin are different; regardless of the activation pathway, once triggered, the resultant DIC-type pathophysiology remains the same.

Pathophysiology

The pathophysiology of DIC, once a triggering event has been provided, is summarized in Figure 6–2. After the coagulation system has been activated and both thrombin and plasmin circulate systemically, the pathophysiology of DIC is relatively constant in all disorders. When thrombin circulates systemically, it behaves as it would locally and begins to cleave fibrinopeptides A and B from fibrinogen, thus leaving behind fibrin monomer. Most of this fibrin monomer will then polymerize into fibrin (clot) in the microcirculation, leading to microvascular as well as macrovascular thrombosis, interference with blood flow, peripheral ischemia, end organ damage, and other attendant findings.[20,21,218,219,235] As fibrin is deposited in the microcirculation, platelets become trapped and the usual attendant thrombocytopenia typical of DIC follows.[194,260] On the other side of the "circle" depicted in Figure 6–2 it will be noted that plasmin also now circulates systemically and behaves as it normally would locally and begins to cleave the carboxy-terminal end of fibrinogen into FDPs systemically, thus creating the clinically recognized X, Y, D, and E fragments.[191,207,208,274] It should be noted that plasmin also rapidly releases specific peptides, the B-beta 15-42 and related peptides, which also serve as diagnostic molecular markers and will be discussed subsequently. FDP may combine with circulating fibrin monomer before fibrin monomer has polymerized into fibrin. When these degradation products complex with fibrin monomer, fibrin monomer cannot polymerize and therefore becomes solubilized. This complex is referred to as soluble fibrin monomer which is a significant aid in the diagnosis of DIC. The presence of soluble fibrin monomer forms the basis of the paracoagulation reactions, the ethanol gelation test, or the protamine sulfate test.[15,118,163,304] If one adds protamine sul-

fate or ethanol to a citrated tube of patient plasma containing soluble fibrin monomer, the ethanol or protamine sulfate will clear the FDP from fibrin monomer, fibrin monomer will then complex with other fibrin monomer and polymerize; as a result, fibrin strands are formed in the test tube and this is interpreted as a positive protamine sulfate or ethanol gelation test.[67,94,135] Thus, systemically circulating FDPs interfere with fibrin monomer polymerization. This, of course, further impairs hemostasis and leads to hemorrhage. Additional biologic activity of degradation products is that the later fragments have a high affinity for platelet membranes and coat their surfaces. This often creates a very clinically significant platelet function defect.[30,180,252] Thus, when seeing a patient with DIC who has a reasonable platelet count and is only mildly to moderately thrombocytopenic, the clinician should not mistakenly harbor a false sense of security because it must be appreciated that those platelets remaining in the circulation are usually significantly dysfunctional and may lead to clinically significant hemorrhage.

Plasmin, unlike thrombin, is a general

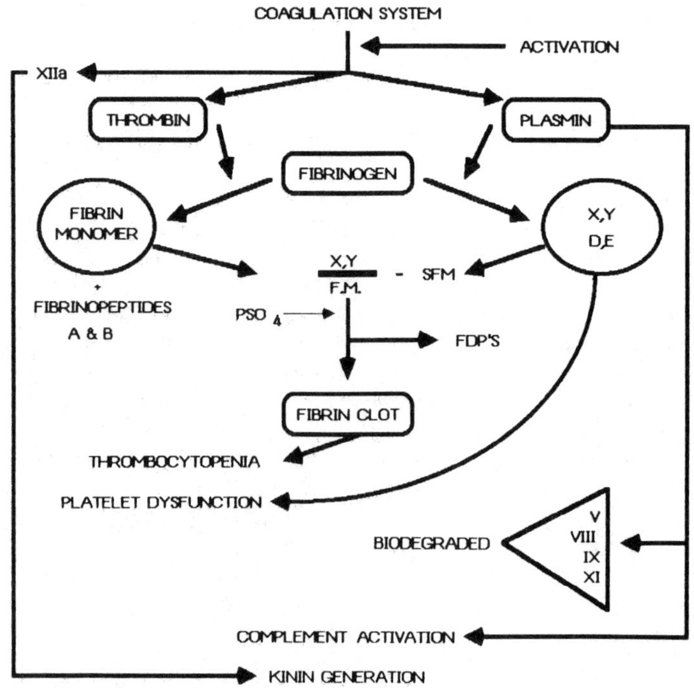

Fig. 6–2. Pathophysiology of DIC.

proteolytic enzyme that has equal affinity for fibrinogen and fibrin.[263,305] In addition, plasmin also effectively biodegrades many clotting factors, including Factors V, VIII, IX, XI, and other plasma proteins, including growth hormone, ACTH, insulin, and perhaps many more.[77,99,254,323] Additionally, as plasmin circulates systemically it often activates both C1 and C3 systemically with the attendant activation of the entire complement sequence leading to C8,9 activation and subsequent cell and platelet lysis.[283,296,332] This is of clinical significance in DIC and related syndromes associated with circulating plasmin, because the attendant red cell lysis will release red cell ADP and red cell membrane phospholipid, thus providing more procoagulant material. In addition, complement-induced platelet lysis will not only cause further thrombocytopenia, but will also provide more platelet procoagulant material. Of additional clinical concern, activation of the complement system will increase vascular permeability, thus leading to hypotension and shock.

Activation of the kinin system is also an important pathophysiologic event with clinical consequences in DIC and related syndromes. With early activation of the coagulation system, as commonly occurs in DIC, there is usually generation of Factor XIIa with the subsequent conversion of prekallikrein to kallikrein and subsequent conversion of high molecular weight kininogen into circulating kinins.[168,307,330,333] This, of course, will also lead to increased vascular permeability, hypotension, and shock.

In summary, as thrombin circulates systemically, the consequences are primarily thrombosis with deposition of fibrin monomer as well as polymerized fibrin in the microcirculation and, at times, large vessels. Concomitant with this, plasmin also circulates systemically. This enyzme primarily accounts for the hemorrhage seen in DIC because of the creation of FDP and the interference of these with fibrin monomer polymerization as well as platelet dysfunction. Additionally, plasmin-induced lysis of numerous aforementioned clotting factors also leads to hemorrhage. By appreciating this circular type of pathophysiology, it is easy to understand why the vast majority of patients with DIC sustain hemorrhage plus thrombosis. Clinicians are often misguided by appreciating only the hemorrhage that occurs in these patients, since this is the most obvious physical finding noted during clinical examination. However, of equal or more importance is the marked degree of microvascular thrombosis and, at times, large vessel thrombosis that is occurring in these patients and leading to altered end organ function, which may be extremely difficult to reverse. Thus, microvascular thrombosis and subsequent interference with blood flow and end organ damage is usually not appreciated until laboratory parameters provide a clue to their presence, for example, impending renal failure, pulmonary failure, elevated muscle-derived enzymes, liver enzymes, bone enzymes, and severely compromised pulmonary function. Thus, it is important to realize that the majority of patients with DIC are not only undergoing significant hemorrhage, but also significant and often diffuse thrombosis.[17,220,264,265] It should again be emphasized that it is usually the thrombosis that is the more irreversible event and more commonly leads to significantly altered morbidity and mortality due to ischemic changes, end organ damage, and potential death of the patient.

Figure 6–3 represents selected pathocybernetic events in DIC, which are depicted for illustrative purposes and only a few isolated events have been chosen. Many others could have been selected to exemplify the all-important point that once a DIC process is initiated the cybernetic nature of the coagulation system and the DIC process itself is such that the process will continue to self-perpetuate until something is done medically to intervene with the procoagulant drive.[300] For example, if one started with a clinical insult resulting in damaged endothelium, damaged endothelium will subsequently convert Factor XII to Factor XIIa with the eventual generation of thrombin and the subsequent generation of fibrin; deposition of fibrin on the endothelium will cause more damaged endothelium. Thus, a self-perpetuating cycle is initiated until stopped. In this selected

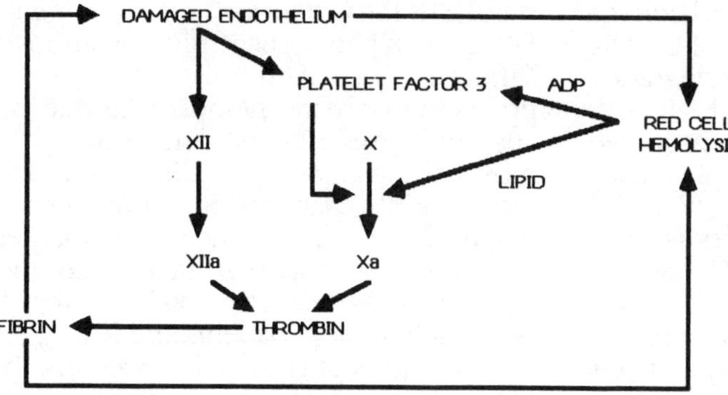

Fig. 6–3. Selected pathocybernetics in DIC.

instance the damaged endothelium will also lead to a platelet release with eventual availability of platelet factor 3 leading to the conversion of Factor X to Factor Xa with the eventual generation of thrombin, more fibrin deposited on the endothelium, and more endothelial damage and more platelet release. Also in this selected instance the damaged endothelium will likely give rise to red cell hemolysis, as will the deposited fibrin, thus giving rise to release of red cell ADP, causing more platelet release, more thrombin generation, further fibrin deposition, further endothelial damage, and further red cell hemolysis. Red cell hemolysis will, of course, also release red cell membrane phospholipid, which may also give rise to eventual Factor Xa generation, thrombin generation, and fibrin deposition, which likewise is associated with more red cell hemolysis and damaged endothelium with attendant red cell hemolysis.

Clinical situations that may give rise to platelet factor 3 release to possibly initiate or, more importantly, to perpetuate a DIC-type episode include the presence of subendothelial collagen, epinephrine, circulating antigen-antibody complexes, endotoxin, thrombin, or complement activation (possibly through previous plasmin generation).[68,91,95,108] It is thought that the availability of platelet factor 3 by any of the aforementioned potential mechanisms is probably more important as an accelerating and self-perpetuating process than a strictly singular etiologic mechanism in the initiating of DIC.

Endotoxin (bacterial coat lipopolysac-charide) is capable of inducing a granulocyte release of procoagulant or coagulation activating enzymes, is capable of directly converting Factor XII to Factor XIIa, may induce a platelet release reaction and may cause endothelial sloughing with subsequent exposure of subendothelial collagen.[10,149,157,221,236,306,341] Any one of these insults may independently initiate an episode of acute DIC; however, what is most likely clinically seen is a summation of several or all of these events.

The clinical consequences of activating Factor XII to Factor XIIa in an episode of DIC is as follows. When Factor XIIa is circulating, there may be activation of the fibrinolytic system via mechanisms previously discussed. Subsequent to this there will be biodegradation of numerous coagulation factors, the clinical manifestation of which will be hemorrhage. Secondly, the generation of Factor XIIa may lead to kinin activation with attendant vasodilation and the resultant clinical manifestations of hypotension and shock.[82,169,170,242,324] Thirdly, as Factor XIIa circulates and activates the fibrinolytic system, there will be subsequent activation of the complement system with cell lysis, vascular changes, and a platelet release reaction.[153,154] Platelet release will likewise provide more coagulant material to self-perpetuate the intravascular clotting process; the vascular changes of complement activation are comprised of increased vascular permeability, again leading to hypotension and shock.

Those clinical situations that may give rise to endothelial damage, endothelial sloughing with exposure of subendothelial collagen and subendothelial basement membrane, and the subsequent activation of Factor XII to Factor XIIa and possible XI to XIa are viremias, presumably through the mechanism of circulating antigen-antibody complex, heat stroke, patients with hyperacute renal allograft rejection, circulating antigen-antibody complexes of any origin, shock and attendant hypoxia and acidosis, endotoxemia, and very importantly ongoing DIC with subsequent vascular damage.[93,149,314,319,338] Many of the pathophysiologic events in DIC, as previously discussed, will give rise to significant endothelial damage with endothelial sloughing and the exposure of subendothelial collagen and basement membrane and subsequent activation of Factor XII to Factor XIIa and possibly Factor XI to Factor XIa thus, again, self-perpetuating the DIC-type process.

Clinical Findings

The general signs and symptoms of DIC can be highly variable and generally consist of fever, hypotension, acidosis, proteinuria, and hypoxia.[20,21,31] These findings are rather general signs and symptoms and may be found in many disorders and are, therefore, not particularly helpful from the diagnostic standpoint. However, more specific signs that are found in patients with DIC and should alert one to the possibility of DIC in the appropriate clinical settings consistent of petechiae and purpura, which are found in the vast majority of patients with DIC, hemorrhagic bullae, acryl cyanosis and, at times, frank gangrene.[20,21,31,32,140,197,222,273,285] In addition, wound bleeding, especially oozing from a surgical or traumatic wound, is an extremely common finding in patients with DIC. Oozing from venipuncture sites or intra-arterial lines is an additional common finding.[21] Large subcutaneous hematomas as well as deep tissue bleeding may also frequently be seen.[21] The average patient with DIC usually bleeds from at least three unrelated sites.[20,21,31,45] For example, the patient may have petechiae and purpura, oozing from intravenous puncture sites, and massive gastrointestinal blood loss or,

as an example, may have petechiae and purpura, massive hemoptysis, and hematuria. At times, other types of bleeding may also occur in deep tissues, including intracranial hemorrhage and compartmental compression syndromes. It should be realized that any combination of types of bleeding sites can be seen, and it is unclear as to why one person will bleed from one site rather than another.

A significant amount of microvascular thrombosis and, at times, large vessel thrombosis may also occur in DIC and may not be clinically obvious unless looked for.[21,31,233,237,294] Table 6–5 gives the incidence of end organ dysfunction in DIC, these findings represent microvascular thrombosis of tissues with resultant ischemia and hypoxia rather than end organ hemorrhage. Those systems that have a high incidence of microvascular thrombosis associated with subsequent end organ dysfunction include cardiac, pulmonary, renal, and central nervous system dysfunction.[21,238] Thrombotic thrombocytopenic purpura (TTP) is commonly associated with central nervous system dysfunction; however, it should be realized that this can occur just as commonly in acute DIC.[248]

Morphologic Findings

Morphologic findings in DIC consist of characteristic but not pathognomonic peripheral smear findings as well as hemorrhage in any organ or combination of organs.[61,310] It is again emphasized that

Table 6–5 End Organ Dysfunction from Microthrombi in Disseminated Intravascular Coagulation

Organ System	Percent Involved*
Skin	70%
Lungs	50%
Kidneys	50%
Pituitary	50%
Liver	35%
Adrenals	30%
Heart	20%

*Microthrombi are found in 50% without shock and in 60% with shock.

any organ may be associated with rather severe hemorrhage in patients with acute or chronic DIC. Early morphologic findings are platelet rich microthrombi.[61,310] These are usually seen in association with intense vasoconstriction presumably due to compounds released from platelets, including biogenic amines, adenine nucleotides, and kinins.[234] These are later replaced by hyaline-rich microthrombi.[61,310] Another early finding is that of fibrin monomer deposition primarily in the reticuloendothelial system; these findings require special staining.[62]

Later findings in patients with acute DIC are the typical fibrin-rich hyaline microthrombi that are thought to replace earlier deposited platelet-rich microthrombi and fibrin monomer deposits.[66,196] In addition, many patients with acute DIC develop typical pulmonary hyaline membranes that account, in part, for the significant degree of pulmonary dysfunction and hypoxemia seen in these patients.[63,75] In this regard it should be noted that pure adult shock lung syndrome is most likely an organ specific DIC-type pathophysiology that usually remains localized to the pulmonary bed.[21] Peripheral smear alterations typically seen in DIC are listed in Table 6-6. Schistocytes are red cell fragments, including atypical so-called "Heilmeyer Helmet cells," which are seen in approximately 50% of patients with acute DIC.[13,72,73,156] The mechanisms for the formation of schistocytes in acute DIC have been elegantly demonstrated by Bull and associates[74,290] who describe fibrin-red cell interactions, which are depicted in Figure 6-4. It is to be emphasized that the absence of schistocytes can certainly not be used to rule out a diagnosis of acute DIC because they only occur in 50%

Table 6-6 Typical Peripheral Smear Alterations in Disseminated Intravascular Coagulation

Schistocytes (red cell fragments)
Reticulocytosis
Polychromatophilia
Leukocytosis with mild shift
Thrombocytopenia
Large young platelets

of patients. The degree of thrombocytopenia that is usually present in most instances of acute DIC is often obvious by examination of the peripheral blood smear.[143,312] In addition, many so-called large bizarre platelets, representing young platelets, are usually seen on the peripheral smear in patients with DIC; this finding most likely simply represents an increased population of young platelets due to increased platelet turnover and decreased platelet survival due to platelet entrapment in microthrombi.[171,172] Figure 6-5 reveals a typical peripheral smear from a patient with acute DIC. In this patient the DIC was secondary to meningococcemia, and approximately 30% of this patient's red cells are fragmented.

Platelet-rich microthrombi are early findings in patients with DIC and are often easily demonstrated in the pulmonary microcirculation where they are usually seen in association with intense vasoconstriction due to vasoconstrictive compounds released from platelets. It is thought that these platelet-rich microthrombi are later replaced by more typical hyaline-rich microthrombi.[61,102,310] Figure 6-6 depicts an early platelet microthrombus found in the pulmonary microcirculation. Note the intense vasoconstriction present. Fibrin monomer may also be precipitated early in DIC, but this is not commonly appreciated because fibrin monomer is not demonstrated with usual staining techniques and requires periodic acid-Schiff (PAS) staining following ethanol fixation of appropriate tissue. Fibrin monomer is most commonly precipitated in the reticuloendothelial system and a study of Figure 6-7 will allow one to appreciate that precipitation of fibrin monomer may cause significant end organ damage due both to primary cellular or tissue damage as well as to microvascular occlusion. In addition, with this precipitation will come impaired reticuloendothelial clearance of FDPs, activated clotting factors, and circulating soluble fibrin monomer.

Typical hyaline microthrombi occurring later in an episode of DIC, and commonly accounting for significant end organ damage, are of three types. Globular hyaline microthrombi may be seen on

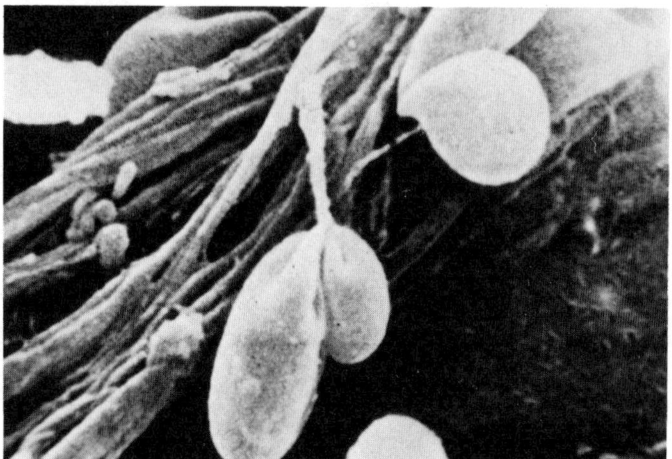

Fig. 6–4. Schistocyte formation. (From: Bull B, Rubenberg M, Dacie J, Brain MC: Microangiopathic hemolytic anemia: Mechanisms of red-cell fragmentation. Br J Haematol 14: 643, 1968. With permission)

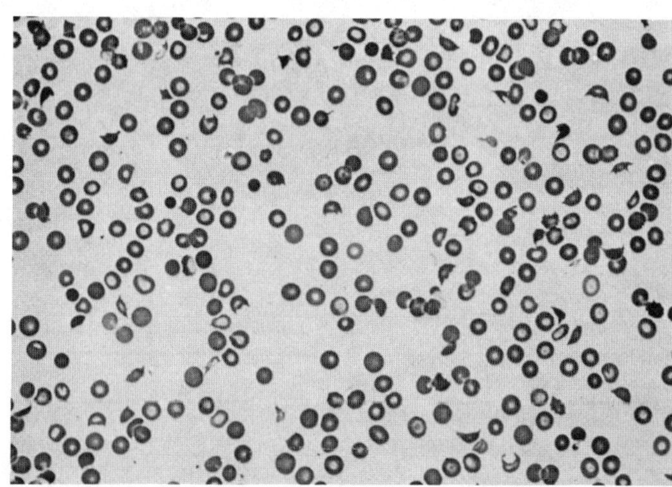

Fig. 6–5. Red cell fragments in DIC.

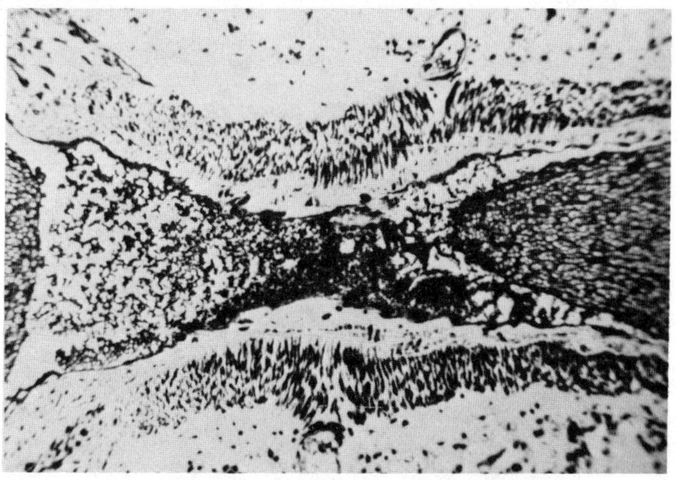

Fig. 6–6. Platelet-rich microthrombus.

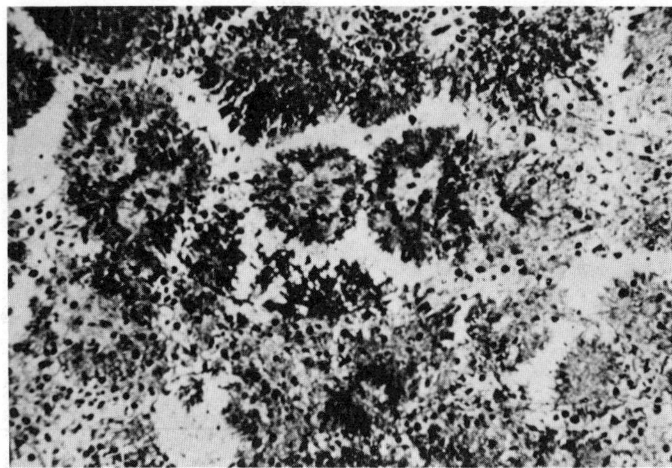

Fig. 6–7. Fibrin monomer precipitation in the reticuloendothelial system (liver).

the peripheral blood smear and are comprised of highly polymerized complexes of FDPs and many intermediates.[61,311] These may be from 4 to 60 μ^3 in volume and may occur singly or in mass and may be noted on a peripheral smear stained with PAS. They are also seen intravascularly but rarely appear to occlude the microcirculation. The second type is the typical intravascular hyaline microthrombus seen by pathologists at postmortem examination in DIC patients.[61,70,239] It should be pointed out, however, that these microthrombi are not pathognomonic of DIC and may be seen in other related disorders, including TTP.[245,248] These intravascular hyaline microthrombi

are homogenous, compact, structures that are oriented parallel to the blood flow and occasionally are noted to contain platelets or white cell fragments. They are easily seen by PAS, trichrome, tryptophan, and fluorescein-labeled antifibrinogen antiserum staining and are readily seen by electron microscopy.[60,126,331] Figure 6–8 depicts globular hyaline microthrombi and Figure 6–9 represents a typical intravascular hyaline microthrombus seen at postmortem examination, in this instance in the pulmonary microcirculation. Finally, pulmonary hyaline membranes are also a form of hyaline microthrombus and consist of highly polymerized complexes of FDPs and all types of intermediates.[211,315]

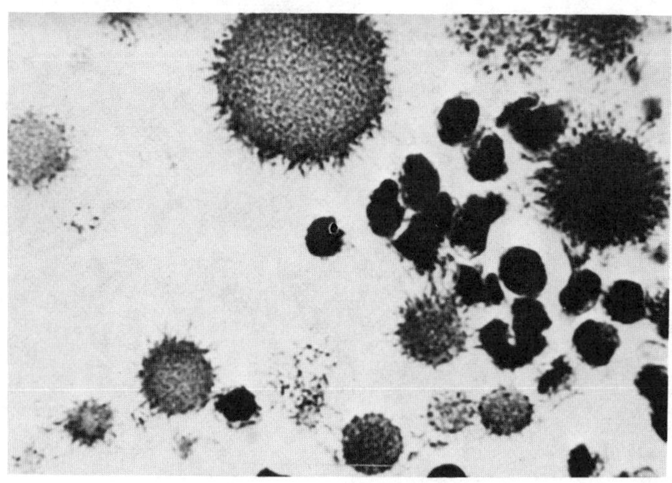

Fig. 6–8. Globular hyaline microthrombi.

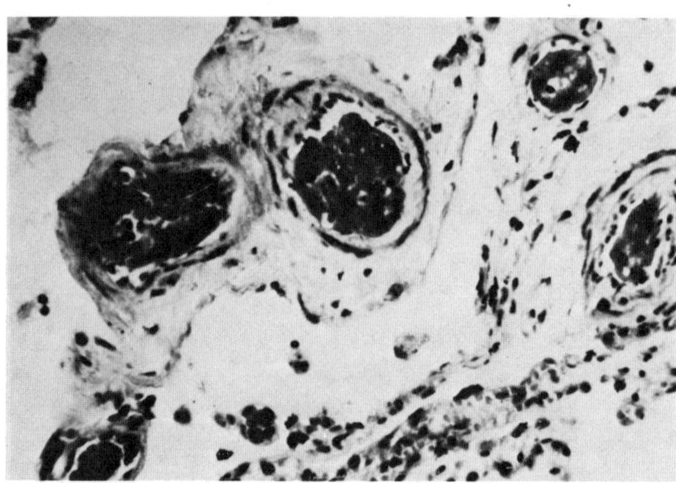

Fig. 6–9. Intravascular hyaline microthrombi.

They are usually seen to cover the alveolar epithelium with a preference for areas that have been denuded of epithelial cells. In addition, the interalveolar capillaries beneath these hyaline membranes often show abnormal vascular permeability with the circulation of endothelial cells, plasma protein precipitation between endothelial borders, and the formation of interstitial edema.

It should be appreciated that many patients with DIC develop these pulmonary hyaline membranes, which may account for significant pulmonary failure, abnormal arterial blood gases and pulmonary function tests, including markedly altered diffusion capacity. In addition, it should be emphasized that so-called pure adult shock-lung syndrome shares similar pathophysiology with acute DIC and in this particular instance the pathophysiology appears to remain localized to the pulmonary microcirculation rather than becoming a systemic process.[141,177] However, the pulmonary hyaline membranes of adult shock-lung syndrome and those seen in DIC are identical. For that matter, the pulmonary hyaline membranes seen in pediatric respiratory distress syndrome are also comprised of the same material: highly polymerized complexes of fibrinogen and fibrin, and FDPs. In this particular clinical situation the pathophysiology also remains much the same as in systemic DIC. This phenomenon has recently been carefully studied and reviewed by Ambrus

and coworkers[5–7] and it appears that in the normal infant during normal delivery, a short period of hypoxia occurs and concomitant with this is endothelial sloughing with the usual precipitation of fibrin that is then removed by subsequent activation of the fibrinolytic system. However, in patients with pediatric respiratory distress syndrome this physiologic event may be altered. In infants born of diabetic mothers the same process occurs, with deposition of polymerized complexes of fibrinogen and fibrin; however, in these infants there are elevated levels of alpha-2-macroglobulins that appear to inhibit the ability of the fibrinolytic system to degrade these deposits and hence a resultant "hyaline membrane."[8]

Similar pathophysiology appears to exist in the premature infant, and in this case there is hypoplasminogenemia and thus a hypoactive fibrinolytic system for activation and therefore fibrinogen and fibrin deposition continues unchecked with no ability to resolve this, and a pulmonary "hyaline membrane" results.[81,335] Understanding the pathophysiology of pediatric respiratory distress syndrome has led to the relatively successful use of plasminogen concentrates in infants with this disease.[5] Figure 6–10 depicts hyaline membranes as well as pulmonary edema in an infant dying from DIC secondary to meningococcemia.

As previously emphasized, DIC is a process associated with hemorrhage and

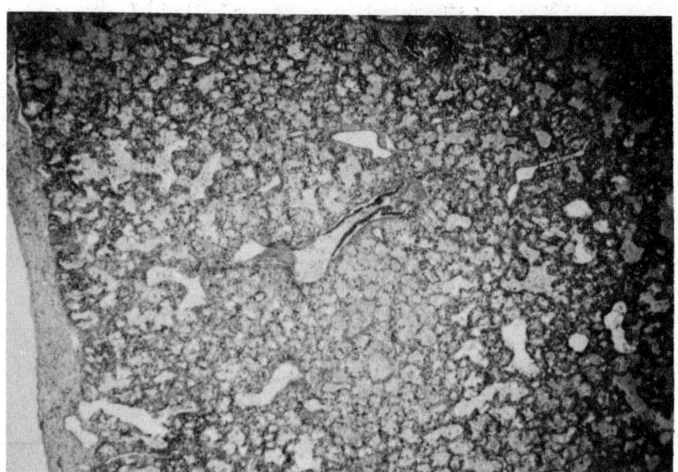

Fig. 6–10. Pulmonary hyaline membranes and congestion in DIC.

thrombosis, although thrombosis is less clinically evident and less commonly appreciated by the clinician until late in a course of DIC or until autopsy is performed. However, hemorrhage may often be successfully contended with in patients with DIC, whereas thrombosis in the microcirculation and macrocirculation may often lead to end organ damage with irreversible ischemic changes that may result in death of a patient. It is therefore useful to examine those parameters that may accelerate or, indeed, cause precipitation of microthrombi and macrothrombi in patients with DIC. Identifiable precipitating causes for acceleration or induction of microthrombi are given in Table 6–7. It will be noticed that important causes are vasomotor reactions, including elevated catecholamines and progressive acidosis.[142,240] In addition, glucocorticoids or ACTH elevation may also contribute to the precipitation of microthrombi in DIC patients, and thus careful thought must be given to the use of steroids in these patients, although in many instances steroid use is indeed warranted.[21,193] In addition, if present, impaired reticuloendothelial clearance (due to fibrin monomer precipitation or the use of steroids) of FDP, circulating soluble fibrin monomer, or activated coagulation factors (especially Factor Xa or thrombin),

could also markedly enhance the precipitation of microthrombi.[21,195] Impaired fibrinolytic system activation may also lead to accelerated fibrin deposition throughout the circulation.[21,223] All of these mechanisms, as well as many interplays between them, may lead to accelerated fibrin monomer precipitation in the microcirculation and macrocirculation with attendant end organ damage that may be irreversible and lead to significant morbidity and mortality.[21] When seeing a patient with DIC, it should be appreciated that these potential mechanisms and their interactions may be operative and should be kept in mind.

Table 6–7 Precipitation of Microthrombi in Disseminated Intravascular Coagulation

Platelets (platelet factor 4)
Granulocytes (release)
Vasomotor Reactions
   Elevated catecholamines
   Acidosis
   Elevated ACTH
   Glucocorticoids
Poor reticuloendothelial clearance of
   Soluble fibrin monomer
   Fibrin(ogen) degradation products
   Activated clotting factors
Impaired fibrinolytic activity

Clinical Findings of Chronic Disseminated Intravascular Coagulation

The clinical findings of chronic DIC are usually significantly different from those in patients with acute DIC. Patients with chronic DIC more commonly have bothersome bleeding and diffuse thromboses rather than acute fulminant life-threatening hemorrhage.[21,261] These patients have been appropriately described as having a "compensated DIC."[86,261] In this instance there is usually an increased turnover and decreased survival of many components of the hemostasis system, including the platelets, fibrinogen, Factor V, and Factor VIII. Because of this, most coagulation laboratory parameters are normal or near normal.[21,86,261] However, patients with chronic DIC almost uniformly have significantly elevated FDPs leading to impairment of fibrin monomer polymerization and a clinically significant platelet function defect resulting from the coating of platelet membranes by FDP. Thus, patients with chronic DIC commonly present with findings of gingival bleeding, easy and spontaneous bruising, large cutaneous ecchymoses, and mild to moderate mucosal membrane bleeding often manifested as genitourinary or gastrointestinal hemorrhage. However, patients may also present with diffuse or singular thromboses that are quite taxing with respect to clinical management.

Laboratory Abnormalities

With the complex pathophysiology depicted previously, the laboratory findings of DIC may be highly variable, complex, and difficult to interpret unless the pathophysiology of this disorder is firmly understood. Likewise, the evaluation of patients with DIC, especially with respect to significant laboratory tests that are useful for aiding in the diagnosis as well as for monitoring efficacy of therapy remains highly confusing and in some instances controversial. To complicate the situation further, many new modalities have become available for assessing the patient with DIC; however, many of these modalities are as yet without enough experience to determine how clinically applicable they may be.[33,109,110,230,231]

The prothrombin time should be abnormal in the vast majority of patients with DIC for multiple reasons. Firstly, the prothrombin time depends on the ultimate conversion of fibrinogen to fibrin, and in DIC there is hypofibrinogenemia and FDP as well as thrombin interference with fibrin monomer polymerization. Additionally, plasmin-induced lysis of Factors V and X, to which the prothrombin time should be sensitive, is often present. In fact, the prothrombin time is prolonged in approximately 75% of patients with acute DIC; in the other 25% of patients the prothrombin time is normal or supernormal. The reasons for this are as follows: a circulating activated clotting factor, such as thrombin or Factor Xa, may accelerate the formation of thrombin and the subsequent conversion of fibrinogen to fibrin in the test system and thus render a normal or supernormal result even though some coagulation factors to which the prothrombin time are sensitive may be extremely low. In addition, early degradation products may be rapidly clottable by thrombin and quickly "gel" the test system, producing a normal or supernormal prothrombin time.[20,21]

The activated partial thromboplastin time (APTT) should likewise be prolonged in acute DIC for multiple reasons. Firstly, there is effective plasmin-induced biodegradation of many clotting factors to which the APTT is sensitive, including Factors V, VIII, IX, and XI. In addition, the PTT, like the prothrombin time, is sensitive to (prolonged by) fibrinogen levels that may be less than 100 mg/dL in patients with DIC. The prothrombin time or APTT begins to prolong at a fibrinogen level of approximately 100 mg/dL or less. Additionally, the APTT should at least theoretically be prolonged because of FDP inhibition of fibrin monomer polymerization. However, the APTT is prolonged in only 50 to 60% of patients with acute DIC, and therefore a normal PTT can certainly not be used to rule out a diagnosis of acute

DIC. The reasons for a supernormal or normal PTT in 40 to 50% of patients are as follows. Firstly, early degradation products may rapidly be thrombin clottable and "gel" the test system, rendering a supernormal result. Secondly, and perhaps more commonly, is that circulating activated clotting factor is usually present in patients with acute DIC and activated clotting factors, especially circulating Factor Xa or circulating thrombin, may bypass the necessity of other clotting factors being measured in the APTT system, thus leading to rapid conversion of fibrinogen to fibrin and a supernormal test.[20,21]

The thrombin time and reptilase time should likewise be prolonged in patients with acute DIC. Both of these tests should be prolonged by the presence of circulating FDPs and interference with fibrin monomer polymerization as well as prolongation from the hypofibrinogenemia commonly present in acute DIC.[36,34–36,181] In fact, both of these tests are generally prolonged in patients with DIC; however, for reasons previously mentioned, they may be normal or supernormal in isolated cases. An additional "bonus test" may be derived from either one or both of these tests by observing the resultant clot for absence or presence of clot lysis. Since many laboratories do not have facilities for assessing the fibrinolytic system, this simple nonquantitative tool may provide significant clinical information. Thus, instead of throwing away the thrombin time or reptilase time derived clot, the tube can be observed after 5 to 10 minutes for evidence of clot dissolution. If the clot is not dissolving by 10 minutes, it may be assumed that the amount of plasmin circulating is not clinically significant; however, if the clot begins to lyse within this period, a clinically significant amount of plasmin is likely to be present.

The platelet count is usually significantly decreased in patients with acute DIC; however, the range may be quite variable and may be as low as 2000 to 3000/mm^3 or greater than 100,000/mm^3. However, in most patients with acute DIC the degree of thrombocytopenia is usually obvious by examination of a peripheral smear and averages about 60,000/mm^3. Virtually all tests of platelet function, in-

cluding the template bleeding time, platelet aggregation, and platelet lumiaggregation, will be abnormal in patients with DIC. This primarily occurs because of FDP coating of platelet membranes; there may be other potential reasons for platelet dysfunction as well, such as partial release of platelet procoagulant materials. Thus, there is no reason for performing tests of platelet function in patients with acute DIC, since abnormal results will invariably be found and add little to the diagnosis. It should be mentioned that no typical aggregation or lumiaggregation patterns are noted in DIC, and a wide variety of different types of defects may be seen in different patients.[21,30,33]

Coagulation factor assays will provide little, if any, clinical useful information in patients with DIC. In the majority with acute DIC there is systemically circulating activated clotting factor present, especially Factors Xa, IXa, and thrombin.[21,37,38] Thus, coagulation factor assays done by the standard APTT-derived or prothrombin time-derived laboratory techniques using deficient substrates will render uninterpretable and meaningless results in patients with DIC. For example, if a Factor VIII assay were attempted in the presence of circulating Factor Xa in a patient with DIC, a high level of Factor VIII would be recorded, since Factor Xa "bypasses" the necessity for Factor VIII:C in the test system[21,187,266,301] and a rapid conversion of fibrinogen to fibrin will be noted; thus a rapid time will be recorded on the typical standard curve and this will be interpreted as a high Factor VIII level when there may, in fact, be no Factor VIII present at all. Thus, factor assays will produce erroneous and meaningless results and are virtually uninterpretable and certainly add little or nothing to the diagnosis of DIC.

FDPs are elevated in 85 to 100% of patients with acute DIC, depending on the series reported.[21,30,33,209,246] It is a common misconception that elevated FDPs are diagnostic of DIC and it should be recalled that these degradation products are only "diagnostic" of plasmin biodegradation of fibrinogen or fibrin, and FDPs are therefore only indicative of the presence of plasmin. Their method of formation was discussed in Chapter 1 and the possibility of false-negative results in some patients with DIC will be discussed subsequently.

The protamine sulfate test or ethanol gelation test for circulating soluble fibrin monomer is almost always positive[15,21,30,136,148,269,346] in acute and chronic DIC and is a highly useful test. However, like the FDP titer, it is not diagnostic because both elevated FDPs and circulating soluble fibrin monomer can be noted in other clinical situations as well, including women using oral contraceptives, patients with pulmonary emboli, selected patients with myocardial infarction, patients with certain selected renal diseases, and patients with arterial or venous thrombotic or thromboembolic events.[270,316] On occasion, the protamine sulfate test or ethanol gelation test may be negative for reasons to be discussed. In these rare instances, after successful therapy, the test may become positive for a short period of time and then revert to negative.[21] The protamine sulfate test as described by Kidder and associates[176] appears to be the most sensitive and clinically applicable test for circulating soluble fibrin and is the one used by my laboratory.

The antithrombin III (AT III) determination has become a key test for aiding the diagnosis and monitoring of therapy in patients with acute and chronic DIC.[39,40,159] In DIC there is almost always an overwhelming generation of activated clotting factors (serine proteases) during the activation (triggering) process as well as during the ongoing intravascular coagulation event. When this occurs, there is an irreversible complexing of some circulating activating clotting factor with AT III, thus leading to significant decreases of functional AT III in the majority of patients with acute and chronic DIC.[2,40,41,145,256,302] As will be discussed in subsequent sections, the determination of an AT III assay provides one of the few reliable modalities for monitoring efficacy of anticoagulant therapy in patients with DIC. Several recent studies have compared the clinical applicability of various AT III methods and, based on these studies, synthetic substrate assay methods are clearly

the method of choice.[42,59,111] Immunologic assays for AT III ignore biologic function and may be normal or low. Just because AT III is complexed with a serine protease does not necessarily mean the antigenic determinants, as measured by immunologic assays, are no longer present. Thus, immunologic assays for AT III in patients with DIC should not be used.[21]

Increased platelet turnover and decreased platelet survival will usually be seen in patients with DIC.[183,345] However, since thrombocytopenia is often present, this method of following patients may be of questionable significance, especially in severely thrombocytopenic patients. It has been found that simple methods using automated electronic counting techniques have proved useful in monitoring efficacy of therapy in patients with chronic DIC provided the platelet count is greater than $80,000/mm^3$.[43] Platelet factor 4 levels and beta-thromboglobulin levels are newer assay techniques that are markers of overall platelet reactivity and release. As such, several recent reports have suggested that either one of these two modalities may be highly useful in aiding in a diagnosis of DIC as well as in monitoring efficacy of therapy with respect to blunting or causing cessation of the intravascular clotting process.[43,115,203,212,343,344] Both assays are now readily available for the clinical laboratory and each has its attendant advantages and disadvantages. Both platelet factor 4 and beta-thromboglobulin are elevated in the vast majority of instances of DIC; however, it should be readily appreciated that neither of these modalities are diagnostic of DIC because they may be elevated in a wide variety of intravascular coagulation disorders, including pulmonary emboli, acute myocardial infarction, deep vein thrombosis, and in many disorders associated with microvascular disease, such as diabetes and autoimmune disorders.[204,253] However, if they are noted to be elevated in the patient with DIC and then decrease after the institution of specific therapy, this may provide a useful sign that therapy has been successful in either blunting or stopping the intravascular clotting process.

Fibrinopeptide A is commonly elevated in patients with DIC and is an overall assessment of hemostasis, much like platelet factor 4 and beta-thromboglobulin levels. The presence of fibrinopeptide A is "diagnostic" of the presence of thrombin acting on fibrinogen. Fibrinopeptide A determinations may be of aid in assessing efficacy of therapy, as has been suggested in several studies.[71,90,100,179,233,255] However, the determination of fibrinopeptide A is presently laborious for the routine clinical laboratory and is not diagnostic of DIC, since it may be found elevated in a wide variety of other microvascular or macrovascular thrombotic events, as previously discussed. However, the noting of high fibrinopeptide A levels followed by dropping of these levels with the institution of therapy may be a good prognostic sign with respect to stopping or blunting the intravascular clotting process. A newer modality, also available by radioimmunoassay, is the B-beta 15-42 and related peptide determination,[112,113,275] which if elevated may, when performed in conjunction with concomitant fibrinopeptide A levels, add greatly to the differential diagnosis of DIC versus primary lysis. As previously discussed, plasmin will rapidly cleave B-beta peptides 1 through 118, 1 through 42, and 15 through 42 (after thrombin has cleaved fibrinopeptide B or amino acid sequence 1 through 14) off of the B-beta chain of fibrinogen. Thus, the elevation of B-beta 15-42 and related peptides in the absence of fibrinopeptide A is strong evidence for primary fibrinolysis, whereas the elevation of both fibrinopeptide A and B-beta 15-42 related peptides is strong evidence of DIC.

Fibrinolytic system assays are now readily available to the clinical laboratory and provide highly useful information in patients with DIC. Typically, there are decreased plasminogen levels and circulating plasmin present.[3,20,21,281,283] The presence or absence of a secondary fibrinolytic response is of clinical value in predicting the degree of potential microvascular thrombosis and resultant irreversible end organ damage in patients. If there is inadequate or absent activation of the fibrinolytic system, the degree of morbidity and mortality due to end organ damage may be expected to be greater. The degree of fibrinolytic system activation can be assessed by mea-

suring plasminogen and plasmin levels by currently available synthetic substrate techniques.[78,124,192,317,329] In this regard, the euglobulin lysis time provides little or no clinically useful information with respect to assessing the fibrinolytic system in clinical disorders, including DIC.[21,182,225] The preparation of a euglobulin fraction, by definition, destroys fibrinolytic inhibitors and thus a positive result is of questionable clinical meaning and may simply represent an artifact. Thus, this test should not be used in clinical medicine. The measurement of fibrinolytic inhibitors, including fast-acting alpha-2-antiplasmin[83,34,103,137,327] and slow-acting alpha-2-macroglobulin[146,243,262] may also be of help in assessing the overall fibrinolytic system in DIC patients. If these two fibrinolytic system inhibitors are markedly elevated, there may be an inadequate fibrinolytic response and resultant enhanced fibrin monomer precipitation, fibrin deposition, and microvascular or macrovascular thrombosis. Recently, assays for tissue (endothelial) plasminogen activator have become available; as more experience becomes available this determination may also become useful in DIC patients.

Fibrinogen chromatography may provide a new and sensitive modality for assessing DIC patients and may prove useful for both aiding in a diagnosis as well as for allowing detailed monitoring of efficacy of therapy in these patients.[3,11,119,120,250] Although this modality is currently only used in large centers specializing in thrombohemorrhagic disorders, it has provided quite impressive data and may become clinically applicable in the future, as will be discussed subsequently.

By understanding the pathophysiology of DIC, it is quite clear that most tests of hemostasis will be highly altered and thus most common laboratory tests will be significantly abnormal.[14,188,205,309] It is therefore useful to determine which tests are of practical significance with respect to providing a high degree of reliability as well as availability in assessing patients with DIC. Tests useful for aiding in a diagnosis of DIC are given in Table 6–8 (tests routinely used for both aiding in a diagnosis of DIC and monitoring efficacy of therapy are asterisked). In general, I do

Table 6–8 Laboratory Evaluation of Acute Disseminated Intravascular Coagulation

Prolonged prothrombin time
Prolonged partial thromboplastin time
Prolonged thrombin time
Prolonged reptilase time
Elevated fibrin(ogen) degradation products*
Positive protamine sulfate test*
Decreased antithrombin III*
Thrombocytopenia*
Schistocytosis*
Leukocytosis
Elevated platelet factor 4*
Elevated beta-thromboglobulin
Elevated fibrinopeptide A*
Elevated B-beta 15–42 related peptides*
Low plasminogen levels*
Circulating plasmin*
Abnormal fibrinogen chromatograms

*Most useful and reliable tests at present.

not indulge in "DIC panels" and prefer to let the particular clinical situation in conjunction with clinical judgment dictate which laboratory tests are to be obtained both initially and subsequent to therapy.[21,36,37,44] However, if a true "DIC panel" were to be devised, those tests which are asterisked would be the recommended current tests for aiding in the diagnosis and monitoring efficacy of therapy because they are readily available and reasonably reliable when evaluated together. However, it must be stressed that none of these tests are diagnostic of DIC and, as in all areas of clinical medicine, laboratory modalities must be evaluated in the *appropriate clinical setting*. In addition, most of these laboratory tests are certainly not specific. The presence of soluble monomer is one of the more specific tests, but certainly not diagnostic. If circulating soluble fibrin monomer is present, as detected by the protamine sulfate test or ethanol gelation test, this is strong evidence that thrombin and plasmin have circulated. Since fibrin monomer is created by the presence of thrombin and fibrin monomer has to then be solubilized by complexing with FDPs created by plasmin, this test determines the presence of both enzymes. The presence of gamma-gamma dimers is likewise a relatively specific, although not diagnostic, test. The presence of gamma chains suggests the presence of plasmin, and if these gamma

chains have been cross-linked by Factor XIIIa, thus creating dimers, this is suggestive of the presence of thrombin, which is the primary activation enzyme for Factor XIIIa.[202] Fibrinogen chromatography also provides a rather specific, although not diagnostic, test for the presence of the enzymes plasmin and thrombin.

Table 6–9 lists the biologic AT III levels in a series of patients with acute and chronic DIC.[46] It will be noted that the vast majority of patients display significant decreases in AT III levels at the time of diagnosis. One exception to this is patients with disseminated malignancy and concomitant DIC. In some instances it appears that AT III as an alpha-2-globulin behaves as an acute phase reactant and may be consumed (complexed) to normal or near normal levels in patients with disseminated malignancy and concomitant DIC.[21,23,24,47,48] However, in most all other instances of acute or chronic DIC, this serine protease inhibitor appears to be significantly and rapidly decreased. In addition, protein C as well as fibronectin levels are decreased in patients with DIC, although their diagnostic efficacy as well as usefulness to monitor therapeutic efficacy remains to be established.[106,134]

As previously discussed, fibrinogen is comprised of an A-alpha, B-beta, and gamma chain, and plasmin first digests along the carboxy terminal of the A-alpha chain, giving rise to Fragment X. Following this, there is asymmetrical digestion by plasmin along the amino-terminal end

Table 6–9 Antithrombin III Levels in Disseminated Intravascular Coagulation

Patient	AT III (%)	Type of DIC
1	36	Chronic
2	81	Chronic
3	36	Chronic
4	65	Chronic
5	85	Chronic
6	32	Chronic
7	52	Chronic
8	65	Acute
9	50	Acute
10	137	Acute
11	75	Acute
12	31	Acute
13	85	Acute

of all three chains, giving rise to a fragment Y and a Fragment D. Subsequently, Fragment Y is further asymmetrically digested on the opposing amino-terminal portion, giving rise to another Fragment D and a Fragment E, or so-called N-terminal disulfide knot. Figure 1–30 reveals that Fragments X and Y still contain fibrinopeptides, and they are thus thrombin clottable. Understanding this and the method of plasmin-induced digestion allows an understanding of why, in selected instances, in acute or chronic DIC patients FDP titers may be negative. The currently available FDP determinations utilize latex particles that are "antifibrinogen" and therefore thrombin clot tubes are supplied to clot out fibrinogen so that latex particles will not react with fibrinogen and erroneously measure fibrinogen rather than its degradation products.[241] However, fibrinogen and its degradation products have common antigenic determinants.[244] When these thrombin clot-tubes are used, not only is fibrinogen removed from the system but also Fragment X and Fragment Y. For this reason currently available FDP methods measure Fragments D and E. Thus, in some instances of DIC when there may be minimal secondary fibrinolytic responses and minimal plasmin circulating, there may only be degradation to the X fragment stage or some intermediate between fibrin(ogen) and Fragment X. In this instance there may be nothing for the test to measure, since Fragment X and its intermediates may be removed from the test system by the thrombin clot tubes used. Alternatively, in instances of acute DIC in which there is a massive secondary fibrinolytic activation and overwhelming amounts of plasmin circulating, there may be degradation past the D and E stages. Fragments D and E are the last degradation products that have antigenic determinants that are capable of being detected by the currently available commercial FDP titer kits. An additional problem is that of massive release of granulocyte enzymes, collagenases and elastases, which may also degrade all available D and E fragments and again render negative FDP titers in patients with acute DIC.[49] Thus, the presence of negative FDP titers cannot be used

to rule out a diagnosis of acute or chronic DIC. Despite these difficulties, FDP titers are almost always elevated in DIC patients.

Table 6–10 depicts those subspecies of fibrinogen and its degradation products that can be readily detected by fibrinogen chromatography. If there is an increase in high molecular weight fibrinogen complexes the presence of thrombin can be assumed. Alternatively, when noticing an increase in concentration of early fibrinogen "first derivitive," it can be assumed that plasmin is present. The concentrations of these two derivitives in conjunction with elevated FDP titers can lead to significant information with respect to aiding in a diagnosis and monitoring of therapy in DIC. For example, if thrombin plus plasmin are circulating in early DIC, both high molecular weight fibrinogen complexes and fibrinogen "first derivitive" will be seen. As the thrombotic events begin to subside, high molecular weight polymerized complexes will begin to decrease and as the fibrinolytic system becomes activated and plasmin begins to biodegrade fibrinogen and fibrin deposited in the microcirculation, fibrinogen "first derivitive" concentrations and FDPs will begin to increase, providing a sensitive method of monitoring efficacy of therapy. Clinical information provided by fibrinogen chromatography is summarized in Table 6–11.

Typical laboratory findings of chronic DIC are significantly different from those seen in acute DIC; many usual tests of hemostasis are normal or near normal and typical findings in chronic DIC are listed in Table 6–12. Although the platelet count

Table 6–10 Fibrinogen Derivatives Measured by Fibrinogen Chromatography

Fibrin Monomer: Fibrinogen minus fibrinopeptides A and B (Molecular weight, 320,000 daltons)

Fibrinogen dimer: Fibrinogen plus fibrin monomer (molecular weight, 650,000 daltons)

Fibrinogen polymer: Fibrinogen plus various fibrin(ogen) fragments (molecular weight, 400,000 to 1,000,000 daltons)

Fibrinogen "first derivitive": Minimal cleavage by plasmin (molecular weight, 267,000 daltons)

Fibrin(ogen) degradation products:
  Moderate cleavage by plasmin

Table 6–11 Clinical Monitoring with Fibrinogen Chromatography in Disseminated Intravascular Coagulation

Thrombosis (thrombin generation)
  Increased fibrin monomer levels
  Increased fibrin(ogen) complexes
  Increased fibrin(ogen) polymer
Thrombus resolution (plasmin circulation)
  Increased fibrinogen "first derivitive"
  Increased fibrin(ogen) degradation products
  Decreased fibrin monomer
  Decreased fibrin(ogen) complexes
  Decreased fibrin(ogen) polymer

Table 6–12 Laboratory Evaluation of Chronic Disseminated Intravascular Coagulation

Platelet count: Usually normal or boarderline
Fibrinogen: Normal or elevated
Factor VIII: C: Normal or elevated
Prothrombin time: Normal or fast
Activated PTT: Normal or fast
Schistocytes: Present in 90%
FDPs: Usually elevated
Protamine sulfate test: Usually positive
Fibrinopeptide A: Usually elevated
Plasminogen: Usually decreased
Plasmin: Usually present

is usually within normal limits or borderline in the patient with chronic DIC, most develop decreased platelet survival and increased turnover of platelets due to platelet consumption. This is often referred to as a "compensated state." Like the platelet count, fibrinogen levels are usually "compensated"; there is increased turnover and decreased survival of fibrinogen as well as Factor V, Factor VIII, and other coagulation proteins. Fibrinogen levels may be significantly elevated in chronic DIC because fibrinogen may behave as an acute phase reactant in many disorders associated with chronic DIC, including malignancy, autoimmune disorders, and chronic inflammatory diseases. For similar reasons, Factor VIII and Factor V levels may be normal or elevated in patients with chronic DIC, with increased turnover and decreased survival. The prothrombin time and APTT are usually within normal limits or supernormal in the patient with chronic DIC for reasons previously discussed. Red cell fragments or

schistocytes are present in almost all patients with chronic DIC, but are only present in 50% of the patients with acute DIC. This is most likely because of the nature of the underlying disease processes giving rise to chronic DIC, such as malignancy and related disorders. FDPs are almost always elevated in patients with chronic DIC and are quite useful for aiding in a diagnosis. The elevation of these fragments accounts for much of the pathophysiology and low-grade hemorrhage seen in patients with chronic DIC because of the platelet dysfunction that they induce. Soluble fibrin monomer is also commonly detected in patients with chronic DIC and, like the FDP titer, can be quite helpful and is a relatively specific finding. Often there is also elevated fibrinopeptide A, beta-thromboglobulin, platelet factor 4, and B-beta 15-42 related peptides in patients with chronic DIC. Their diagnostic efficacy remains to be determined, but looks promising, and the use of these assays in monitoring efficacy of therapy also remains to be determined, although they may prove quite helpful. Circulating plasmin associated with hypoplasminogenemia is also a common finding of patients with chronic DIC. In the appropriate clinical setting, the noting of elevated FDP, a positive protamine sulfate test, elevated fibrinopeptide A, elevated B-beta 15-42 peptides, and hypoplasminogenemia is strongly suggestive of chronic DIC.

Table 6–13 reveals average laboratory values, using commonly available laboratory modalities, in a series of 48 patients with acute DIC.[50] Average values for pretreatment and post-treatment are given,

Table 6–13 Average Laboratory Values in Acute Disseminated Intravascular Coagulation

	Pre-therapy	Post-therapy
Prothrombin	16.8 sec	13.6 sec
Activated PTT	55.8 sec	42.4 sec
Reptilase time	26.8 sec	18.8 sec
Thrombin time	23.8 sec	15.6 sec
FDP level	>40	>40
Platelets	64,600	204,000
Protamine sulfate	+	+
Fibrinogen	129 mg/dL	221 mg/dL
AT III	57.8%	101.4%

and post-treatment values were derived 4 to 6 hours after delivering therapy that was thought to stop or significantly blunt the intravascular clotting process. It will be noted that the prothrombin time and PTT are borderline prolonged. It is also noted that in the vast majority of patients these two tests are corrected to well within normal limits after the delivery of effective therapy. In addition, the average platelet count was 64,600/cmm at the time of making the diagnosis and 204,000/cmm after delivering of effective therapy. The average fibrinogen level was 129 mg% before therapy and 221 mg% after therapy.

Also of significance is the noting of AT III levels before and after therapy, which will be discussed in more detail subsequently. In this particular series of patients the average biologic AT III level was 58% at the time of making a diagnosis and well within normal range 4 to 6 hours after therapy which was thought to cause cessation or significant blunting of the intravascular clotting process.

Laboratory testing and the interpretation of the laboratory results with respect to aiding in the diagnosis and monitoring of therapy in patients with acute DIC remain highly confusing and, in fact, controversial, since studies of very few patient series have been published. The reliability of laboratory testing in patients with acute DIC is given in Table 6–14.[50] The percentage of abnormal results pretreatment and the percentage of those remaining abnormal post-treatment are depicted for each test. It will be noticed that in this series of patients, FDPs were elevated in 100% of patients at the time of making a diagnosis, but remained elevated in 25% of patients after the delivering of effective therapy; thus, FDP determinations are of significant diagnostic value but are of only limited value with respect to monitoring efficacy of therapy.

The AT III level was noted to be decreased in 97% of patients at the time of making a diagnosis and was only decreased in 16% of patients after delivering of therapy which was thought to be successful at stopping the intravascular clotting process. Thus, the AT III level appears to be quite useful for both aiding in the diagnosis as well as providing information

Table 6–14   Reliability of Laboratory Tests in Acute Disseminated Intravascular Coagulation

Test	Pre-therapy (% Abnormal)	Post-therapy (% Abnormal)
FDP level	100%	24%
AT III	97%	16%
Platelets	97%	34%
Protamine sulfate	92%	18%
Thrombin time	81%	32%
Fibrinogen	79%	16%
Prothrombin	76%	58%
APTT	63%	24%
Reptilase time	58%	8%

*Listed in descending order of reliability.

regarding cessation of the intravascular clotting process. It can be concluded from this study that the most reliable commonly used laboratory tests for aiding in a diagnosis of DIC and for monitoring efficacy of therapy in acute DIC are the FDP titer, the AT III level, the platelet count, the presence of soluble fibrin monomer, followed by the thrombin time, fibrinogen level, prothrombin time, PTT, and reptilase time, all of which appear to be significantly unreliable. It should be noted in this series of patients that the APTT was only prolonged in 63% of patients at the time of rendering a diagnosis of acute DIC, thus emphasizing that the APTT is not a reliable test for aiding in a diagnosis of DIC or for monitoring of therapy.

Table 6–15 summarizes average pretreatment and post-treatment values for commonly available laboratory modalities in a group of patients with chronic DIC.[21,49,50] It will be noted that the prothrombin time and APTT are even less reliable as diagnostic aids in chronic DIC, as are the fibrinogen level and platelet count. The AT III level is also less reliable in diagnosing chronic DIC; however, it appears to be almost as useful for monitoring efficacy of therapy as it is in acute DIC.

Table 6–16 gives the percentage of patients demonstrating an abnormal laboratory test at the time of making a diagnosis (pretherapy) and the percentage of those tests remaining abnormal after it was clinically deemed that the intravascular clotting process had been successfully stopped. It will be noticed that the FDP titer was elevated in all patients; how-

Table 6–15 Average Laboratory Values in Chronic Disseminated Intravascular Coagulation

Test	Pre-therapy	Post-therapy
Prothrombin time	14.4 sec	12.6 sec
APTT	43.9 sec	34.5 sec
Reptilase time	27.8 sec	18.2 sec
Thrombin time	17.7 sec	11.9 sec
FDP level	>40	>40
Platelets	190,000	254,000
Protamine sulfate	+	+
Fibrinogen	231 mg/dL	333 mg/dL
AT III	83.9%	116.8%

Table 6–16 Reliability of Laboratory Tests in Chronic Disseminated Intravascular Coagulation

Test*	Pre-therapy (% Abnormal)	Post-therapy (% Abnormal)
FDP Level	100%	50%
Protamine sulfate	80%	20%
Prothrombin	80%	30%
AT III	70%	10%
Reptilase time	70%	0%
Platelets	50%	30%
Fibrinogen	30%	0%
APTT	30%	10%
Thrombin time	30%	0%

*Listed in descending order of reliability.

Table 6–17 Reliability of Laboratory Tests in All Types of Disseminated Intravascular Coagulation

Test*	Pre-therapy (% Abnormal)	Post-therapy (% Abnormal)
FDP, elevated	100	31
AT III, decreased	89	8
Platelets, low	89	18
Protamine test, positive	89	10
Prothrombin test, long	82	47
Thrombin time, long	76	18
Fibrinogen, low	71	5
Reptilase time, long	66	58
APTT, long	63	21

*Listed in descending order of reliability.

Table 6–18 Laboratory Modalities Available for the Evaluation of Disseminated Intravascular Coagulation

Old Methods Manual	New Methods Automated
Prothrombin	AT III*
APTT	Plasminogen*
Thrombin time	Plasminogen activator*
Reptilase time	Plasmin*
Platelet count	Alpha-2-Antiplasmin*
Fibrinogen level	Fibrinogen[†]
Soluble fibrin monomer	Fibrinopeptide A[‡]
(protamine or ethanol)	Fibrinopeptide B[‡]
FDP titer	B-beta 15–42 peptides[‡]
Blood smear	Fibronectin[†]
Factor assays	Fibrinogen
(not useful)	chromatography
	Platelet survival
	Platelet factor 4[‡]
	Beta-thromboglobulin[‡]
	Prostaglandin Derivatives[‡]

* Synthetic substrate.
[†] Immunoassay and ELISA. These tests have not been clinically available long enough to indicate their usefulness in diagnosing and monitoring efficacy of therapy.
[‡] Radioimmunoassay.

bin time are of little diagnostic reliability in chronic DIC. Table 6–17 depicts the probability of pretreatment and post-treatment coagulation abnormalities in all forms of DIC.

It appears that the noting of elevated FDPs, a depressed AT III level in conjunction with thrombocytopenia, and a positive protamine sulfate test or ethanol gelation test appear to be the most reliable laboratory indices for aiding in and con-

ever, the titer remained elevated in 50% of patients after therapy. Likewise, soluble fibrin monomer was present in 80% of patients with chronic DIC but remained circulating in 20% of patients after successful therapy had been delivered. The prothrombin time appears to be more useful in chronic than acute DIC. The AT III level is of less diagnostic value (as it is only decreased in 70% of chronic DIC patients), but after therapy remained depressed in only 10%, suggesting that it is a useful monitoring modality. The platelet count, fibrinogen level, APTT, and thrombin time do not appear to be of useful diagnostic significance in chronic DIC. Thus, the reliability of commonly available laboratory tests for aiding in a diagnosis and monitoring therapy in chronic DIC are the FDP product titer, the presence of soluble fibrin monomer, the prothrombin time, and the AT III determination.[21,36,37,50,51] The reptilase time, platelet count, fibrinogen level, APTT, and throm-

Table 6-19 Molecular Marker Profiling in the Differential Diagnosis of Disseminated Intravascular Coagulation Type Syndromes Versus Thrombotic Thrombocytopenic Purpura

Marker	DIC	Primary Lysis
Fibrinopeptide A	Elevated	Normal
Fibrinopeptide B	Elevated	Normal
B-beta 15-42 peptide	Elevated	Normal
B-beta 1-42 peptide	Elevated	Elevated
B-beta 1-118 peptide	Elevated	Elevated
Platelet factor 4	Elevated	Normal
Beta-thromboglobulin	Elevated	Normal

firming a diagnosis of DIC and for helping to determine the success of therapy.[21,36,37,49-51] Likewise, other traditional tests, including the prothrombin time, thrombin time, fibrinogen level, reptilase time, and PTT are less reliable as diagnostic or therapeutic indices. Table 6-18 compares older and newer modalities that may be useful in diagnosing and monitoring therapy in DIC.[21,33] Newer methods are totally automated or at least automatable, and when their diagnostic efficacy is proved, they may aid greatly in providing data for diagnosis as well as for monitoring efficacy of therapy. Molecular marker profiling for DIC has now become available and is fully automatable.[52,53,114] These molecular markers are not only useful for diagnosing DIC, but are also useful for providing a differential diagnosis of DIC versus primary fibrinolysis or TTP. The differential diagnosis of DIC versus TTP by molecular marker profiling was discussed in Chapter 4; the differential diagnosis of DIC versus primary fibrinolysis by automated molecular marker profiling is summarized in Table 6-19. Many other similar disorders, some systemic and some organ specific or multiorgan specific, are listed in Table 6-20.

Therapy of Disseminated Intravascular Coagulation

Acute

The treatment of acute and chronic DIC remains confusing to many and, indeed, controversial. Concomitant with this controversy and confusion is the general feel-

Table 6-20 Conditions Similar to Disseminated Intravascular Coagulation

Thrombotic thrombocytopenic purpura
Pediatric respiratory distress syndrome
Adult respiratory distress syndrome (shock lung)
Hemolytic-uremic syndrome
Malignant hypertension
Preeclampsia or eclampsia
Glomerulonephritis
Collagen vascular disorders
Circulating immune complex disorders
Serum sickness
Cavernous hemangioma
Hemangio(endothelio)sarcoma
Traumatic arteriovenous fistula
Vasculitis
Rocky Mountain spotted fever
Mycoplasma infections
"Waring blender" syndrome

ing that therapy is fruitless and most patients succumb to the process. However, most published comments about therapy are based on fiction rather than fact and emotion rather than clinical judgment. The reasons for this are because very few objective series of patients with DIC with respect to therapy given, morbidity, mortality, and survival, have been published. Many clinicians argue vehemently against the use of heparin in acute or chronic DIC despite the surprising lack of published case reports or series in the literature regarding the adverse effects of heparin in DIC.[150,198,201] Likewise, many argue strongly in favor of the use of heparin in DIC; however, there is, likewise, a surprising lack of published reports demonstrating positive effects of heparin.[88,127,151] It is my experience that if logical aggressive and sequential therapy is undertaken in the patient with DIC, morbidity and mortality are not as likely as suspected.[21,36,37,50] Clinicians and investigators should develop judgment regarding therapy based on experience and published series of patients and documentation rather than opinion and myth. It is to be hoped that the future will offer more guidelines than are available at the present time with respect to successes and failures with various forms of therapy.

My approach to therapy in acute DIC is somewhat vigorous and is summarized in Table 6–21. Although this approach is rather aggressive, it has been associated with a high survival rate (76%) and low morbidity in patients with classic acute DIC.[21,36,37,50] The most important therapeutic modality to be delivered to a patient with acute DIC is that of an aggressive but reasonable therapeutic approach to remove or treat the triggering disease process that is thought to be responsible for DIC.[2,4,36,37,50,232] This is sometimes impossible, but therapy may, in some instances, stop or at least significantly blunt the intravascular clotting process. If, however, there are no attempts to treat the triggering event and pathophysiology, subsequent attempts at anticoagulant therapy, including heparin, will rarely, if ever,

Table 6–21 Sequential Therapy of Acute Disseminated Intravascular Coagulation

Treat or remove the triggering process
  Evacuate uterus
  Antibiotics
  Control shock
  Volume replacement
  Maintain blood pressure
  Steroids?
  Antineoplastic therapy
  Other indicated therapy
Stop intravascular clotting process
  Subcutaneous heparin
  Intravenous heparin?
  Antiplatelet agents
  AT III concentrate therapy
Component therapy as indicated
  Platelet concentrates
  Packed red cells (washed)
  AT III concentrate
  Fresh frozen plasma
  Cryoprecipitate (fibrinogen)
  Prothrombin complex
Inhibit residual fibrino(geno)lysis
  Aminocaproic acid

alleviate the DIC process. However, attempts to treat the underlying disease process does give the patient a reasonable chance of responding to therapy designed to stop the intravascular clotting process.

The removal of the triggering pathophysiology may stop the disease process, and the classic example of this is an obstetric accident. Simply evacuating the uterus or in rare instances hysterectomy will usually rapidly stop the intravascular clotting process[65,186] without the need for anticoagulant therapy. Although it is often difficult to convince the obstetrician or gynecologist to take a hemorrhaging hypofibrinogenemic patient to the operating room, the results are rewarding when this approach is pursued. The results are usually immediate and dramatic. More commonly, however, therapy of the underlying process will at least blunt the process enough so that the patient may respond to anticoagulant therapy, as occurs in septicemia. The successful treatment of septicemia will blunt the process in many patients, thus giving them the opportunity to respond to anticoagulant therapy, and alleviating triggering pathophysiology may actually stop the intravascular clotting process. In septicemia, specific antibiotic therapy, alleviation of shock, volume replacement, the potential use of steroids, and other therapy to maintain hemodynamics will often cause significant blunting and on some occasions may actually stop the DIC process.

Each case must, of course, be evaluated on its own merit, depending on the clinical situation and what the clinician feels to be the significant dominant triggering event. However, the key point is that attempts to treat the triggering event are the most important therapeutic modality that may be delivered to the patient with DIC. The majority of patients, except those with DIC secondary to obstetric accidents or massive liver failure, will subsequently require anticoagulant therapy of some form. The use of subcutaneous low-dose heparin appears to be highly effective and has been my choice of anticoagulant therapy for the last 9 years.[21,36,37,50] Anticoagulant therapy is indicated if the patient continues to bleed or clot significantly for approximately 4 hours after the initiation of therapy to stop or blunt the triggering pathophysiologic event. This time period is somewhat empirical and depends on the sites and severity of bleeding. When the patient continues to bleed in this situation, subcutaneous calcium heparin is administered at 80 U/kg every 4 to 6 hours as the clinical situation, site, severity of bleeding and thrombosis, and patient size dictates. It has been noted that low-dose subcutaneous heparin appears to be as effective or possibly more effective than larger doses of intravenous heparin in DIC.[19,21,36,37,50,51,54,164] With this approach, one often notes cessation of AT III consumption, lowering of FDPs, and increases in fibrinogen levels and slow or rapid correction of other abnormal laboratory modalities of acute DIC in 3 to 4 hours, followed shortly thereafter by blunting or cessation of clinically significant hemorrhage and thrombosis. The use of subcutaneous low-dose heparin, rather than intravenous heparin appears reasonable for several reasons: (1) if the patient fails to respond, larger doses of heparin can always be administered if deemed appropriate; (2) low-dose subcutaneous heparin therapy is associated with minimal or no chance of increasing the patient's risk of hemorrhage; and (3) most importantly, the use of low-dose subcutaneous heparin has been as efficacious as large-dose heparin therapy and is associated with a high percentage of patient survival when used in conjunction with other therapeutic modalities.[21,36,37,50]

In light of current understanding of the heparin-AT III-serine protease-thrombin-fibrinogen axis, low-dose subcutaneous heparin, from a theoretical standpoint as well as in published reports, is thought to be equal or more effective than larger intravenous doses of USP heparin.[19,54,164] This will be discussed in appropriate chapters. Other anticoagulant modalities that are available, depending on the clinician's experience, are those of intravenous heparin, the use of combination antiplatelet agents, or the use of AT III concentrates. Those clinicians using intravenous heparin therapy for acute DIC most commonly deliver between 20,000 and 30,000 U/24 hours by constant infusion, and this also may be associated with significant blunting or cessation of the intravascular clotting process. Combination antiplatelet agents are far less commonly effective in acute DIC, but on occasion may be called for as the specific clinical situation dictates and will be discussed later. Acute DIC has been successfully treated with investigational AT III concentrates in small groups of patients by several investigators, and preliminary experience would suggest these to be quite effective.[21,40,55,167,328] From a theoretical standpoint, AT III concentrates should be highly effective in treating acute DIC and it is to be hoped that this therapeutic fraction may become available for such use in the near future, and that there will be large-scale clinical trials using this investigational modality to treat this potentially catastrophic disease. With respect to heparin, it is my opinion that subcutaneous heparin, or heparin in any dose, is contraindicated in patients with acute DIC and central nervous system insults of any type, patients with acute DIC associated with fulminant liver failure, and in most instances of obstetric accidents.

Approximately 75% of patients will respond to the two previously outlined sequential therapeutic steps. However, if patients continue to bleed after initiating reasonable attempts to treat the triggering pathophysiology thought to be responsible for DIC and after initiating anticoagulant therapy, the most likely cause of continued bleeding is component depletion. In this instance, the exact components missing and clinically thought to be contributing to hemorrhage should be defined as precisely as possible. The delivery of certain components is associated with attendant hazards in patients with ongoing DIC and as a general guideline only concentrates and components that are devoid of fibrinogen should be delivered to a patient with ongoing DIC, which is manifested by continued severe depression of the AT III level. If however, the AT III level, or other specific monitoring modality that the clinician chooses to use is returning to normal and associated with a potential response, it can be assumed that the intravascular clotting process has been controlled and in this instance any component or concentrate deemed necessary can safely be given. In general, the only components that are generally safe in patients with an active uncontrolled DIC process are packed red cells, platelet concentrates, AT III concentrates, and nonclotting protein containing volume expanders, such as plasma protein fraction, albumin, and hydroxyethyl starch. If a patient continues to bleed after successful anticoagulant therapy and cessation of the DIC process, as manifested by correcting AT III levels, then any component deemed depleted to the point of contributing with a high degree of probability to continued hemorrhage is safe to give to the patient. However, it should be emphasized that components containing clotting factors or fibrinogen are, in general, not safe for patients with ongoing DIC and the use of fresh frozen plasma and fresh whole blood may be associated with enhanced hemorrhage and thrombosis in a patient with active DIC to whom these components are unwisely administered.[21,36,37,57] Not only has this been seen clinically but would be expected from a theoretical standpoint when understanding the pathophysiology of DIC. If whole blood, fresh frozen plasma, or cryoprecipitate is given to a patient with ongoing DIC, it is to be expected that plasmin will readily biodegrade most, if not all, of the coagulation factors supplied. This event in itself may not be particularly harmful, but is certainly not helpful.

Of more significance is that these components contain fibrinogen and are associated with a great potential for creation of even higher levels of FDPs, which will further impair hemostasis by interference with fibrin monomer polymerization, further impair already compromised platelet function, and will lead to enhanced microvascular deposition and subsequent thrombocytopenia. Thus, a reasonable approach is to assess the patient after anticoagulant therapy and continued bleeding; if the AT III level, or other selected monitoring modality has returned to normal or near normal, any component deemed significantly depleted and likely to be contributing to continued hemorrhage is reasonable to use. Alternatively, if the patient continues to bleed after anticoagulant therapy has been delivered and the AT III

level and other modalities used to monitor the patient remain abnormal, it is highly likely that the intravascular clotting process has not been controlled and continues. In this instance the component should be restricted to packed red cells, platelets, volume expanders, and, if available, AT III. By adhering to these three sequential aggressive steps, greater than 95% of patients will stop hemorrhaging if they are, in fact, going to survive.

The potentially disastrous consequences of using fibrinogen-containing components, in this case plasma, in a patient with acute ongoing DIC are summarized in Figure 6–11. Although the clotting factors initially improved, hemorrhage became worse and the patient exsanguinated. In those rare instances in which bleeding continues after the aforementioned three sequential steps are initiated, the fourth step in the therapy of acute DIC is to consider inhibition of the fibrinolytic system. This step is needed in approximately 3% of patients only. In some rare instances, even though the intravascular coagulation process has been alleviated, the patient may continue to bleed because for unexplained reasons secondary fibrinolysis has continued with the concomitant biodegradation of the usual plasma protein targets of plasmin. In this rare instance, and it must be emphasized that this is necessary in less than 3 to 5% of all patients with acute DIC, antifibrinolytic therapy may be indicated.

However, it should be emphasized that antifibrinolytic therapy should never be delivered to patients with ongoing DIC who desperately need the fibrinolytic system to keep the microcirculation as clear of microthrombi as possible.[2,36,37] Thus, antifibrinolytic therapy should never be delivered unless the first three sequential steps have been resorted to and it has been well documented from the laboratory and clinical standpoint that the intravascular coagulation process has been terminated by noting correction of biologic AT III levels or other modalities used by the clinician to monitor the event. In addition, antifibrinolytic therapy should never be used unless not only the cessation of DIC has been documented, but also the presence of significant amounts

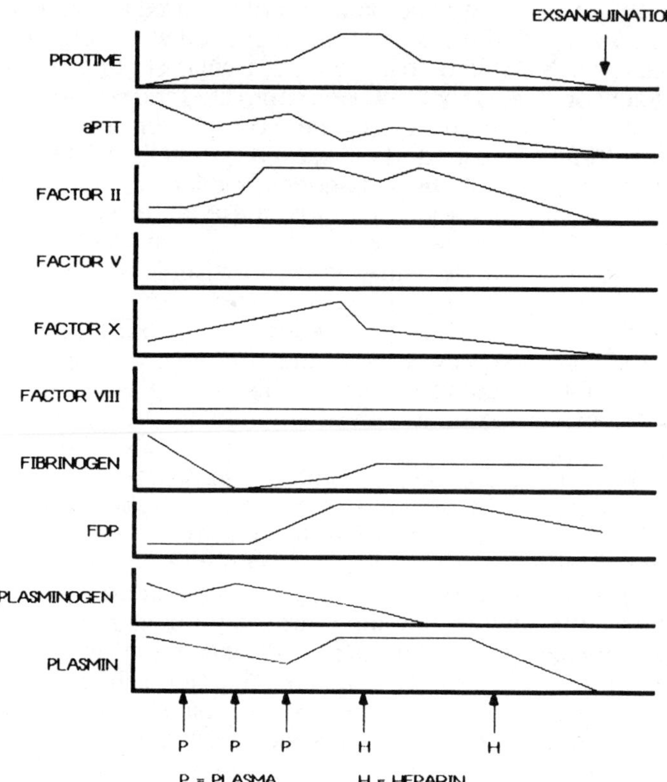

Fig. 6–11. Consequences of plasma therapy in ongoing DIC.

of plasmin have been documented in the laboratory. In those rare instances in which antifibrinolytic therapy is indicated, epsilon-aminocaproic acid is given as an initial 5 to 10 slow intravenous push followed by 2 to 4 g/hour for 24 hours or until bleeding ceases. This agent should be used with great caution, since it may cause ventricular arrhythmias, severe hypotension, and severe hypokalemia.[133,224,247] In addition, it should be realized that if epsilon-aminocaproic acid, or any fibrinolytic inhibitor, is used in a patient with ongoing DIC, it may cause enhanced precipitation of fibrin in the microcirculation and macrocirculation and lead to often fatal disseminated thrombosis.

Table 6–22 gives a series of patients with chronic and acute DIC to demonstrate how AT III levels may be used as an aid in the diagnosis and may be used to monitor potential efficacy of therapy.[21,36,37,57] It will be noted that in the vast majority of patients depicted, the biologic AT III levels are significantly de-

pressed at the time of making a diagnosis. The exceptions are patients noted to have disseminated malignancy. Thus, in a patient with acute or chronic DIC and normal or high AT III levels, disseminated underlying malignancy should be seriously considered and searched for.[24] However, in almost all individuals receiving successful therapy there is an associated rapid return to normal or near normal biologic AT III levels. Even in those instances when the AT III levels are normal or elevated in association with malignancy, the delivery of effective therapy is associated with significant further increases in the AT III level. When the AT III level is noted to increase to normal or near normal levels after therapy, it can be assumed with reasonable certainty that the intravascular coagulation process has undergone cessation or significant blunting.

More clinical experience may demonstrate that drastic dropping of previously elevated fibrinopeptide A, beta-thromboglobulin, or platelet factor 4 levels may

Table 6–22 Monitoring of AT III During Therapy In Disseminated Intravascular Coagulation

| | AT III | | |
| | Before | After | |
Patient	Therapy	Therapy	Therapy
1	90	130	Antiplatelet
2	105	176	Antiplatelet
3	80	97	Antiplatelet
4	65	99	Antiplatelet
5	60	98	Antiplatelet
6	77	100	Antiplatelet
7	66	104	Antiplatelet
8	80	160	Antiplatelet
9	145	163	Antiplatelet
10	47	104	Intravenous heparin
11	68	93	Intravenous heparin
12	36	103	Intravenous heparin
13	73	124	Intravenous heparin
14	50	90	Subcutaneous heparin
15	75	107	Subcutaneous heparin
16	50	98	Subcutaneous heparin
17	75	93	Subcutaneous heparin
18	137	167	Subcutaneous heparin
19	31	86	Subcutaneous heparin
20	76	105	Subcutaneous heparin
21	68	98	Subcutaneous heparin
22	47	68	Subcutaneous heparin
23	80	114	Subcutaneous heparin
24	58	100	Subcutaneous heparin
25	12	110	Subcutaneous heparin
26	80	148	Subcutaneous heparin
27	72	115	Subcutaneous heparin
28	65	95	Subcutaneous heparin
29	65	128	Subcutaneous heparin
30	55	76	Subcutaneous heparin

Table 6–23 Low-Dose Heparin Therapy in Disseminated Intravascular Coagulation

| | Pre Therapy | After Post Therapy | Therapy |
Test		4 Hours	8 Hours
Fibrinogen	68 mg/dL	104 mg/dL	450 mg/dL
Platelets	48,000	270,000	270,000
Thrombin time	22 sec	22 sec	20 sec
Reptilase time	20 sec	16 sec	24 sec
Prothrombin	16 sec	14.8 sec	12 sec
A PTT	48 sec	36 sec	36 sec
FDP level	>40	>40	<10
Protamine test	+	+	0
AT III	60%	76%	185%

Table 6–24 AT III Concentrate Therapy in Disseminated Intravascular Coagulation

| | Pre Therapy | After Post Therapy | Therapy |
Test		12 Hours	24 Hours
Fibrinogen	30 mg/dL	110 mg/dL	150 mg/dL
Platelets	62,000	90,000	128,000
Thrombin time	30 sec	18 sec	16 sec
Reptilase time	38 sec	18 sec	18 sec
Prothrombin	18 sec	13 sec	12 sec
A PTT	62 sec	59 sec	38 sec
FDP level	>40	>10	<10
Protamine test	+	+	0
AT III	48%	102%	115%

be of equal efficacy in assessing response to therapeutic manipulation in patients with DIC. Table 6–23 gives the results in a patient with acute DIC who was treated with miniheparin.[21,37] The pretherapy and post-therapy laboratory values are given; within 4 hours there was general correction of laboratory modalities and this was associated with cessation of clinical hemorrhage. Table 6–24 gives the results in a patient treated with an investigational AT III concentrate, and in this instance the patient not only stopped bleeding and thrombosing, but also survived the DIC process with minimal morbidity.[55]

Chronic

Therapy of chronic DIC is approached much differently than that for acute DIC and is summarized in Table 6–25. The majority of patients with chronic DIC do not have life-threatening hemorrhage, but rather have bothersome hemorrhage that is often associated with diffuse superficial or deep vein thrombosis and thromboembolus.[103,261] As with acute DIC, the most important therapeutic modality for a patient with chronic DIC is therapy for the underlying disease process; in many instances, this will cause cessation of the intravascular clotting process and alleviation of hemorrhage and thrombosis. If treatment for the triggering disease process does not stop the intravascular coagulation process, at least it will often significantly blunt it to a degree in which bothersome bleeding or thrombosis may cease to be a clinical problem. If this first step is vigorously attempted and hemorrhage or thrombosis or thromboembolus continues, then anticoagulant therapy is

Table 6–25 Sequential Therapy of Chronic Disseminated Intravascular Coagulation

Therapy for the triggering disease process
Any indicated therapy
Anticoagulant therapy when indicated
Antiplatelet drugs
Subcutaneous heparin
No warfarins
Component therapy
Rarely indicated
Inhibit residual fibrino(geno)lysis
Aminocaproic acid rarely indicated

indicated. However, since chronic DIC patients usually do not have life-threatening hemorrhage, anticoagulant therapy need not be vigorous in many instances. In fact, vigorous therapy may be contraindicated, as in selected instances of malignancy, especially those with intracranial metastases.[21,58,128] Combination antiplatelet therapy is often successful in stopping a chronic DIC provided that attempts to treat the triggering pathophysiology have also been instituted. A combination of two antiplatelet agents with independent mechanisms of action are often needed, and the three agents clinically available and commonly used are acetylsalicylic acid plus dipyridamole or sulfinpyrazone plus dipyridamole. A combination of acetysalicylic acid, 600 mg orally twice daily, in conjunction with 30 mL of liquid antacid, plus dipyridamole, 50 mg orally four times a day, will often stop the process within 24 to 30 hours, as demonstrated by generalized correction of laboratory parameters and the cessation of bleeding or thrombosis. Alternatively, the use of sulfinpyrazone, 200 mg orally three times a day, in conjunction with 30 mL of liquid antacid, plus dipyridamole, 50 mg orally four times a day, may be used.[144,336]

Both acetylsalicylic acid and sulfinpyrazone are cyclo-oxygenase inhibitors leading to a decreased synthesis of thromboxane A_2; it is often without avail to use both of these agents in combination, since they both have the same mechanism of action.[249] Dipyridamole, however, is an inhibitor of phosphodiesterase, leading to increased concentrations of intraplatelet cyclic adenosine monophosphate[152] and

therefore the ideal combination appears to be acetylsalicylic acid plus dipyridamole or sulfinpyrazone plus dipyridamole. Miniheparin, or intravenous heparin, is rarely indicated in patients with chronic DIC; however, low-dose subcutaneous heparin therapy should be considered in patients with chronic DIC who appear to be evolving into a more subacute or acute DIC process or who are developing active thrombotic or thromboembolic problems. Replacement therapy is rarely, if ever, indicated in the patient with chronic DIC unless the patient demonstrates component depletion from other triggering mechanisms, such as the patient with chronic DIC and malignancy who also demonstrates thrombocytopenia because of therapy, bone marrow replacement, hypersplenism, or other mechanisms. Inhibition of the fibrinolytic system with epsilon-aminocaproic acid is also rarely, if ever, indicated in patients with chronic DIC.

Therapy in the Patient with Malignancy

Successful therapy of DIC in the patient with malignancy represents a major clinical challenge and is summarized in Table 6–26. Effective therapy is multiphasic and must be approached in a logical, sequential manner if the process is to be controlled. The first and most important modality to be given is to treat the malignancy itself, since this is providing the trigger for the intravascular coagulation process. Therapy may be surgical, radiotherapeutic, or chemotherapeutic as the clinical situation warrants. Treatment of the specific tumor is often associated with cessation or significant improvement in DIC and until antineoplastic therapy is instituted, subsequent therapy of bleeding or thrombosis is often unsuccessful.[21,23,24,37,58] A classic example of response to antineoplastic drugs is seen in the patient with prostatic carcinoma.[69,257] These patients often show a marked improvement of the hemorrhagic or thrombotic or throm-

Table 6–26 Therapy of Disseminated Intravascular Coagulation in Malignancy

Treat the malignancy
  Surgery as indicated
  Radiation as indicated
  Chemotherapy or hormonal therapy as indicated
Stop intravascular clotting process
  Antiplatelet drug therapy
  Subcutaneous heparin*
  Intravenous heparin*
Component therapy as indicated
  Platelet concentrates
  Packed red cells (washed)
  Fresh frozen plasma
  AT III concentrates
Inhibit residual fibrino(geno)lysis
  Rarely, if ever, indicated

*Contraindicated with central nervous system metastases.

boembolic problems with the institution of diethylstilbesterol therapy or cytotoxic chemotherapy as indicated. This phenomenon may be noted in other tumors as well when antineoplastic therapy is started. In addition, the use of antiplatelet agents, especially in the form of aspirin plus dipyridamole, as previously outlined, has been associated with correction of altered laboratory tests suggestive of DIC, including normalization of fibrinogen and platelet survival in patients with malignancy and chronic DIC. However, patients with malignancy are also notoriously resistant to anticoagulant therapy or successful therapy with respect to stopping minor to moderate bleeding and thrombotic episodes as well as major thrombotic and thromboembolic episodes, all of which are commonly due to a chronic DIC-type process.[21,23,24,58]

Tables 6–27 and 6–28 report, in a series of patients with DIC, the laboratory findings at the time of making the diagnosis and after successful therapy. In addition, the specific type of anticoagulant therapy and the triggering pathophysiologic event are given.[57] Particular attention should be focused on the AT III level as a predictor of monitoring efficacy of successful therapy in stopping the intravascular clotting process. A series of 48 patients who exemplified the incidence of hemorrhage or clinical thrombosis in acute and chronic DIC[21,50] (Table 6–29) was chosen because the laboratory testing was done by one individual and thought to be reasonably uniform. In patients with acute DIC slightly more than 50% had clinical or clinical and laboratory evidence of microvascular and macrovascular thrombosis and all patients had hemorrhage. In ten patients with chronic DIC eight had clinical or clinical and laboratory evidence of thrombosis and all patients had hemorrhage. In this same group survival in patients with chronic DIC was 100% with respect to the DIC process. In addition, patients with acute DIC in this series treated with aggressive therapy, as previously outlined, demonstrated an overall survival of 76%. Thus, the syndrome of DIC need not be universally associated with a high mortality rate, as has previously been generally believed.

Summary

Current concepts of the etiology, pathophysiology, diagnosis, and management of classic acute and chronic DIC have been discussed. Considerable attention has been devoted to interrelationships that have remained confusing. Only by clearly understanding these pathophysiologic interrelationships can the clinician and laboratorian appreciate the divergent and wide clinical spectrum of often confusing clinical and laboratory findings in patients with DIC. Many of the therapeutic decisions to be made in these patients remain controversial and will remain so until more series of patients are published with respect to specific therapeutic modalities, and survival patterns. Subsequent chapters will outline syndromes that are superficially confused with DIC. In this regard it should be reemphasized that many syndromes that remain organ-specific share common pathophysiology with DIC but are identified as an independent disease entity, such as HUS, adult shock lung syndrome, eclampsia, and other isolated organ-specific disorders.

Table 6–27 Laboratory Findings in Patients with DIC at Time of Diagnosis

	Pro-thrombin Time (sec)	Partial Thrombo-plastin Time (sec)	Rep-tilase Time (sec)	Thrombin Time (sec)	Fibrin-(ogen) Degra-dation Products (mg/dL)	Platelets (×1,000)	Prota-mine Sulfate	Fibrin-ogen (mg/dL)	AT III (%)	Therapy*
Patient 1	16.2	32.4	18	11	> 40	98	+	475	90	ASA/dipyridamole
Patient 2	15.8	48.6	24	14	> 40	455	+	240	105	ASA/dipyridamole
Patient 3	11.2	31.7	23	33	> 40	302	+	650	80	ASA/dipyridamole
Patient 4	12.3	68.8	36	28	> 10 > 40	77	+	105	65	ASA/dipyridamole
Patient 5	14.1	28.4	30	14	> 40	58	+	328	80	ASA/dipyridamole
Patient 6	14.6	52.5	29	8	> 40	380	0	127	145	ASA/dipyridamole
Patient 7	15.2	65.7	17	12	> 80	205	+	92	66	ASA/dipyridamole
Patient 8	13.7	25.0	60	33	> 10 > 40	58	+	460	80	ASA/dipyridamole
Patient 9	18.2	70.7	52	28	> 40	70	+	75	137	Miniheparin
Patient 10	22.0	64.4	41	18	> 40	32	+	43	31	Miniheparin
Patient 11	16.3	38.0	12	21	> 80	105	+	108	76	Miniheparin
Patient 12	14.8	51.5	16	16	> 40	28	+	156	68	Miniheparin
Patient 13	15.2	62.7	26	14	> 10 > 40	56	+	42	80	Miniheparin
Patient 14	19.0	74.7	38	34	> 40	72	+	115	55	Miniheparin
Patient 15	14.4	54.4	29	28	> 40	30	0	215	33	Miniheparin
Patient 16	12.8	48.0	19	28	> 40	16	+	105	77	Miniheparin
Patient 17	17.6	38.4	21	18	> 40	78	+	128	68	Heparin
Patient 18	16.4	27.1	18	16	> 40	92	+	144	75	Miniheparin
Patient 19	21.0	61.6	26	19	> 80	120	+	97	17	Miniheparin
Patient 20	18.4	74.8	36	22	> 80	17	+	82	64	Miniheparin
Patient 21	16.4	55.2	30	38	> 80	63	+	44	73	Heparin
Patient 22	14.0	61.2	12	66	> 40	41	+	68	50	Miniheparin
Patient 23	12.6	38.9	34	37	> 80	97	+	110	58	Miniheparin
Patient 24	13.6	49.0	48	18	> 10 > 40	114	+	137	47	Heparin
Patient 25	14.8	63.4	23	22	> 40	72	0	144	50	Miniheparin
Patient 26	16.2	58.9	22	24	> 40	70	0	74	36	Heparin
Patient 27	18.4	74.0	28	12	> 80	29	+	168	60	Miniheparin
Patient 28	11.8	52.5	32	18	> 40	58	+	117	56	Miniheparin
Patient 29	17.4	66.4	23	16	> 40	38	+	79	21	Miniheparin
Patient 30	16.4	73.9	44	24	> 40	104	+	122	80	Miniheparin
Patient 31	11.2	59.0	18	33	> 40	131	+	146	72	Miniheparin
Patient 32	14.8	63.7	24	18	> 80	63	+	90	65	Miniheparin
Patient 33	12.6	89.0	33	63	> 40	20	+	78	75	Miniheparin
Patient 34	14.2	32.4	14	10	> 40	140	+	215	77	ASA/dipyridamole
Patient 35	16.4	59.4	16	23	> 40	18	+	168	12	Miniheparin
Patient 36	15.2	48.4	28	22	> 80	74	+	118	65	Miniheparin
Patient 37	14.4	28.8	18	11	> 10 > 40	102	+	265	60	ASA/dipyridamole
Patient 38	14.8	55.9	36	43	> 40	97	+	68	73	D & C
Average	15.4	53.9	27.7	24.0		95.5		156	66.4	
Normal	9–13	32–49	< 22	< 15	< 10	150–450	0	149–341	85–116	
% of patients who had abnormalities	82%	63%	66%	76%	100%	89%	89%	71%	89%	

*Acetylsalicylic acid (ASA) was given in a dosage of 600 mg orally twice daily, dipyridamole, 50 mg twice daily, miniheparin, 2500 to 5000 U subcutaneously every 8 to 12 hours, heparin, 20,000 to 30,000 U/24 hours by constant infusion. D & C: dilation and curettage.

Table 6-28 Laboratory Findings in Patients with DIC after Successful Therapy*

	Prothrombin Time (sec)	Partial Thromboplastin Time (sec)	Reptilase Time (sec)	Thrombin Time (sec)	Fibrin(ogen) Degradation Products (mg/dL)	Platelets (×1,000)	Protamine Sulfate	Fibrinogen (mg/dL)	AT III (%)	Diagnosis (Trigger)
Patient 1	13.0	30.0	18	9	> 10< 10	228	0	420	130	Malignancy
Patient 2	12.4	29.0	17	11	> 10< 40	400	0	300	176	Malignancy
Patient 3	12.0	28.8	15	8	< 10	400	0	290	97	Malignancy
Patient 4	12.0	29.9	15	12	> 10< 40	188	+	248	99	Malignancy
Patient 5	11.9	28.4	21	14	> 10< 40	128	0	405	160	Malignancy
Patient 6	13.8	34.4	22	14	> 10< 40	360	0	268	163	Malignancy
Patient 7	12.8	38.8	18	13	< 10	350	0	240	104	Malignancy
Patient 8	13.8	25.2	17	14	< 10	205	0	310	160	Malignancy
Patient 9	14.6	40.1	21	9	< 10	128	0	241	167	Malignancy
Patient 10	14.0	38.7	19	8	< 10	134	0	190	86	Malignancy/sepsis
Patient 11	12.5	38.2	14	16	< 10	225	0	244	105	Malignancy/sepsis
Patient 12	14.5	41.7	15	20	< 10	168	0	350	98	Malignancy/sepsis
Patient 13	11.9	48.0	22	14	< 10	155	0	168	114	Malignancy/sepsis
Patient 14	14.0	54.4	19	14	< 10	124	0	240	76	Malignancy/sepsis
Patient 15	13.8	32.7	16	12	< 10	150	0	368	58	Malignancy/sepsis
Patient 16	12.8	33.0	14	9	< 10	105	0	241	191	Malignancy/sepsis
Patient 17	11.9	54.8	21	28	< 10	250	0	256	93	Shock/arrest
Patient 18	14.0	30.1	19	14	< 10	355	0	176	107	Shock/arrest
Patient 19	11.9	51.2	28	20	> 40	350	+	154	93	Shock/arrest
Patient 20	14.0	33.0	21	14	< 10	98	0	105	131	Shock/hemolysis
Patient 21	14.4	64.2	18	21	> 10< 40	263	0	210	124	Shock/hemolysis
Patient 22	14.2	41.7	16	13	< 10	168	0	156	98	Shock/hemolysis
Patient 23	13.0	38.6	15	15	< 10	403	0	216	100	Shock/transplant recipient
Patient 24	11.8	68.2	19	39	< 10	215	0	168	104	Shock/sepsis
Patient 25	14.4	30.9	19	7	< 10	290	+	205	90	Shock
Patient 26	13.2	59.9	17	34	> 10 <40	156	0	312	103	Shock
Patient 27	15.0	50.2	14	13	> 10 <40	190	0	183	123	Shock
Patient 28	11.8	41.1	20	11	< 10	138	0	208	127	Shock
Patient 29	15.4	33.7	19	14	< 10	207	0	160	73	Shock
Patient 30	16.0	34.0	23	12	< 10	256	0	214	148	Hereditary hemorrhagic telangiectasia
Patient 31	11.4	43.1	16	15	> 10 <40	360	0	315	115	Hereditary hemorrhagic telangiectasia
Patient 32	12.0	29.8	20	9	> 10 <40	244	0	222	128	Hereditary hemorrhagic telangiectasia
Patient 33	12.3	43.7	19	8	< 10	120	0	169	93	Kasabach-Merritt
Patient 34	14.4	32.0	16	11	> 10 <40	468	+	215	100	Collagen vascular disorders
Patient 35	15.0	40.9	13	15	< 10	240	0	97	100	Collagen vascular disorders
Patient 36	15.4	45.0	18	13	< 10	323	0	214	95	Hip fracture
Patient 37	12.0	29.0	20	11	< 10	430	0	305	98	Polycythemia vera
Patient 38	11.0	32.4	19	14	< 10	375	0	300	100	Missed abortion
Averages	13.6	39.4[†]	18.2	14.4[†]		246		241	114	
Normal		35.8[†]		12.5[†]						
	9–13	32–49	< 22	< 15	< 10	150–450	0	149–341	85–116	
% of patients who had abnormalities	47%	21% / 10%[‡]	5%	13%[†] / 8%[‡]	31%	18%	10%	5%	8%	
% of patients for whom pretreatment abnormalities were corrected	35%	42%	61%	58%	69%	71%	79%	66%	81%	

*All values for patients with chronic DIC were measured 24 to 36 hours after initiation of therapy (aspirin and dipyridamole). All values for patients with acute DIC were measured 4 to 6 hours after initiation of therapy (miniheparin or heparin).
[†]Includes values for four patients still being given heparin therapy.
[‡]Excludes values for four patients still being given heparin therapy.

Table 6-29 Hemorrhage or Thrombosis or Survival
in Disseminated Intravascular Coagulation

Type DIC	Hemorrhage (%)	Thrombosis (%)	Survival (%)
Acute	100	53	74
Chronic	100	80	100
Total	100	58	79

* Data from 48 patients.

References

1. Abildgaard CF, Corrigan JJ, Seeler RA, Simone JV, Schulman I: Meningiococcemia associated with intravascular coagulation. Pediatrics 40: 78, 1967.
2. Abildgaard U, Graven K, Godal HC: Assay of progressive antithrombin in plasma. Throm Diath Haemorrh 24:224, 1970.
3. Alkjaersig H, Roy L, Fletcher AP: Analysis of gel exclusion chromatographic data by plasma fibrinogen chromatography. Thromb Res 3: 525, 1973.
4. Al-Mondhiry H: Disseminated intravascular coagulation: experience in a major cancer center. Thromb Diath Haemorrh 34:181, 1975.
5. Ambrus CM, Choi TS, Weintraub DH, Eisonberg B, Staub HP, Courey NG, Foote RJ, Goperlund D, Moesch RV, Ray M, Bross I, Jung OS, Mink IB, Ambrus JL: Studies on the prevention of respiratory distress syndrome of infants due to hyaline membrane disease with plasminogen. Semin Thromb Hemost 2:42, 1975.
6. Ambrus CM, Weintraub AH, Dunphy D, Dowd JE, Pickren JW, Niswander KR, Ambrus JL: Studies on hyaline membrane disease. I. the fibrinolysis system in pathogenesis and therapy. Pediatrics 32:10, 1963.
7. Ambrus CM, Pickren JW, Weintraub DH, Niswander KR, Ambrus JL, Rodbard D, Levy JL: Studies on hyaline membrane disease; oxygen induced hyaline membrane disease in guinea pigs. Biol Neonate 12:246, 1968.
8. Ambrus CM, Ambrus JL, Weintraub DH, Foote RJ, Courey NG, Niswander KR: Thrombolytic therapy in hyaline membrane disease. Thromb Diath Haemorrh. (Suppl) 47:269, 1971.
9. Amundsen MA, Spittell JA, Thompson JH: Hypercoagulability associated with malignant disease and with the postoperative state. Ann Intern Med 58:608, 1963.
10. Apitz K: A study of the generalized Schwartzman phenomenon. J Immunol 29:255, 1935.
11. Arneson H: Characterization of fibrinogen and fibrin degradation products by isoelectric focusing in polyacrylamide gel. Thromb Res 4:861, 1974.
12. Backman F: The paradoxes of disseminated intravascular coagulation. Hosp Pract 6:113, 1971.
13. Baker LR, Rubenberg ML, Dacie JV, Brain MC: Fibrinogen catabolism in microangiopathic hemolytic anemia. Br J Haematol 14:617, 1968.
15. Bang NU, Chang M: Soluble fibrin complexes. Semin Thromb Hemost 1:91, 1974.
16. Beller FK: Experimental animal models for the production of disseminated intravascular coagulation. In Bang N, Beller FK, Deutsch E, Mammen EF (Eds): Thrombosis and Bleeding Disorders. Academic Press, New York, 1971, p 514.
17. Beller FK, Theiss W: Fibrin derivitives, plasma hemoglobin and glomerular fibrin deposition in experimental intravascular coagulation. Thromb Diath Haemorrh 29:363, 1973.
18. Bennett RM: Proc Tutorial in Hematopathology. H Rappaport (Ed), University of Chicago Press, Pasadena, 1980.
19. Bentley PG, Kakkar VV, Scully MF, MacGregor IR, Webb P, Chan P, Jones H: An objective study of alternative methods of heparin administration. Thromb Res 18:177, 1980.
20. Bick RL, Adams T: Disseminated intravascular coagulation: Etiology, pathophysiology, diagnosis, and management. Med Counterpoint 6:38, 1974.
21. Bick RL: Disseminated intravascular coagulation. In Bick RL (Ed): Disseminated Intravascular Coagulation and Related Syndromes. CRC Press, Boca Raton, FL, 1983, p 31.
22. Bick RL: Hypercoagulability and thrombosis. In Murano G, Bick RL (Eds): Basic Concepts of Hemostasis and Thrombosis. CRC Press, Boca Raton, FL, 1980, p 237.
23. Bick RL: Alterations of hemostasis associated with malignancy. In Murano G, Bick RL (Eds): Basic Concepts of Hemostasis and Thrombosis. CRC Press, Boca Raton, FL, 1980, p 213.
24. Bick RL: Alterations of hemostasis associated

with malignancy: Etiology, pathophysiology, diagnosis, and management. Semin Thromb Hemost 5:1, 1978.

25. Bick RL: Vascular disorders associated with thrombohemorrhagic phenomena. Semin Thromb Hemost 5:167, 1979.

26. Bick RL: Hereditary hemorrhagic telangiectasia and disseminated intravascular coagulation: A new clinical syndrome. Ann NY Acad Sci 370:851, 1981.

27. Bick RL: Vascular disorders. In Murano G, Bick RL (Eds): Basic Concepts of Hemostasis and Thrombosis. CRC Press, Boca Raton, FL, 1980, p 89.

28. Bick RL: Hereditary hemorrhagic telangiectasia and disseminated intravascular coagulation: A new clinical syndrome. Vasc Surg 15: 394, 1981.

29. Bick RL: Alterations of hemostasis associated with surgery, cardiopulmonary bypass surgery, and prosthetic devices. In Ratnoff OD, Forbes C (Eds): Disorders of Hemostasis. Grune & Stratton, New York, 1984.

30. Bick RL: The clinical significance of fibrinogen degradation products. Semin Thromb Hemost 8:302, 1982.

31. Bick RL: Disseminated Intravascular Coagulation and Related Syndromes. Manual 5570, American Society of Clinical Pathology, Chicago, 1979, p 14.

32. Bick RL: Difficult Diagnostic Problems in Hemostasis and Thrombosis. Manual 5549, American Society of Clinical Pathology, Chicago, 1980, p 1.

33. Bick RL: Clinical hemostasis practice: The major impact of laboratory automation. Semin Thromb Hemost 9:139, 1983.

34. Bick RL: Disseminated intravascular coagulation: Pathophysiology and diagnosis. Pract Cardiol 7:145, 1981.

35. Bick RL: Clinical significance of fibrino-(geno)lytic degradation product (FDP) testing. Lab Lore 9:683, 1981.

36. Bick RL: Disseminated intravascular coagulation. In Fareed J, Messmore HL, Fenton J, Brinkhous KM (Eds): Perspectives in Hemostasis. Pergamon Press, New York, 1981, p 121.

37. Bick RL: Disseminated intravascular coagulation and related syndromes. In Murano G, Bick RL (Eds): Basic Concepts of Hemostasis and Thrombosis. CRC Press, Boca Raton, FL, 1980, p 163.

38. Bick RL: Pathophysiology of disseminated intravascular coagulation. In Bick RL (Ed): Clinical Significance of FDP Testing. Health Sciences Consortium Press, Chapel Hill, 1981.

39. Bick RL, Dukes ML, Wilson WL, Fekete L: Antithrombin III (AT-III) as a diagnostic aid in disseminated intravascular coagulation. Thromb Res 10:721, 1977.

40. Bick RL: Clinical relevance of antithrombin III. Semin Thromb Hemost 8:276, 1982.

41. Bick RL, Kovacs I, Fekete LF: A new two-stage functional assay for antithrombin-III: Clinical and laboratory evaluation. Thromb Res 8:745, 1976.

42. Bick RL, McClain BJ: A clinical comparison of chromogenic, fluorometric, and natural (fibrinogen) substrates for determination of antithrombin-III. Thromb Haemost 46:364, 1981.

43. Bick RL, McClain BJ: Sequential platelet size distribution profiling for assessing platelet survival and response to antiplatelet drugs. Blood 58:230, 1981.

44. Bick RL: Disseminated intravascular coagulation and related syndromes.II. Pract Cardiol 7:152, 1981.

45. Bick RL, Shanbrom E: A systematic approach to the diagnosis of bleeding disorders. Med Counterpoint 4:28, 1972.

46. Bick RL, Kovacs I, Fekete LF: A two-stage functional assay for antithrombin III: Clinical and laboratory evaluation. Thromb Res 8:745, 1976.

47. Bick RL: Acquired circulating anticoagulants and defective hemostasis in malignant paraprotein disorders. In Murano G, Bick RL (Eds): Basic Concepts of Hemostasis and Thrombosis. CRC Press, Boca Raton, FL, 1980, p 205.

48. Bick RL: Malignancy's effect on hemostasis: Complex questions finding answers. Diagn Dialog 2:1, 1980.

49. Bick RL: Disseminated intravascular coagulation and related syndromes. Am J Hematol 5:265, 1978.

50. Bick RL: Disseminated intravascular coagulation: A clinical/laboratory study of 48 patients. Ann NY Acad Sci 370:843, 1981.

51. Bick RL: Disseminated intravascular coagulation: Clinical/laboratory correlations. Am J Clin Pathol 77:244, 1982.

52. Bick RL, Fareed J, Squillaci G, Walenga J, Bermes EW, Messmore HL: Molecular markers of hemostatic processes. Implications in diagnostic and therapeutic management of thrombotic and hemorrhagic disorders. Fed Proc 42:1031, 1983.

53. Bick RL, Fareed J, Walenga J, Bermes EW: Automation in coagulation testing. Clin Chem 29:1196, 1983.

54. Bick RL: Monitoring heparin therapy. Diagn Dialog 1:1, 1979.

55. Bick RL, Fekete LF, Wilson WL: Treatment of disseminated intravascular coagulation with antithrombin III. Trans Am Soc Hematol, 1976, p 167.

56. Bick RL, Schmalhorst WR, Fekete LF: Disseminated intravascular coagulation and blood

component therapy. Transfusion 16:361, 1976.

57. Bick RL, Bick MB, Fekete LF: Antithrombin III patterns in disseminated intravascular coagulation. Am J Clin Pathol 73:577, 1980.

58. Bick RL: Treatment of bleeding and thrombosis in the patient with cancer. In Nealon T (Ed): Management of the Patient with Cancer. W.B. Saunders, Philadelphia, 1976, p 48.

59. Bishop RC, Hudson PM, Mitchell G, Pochron SP: Use of fluorogenic substrates for the assay of antithrombin III and heparin. Ann NY Acad Sci 370:720, 1981.

60. Blaisdell FW, Stallone RJ: The mechanism of pulmonary damage following traumatic shock. Surg Gynecol Obstet 130:15, 1970.

61. Bleyl U: Morphologic diagnosis of disseminated intravascular coagulation: Histologic, histochemical, and electron-microscopic studies. Semin Thromb Hemost 3:247, 1977.

62. Bleyl A, Kuhn W, Graeff H: Reticulo-endotheliale clearance intravascaler. Fibrinmonere in der milz. Thromb Diath Haemorrh 22:87, 1969.

63. Bleyl U, Busing CM, Kremplen B: Pulmonale hyaline membranen und perinataler kreislaufschock. Virchow Arch [Pathol Anat] 348:187, 1969.

64. Bonnar J, McNicol GP, Douglas AS: Coagulation and fibrinolytic systems in pre-eclampsia and eclampsia. Br Med J 1:12, 1971.

65. Bonnar J: Blood coagulation and fibrinolysis in obstetrics. Clin Hematol 2:213, 1973.

66. Boyd JF: Disseminated fibrin-thromboembolism among neonates dying within 48 hours of birth. Arch Dis Child 42:401, 1967.

67. Breen FA, Tullis JZ: Ethanol gelation, a rapid screening test for intravascular coagulation. Ann Intern Med 69:1197, 1968.

68. Brown DL, Lachmann PJ: The behavior of complement and platelets in lethal endotoxin shock in rabbits. Int Arch Allergy Appl Immunol 45:193, 1973.

69. Brown RC, Campbell DC, Thompson JH: Increased fibrinolysis with malignant disease. Arch Intern Med 109:129, 1962.

70. Brozovic M: Acquired disorders of blood coagulation. In Bloom A, Thomas DP (Eds): Hemostasis and Thrombosis. Churchill Livingstone, New York, 1981, p 411.

71. Budzynski AZ, Marder VJ: Determination of human fibrinopeptide A by radioimmunoassay in purified systems and in the blood. Thromb Diath Haemorrh. 34:709, 1975.

72. Bull B, Kuhn IN: The production of schistocytes by fibrin strands (a scanning electron microscope study). Blood 35:104, 1970.

73. Bull B, Brain MC: Experimental models of microangiopathic hemolytic anemia. Proc R Soc Med 61:1134, 1968.

74. Bull B, Rubenberg M, Dacie J, Brain MC: Microangiopathic hemolytic anemia: Mechanisms of red-cell fragmentation. Br J Haematol 14:643, 1968.

75. Busing CM, Bleyl U, Dohnert G: Pulmonary hyaline membranes in the rabbit after thrombin infusion. IVth International Congress on Haemostasis, Vienna, 1973.

76. Carvalho AC, Lees RS, Vaillancourt RA, Cabral RB, Weinberg RM, Coleman RW: Intravascular coagulation in hyperlipidemia. Thromb Res 8:843, 1976.

77. Chesterman CN: The fibrinolytic system and haemostasis. Thromb Diath Haemorrh 34:308, 1975.

78. Clavin SA, Bobbitt JL, Shuman RT, Smithwick EL: Use of peptidyl-4-methoxy-2-naphthylamides to assay plasmin. Anal Biochem 80:355, 1977.

79. Cline MJ, Melmon KL, Davis WC, Williams HE: Mechanism of endotoxin interaction with leukocytes. Br J Haematol 15:539, 1968.

80. Cohen E, Ballard CA: Consumptive coagulopathy associated with intraamniotic saline instillation and the effect of oxytocin. Obstet Gynecol 43:300, 1974.

81. Cohen MM, Weintraub DS, Lilienfeld AM: The relationship of pulmonary hyaline membrane to certain factors in pregnancy and delivery. Pediatrics 26:42, 1960.

82. Coleman RW, Shapira M, Scott CF: Regulation of the formation and inhibition of human plasma kallikrein. Ann NY Acad Sci 370:261, 1981.

83. Collen D, DeCock F, Verstraete M: Immunological distinction between anti-plasmin and X-1-anti-trypsin. Thromb Res 7:245, 1975.

84. Collen P: identification and some properties of a new fast-acting plasmin inhibitor in human plasma. Eur J Biochem 69:209, 1976.

85. Collins GJ, Heymann RL, Zajtchuk R: Hypercoagulability in patients with peripheral vascular disease. Am J Surg 130:2, 1975.

86. Cooper HA, Bowie EJW, Didisheim P: Paradoxic changes in platelets and fibrinogen in chronically induced intravascular coagulation. Mayo Clin Proc 46:521, 1971.

87. Corrigan JJ: Changes in the blood coagulation system associated with septicemia. N Engl J Med 279:851, 1968.

88. Corrigan JJ, Jordan CM: Heparin therapy in septicemia with disseminated intravascular coagulation. Effect on mortality and correction of hemostatic defects. N Engl J Med 283:778, 1970.

89. Cronberg S, Skansberg P, Nivenios-Larsson K: Disseminated intravascular coagulation in septicemia caused by beta-hemolytic streptococci. Thromb Res 3:405, 1973.

90. Cronlund M, Hardin J, Burton J, Lee L, Haber I, Bloch KJ: Fibrinopeptide-A in plasma of nor-

mal subjects and patients with disseminated intravascular coagulation and systemic lupus erythematosus. J Clin Invest 58:142, 1976.

91. Davey MG, Luscher EF: Release reactions of human platelets induced by thrombin and other agents. Biochim Biophys Acta 165:490, 1968.

92. Davis RB, Theologides A, Kennedy BJ: Comparative studies of blood coagulation and platelet aggregation in patients with cancer and nonmalignant disease. Ann Intern Med 71:67, 1969.

93. Dennis LH, Reisberg BE, Crosbie J, Crozier D, Conrad ME: The original haemorrhagic fever: Yellow fever. Br J Haematol 17:455, 1969.

94. Derechin M, Szuchet S: Gelation phenomena in degraded fibrinogen and fibrin. Arch Biochem Biophys 87:100, 1960.

95. Des Prez RM, Horowitz HI, Hook EW: Effects of bacterial endotoxin on rabbit platelets. I. Platelet aggregation and release of platelet factors in vitro. J Exp Med 114:857, 1961.

96. DeVries WI, Braat-van Straaten MAJ, Muller E, Wettermark M: Antiplasmin deficiency in polycythaemia: A form of thrombopathy. Thromb Diath Haemorrh 6:445, 1961.

97. Deykin D: The clinical challenge of disseminated intravascular coagulation. N Engl J Med 283:636, 1970.

98. Dobbs RM, Barber JA, Weigel JW, Bergin JE: Clotting predisposition in carcinoma of the prostate. J Urol 123:706, 1980.

99. Donaldson V: Effect of plasmin in vitro on clotting factors in plasma. J Lab Clin Med 56:644, 1960.

100. Douglas JT, Shah M, Lowe GDO, Prentice CRM: Fibrinopeptide-A and beta-thromboglobulin levels in pre-eclampsia and hypertensive pregnancy. Thromb Haemost 46:8, 1981.

101. Dubber AHC, McNicol GP, Douglas AS: Acquired hypofibrinogenemia; the "defibrination syndrome". A study of seven patients. Scott Med J 12:138, 1967.

102. Eckhardt T, Muller-Berghous G: The role of blood platelets in the precipitation of soluble fibrin endotoxin. Scand J Haematol 14:181, 1975.

103. Edwards EA: Migrating thrombophlebitis associated with carcinoma. N Engl J Med 240:1031, 1949.

104. Edy J, Collen D, Verstraete M: Quantitation of the plasma protease inhibitor antiplasmin with the chromogenic substrate (S-2251). In Davidson JF, Rowan RM, Samama MM, Desnoyers PC (Eds): Chemical Fibrinolysis and Thrombolysis. Raven Press, New York, 1978, p 315.

105. Egeberg O: Blood coagulation and intravascular hemolysis. Scand J Clin Lab Invest 14:217, 1962.

106. Esmon CT: Protein-C: Biochemistry, physiology, and clinical implications. Blood 62:1155, 1983.

107. Evanson SA, Elgjo RF, Shepro D: Platelets, endothelium, and the triggering mechanisms of intravascular coagulation. Thromb Diath Haemorrh 24:207, 1973.

108. Evenson SA, Jeremic M: Platelets and the triggering mechanism of intravascular coagulation. Br J Haematol 19:33, 1970.

109. Fareed J, Messmore HL, Bermes EW: New perspectives in coagulation testing. Clin Chem 26:1380, 1980.

110. Fareed J: New methods in hemostatic testing. In Fareed J, Messmore HL, Fenton J, Brinkhous KM (Eds): Perspectives in Hemostasis. Pergamon Press, New York, 1981, p 310.

111. Fareed J, Messmore HL, Walenga JM, Bermes EW, Bick RL: Laboratory evaluation of antithrombin III: A critical overview of currently available methods for antithrombin III measurements. Semin Thromb Hemost 8:288, 1982.

112. Fareed J, Bick RL, Walenga J, Messmore HL, Bermes EW: Clinical and experimental studies using a modified radioimmunoassay for B-beta 15-42 related peptides. Thromb Haemost 50:300, 1983.

113. Fareed J, Bick RL, Squillaci G, Walenga J, Messmore HL, Bermes EW: Clinical and experimental utilization of a modified radioimmunoassay for B-beta 15-42 related peptides. Clin Chem 29:1161, 1983.

114. Fareed J, Walenga J, Bick RL, Bermes EW, Messmore HL: Impact of automation on the quantitation of low molecular weight markers of hemostatic defects. Semin Thromb Hemost 9:355, 1983.

115. Farrel RJ, Duffy MJ, Duffy GJ: Elevated plasma beta-thromboglobulin in patients with malignancy. Thromb Haemost 42:143, 1979.

117. Fleishman AI, Bierenbaum ML, Stier A, Somol H, Watson PB: In vivo platelet function in diabetes mellitus. Thromb Res 9:467, 1976.

118. Fletcher AP, Alkjaersig N, Fisher S, Sherry S: The proteolysis of fibrinogen by plasmin: The identification of thrombin-clottable fibrinogen derivatives which polymerize abnormally. J Lab Clin Med 68:780, 1966.

119. Fletcher AP, Alkjaersig N: Blood hypercoagulability, intravascular coagulation, and thrombosis: New diagnostic concepts. Thromb Diath Haemorrh (Suppl) 45:389, 1974.

120. Fletcher AP, Alkjaersig HK: Gel chromatogrphy of fibrinogen in the diagnosis of prethrombotic states. In Neri-Sernari GG, Prentice CRM (Eds): Haemostasis and Thrombosis. Academic Press, London, 1979, p 113.

121. Flute PT: Intravascular coagulation. Postgrad Med J 48:346, 1972.
122. Folkman J: Tumor angiogenesis: Therapeutic implications. N Engl J Med 285:1182, 1971.
123. Folkman J, Coltran RS: Relation of capillary proliferation to tumor growth. Int Rev Exp Pathol 16:167, 1976.
124. Gaffney PJ, Philo RD: A commentary of new methodology in haemostasis using chromogenic substrates. In Fareed J, Messmore JL, Fenton J, Brinkhous KM (Eds): Perspectives in Hemostasis. Pergamon Press, New York, 1981, p 405.
125. Gagel C, Linder M, Muller-berghous G, Lasch H: Virus infection and blood coagulation. Thromb Diath Haemorrh. 23:1, 1970.
126. Gitlin D, Craig JM: The nature of the hyaline membrane in asphyxia of the newborn. Pediatrics 17:64, 1956.
127. Good RA, Thomas L: Studies on the generalized Schwartzman reaction: Prevention of the local and generalized Schwartzman reactions with heparin. J Exp Med 97:871, 1953.
128. Goodnight SH: Bleeding and intravascular clotting in malignancy: A review. Ann NY Acad Sci 230:271, 1974.
129. Gore I: Thrombin and pancreatic carcinoma. Am J Pathol 29:1093, 1953.
130. Gralnick HR, Tan HK: Acute promyelocytic leukemia: A model for understanding the role of the malignant cell in hemostasis. Hum Pathol 5:661, 1974.
131. Gralnick HR, Bagley J, Abrell E: Heparin treatment for the hemorrhagic diathesis of acute promyelocytic leukemia. Am J Med 52:167, 1974.
132. Gralnick HR: Cancer cell procoagulant activity. In Donati MB, Davidson JF, Garattini S (Eds):Malignancy and the Hemostatic System, Raven Press, New York, 1981, p 57.
133. Gralnick HR, Greipp P: Thrombosis with epsilon-aminocaproic acid therapy. Am J Clin Pathol 56:151, 1971.
134. Griffin JH: Clinical studies of protein C. Semin Thromb Hemost 10:162, 1984.
135. Gurewich V, Hutchinson E: Detection of intravascular coagulation by protamine sulfate and ethanol gelation tests. Thromb Res 2:539, 1973.
136. Gurewich V, Lipinsky B, Lipinska I: A comparative study of precipitation and paracoagulation by protamine sulfate and ethanol gelation tests. Thromb Res 2:539, 1973.
137. Gyzander E, Friberger P, Myrwold H, Noppa H, Olsson R, Teger-Nilsson AC, Walmo L: Antiplasmin determination by means of the plasmin specific substrate S-2251: Methodology studies and some clinical applications. In Witt I (Ed): New Methods for the Analysis of Coagulation Using Chromogenic Substrates. Walter deGruyter, Berlin, 1977, p 229.
138. Hafter R, Graeff H: Molecular aspects of defibrination in a reptilase-treated case of "dead-fetus syndrome". Thromb Res 7:391, 1975.
139. Haragawa N, Watanabe N, Nagata H, Murao M: Analysis of the disappearance curve of labeled fibrinogen at the time of hypofibrinogenemia in rabbits with acute or chronic intravascular coagulation. Thromb Haemost 50:49, 1976.
140. Hardaway R: Disseminated intravascular coagulation in shock. Thromb Diath Haemorrh (Suppl) 36:159, 1967.
141. Hardaway RM: Acute respiratory distress syndrome and disseminated intravascular coagulation. South Med J 71:596, 1978.
142. Hardaway RM: Syndromes of Disseminated Intravascular Coagulation with Special Reference to Shock and Hemorrhage. Charles C Thomas, Springfield, Ill, 1966.
143. Harker L, Slichter S: Platelet and fibrinogen consumption in man. N Engl J Med 287:999, 1972.
144. Harker LA, Hirsh J, Gent M, Yenton E: Critical evaluation of platelet inhibiting drugs in thrombotic disease. Prog Hematol 9:229, 1975.
145. Harpel PC, Rosenberg RD: Alpha-2-macroglobulin and antithrombin-heparin cofactor: Modulators of hemostasis and inflammatory reactions. Prog Hemost Thromb 3:145, 1976.
146. Harpel PC, Mosesson MW, Cooper NR: Studies on the structure and function of α-2-macroglobulin and C1 inactivator. In Reich E, Rifkin DB, Shaw E (Eds): Proteases and Biological Control. Cold Spring Harbor Symposium, Cold Spring Harbor, New York, 1975, p 387.
147. Hartman RC, Jenkins DE: Proxysmal nocturnal hemoglobinuria: Current concepts of certain pathophysiological features. Blood 25:850, 1965.
148. Hedner U, Nilsson IM: Parallel determinations of FDP and fibrin monomers with various methods. Thromb Diath Haemorrh 28:268, 1972.
149. Heene D, Hoffmann-Fezer G, Hoffmann R, Weiss E, Muller-Berghous G, Lasch HG: Coagulation disorders in acute hog cholera. Beitr Pathol 144:259, 1931.
150. Heene DL: Blood coagulation mechanism and endotoxins: Hemostatic defect in septic shock. In Urbaschek B (Ed): Gram-Negative Bacterial Infections and Mode of Endotoxin Actions. Springer-Verlag, Vienna, 1975, p 367.
151. Heene DL: Disseminated intravascular coagulation: Evaluation of therapeutic approaches. Semin Thromb Hemost 3:291, 1977.
152. Henry RL: Platelet function in hemostasis. In Murano G, Bick RL (Eds): Basic Concepts of Hemostasis and Thrombosis. CRC Press, Boca Raton, FL, 1980, p 17.

153. Henson PM: The adherence of leukocytes and platelets induced by fixed IgG antibody or complement. Immunology 16:107, 1969.

154. Henson PM: Complement-dependent platelet and polymorphonuclear leukocyte reactions. Transplant Proc 6:27, 1963.

155. Heyes H, Hilgard P, Theiss W: Induction of disseminated intravascular coagulation by endotoxin and saline loading in rats. I. The influence on fibrinogen turnover and plasma parameters. Thromb Res 7:37, 1975.

156. Heyes H, Kohle W, Slijerpcevic B: The appearance of schistocytes in the peripheral blood in correlation to degree of disseminated intravascular coagulation. Haemostasis 5:66, 1976.

157. Hjort PF, Rapaport SI: The Schwartzman reaction: Pathogenic mechanism and clinical manifestations. Annu Rev Med 16:135, 1965.

158. Holder LA, Malin LL, Fox CL: Hypercoagulability after thermal injuries. Surgery 54:316, 1963.

159. Huseby RM, Smith RE: Synthetic oligopeptide substrates: Their diagnostic application in blood coagulation, fibrinolysis, and other pathological states. Semin Thromb Hemost 6:173, 1980.

160. Inceman S, Tangun Y: Chronic defibrination syndrome due to a giant hemagioma associated with microangiopathic hemolytic anemia. Am J Med 46:997, 1969.

161. Innerfield I, Anrist A, Benjamin JW: Plasma antithrombin patterns in disturbances of the pancreas. Gastroenterology 19:843, 1951.

162. Jacobson RJ, Sandler SF, Rath CE: Systemic amyloidosis associated with microangiopathic hemolytic anemia and Factor X (Stuart Factor) deficiency. S Afr Med J 46:1634, 1972.

163. Jacobson E, Ly B, Kieulf P: Incorporation of fibrinogen with soluble fibrin complexes. Thromb Res 4:499, 1974.

164. Jaques LB: The premises involved in the clinical use of heparin. Semin Thromb Hemost 4:275, 1978.

165. Johnson JF, Seegers WH, Braden RG: Plasma AC-globulin changes in placenta abruptio. Am J Clin Pathol 22:322, 1952.

166. Johnson AJ, Mersky C: Diagnosis of diffuse intravascular clotting: Its relation to secondary fibrinolysis and treatment with heparin. Thromb Diath Haemorrh (Suppl) 20:161, 1966.

167. Kakkar VV: The clinical use of anti-thrombin III. Thromb Haemost 42:265, 1979.

168. Kaplan A, Meier H, Mandel R: The Hageman factor dependent pathways of coagulation, fibrinolysis, and kinin generation. Semin Thromb Hemost 3:6, 1976.

169. Kaplan AP, Silverberg M, Dunn JT, Miller G: Mechanisms for Hageman factor activation and role of HMW kininogen as a coagulation cofactor. Ann NY Acad Sci 370:253, 1981.

170. Kaplan AP: The Hageman factor dependent pathways of human plasma. Microvasc Res 8:97, 1974.

171. Karpatkin S, Khan Q, Freedman M: Heterogeneity of platelet function correction with platelet volume. Am J Med 64:542, 1978.

172. Karpatkin S: Heterogeneity of human platelets. VI. Correlation of platelet function with platelet volume. Blood 51:307, 1978.

173. Kasabach HH, Merritt KK: Capillary hemangioma with extensive purpura—report of a case. Am J Dis Child 59:1063, 1940.

174. Katz J, Krawitz S, Sachs PV, Levin SE, Thompson P, Levin J, Metz J: Platelet, erythrocytes, and fibrinogen kinetics in the hemolyticuremic syndrome of infancy. J Pediatr 83:739, 1973.

175. Kaxmier FJ, Didisheim P, Fairbanks VK, Ludwig J, Payne WS, Bowie EJW: Intravascular coagulation and arterial disease. Thromb Diath Haemorrh (Suppl) 36:295, 1969.

176. Kidder WR, Logan LJ, Rapaport SI, Patch MJ: The plasma protamine paracoagulation test: Clinical and laboratory evaluation. AM J Clin Pathol 58:675, 1972.

177. Killough J: Protective mechanisms of the lungs: Pulmonary diseases, pleural diseases. In Sodeman WA, Sodeman TM (Eds): Mechanism of Disease. W.B. Saunders, Philadelphia, 1979, p 459.

178. Kisker CT, Rush R: Detection of intravascular coagulation. J Clin Invest 50:2235, 1971.

179. Kockum C: Radioimmunoassay of fibrinopeptide-A—clinical applications. Thromb Res 8:225, 1976.

180. Kopec M, Wegrzynowiczy Z, Budzynski A, Latallo Z, Lipinski B, Kowalski E: Interaction of fibrinogen degradation products with platelets. Exp Biol Med 3:73, 1968.

181. Kowalski E: Figrinogen derivatives and their biological activities. Semin Hematol 5:45, 1968.

182. Kowalski E, Kopec M, Niewiarowski S: An evaluation of the euglobulin method for the determination of fibrinolysis. J Clin Pathol 12:215, 1959.

183. Kraytman M: Platelet size in thrombocytopenias and thrombocytosis of various origin. Blood 41:587, 1973.

184. Krevins JR, Jackson DP, Cowley CL, Hartman RC: The nature of the hemorrhagic disorder accompanying hemolytic transfusion reactions in man. Blood 12:834, 1957.

185. Kudryk B, Robinson D, Netre C, Hessel B, Blomback M: Measurement in human blood of fibrinogen/fibrin fragments containing the B-beta 15-42 sequence. Thromb Res 25:277, 1982.

186. Kuhn W, Graeft H: Gerinnungsstorungen in der Geburtshilfe. Thieme Verlag, Stuttgart, 1977, p 90.

187. Kurcznski EM, Penner JA: Activated prothrombin concentrate for patients with Factor VIII inhibitors. N Engl J Med 291:164, 1974.

188. Kwaan HC: Disseminated intravascular coagulation. Med Clin North Am 56:177, 1972.

189. Langdell RD, Hedgpeth EM: A study of the role of hemolysis in the hemostatic defect of transfusion reactions. Thromb Diath Haemorrh 3:566, 1959.

190. Lasch HG, Henne DL, Huth K, Sandritter W: Pathophysiology, clinical manifestations, and therapy of consumptive-coagulopathy. Am J Cardiol 20:381, 1967.

191. Latallo ZS: Products of fibrin(ogen) proteolysis. Thromb Diath Haemorrh (Suppl) 24:145, 1973.

192. Latallo ZS, Teisseyre E, Lopaciuk S: Evaluation of a fibrinolytic profile of plasma using chromogenic substrates. In Scully MF, Kakkar VV (Eds): Chromogenic Peptide Substrates. Churchill Livingstone, London, 1979, p 262.

193. Latour JG, Prejean JB, Margaretten W: Corticosteroids and the generalized Schwartzman reaction. Mechanisms of sensitization in the rabbit. Am J Pathol 65:189, 1971.

194. Lee D, Brown D, Baker L, Littlejohns D, Roberts D: Hematological complications of chlorate poisoning. Br Med J 2:31, 1970.

195. Lee L: Reticuloendothelial clearance of circulating fibrin in the pathogenesis of the generalized Schwartzman reaction. J Exp Med 115:1065, 1962.

196. Lendrum AC, Fraser DC, Slidders W, Henderson R: Studies on the character and staining of fibrin. J Clin Pathol 15:401, 1962.

197. Lerner RG: The defibrination syndrome. Med Clin North Am 60:871, 1976.

198. Leroy J, Lamagnere JD, Mercier C: La Coagulopathic de consommation au cours des purpuras fulminans et son traitment (10 observations). Sem Hop Paris 50:843, 1974.

199. Lisiewicz J: Mechanisms of hemorrhage in leukemias. Semin Thromb Hemost 4:241, 1978.

200. Lisiewicz J: Acute leukemias. In Hemorrhage in Leukemias. Polish Medical Publishers, Warsaw, 1976, p 51.

201. Lo SS, Hitzig WH, Frick PG: Clinical experience with anticoagulant therapy in the management of disseminated intravascular coagulation in children. Acta Haematol 45:1, 1971.

202. Lorand L: Fibrinoligase: The fibrin-stabilizing factor system of blood plasma. Ann NY Acad Sci 202:6, 1972.

203. Lundham CA, Cash JD: B-thromboglobulin: A new tool for the diagnosis of hypercoagulability. In Neri-Sernari GG, Prentice CRM (Eds): Hemostasis and Thrombosis. Academic Press, London, 1979, p 159.

204. Lundham CA, Allen N, Bradford RB, Dowdle R, Bentley N, Bloom AL: B-thromboglobulin and platelet survival in patients with rheumatic diseases and prosthetic heart valves and their treatment with sulfinpyrazone. Thromb Haemost 42:329, 1979.

205. Maki M, Sasaki K, Sata S: Methods for differential diagnosis of consumptive coagulopathy. Tohoku J Exp Med 99:347, 1969.

206. Malofiejew M: Kallikrein-like activity in human myometrium, placenta, and amniotic fluid. Biochem Pharmacol 22:123, 1973.

207. Marder VJ, Shulman HR, Carroll WR: High molecular weight derivatives of human fibrinogen produced by plasmin. I. Physicochemical and immunological characterization. J Biol Chem 244:2111, 1969.

208. Marder VJ, Budzynski AZ, James HL: High molecular weight derivatives of human fibrinogen produced by plasmin. III. Their NH_2-terminal amino acids and comparison of the "NH_2-terminal amino disulfide knot." J Biol Chem 247:4775, 1972.

209. Marder VJ, Matchett M, Sherry S: Detection of serum fibrinogen and fibrin degradation products: Comparison of six techniques using purified products and application in clinical studies. Am J Med 51:71, 1971.

210. Martin AM, Soloway HB, Simmons RL: Pathologic Anatomy of the lungs following shock and trauma. J Trauma 8:687, 1968.

211. Martin AM, Soloway HB, Simmons RL: Pathologic anatomy of the lungs following shock and trauma. J Trauma 8:687, 1968.

212. Matsuda T, Seki T, Ogawara M, Miura R, Yokouchi M, Murakami M: Comparison between plasma levels of βthromboglobulin and platelet factor 4 in various diseases. Thromb Haemost 42:288, 1979.

213. McGehee WG, Rapaport SI, Hjort PF: Intravascular coagulation in fulminant meningiococcaemia. Ann Intern Med 67:250, 1967.

214. McKay DG, Shapiro SS: Alterations in the blood coagulation system induced by bacterial endotoxin I: In vitro (generalized Schwartzman reaction). J Exp Med 107:353, 1958.

215. McKay DG, Margaretten W: Disseminated intravascular coagulation in virus diseases. Arch Intern Med 120:129, 1967.

216. McKay DG: Progress in disseminated intravascular coagulation. Calif Med 111:186, 1969.

217. McKay DG: Disseminated intravascular coagulation: An intermediary mechanism of disease. Harper & Row, New York, 1965.

218. McKay DG, Gitlin D, Graig JM: Immunochemical demonstration of fibrin in the generalized Schwartzman reaction. Arch Pathol 67:270, 1969.

219. McKay DG, Csavossy W Margaretten I: An electron microscope study of the effects of bacterial endotoxin on the blood-vascular system. Lab Invest 15:1815, 1966.

220. McKay DG, Linder MM, Cruse VK: Mechanisms of thrombosis of the microcirculation. Am J Pathol 63:231, 1971.

221. McKay DG, Cszvossy W, Margaretten I: An electron microscopic study of endotoxin shock in rhesus monkeys. Surg Gynecol Obstet 125:825, 1967.

222. McKay DG: Tissue damage in disseminated intravascular coagulation: Mechanisms of localization of thrombi in the microcirculation. Thromb Diath Haemorrh (Suppl) 36:67, 1969.

223. McKay DG, Muller-Berghous G: Therapeutic implications of disseminated intravascular coagulation. Am J Cardiol 20:392, 1967.

224. McNicol GP, Douglas AS: Thrombolytic therapy and fibrinolytic inhibitors. In Biggs R (Ed): Human Blood Coagulation, Haemostasis, and Thrombosis. Oxford University Press, London, 1972, p 393.

225. Menon IS: A study of the possible correlation of euglobulin lysis time and dilute blood clot lysis time in the determination of fibrinolytic activity. Lab Pract 17:334, 1968.

226. Mersky C, Johnson AJ, Kleiner GJ, Wohl H: The defibrination syndrome: Clinical features and laboratory diagnosis. Br J Haematol 13:528, 1967.

227. Mersky C: Altered blood coagulability in patients with malignant tumors. Ann NY Acad Sci 23:289, 1974.

228. Mersky C: Defibrination syndrome. In Biggs R (Ed): Human Blood Coagulation. Blackwell Scientific, London, 1976, p 492.

229. Mertins BF, Greene LF, Bowie EJW, Elueback LR, Owen CA: Fibrinolytic split products and ethanol gelation test in pre-operative evaluation of patients with prostatic disease. Mayo Clin Proc 49:642, 1974.

230. Messmore HL, Fareed J, Kniffin J, Squillacia G, Walenga J: Synthetic substrate assays of the coagulation enzymes and their inhibitors. Comparision with clotting and immunologic method for clinical and experimental usage. Ann NY Acad Sci 370:785, 1981.

231. Messmore HL: Automation in coagulation testing: Clinical applications. Semin Thromb Hemost 9:335, 1983.

232. Minna JD, Robboy S, Coleman RW: Clinical approach to a patient with suspected DIC. In Minna JD, Robboy S, Coleman RW (Eds): Disseminated Intravascular Coagulation. Charles C Thomas, Springfield, Ill, 1974, p 167.

233. Mombelli G, Roux A, Haelberli AW, Straub PW: Comparison of 125-I fibrinogen kinetics and fibrinopeptide A in patients with disseminated neoplasia. Thromb Haemost 46:9, 1981.

234. Morris JA, Smith RW, Assali NS: Hemodynamic action of vaso-pressor and vaso-depressor agents in endotoxin shock. Am J Obstet Gynecol 91:491, 1965.

235. Muller-Berghaus G, Roka L, Lasch HG: Induction of glomerular microclot formation of fibrin monomer infusion. Thromb Diath Haemorrh 29:275, 1973.

236. Muller-Berghous G, Hocke M: Effect of endotoxin on the formation of microthrombi from circulating fibrin monomer complexes in the absence of thrombin generation. Thromb Res 1:541, 1972.

237. Muller-Berghous G, Lasch HG: Microcirculatory disturbances induced by generalized intravascular coagulation. In Born GVR (Ed): Handbook of Experimental Pharmacology. Springer Verlag, Berlin, 1975, p 429.

238. Muller-Berghous G: Pathophysiology of generalized intravascular coagulation. Semin Thromb Hemost 3:209, 1977.

239. Muller-Berghous G, Lasch HG: Consumption of Hageman factor activity in the generalized Schwartzman reaction induced by liquid. Its prevention by inhibition of Hageman factor activation. Thromb Diath Haemorrh 23:386, 1970.

240. Muller-Berghous G, Mann B: Precipitation of ancrod-induced soluble fibrin by aprotinin and norepinephrine. Thromb Res 2:305, 1973.

241. Murakami M: A new method of fibrinolysis measurement. Acta Haematol Jpn 28:341, 1965.

242. Murano G: "The Hageman Connection": interrelationships between complement, kinins, and coagulation. Am J Hematol 4:409, 1978.

243. Murano G: Plasma protein function in hemostasis. In Murano G, Bick RL (Eds): Basic Concepts of Hemostasis and Thrombosis. CRC Press, Boca Raton, FL, 1980, p 43.

244. Murano G: The molecular structure of fibrinogen. Semin Thromb Hemost 1:1, 1974.

245. Mustard JF, Packham MA, Kinlough-Rathbone RL: Mechanisms in thrombosis. In Bloom AL, Thomas DP (Eds): Haemostasis and Thrombosis. Churchill Livingstone, New York, 1981, p 503.

246. Myers AR, Bloch KJ, Coleman RW: A comparative study of four methods for detecting fibrinogen degradation products in patients with various diseases. N Engl J Med 283:663, 1970.

247. Naeye RL: Thrombolytic state after hemorrhagic diathesis, possible complications of therapy with epsilon-aminocaproic acid. Blood 19:694, 1962.

248. Nalbandian RM, Henry RL, Bick RL: Thrombotic thrombocytopenic purpura. Semin Thromb Hemost 5:216, 1979.

249. Nalbandian RM, Henry RL: Platelet-endothelial cell interactions: Metabolic maps of structures and actions of prostaglandins, prostacyclin, thromboxane, and cyclic AMP. Semin Thromb Hemost 5:87, 1978.

250. Neri-Sernari GG, Gensini GF, Abbate R: High molecular weight fibrinogen complexes in the assessment of hypercoagulability. In Neri-Sernari GG, Prentice CRM (Eds): Hemostasis and Thrombosis. Academic Press, London, 1979, p 123.

251. Niewiarwski S, Bandowski E, Rogowicka I: Studies in the absorption and activation of Hageman Factor (Factor XII) by collagen and elastin. Thromb Diath Haemorrh 24:387, 1965.

252. Niewiarowski S, Regoeczi E, Stewart G, Senyi A, Mustard J: Platelet interaction with polymerizing fibrin. J Clin Invest 51:685, 1972.

253. Niewiarowski S, Guzzo J, Rav AK, Berman I, James P: Increased levels of low-affinity platelet factor 4 in plasma and urine of patients with chronic renal failure. Thromb Haemost 42:416, 1979.

254. Nilsson IM: Local fibrinolysis as a mechanism for haemorrhage. Thromb Diath Haemorh 34:623, 1975.

255. Nossel HL, Ti M, Kaplan KL, Spandonis K, Butler TVD: The generation of fibrinopeptide-A in clinical blood samples—evidence for thrombin activity. J Clin Invest 58:1136, 1976.

256. Odegard OR, Lie M, Abildgaard U: Heparin cofactor activity measured with an amidolytic method. Thromb Res 6:287, 1975.

257. Omar JB, Saxena H, Mitel HS: Fibrinolytic activity in malignant diseases. J Assoc Physicians India 19:293, 1971.

258. Owen CA, Oels H, Bowie EJW, Didisheim P, Thompson JH: Chronic intravascular coagulation syndrome. Thromb Diath Haemorrh (Suppl) 36:197, 1969.

259. Owen CA, Bowie EJW: Chronic intravascular coagulation fibrinolysis (ICF) syndromes (DIC). Semin Thromb Hemost 3:268, 1977.

260. Owen CA, Bowie EJW, Cooper HA: Turnover of fibrinogen and platelets in dogs undergoing induced intravascular coagulation. Thromb Res 2:251, 1973.

261. Parvez Z, Moncada R: Immunological vs functional methods for the evaluation of serine protease inhibitors. In Fareed J, Messmore HL, Fenton J, Brinkhous KM (Eds): Perspectives in Hemostasis. Pergamon Press, New York, 1981, p 355.

262. Pechet L: Fibrinolysis. N Engl J Med 273:96, 1965.

263. Penick GD, Roberts HR, Webster WP, Brinkhous KM: Hemorrhagic states secondary to intravascular clotting. Arch Pathol 66:708, 1958.

264. Penick GD, Roberts HR: Intravascular clotting: Focal and systemic. Int Rev Exp Pathol 3:269, 1964.

265. Penner JA, Kelly PE: Management of patients with Factor VIII or IX inhibitors. Semin Thromb Hemost 1:386, 1975.

266. Pergament ML, Swaim WR, Blackard CE: Disseminated intravascular coagulation in the urologic patient. J Urol 116:1, 1976.

267. Perry S: Coagulation defects in leukemia. J Lab Clin Med 50:229, 1957.

268. Phillips L, Skrodelis V: Intravascular coagulation in obstetric complications: Fibrin monomer and fibrin split products. In Sorneri GG, Prentice CRM (Eds): Haemostasis and Thrombosis. Academic Press, New York, 1979, p 551.

269. Pindyck J. Lichtman NC, Kohl SG: Cryofibrinogenemia in women using oral contraceptives. Lancet 1:51, 1970.

270. Pineo GF, Regoeczi E, Haton MW, Brain ML: The activation of coagulation by extracts of mucin: A possible pathway of intravascular coagulation accompanying adenocarcinoma. J Lab Clin Med 82:255, 1976.

271. Pineo GF, Brain MC, Gallus AS, Hirsch J, Hatton MW, Regoeczi E: Tumors, mucus production, and hypercoagulability. Ann NY Acad Sci 230:262, 1974.

272. Pitner W: Disseminated intravascular coagulation. Semin Hematol 8:65, 1971.

273. Plow EF, Hougie C, Edgington TS: Immunochemical and molecular investigations of fibrinogen cleavage fragments. In Plooer L (Ed): Recent Advances in Thrombosis. Churchill Livingstone, London, 1973, p 203.

274. Plow EF, Edgington TS: Surface markers of fibrinogen and its physiologic derivatives related by antibody probes. Semin Thromb Hemost 8:36, 1982.

275. Pritchard A, Cunningham G, Mason MA: Coagulation changes in eclampsia; their frequency and pathogenesis. Am J Obstet Gynecol 124:855, 1970.

276. Quick AJ, Georgatsos JG, Hussey CV: The clotting activity of human erythrocytes: Theoretic and clinical implications. Am J Med 228:207, 1954.

277. Rand JJ, Maloney WE, Sise HS: Coagulation defects in acute promyelocytic leukemia. Arch Intern Med 123:39, 1969.

278. Rapaport SI, Chapman CG: Coexistant hypercoagulability and hypofibrinogenemia in a patient with prostatic carcinoma. Am J Med 27:144, 1959.

279. Ratnoff OD, Pritchard JA, Calopy JA: Hemorrhagic states during pregnancy. I. N Engl J Med 253:63, 1955.

280. Ratnoff OD, Pritchard JA, Colopy JA: Hemorrhagic states during pregnancy. II. N Engl J Med 253:97, 1955.

281. Ratnoff OD, Nebehay WG: Multiple coagulative defects in a patient with the Waterhouse-Friderichsen syndrome. Ann Intern Med 56:627, 1962.

282. Ratnoff OD, Haff GB: The conversion of Cils

to C1' esterase by plasmin and trypsin. J Exp Med 125:337, 1961.

283. Robbins JE, Stetson CA: An effect of antibody-antigen interaction in blood coagulation. J Exp Med 109:1, 1959.

284. Robboy SJ, Coleman RW, Minna JD: Pathology of disseminated intravascular coagulation (DIC). Analysis of 26 cases. Hum Pathol 3:327, 1972.

285. Roberts JM, May WJ: Consumption coagulopathy in severe pre-eclampsia. Obstet Gynecol 48:163, 1976.

286. Rodriquez-Erdman F: Bleeding due to increased intravascular blood coagulation: Hemorrhagic syndromes caused by consumption of blood-clotting factors (consumption coagulopathies). N Engl J Med 273:1370, 1965.

287. Rohner RF, Prior JT, Sipple JH: Mucinous malignancies, venous thrombosis, and termina endocarditis with emboli: A syndrome. Cancer 19:1805, 1966.

288. Rubenberg WL, Baker LR, McBride JA, Sevitt JA, Brain WL: Intravascular coagulation in a case of Clostridium perfringens septicemia: Treatment by exchange transfusion and heparin. Br Med J 3:271, 1967.

289. Rubenberg M, Regoeczi E, Bull B, Darcie J, Brain MC: Microangiopathic hemolytic anemia: The experimental production of hemolysis and red-cell fragmentation by defibrination in vivo. Br J Haematol 74:627, 1968.

290. Ryan TJ: Coagulation and fibrinolysis. In Ryan TJ (Ed): Microvascular Injury. W.B. Saunders, Philadelphia, 1976, p 221.

291. Saliba MJ, Demsey WL, Kruggel JL: Large burns in humans: Treatment with heparin. JAMA 225:261, 1973.

292. Salmon SJ, Lambert PH, Louis J: Pathogenesis of the intravascular coagulation syndrome induced by immunological reactions. Thromb Diath Haemorrh 45:161, 1971.

293. Sandritter W, Lasch NG: Pathologic aspects of shock. Arch Exp Pathol 3:86, 1967.

294. Schnetzer GW, Penner JA: Chronic intravascular coagulation syndrome associated with atherosclerotic aortic aneurysm. South Med J 66:264, 1973.

295. Schreiber AD, Austen KF: Interrelationships of the fibrinolytic, coagulation, kinin generation, and complement systems. Semin Hematol 6:593, 1973.

296. Seegers WH: Factors in the control of bleeding. Cincinnati J Med 31:395, 1950.

297. Seegers WH, Schneider CL: The nature of the blood coagulation mechansim and its relationship to some unsolved problems in obstetrics and gynecology. Trans Int and 4th Amer Cong Obstet Gynecol 61A:469, 1951.

298. Seegers WH: Coagulation of the blood. Harvey Lect 48:180, 1952.

299. Seegers WH: Use and regulation of blood clotting mechanisms. In Seegers WH (Ed): Blood Clotting Enzymology. Academic Press, New York, 1971, p 1.

300. Seegers WH, Marceniak E: Autoprothrombin C in irregular blood clotting. Thromb Diath Haemorrh 8:81, 1962.

301. Seegers WH: Antithrombin III: Theory and clinical applications. Am J Clin Pathol 69:367, 1968.

302. Semeraro N, Donati MB: Pathways of blood clotting initiation by cancer cells. In Donati MB, Davidson JF, Garattini S (Eds): Malignancy and the Hemostatic System. Raven Press, New York, 1981, p 65.

303. Shainoff JR, Page IH: Significance of cryoprofibrin in fibrinogen-fibrin conversion. J Exp Med 116:687, 1962.

304. Sharp AA: Pathological fibrinolysis. Br Med Bull 20:240, 1964.

305. Shen SM, Rapaport SI, Feinstein DI: Intravascular clotting after endotoxin in rabbits with impaired intrinsic clotting produced by a factor VIII antibody. Blood 42:523, 1973.

306. Sherry S: The kallikrein system: A basic defense mechanism. Hosp Pract 5:75, 1970.

307. Silverstein MH: Agnogenic myeloid metaplasia. Publishing Sciences Group, Acton, Mass, 1975, p 10.

308. Simpson JG, Stalker AL: The concept of disseminated intravascular coagulation. Clin Haematol 2:189, 1973.

309. Skjorten F: Hyaline microthrombi in an autopsy material. A quantitative study with discussion of the relationship to small vessels thrombosis. Acta Pathol Microbiol Scand 76:361, 1969.

310. Skjorten F: Bilateral renal cortical necrosis and the generalized Schwartzman reaction. Acta Pathol Microbiol Scand 65:405, 1964.

311. Slaastad RA, Godal NC: Coagulation profile and ehtanol gelation test with special reference to components consumed during coagulation. Scand J Haematol 16:25, 1976.

312. Slickter SJ, Harker LA: Hemostasis in malignancy. Ann NY Acad Sci 230:252, 1974.

313. Sohal RS, Sun SC, Colcolough HL, Burch GE: Heat stroke: An electron microscopic study of endothelial cell damage and disseminated intravascular coagulation. Arch Intern Med 122:43, 1968.

314. Soloway HB, Castillo Y, Martin AM: Adult hyaline membrane disease. Ann Surg 168:937, 1968.

315. Sonnabend D, Cooper D, Fiddes P, Penny R: Fibrin degradation products in thromboembolic disease. Pathology 4:47, 1972.

316. Soria CS, Samama M: A plasminogen assay using a chromogenic synthetic substrate: Results from clinical work and from studies of

thrombolysis. In Davidson JF, Rowan RM, Samama MM, Desnoyers PC (Eds): Progress in Chemical Fibrinolysis and Thrombolysis. Raven Press, New York, 1978, p 337.

317. Spivack JL, Sprangler DB, Bell WR: Defibrination after intraamniotic injection of hypertonic saline. N Engl J Med 287:321, 1972.

318. Starzl TE, Boehmig NJ, Amemiya N, Wilson CB, Dixon FJ, Giles GR, Simpson KM, Halgrimson CG: Clotting changes including disseminated intravascular coagulation during rapid renal-allograft rejection. N Engl J Med 283:383, 1970.

319. Steichele DF: Consumptive coagulopathy in obstetrics and gynecology. Thromb Diath Haemorrh (Suppl) 36:177, 1969.

320. Steiner PE, Lushbough CC: Maternal pulmonary embolism by amniotic fluid as a cause of shock and unexplained deaths in obstetrics. JAMA 117:1245, 1941.

321. Stevenson CS, Braden RG, Schneider CL, Johnson JF, Seegers WH: Hemorrhagic diathesis in abruptio placentae with particular reference to the indications for cesarean section. Am J Obstet Gynec 65:88, 1953.

322. Stormorken H: Relation of the fibrinolytic to other biological systems. Thromb Diath Haemorrh 34:378, 1975.

323. Stormorken H: Interrelationships between the coagulation, the fibrinolytic, and the kallikrein-kinin systems. In Meri-Sernari GG, Prentice CRM (Eds): Haemostasis and Thrombosis. Academic Press, London, 1979, p 203.

324. Sun NC, Bowie EJW, Kazmier FJ, Elueback LR, Owen CA: Blood coagulation studies in patients with cancer. Mayo Clin Proc 49:636, 1974.

325. Surgenor DM: Erythrocytes and blood coagulation. Thromb Diath Haemorrh 32:247, 1974.

326. Teger-Nilsson AC, Gryzander E, Hedner U, Myrwold H, Noppa H, Olsson R, Walmo L: Antiplasmin and other natural inhibitors of fibrinolysis in clinical material. In Davidson FJ, Rowan RM, Samama MM, Desnoyers PC (Eds): Progress in Chemical Fibrinolysis and Thrombolysis. Raven Press, New York, 1978, p 327.

327. Thaler E, Lechner K: Antithrombin III deficiency and thromboembolism. Clin Hematol 10:369, 1981.

328. Triplett DA, Harms C, Hermelin L, Huseby RM, Mitchell GA, Pochron SP: Clinical studies of the use of fluorogenic substrate assay method for the determination of plasminogen. Thromb Haemost 42:50, 1979.

329. Ulevich R, Cochran C, Revak S, Morrison D, Johnson A: The structural and enzymatic properties of the Hageman Factor-activated pathways. In Reich E, Rifkin D, Shaw E (Eds): Proteases and Biological Control. Cold Spring Harbor, New York, 1975, p 85.

330. Van Breeman VL, Heustein HB, Bruns PD: Pulmonary hyaline membranes studied with the electron microscope. Am J Pathol 33:769, 1957.

331. Ward PA: A plasmin split fragment of C-3 as a new chemotactic factor. J Exp Med 126:189, 1967.

332. Waxman B, Gambrin R: Use of heparin in disseminated intravascular coagulation. Am J Obstet Gynecol 112:434, 1972.

333. Webster ME: Human plasma kallikrein, its activation and pathological role. Fed Proc 27:84, 1968.

334. Weintraub DB, Ambrus JL, Ambrus CM: Studies on hyaline membrane disease: Diagnostic and prognostic problems. Pediatrics 38:244, 1966.

335. Weiss HJ: The pharmacology of platelet inhibition. Prog Hemost Thromb 1:199, 1972.

336. Wilner GD, Nossell HL, Leroy EI: Activation of Hageman factor by collagen. J Clin Invest 47:2608, 1968.

337. Wilson WL: Malignancy and anticoagulation. In Murano G, Bick RL (Eds): Basic Concepts of Hemostasis and Thrombosis. CRC Press, Boca Raton, FL, 1980, p 227.

338. Winkestein A, Songster CL, Caras TS: Fulminant meningiococcemia and disseminated intravascular coagulation. Arch Intern Med 124:55, 1969.

339. Wong TC: A study on the generalized Schwartzman reaction in pregnant rats induced by bacterial endotoxin. Am J Obstet Gynecol 84:786, 1962.

340. Yoshikawa T, Tanka R, Guze LB: Infection and disseminated intravascular coagulation. Medicine (Baltimore) 50:237, 1971.

341. Zahavi J, Kakkar VV: B-thromboglobulin—a specific marker of in vivo platelet release reaction. Thromb Haemost 44:23, 1980.

342. Zieman M, Friedrich I, Beddin HK: Activated platelets and platelet function in traumatic septic and haemorrhagic pre-shock conditions. Thromb Haemost 42:410, 1979.

343. Zieve PM, Levin J: Disseminated intravascular coagulation. In Zieve PD, Levin J (Eds): Disorders of Hemostasis. W.B. Saunders, Philadelphia, 1976, p 71.

344. Zirlinsky A, Aitman R, Rouvier J: Comparison between a modified ethanol gelation test and protamine sulfate test: Experimental studies. Thromb Haemost 36:165, 1976.

7
Liver Disease

Patients with acute and chronic liver disease experience significant hemorrhage, which represents a major challenge in clinical care, taxes the laboratory and local blood bank facilities, and is often the terminal event in these patients.[2,53] Alterations of hemostasis that occur in patients with liver disease both acute and chronic and of any etiology are complex and extremely multifaceted.

Classically, it has been taught that hemorrhage in chronic liver disease is due to defective hepatocyte synthesis of the vitamin K dependent prothrombin complex factors, Factors II, VII, IX, and X.[37] However, numerous additional alterations of hemostasis, including primary hyperfibrinolysis, platelet function defects, and thrombocytopenia must be appreciated in order to render effective therapy.[6,7] Disseminated intravascular coagulation (DIC) may play a role as chronic liver disease becomes terminal.[6,7] However, DIC is more commonly of etiologic significance in acute hepatic failure of many etiologies as well as in biliary stasis, as will be discussed. The most common sequence of events in patients with chronic liver disease is the development of localized bleeding, usually from a ruptured esophageal varix, peptic ulcer disease, or hemorrhagic gastritis.[3] These bleeding episodes then tend to cascade into massive hemorrhage, which is poorly responsive to the usual therapeutic modalities of Sengstaken-Blakemore tamponade, massive transfusions with whole blood, fresh frozen plasma, plasma expanders, and vasopressin infusion. The usually unsuccessful control of hemorrhage in patients with chronic liver disease is often due to the fact that although many hemostasis defects are corrected, primarily defects in the prothrombin complex factors, many other defects are left essentially unattended, and effective hemostasis cannot be adequately achieved. Alterations of hemostasis occurring in acute and chronic liver disease are summarized in Table 7–1.

Coagulation Protein Changes (Impaired Synthesis)

The hepatocyte is responsible for synthesizing Factors I, II, V, VII, VIII:C, IX, X, XI, XII, and XIII, prekallikrein (Fletcher factor), high molecular weight kininogen (Fitzgerald, Flaujeac, Williams, Reid, and Fujiwara factors), as well as antithrombin III, alpha-2-macroglobulin, alpha-2-antiplasmin, and plasminogen.[2,77] However, there may be other sites of synthesis for Factor VIII:C, plasminogen, and Factor XIII.[5,59] The patient with chronic liver disease commonly demonstrates an early and significant decreased hepatic synthesis of the prothrombin complex factors (II, VII, IX, and X) as well as fibrinogen, Factor V, XI, XII, prekallikrein, high molecular

Table 7–1 Alterations of Hemostasis in Liver Disease

Acute
Defective (PIVKA*) synthesis
Disseminated intravascular coagulation
Thrombocytopenia
Platelet function defects
Decreased synthesis
Chronic
Defective synthesis
Primary fibrino(geno)lysis
Thrombocytopenia
Platelet function defects
Vascular defects (poorly defined)
Disseminated intravascular coagulation (usually only at terminal stage)

* PIVKA: proteins induced by vitamin K absence or antagonists.

weight kininogen, antithrombin III, alpha-2-antiplasmin, and plasminogen.[6,7,53,77] However, the degree of decrease in each of these factors is going to be somewhat dependent on the degree of primary fibrinolysis present, the degree of elevation of those factors that may behave as acute phase reactants, including antithrombin III, fibrinogen, Factor V, Factor VIII:C, and alpha-2-macroglobulin. Thus, the coagulation factor changes will be a clinical summation of many multifactorial events occurring.[6,7] In addition, patients with chronic liver disease demonstrate some degree of abnormal carboxylation leading to synthesis of abnormal Factors II, VII, IX, and X or the synthesis of proteins induced by vitamin K absence or Antagonists (PIVKA).[36,69] The decrease in Factor VII best correlates with the prothombin time determination; however, the decreases in Factors IX and X best correlate with predisposition to clinical hemorrhage.

The patient with chronic liver disease may also synthesize defective fibrinogen leading to a pseudodysfibrinogenemia; this can come about through numerous mechanisms, including not only the synthesis of an abnormal fibrinogen by the hepatocyte, but also by fibrinogen being mildly plasmin degraded into a high-solubility, low-thrombin clottability type of abnormal fibrinogen; in addition, fibrinogen may complex with split products and become dysfunctional.[6-8] Thus, a dysfibrinogenemia or pseudodysfibrinogenemia may occur via numerous multifaceted mechanisms. However, if significant primary fibrinolysis is not present, the degree of hypofibrinogenemia is usually not of clinical significance with respect to hemorrhage. As noted, normal or increased fibrinogen levels may also be seen in patients with chronic liver disease, since fibrinogen may behave as an acute phase reactant. As previously mentioned, the degree of primary fibrinolysis as well as other defects will also be multifaceted determinants of the levels of all of the aforementioned clotting factors that are synthesized by the hepatocyte.

Thus, many patients with chronic liver disease will have an acquired dysfibrinogenemia reflected by abnormal fibrin monomer polymerization resulting in prolonged thrombin times or reptilase times. This may be due to many multifaceted events, including abnormal carbohydrate content of fibrinogen.[42,52] As liver disease becomes "end-stage" there may also be decreased sythesis of Factors V and VIII:C; alternatively, these factors may be markedly decreased, simply due to significant activation of the fibrinolytic system and circulating plasminemia. However, early in the course of chronic liver disease, these two factors may actually be elevated. The synthesis of prekallikrein and high molecular weight kininogen is also decreased. Although the clinical significance of this defect, if any, remains unclear. Patients with chronic liver disease of any etiology usually demonstrate significantly decreased levels of antithrombin III and the pathophysiology of this remains unclear and may represent either a true decreased synthesis or the synthesis of a dysfunctional antithrombin III molecule.[1,25] In addition, if DIC becomes a manifestation of end stage chronic liver disease or if the patient has acute liver failure due to viral hepatitis, acute hepatitis of any infectious etiology, or liver failure due to acute hepatic failure which is drug-induced or toxin- or chemical-induced, a DIC-type syndrome may also develop, and then the typical findings of this fulminant syndrome, as discussed in Chapter 6, may be operative.[9,22,29,53,64,65,70] Some patients may have high or high normal antithrombin III levels if DIC is not present.[10] This alpha-2-globulin, like fibrinogen, may also behave as an acute phase reactant.[11] The clinical significance of antithrombin III findings in chronic liver disease remain unclear with respect to clinical development of hypercoagulability or thrombosis.

Patients with acute hepatic failure of any etiology, especially viral-induced, drug-induced, or toxin- or chemical-induced may develop a DIC-type syndrome with the findings as previously depicted being present.[9,22,29,53,64,65,70] In addition, patients developing long-term intrahepatic or extrahepatic cholestasis by biliary obstruction commonly develop decreased synthesis of the vitamin K dependent factors due to the inability of vitamin K to be utilized.[26,28,54,63,65] Vitamin K is lipid soluble and thus may be malabsorbed in these obstructive type syndromes. Thus, these patients will commonly demonstrate abnormal synthesis (PIVKA synthesis) of Factors II, VII, IX, and X[36,64,65,69] However, patients may also, on occasion, develop an acute fulminant DIC-type syndrome as discussed in Chapter 6. Impaired synthesis-type defects in chronic liver disease are summarized in Table 7–2. Common defects of hemostasis occurring in acute hepatic failure and cholestatic liver disease are summarized in Table 7–3. Older and newer laboratory modalities for assessing defective coagulation proteins in liver disease are summarized in Table 7–4.

Table 7–2 Impaired Synthesis in Chronic Liver Disease

Decreased synthesis of prothrombin complex
  Factor II
  Factor VII
  Factor IX
  Factor X
Defective (PIVKA) synthesis of prothrombin complex
  PIVKA Factor II
  PIVKA Factor VII
  PIVKA Factor IX
  PIVKA Factor X
  PIVKA Protein C?
Decreased synthesis of
  Fibrinogen
  Factor V
  Factor VIII:C
  Factor XI
  Factor XII
  Factor XIII
  Prekallikrein
  High molecular weight kininogen
  Antithrombin III
  Protein C
  Protein S
  Plasminogen
  Alpha-2-antiplasmin
  Alpha-2-macroglobulin

Table 7–3 Defects in Hemostasis in Acute Hepatic Failure and Cholestasis

Acute hepatic failure
  Decreased or defective synthesis
  Thrombocytopenia
  Disseminated intravascular coagulation
Intrahepatic or extrahepatic cholestasis
  Defective (PIVKA) synthesis
  Disseminated intravascular coagulation

Table 7–4 Laboratory Evaluation of Defective Synthesis in Liver Disease

Older Methods (Manual)	Newer Methods (Automated)
Prothrombin time	Extrinsic pathway generated thrombin*
Partial thromboplastin time	Intrinsic pathway generated thrombin[†]
Factor II assay	Biologic Factor II[‡]
Factor VII assay	Biologic Factor VII[‡]
Factor IX assay	Biologic Factor IX[‡]
Factor X assay	Biologic Factor X[‡]
Fibrinogen assay	Biologic fibrinogen[§]
	Immunologic Factor II[§]
	Immunologic Factor VII[§]
	Immunologic Factor IX[§]
	Immunologic Factor X[§]
	Immunologic Fibrinogen[§]

* Synthetic substrate equivalent of prothrombin time.
[†] Synthetic substrate equivalent of partial thromboplastin time.
[‡] Synthetic substrate (chromogenic or fluorogenic).
[§] ELISA, radioimmunoassay, laser nephelometer.

Enhanced Destruction (Primary Fibrinolysis)

The physiology of the fibrinolytic system was discussed in Chapter 1; this section will be concerned with pathologic fibrinolysis as it relates to liver disease. Enhanced destruction-type defects in liver disease are summarized in Table 7–5. In many, if not most, instances of pathologic activation of the fibrinolytic system the precise mechanisms remain unclear.[6–8] Additionally, many proposed mechanisms are only theoretical. If details of pathologic activation mechanisms are known, they are included in the appropriate disease-related discussions of this book. Potential pathologic activation mechanisms are as follows: (1) Elevated plasminogen levels may lead to pathologic activation of the fibrinolytic system, although in most instances of "hyperplasminogenemia" there is no such activation; (2) decreased inhibitors of the fibrinolytic system, primarily alpha-2-antiplasmin and alpha-2-macroglobulin, may lead to pathologic activation,[53] which may be, in part, responsible for primary activation processes in liver disease and liver failure; (3) increased plasminogen activators may cause pathologic activa-

Table 7–5 Enhanced Destruction (Pathologic Fibrinolysis) in Chronic Liver Disease

Plasmin biodegradation
Hypofibrinogenemia
Dysfibrinogenemia
Factor V
Factor VIII:C
Factor XI
Factor XII
Other plasma proteins (ACTH, insulin, growth hormone)
Fibrin(ogen) degradation products
Dysfibrinogenemia
Defective fibrin monomer polymerization
Platelet function defects
Hyperpyrexia
Plasmin-induced activation
Factor XII activation
Complement activation (C1 and C3)
Prekallikrein activation
Kinin generation

tion; this mechanism, via poor hepatic clearance of activators, appears to be operative in hepatic cirrhosis; (4) decreased "activation" inhibitors may be responsible for pathologic fibrinolytic system activation, although, this is presently only a hypothetical mechanism, (5) exposure of blood and fibrinolytic system enzymes to foreign surfaces or abnormal vasculature may lead to activation, and both of these may account for pathologic activation during cardiopulmonary bypass,[17,19] and the last may be operative in some instances of secondary activation in DIC.[9,22] With respect to activation of the fibrinolytic system during cardiopulmonary bypass, another mechanism now known to be operative is that of Factor XII activation and subsequent activation of the fibrinolytic system; (6) drugs may serve to activate the fibrinolytic system by unclear mechanisms, and certain antineoplastic agents, anabolic steroids, and nicotinic acid are known to possess this property;[51,75] (7) tumor-derived enzymes and extracts have been shown to be capable of activating the plasminogen-plasmin system; this may clearly lead to primary fibrinolytic syndromes in certain selected malignancies;[18,21] (8) pathologic activation of the Hageman factor or of endothelial plasminogen activator may account for the secondary activation (release) of fibrino-

lysis in DIC-type syndromes;[9,20,22,23] and (9) streptokinase and urokinase are pharmacologic activators and are currently used clinically to induce a therapeutic thrombolytic state.[38]

Thrombolytic therapy will be discussed in Chapter 14. Potential activation mechanisms are summarized in Table 7–6, and pathologic activation pathways are summarized in Figure 7–1.

Biological Effects of Fibrin(ogen) Degradation Products on Hemostasis

As plasmin begins to lyse fibrinogen and fibrin, the carboxy-terminal end of the A-alpha chain is destroyed (removed) first. This process then continues to destruction of the B-beta chain, and finally the gamma chain is digested. This process of sequential digestion is responsible for the formation of the four major clinically recognized degradation products, the X, Y, D, and E fragments, referred to as fibrin(ogen) degradation products (FDPs) or fibrin(ogen) split products.[56,58] During any type of intravascular fibrino(geno)-lysis, whether it be a primary or secondary event or therapeutically induced, the titer of these four degradation products become significantly increased as the rate of formation exceeds the ability of the reticuloen-

Table 7–6 Activation Pathways for Pathologic Primary Fibrinolysis

Elevated plasminogen
Decreased fibrinolytic inhibitors (alpha-2-antiplasmin or alpha-2-macroglobulin)
Increased plasminogen activators (endothelial or plasma)
Decreased activation inhibitors
Exposure of fibrinolytic components to foreign surfaces or abnormal vasculature
Drug-induced activation of fibrinolysis (streptokinase, urokinase, anabolic steroids, and nicotinic acid)
Tumor-derived materials or enzymes
Factor XII activation
Pathologic endothelial plasminogen activator activity
Therapeutic thrombolysis

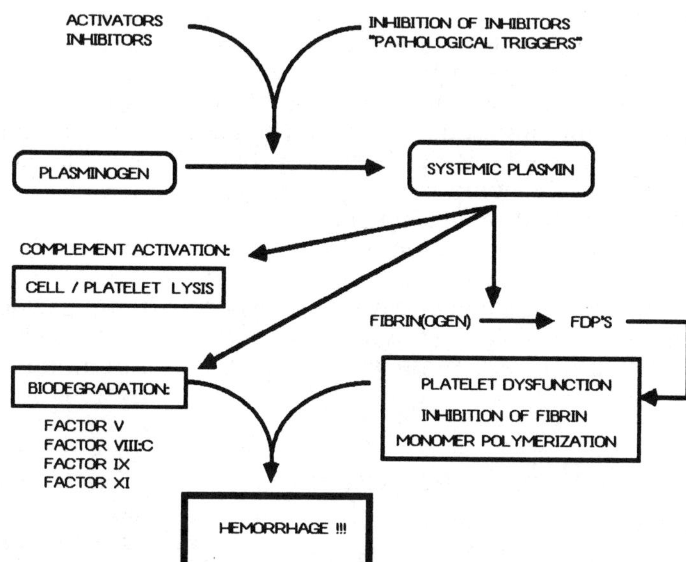

Fig. 7–1. Pathologic activation of the fibrinolytic system.

dothelial system to clear them from the circulation.[66] Thus, the titer can be used as an *indirect approximation* of the extent of fibrino(geno)lysis occurring. The scheme of fibrin(ogen) degradation by plasmin is depicted in Figure 1–30. These four degradation products exert significant biologic effects, many of which have major deleterious consequences in hemostasis and may significantly enhance hemorrhage. Fragment X exerts a very potent antithrombin action by still being clottable by thrombin, although much more slowly than is intact fibrinogen. The Y fragment is derived from fragment X and appears to be a very short-lived intermediate. The formation of this derivitive involves cleavage of peptides from the aminoterminal portion of the B-beta chains followed by asymmetrical splitting of the three chains at one side of the partly degraded dimer. The Y derivitive, like the X derivitive, also prolongs the thrombin time when added to fibrinogen. In addition, both X and Y fragments may form soluble fibrin monomer complexes, as was discussed in detail in Chapter 6.

Since one of the polymerization sites is located on the D area (others are located on the E area), it is understandable that in the presence of these fragments polymerization will be abnormal, since these fragments may complex with fibrin monomer and give rise to interference with fibrin monomer polymerization. Further digestion of the Y fragment gives rise to a second D fragment and one final E fragment. Fragment D also interferes with normal polymerizaion. However, anticoagulant activity of fragment E has not been determined with certainty. As an additional insult to hemostasis, all four of these fragments demonstrate an affinity for platelet membranes, thus coating the platelet membranes and rendering platelets dysfunctional. This often causes a clinically significant platelet function defect, as will be discussed subsequently.[8,48,50] Fragments D and E appear to be the most pronounced in this action. Additionally, there is evidence to suggest that FDPs may account for, at least in some instances, hyperpyrexia seen in hemorrhagic and thrombotic disorders.

An additional early activity of plasmin is to split B-beta 15–42 and related peptides from the B-beta chain; the noting of these peptides in conjunction with the presence or absence of fibrinopeptide A is of marked benefit in offering a differential diagnosis between DIC-type syndromes with secondary fibrinolysis and primary activation of the fibrinolytic system.[12,13] This will be discussed in the laboratory diagnosis section.

In summary, as FDPs are formed from the plasmin-induced lysis of fibrinogen and fibrin, the biologic effects are: (1) inhibition of the hemostasis system by interference with fibrin monomer polymerization; (2) an antithrombin effect; and (3) interference with platelet function. In addition, these fragments·may induce hyperpyrexia. The biologic consequences of circulating FDPs are summarized in Table 7–7.

Clinical and Laboratory Consequences of Abnormal Fibrinolytic Activation

The clinical and laboratory manifestations of pathologic fibrinolytic system activation are summarized in Figure 7–1. During pathologic fibrinolytic activation, plasmin-induced degradation of fibrinogen and fibrin rapidly creates FDPs the X, Y, D, and E fragments. These fragments interfere with fibrin monomer polymerization, induce a platelet function defect, and are associated with hypofibrinogenemia or dysfibrinogenemia. The net

Table 7–7 Biologic Significance of Circulating Fibrin(ogen) Degradation Products

Hemostasis manifestations
  Interference with fibrin monomer polymerization
  Platelet function defects
  Inhibition of thrombin
  Dysfibrinogenemia
  Hyperpyrexia
Laboratory manifestations
  Prolonged prothrombin time
  Prolonged activated partial thromboplastin time
  Prolonged thrombin time
  Prolonged reptilase time
  Hypofibrinogenemia
  Elevated FDPs
  Abnormal clot retraction
  Prolonged template bleeding time
  Abnormal platelet aggregation

clinical result of these three events will be hemorrhage.[6–8]

The hallmark laboratory finding of plasmin-induced lysis of fibrinogen or fibrin is the noting of an elevated titer of FDPs and elevated B-beta 15–42 and related peptides.[12] Laboratory manifestations of defective fibrin monomer polymerization are a prolonged thrombin time, a prolonged reptilase time, faulty clot retraction, and occasional prolongation of the prothrombin time and activated partial thromboplastin time.[6–8,12] In addition, hypoplasminogenemia and circulating plasmin may be found; both of these proteins are readily assayed by synthetic substrate technique. An additional potential aid for the assessment of pathologic fibrinolysis are synthetic substrate-based assays for tissue (endothelial) plasminogen activator activity.[12]

FDP-induced platelet function defects will be discussed subsequently but are manifested in the laboratory as a prolonged template bleeding time and abnormal platelet aggregation and lumiaggregation, although the patterns may not be consistent with respect to the type of abnormal patterns seen.[12] The laboratory findings of hypofibrinogenemia or dysfibrinogenemia induced by FDPs will be prolongation of the thrombin time, prolongation of the reptilase time, and the noting of low fibrinogen levels by clotting assay, immunologic assay, or protein determination techniques.[6–9,12,22]

Since plasmin is a nonspecific proteolytic enzyme, it also degrades many of the coagulation factors, as has been discussed. The primary factors that are degraded, besides fibrinogen (Factor I) are Factors V, VIII, IX, and XI.[6–8] This may be pronounced and the clinical manifestation will be hemorrhage.[6–8] The laboratory consequences of plasmin-induced coagulation factor degradation are prolongation of the prothrombin time, prolongation of the activated partial thromboplastin time, and abnormalities found on specific factor assays, such as low Factor V, Factor VIII, and other factors.[12] Another consequence of circulating plasmin is potentially that of complement activation, a commonly neglected or ignored clinical aspect of primary activation of the fibrinolytic system.[59] The clinical manifestations of this activation pathway are increased vascular permeability leading to third spacing, hypotension, and shock; in addition, there are cellular membrane alterations leading to cell lysis, including red cell lysis and platelet lysis, both associated with release of procoagulant material.[9,22] This may be noted by abnormal complement assays, usually manifested as a decreased C3 level and decreased total hemolytic complement, and laboratory evidence of mild to moderate red cell hemolysis (low haptoglobin, elevated serum, and urine iron levels, indirect hyperbilirubinemia, and elevated reticulocyte count).[9,22]

A less common potential event subsequent to activation of the fibrinolytic system is kinin generation.[59] More commonly, the prekallikrein and then kinin system is activated by mechanisms common to or previous to fibrinolytic system activation. The clinical consequences of kinin system activation are increased vascular permeability and vasodilation leading to hypotension and shock.[9,22] Few clinical laboratory tools are yet available to document activation of the kinin system. The biologic consequences of pathologic activation of the fibrinolytic system are summarized in Table 7–8.

Until recently, primary activation of the fibrinolytic system was considered uncommon and the only situations in which clinical fibrinolysis existed were assumed to be those secondary to DIC-type syndromes. However, these considerations were formulated in an era when there were insufficient clinical laboratory tools to assess fibrinolytic activity in patients with disease. Early work in clinical fibrinolysis was limited to the use of the euglobulin lysis time, which is of questionable clinical significance in assessing clinical fibrinolytic activity.[49,57] With the advent of newer and more sophisticated techniques such as the determination of FDPs and plasminogen, plasmin, alpha-2-antiplasmin, and endothelial plasminogen activator assays, it is now recognized that primary activation of the fibrinolytic system is a relatively common clinical event.[6–8] New assays for assessment of the fibrinoly-

Table 7–8 Clinical Consequences of Pathologic Fibrinolytic System Activation

Plasmin-induced biodegradation of clotting factors
  Hemorrhage
Plasmin-induced activation of complement
  Platelet lysis (procoagulant release)
  Red blood cell lysis (procoagulant release)
  Hemorrhage
  Hypotension
  Shock
  End organ damage
Plasmin-induced activation of kinins
  Hypotension
  Shock
  End organ damage

tic system in addition to those just mentioned are alpha-2-macroglobulin and B-beta 15–42 and related peptides.

The conditions in which primary activation of the fibrinolytic system may occur are generally well defined and include chronic liver disease, cardiopulmonary bypass surgery, and malignancy.[6–8,21] The majority of patients with chronic liver disease experience a hyperfibrino(geno)lytic syndrome due to increased quantities of circulating plasmin.[6–8,62] Primary hypofibrino(geno)lysis (circulating plasmin) causes numerous hemostatic defects, as previously discussed. Hypofibrinogenemia and pseudodysfibrinogenemia are manifested in several forms; one is the creation of high-soluability, low-thrombin clottability fibrinogen subspecies.[58] This represents fibrinogen that has undergone minimal cleavage by plasmin. Because of the fibrino(geno)lysis, patients with chronic liver disease demonstrate elevated FDPs.[6–8] The early degradation products complex with fibrinogen and thus interfere with fibrin monomer polymerization, leading to a pseudodysfibrinogenemia. FDPs also cause a significant platelet function defect, as will be discussed. Circulating plasmin digests Factors V, VIII, IX, and XI, further propagating hemorrhage.[6,7] These additional fibrino(geno)lytic insults to hemostasis must always be borne in mind when clinical care is being rendered to the patient with chronic liver disease.

Laboratory Manifestations of Primary Fibrinolysis

The consequences of circulating plasmin have previously been discussed in detail.[6–8,12,13] The hallmark finding is elevated FDPs. In association with elevated FDPs there is a severe platelet function defect, plasmin-induced degradation of clotting factors, and elevation of B-beta 15–42 and related peptides.

Global tests of hemostasis, such as the prothrombin time and activated partial thromboplastin time, are often prolonged due to the presence of FDPs, degradation of clotting Factors V, VIII, IX, and XI, and FDP-induced defective fibrin monomer polymerization. The thrombin time and reptilase time are usually prolonged due to FDP interference with fibrin monomer polymerization, plasmin-induced hypofibrinogenemia or dysfibrinogenemia, and defective fibrin monomer polymerization. Specific factor assays usually reveal low levels of Factors V, VIII, IX, and XI due to degradation, but these assays add little to a specific diagnosis. Assays for soluble fibrin monomer are almost always negative, since no significant fibrin monomer is formed in the absence of thrombin. Little or no antithrombin III consumption is present; however, this test may not be of diagnostic significance, since antithrombin III levels, as previously discussed, are commonly low due to defective synthesis in patients with liver disease. In addition, antithrombin III levels may be significantly decreased in patients with acute liver failure if developing a DIC-type syndrome. Thus, antithrombin III levels in liver disease are sometimes not of differential diagnostic significance.

The presence or absence of thrombocytopenia is variable and depends on the etiology of liver disease. Thrombocytopenia, as will be discussed, is not a good differential diagnostic tool in patients with chronic liver disease or in patients with acute hepatic insult who develop DIC and subsequent thrombocytopenia. Thus, thrombocytopenia is highly variable, depending on the underlying type of liver disease and, at times, may not be a reliable diagnostic test for distinguishing between primary fibrino(geno)lysis and DIC-type syndromes. It should be recalled that primary lysis itself will not induce thrombocytopenia, but many hepatic disorders are commonly associated with thrombocytopenia by independent mechanisms.

In summary, the key to a laboratory diagnosis of primary fibrino(geno)lysis in liver disease is to note elevated FDPs, elevated B-beta 15–42 related peptides, normal fibrinopepetide A levels, a usually negative paracoagulation reaction, hypofibrinogenemia, and the demonstration of hypoplasminogenemia and elevated plasmin levels.[6,7,12,13] Decreased levels of alpha-2-antiplasmin will usually be found. Antithrombin III levels and platelet counts may or may not be of benefit, depending on the underlying disease process, as previously discussed. In the majority of cases of primary lysis, FDP will be elevated, the B-beta 15–42 related peptides, will be elevated, fibrinopeptide A will be normal, and the protamine sulfate or ethanolgelatin test will usually be negative.[12–14] In most instances of DIC the FDPs, B-beta 15–42 peptides, and fibrinopeptide A or B levels will be elevated, and the protamine sulfate or ethanol gelation test will be positive; plasminogen and alpha-2-antiplasmin will be depressed, circulating plasmin may be demonstrated, and antithrombin III levels will be markedly decreased.[9,12,22] Newer and older methods for the laboratory assessment of primary fibrino(geno)lysis are depicted in Table 7–9. Molecular marker profiling for rendering a differential diagnosis between DIC and primary fibrino(geno)lysis is depicted in Table 7–10.

Thus, it is extremely important to recall that primary activation of the fibrinolytic system occurs in many instances of chronic liver disease and this defect in hemostasis must, like other defects, be looked for in the patient with liver disease and hemorrhage assessed from the laboratory standpoint and treated appropriately if present. The usual therapy for primary fibrinolysis is the use of episilon-aminocaproic acid as 5 to 10 g slow intravenous push followed by 1 to 2 g/hour for 24 hours or until fibrinolysis and subsequent hemorrhage cease.[6,7]

Table 7–9 Laboratory Evaluation of Fibrino(geno)lysis

Older Methods (Manual)	Newer Methods (Automated)
Prothrombin time	Extrinsic pathway generated thrombin*
Activated partial thromboplastin time	Intrinsic pathway generated thrombin*
Thrombin time	
Reptilase time	Antithrombin III*
FDPs	Fibrinopeptide A[†]
Fibrinogen	Plasminogen*
Euglobulin lysis time	Plasmin*
	Plasminogen activator*
	Alpha-2-antiplasmin*
	Alpha-2-macroglobulin*
	FDPs[†]
	Fibrinogen[†]
	B-beta 15-42 peptides[†]

* Synthetic substrate.
[†] ELISA, radioimmunoassy, laser nephelometry.

Table 7–10 Molecular Market Profiling in the Differential Diagnosis of Disseminated Intravascular Coagulation-Type Syndromes Versus Primary Fibrino(geno)lytic Syndromes

Marker	DIC	Primary Lysis
Fibrinopeptide A	Elevated	Normal
Fibrinopeptide B	Elevated	Normal
B-beta 15-42 peptide	Elevated	Normal
B-beta 1-42 peptide	Elevated	Elevated
B-beta 1-118 peptide	Elevated	Elevated
Platelet factor 4	Elevated	Normal
Beta-thromboglobulin	Elevated	Normal

Platelet Defects

Thrombocytopenia

Thrombocytopenia is seen in up to 35% of patients with chronic liver disease (cirrhosis) of diverse etiologies.[6,7,61] The most common cause, of course, is portal hypertension with resultant congestive splenomegaly and hypersplenism.[4,74] It should be noted, however, that hypersplenism (increased splenic sequestration of platelets and other cellular elements) need not be always associated with significant splenomegaly. However, in the majority of patients with chronic liver disease the degree of thrombocytopenia correlates reasonably well with the degree of splenomegaly,[40] as does the severity of hepatic damage.[40] This results in decreased platelet survival, but marrow megakaryocytes are usually normal or increased. Portacaval shunts will correct the thrombocytopenia of hypersplenism secondary to portal hypertension in approximately 30% of patients.

Patients with cirrhosis may also have thrombocytopenia secondary to folate deficiency which may arise from poor dietary intake, poor intestinal absorption, or enhanced requirements, such as in the patient with cirrhosis and hemolysis.[46] The archaic use of massive transfusions of banked whole blood to treat hemorrhage associated with liver disease may also significantly add to already existing thrombocytopenia or this practice may independently induce thrombocytopenia.[65] This practice is, of course, to be condemned. Although this supplies volume and oxygen-carrying capacity to the patient, its use in patients with acute or chronic liver disease is generally detrimental to the platelet count and to many other already impaired hemostasis systems and often will lead to enhanced and uncontrollable hemorrhage.[6,7] The more modern approach of component therapy in patients with liver disease and hemorrhage, utilizing washed packed red cells, fresh frozen plasma, and platelet concentrates, has served to ameliorate this problem to a large extent. Thrombocytopenia may also arise as a consequence of DIC in patients with chronic liver disease.[6,7] DIC is usually not associated with cirrhosis until cirrhosis reaches its terminal stage.[6,7] However, the patient with chronic liver disease can certainly develop DIC and associated severe thrombocytopenia if subjected to any of the usual triggers or disease entities, such as septicemia or shock that may induce DIC, as previously discussed in Chapter 6.

Significant thrombocytopenia may also be seen in acute liver failure of viral or drug- or chemical-induced etiology.[38] The thrombocytopenia of acute viral hepatitis and hepatitis seen with mononucleosis or cytomegalovirus may be multifactorial. In these instances there may be an element of DIC contributing to or accounting for thrombocytopenia via previously mentioned mechanisms; there may be a selective suppression of megakaryopoiesis, or the thrombocytopenia may be part of a pancytopenia associated with marrow aplasia, which occasionally occurs in patients with acute hepatic failure.[45,64,71] In acute hepatic failure of viral, drug, chemical or toxin etiology, thrombocytopenia may also result from the development of antiplatelet antibodies or the presence of circulating immune complexes.[47] In clinical practice, the thrombocytopenia of chronic or acute liver disease may be a summary of several or all of the aforementioned mechanisms.

If the patient with chronic liver disease is also an alcoholic, additional mechanisms for the development of thrombocytopenia may also be operative. Thrombocytopenia may be seen in up to 25% of ill patients who are actively drinking;[30,33] 50% of these will have concomitant cirrhosis.[30,33,39] Ethanol appears to be directly toxic to megakaryocytes and may induce peripheral thrombocytopenia by causing ineffective megakaryopoiesis.[30,31,67,72] Additionally, ethanol appears to induce a nonselective peripheral destruction of platelets that is not necessarily due to splenic sequestration.[30,67,72] The reported findings of platelet size distribution profile and platelet survival studies show ethanol to induce an increase in the percent of small circulating platelets and a decrease in platelet survival; these findings are compatible with both ineffective megakaryopoiesis as well as enhanced peripheral destruction.[30,33,67] Folate deficiency associated with ethanol abuse, even in the absence of cirrhosis, may also contribute to or be responsible for thrombocytopenia.[30,31] Thrombocytopenia that is persistent is usually due to portal hypertension, splenomegaly, and associated hypersplenism; however, if due primarily to acute ethanol intoxication, rather than splenic sequestration, the thrombocytopenia will usually abate within 1 to 3 weeks after abstinence.[30,33] In this regard, a rebound thrombocytosis may be seen in up to 30% of patients and in some instances has been thought to be responsible for thrombotic episodes.[30,43]

It has been noted that the template bleeding time is two times prolonged in acute ethanol intoxication and up to five times prolonged in ethanol ingestion plus thrombocytopenia.[30] These findings should be viewed as multifactorial and consist of not only an ethanol-induced or cirrhosis-induced platelet function defect or thrombocytopenia, but also may be due to a vascular defect that may be present in alcoholic and cirrhotic patients.[6,7,15] Causes of thrombocytopenia associated with chronic and acute liver disease and acute hepatic failure and alcohol are summarized in Table 7–11. Platelet function defects and vascular defects seen in patients with liver disease will be discussed in subsequent sections.

Liver transplantation may be associated with thrombocytopenia; this is usually part of a DIC-type syndrome via mechanisms that were discussed in Chapter 6. However, if transplantation rejection is occurring, circulating immune complexes may also contribute to thrombocytopenia. Additionally, of course, circulating immune complexes may also compromise hemostasis by inducing a platelet function defect and vascular defect as well.

Table 7–11 Causes of Thrombocytopenia in Chronic and Acute Liver Disease, Acute Hepatic Failure, and Ethanol Abuse

Chronic liver disease
  Splenomegaly and hypersplenism
  Disseminated intravascular coagulation (terminal disease)
  Massive transfusions (especially whole blood)
  Folate deficiency (malabsorption, diet, hemolysis)
  Concurrent ethanol use
Acute liver disease or acute hepatic failure
  Suppression of megakaryopoiesis (viral, drug, toxin)
  Aplastic anemia (viral, drug, toxin)
  Disseminated intravascular coagulation (may occur early)
  Antiplatelet antibodies (viral, drug, toxin)
  Circulating immune complexes (viral, drug, toxin)
  Liver transplantation rejection
    Disseminated intravascular coagulation
    Circulating immune complexes
Ethanol abuse
  Splenomegaly and hypersplenism
  Ineffective megakeryopoiesis
  Nonselective peripheral destruction
  Folate deficiency
  Rebound thrombocytosis in 30% with abstinence

Many patients with chronic liver disease and ascites are subjected to LeVeen shunting; this may induce a DIC-type syndrome and associated severe thrombocytopenia. This phenomena will be discussed in detail in Chapters 8 and 10.

It is unclear as to what degree thrombocytopenia contributes to hemorrhage in the patient with liver disease; not only are the causes of thrombocytopenia multifaceted, but thrombocytopenia is actually only one of numerous alterations of hemostasis in patients with acute or chronic liver disease. Thus, thrombocytopenia should be thought of as being part of a summation of multifactorial events when hemorrhage is present in these patients. Fortunately, however, thrombocytopenia is a defect that if thought to be of clinical significance in the hemorrhaging patient with liver disease, can usually be readily corrected with the liberal use of platelet concentrates.

Platelet Function Defects

Significant platelet dysfunction also occurs in patients with liver disease, although this hemostatic defect is less commonly appreciated and often goes unrecognized in patients with liver disease and hemorrhage.[6-8] As with thrombocytopenia, causes of platelet dysfunction in patients with liver disease may be multifactorial in origin. The majority of patients with chronic liver disease have primary activation of the fibrinolytic system and resultant elevated circulating FDPs[6-8] These circulating FDPs may severely compromise platelet function, as has been discussed in previous sections. Another reason for platelet dysfunction is the finding of an increase in older platelets, as noted by a decreased mean platelet volume in patients with liver disease; these are presumably less hemostatically active platelets.[67] Patients with both acute and chronic liver disease often demonstrate secondary aggregation defects or storage pool-type aggregation defects manifested as blunted aggregation to collagen, thrombin, and ristocetin, and absent secondary aggregation waves after aggregation with adenosine diphosphate (ADP) and epi-

nephrine.[30,32] In addition, platelet factor 3 release is commonly impaired.[44] Platelet dysfunction in liver disease may be manifestations of altered platelet membrane palmate or stearate metabolism,[73] may result from coating of platelet membranes by FDPs,[8] or may be a combination of these defects; platelet dysfunction may also be a manifestation of many as yet undefined alterations in platelet metabolic pathways.

If the patient with liver disease is an ethanol abuser, platelet function is further compromised. The ingestion of high doses of ethanol, even in the absence of significant liver disease, may induce a storage pool-type defect; decreased storage pool ADP and adenosine triphosphate (ATP) is induced by ethanol alone, and cyclic AMP levels are also reduced by ethanol-induced inhibition of adenylate cyclase.[30,32,34] As an additional insult, ethanol inhibits thromboxane A2 synthesis.[30,32] Ethanol also is known to inhibit monoamine oxidase but causes a 50 to 100% increase in intraplatelet serotonin; the significance of this finding is unknown.[27,30,35,55] Thus, it appears that ethanol itself induces significant changes in intraplatelet metabolism with adenine nucleotides, cyclic AMP, prostaglandins, and thromboxanes. Ethanol ingestion also impairs platelet factor 3 availability; whether this is due to aforementioned alterations or other, undefined effects of ethanol remains unclear. Folate deficiency may also accompany heavy ethanol ingestion in the absence of significant liver disease, and this also may induce a platelet function defect, independent of folate-associated thrombocytopenia.[30,46,65] Morphologic alterations of platelets induced by ethanol, and presumably associated with defects in platelet function, have also been described. These morphologic changes consist of vacuolization of both platelets and megakaryocytes, abnormal platelet granules, microtublar fragmentation, and the presence of giant platelets.[30,32] Platelet function defects, like thrombocytopenia, have also been seen in association with liver transplantation.[24] This is most likely due to coating of platelets by FDPs, resulting from a DIC-type syndrome. As with thrombocytopenia associated with transplantation rejection and resultant circulating immune complexes, these immune complexes will also compromise platelet function because they are potent inducers of a platelet release reaction.

In summary, acute and chronic liver disease is often associated with a severe and clinically significant platelet function defect. This defect is multifactorial and may be due to altered intraplatelet metabolism of the compounds previously discussed, as well as due to the presence of FDPs. If the patient is also an ethanol abuser, these defects will be compounded. In addition, it should be recalled that ethanol itself, in the absence of significant liver disease, may induce a significant platelet function defect. It is of clinical importance to recall that most patients with acute and chronic liver disease do demonstrate significant platelet dysfunction; one cannot assume a false sense of security when seeing a patient with liver disease, hemorrhage, and a normal or near normal platelet count, since the platelets circulating, although normal in number, may be significantly dysfunctional and thus contribute to hemorrhage that has remained unresponsive to infusions of fresh frozen plasma. When seeing patients with liver disease and hemorrhage, platelet dysfunction should be considered, its presence or absence documented by aggregation or lumiaggregation, and, if present, treated with appropriate numbers of platelet concentrates regardless of the platelet count. Mechanisms of platelet function defects in chronic liver disease, and in association with acute liver disease, acute hepatic failure, and ethanol are summarized in Table 7–12.

Vascular Defects

The patient with chronic liver disease often demonstrates poorly defined vascular defects. This has often been ascribed to an estrogen-like effect on the vasculature, because these patients do have abnormal hepatic clearance and resultant hyperestro-

Table 7–12 Causes of Platelet Function Defects in Chronic and Acute Liver Disease, Acute Hepatic Failure, and Ethanol Abuse

Chronic liver disease
 Elevated fibrin(ogen) degradation products
 Older circulating platelets (decreased mean volume) (hemostatically less active)
 Acquired storage pool defect
  Blunted aggregation to
   Thrombin
   Collagen
   Ristocetin
  Absent secondary aggregation to
   Adenosine diphosphate
   Epinephrine
 Impaired platelet factor 3 availability
 Abnormal platelet membrane function (receptor sites) (abnormal palmate and stearate metabolism)
 Folic acid deficiency
Acute liver disease or acute hepatic failure
 Elevated fibrin(ogen) degradation products (if DIC is present)
 Acquired storage pool defect
 Impaired platelet factor 3 availability
Ethanol abuse
 Acquired storage pool defect
 Deranged intraplatelet metabolism
  Decreased adenine nucleotides
  Decreased or impaired cyclic AMP
  Abnormal prostaglandin metabolism
  Decreased or absent thromboxanes
  Abnormal platelet granules
  Fragmented intraplatelet microtubules
 Folic acid deficiency
Hepatic transplantation rejection
 Elevated fibrin(ogen) degradation products (DIC is usual mechanism of rejection)
 Circulating immune complexes (membrane interaction)

genemia. This mechanism as a cause of the commonly seen vascular defect in patients is, however, poorly understood. Regardless of the mechanism(s), the vascular defect may reach clinical significance, especially if the patient is subjected to surgery or trauma. This defect may also contribute to the prolonged template bleeding time seen in patients with chronic liver disease. Thus, it should be appreciated that the noting of prolonged template bleeding times in patients with chronic liver disease may be due to a combination of thrombocytopenia, platelet dysfunction, and a vascular defect.

Disseminated Intravascular Coagulation

DIC rarely, if ever, occurs de novo as a hemostatic defect in the patient with chronic liver disease.[6-9] However, as previously mentioned, it may be operative in acute liver failure, including hepatitis and in patients subjected to LeVeen shunting and with longstanding biliary obstruction and intrahepatic or extrahepatic cholestasis.[28,54,64,65,70] However, the patient with chronic liver disease is a candidate for DIC, as is any other patient, if provided with one of the usual triggering events for this syndrome, such as sepsis, massive transfusions with banked whole blood, transfusion reactions, shock, and other etiologic events that are known to trigger this syndrome. Vascular defects and DIC-type defects associated with acute and chronic liver disease are summarized in Table 7—13.

Laboratory Findings

Most tests of hemostasis, including global screening tests, will be markedly abnormal with significant alterations of hemostasis associated with liver disease. It must be remembered that the laboratory alterations in patients with chronic liver disease will be a summation of not only the underlying type of defect, i.e., acute, chronic, or cholestatic liver disease, but will also be a summary manifestation of all of the aforementioned defects that may be present and operative singly or in any potential combination. Useful laboratory modalities for assessing hemostasis in patients with chronic liver disease are summarized in Table 7–14.[12] The mainstay laboratory test for assessing function of the prothrombin complex factors is the prothrombin time. In significantly decreased or dysfunctional synthesis of Factors II, VII, IX, and X, the prothrombin time will be significantly prolonged.[6,7] It is controversial as to whether the degree of prolongation of the prothrombin time is related to clinical hemorrhage. The decrease in Factor VII closely correlates with prolongation of the prothrombin time; however, decreased or dysfunctional synthesis of Factors IX and X more closely correlate with clinical hemorrhage. The

Table 7–13 Other Defects in Chronic Liver Disease

Vascular defects
  Poorly defined
  Often ascribed to hyperestrogenemia
  In acute liver disease may be due to
    Circulating immune complex (virus, drug, toxin)
    Antiendothelial antibody (virus, drug, toxin)
Disseminated intravascular coagulation
  Usually not until terminal stage
  Most common causes in chronic liver disease
    Massive transfusions
    Sepsis
    Shock
    LeVeen Shunting
    Biliary obstruction or cholestasis

Table 7–14 Evaluation of Hemostasis in Patients with Chronic Liver Disease

Coagulation factor defects
  Prothrombin time or extrinsic pathway generated thrombin
    Decreased synthesis of prothrombin complex
    Defective synthesis of prothrombin complex
    Decreased synthesis of Factor V
  Activated partial thromboplastin time or intrinsic pathway generated thrombin
    Decreased synthesis of other factors
      Factor V
      Factor VIII:C
      Factor XI
      Factor XII
      Factor XIII
      Prekallikrein
      High molecular weight kininogen
Primary fibrino(geno)lysis
  Plasminogen
  Plasmin
  Alpha-2-antiplasmin
  Alpha-2-macroglobulin
  Fibrin(ogen) degradation products
  B-beta 15-42 and related peptides
Platelet function defects
  Template bleeding time
  Platelet lumiaggregation
Thrombocytopenia
  Platelet count
  Spleen scan
Vascular defects
  Template bleeding time

prothrombin time may also be abnormal for additional reasons, such as the presence of elevated FDP or plasmin-induced biodegradation of Factor V. The activated partial thromboplastin time is likewise prolonged in the patient with acute or chronic liver disease. This occurs for reasons similar to those described for the prothrombin time, including plasmin-induced biodegradation of Factor VIII:C and other factors susceptable to plasmin. Specific factor assays will usually reveal low levels: however, values for selected factors may be high or normal, depending on the particular defect operative, the degree of fibrinolysis, and the degree to which several factors have increased as acute phase reactants. Thus, high levels of Factor VIII:C may be found unless significant plasmin is present, in which case low levels of Factor VIII:C, V, and XI may be seen.[6,7] In addition, the degree of lysis may contribute to the degree of decrease in Factor XII, Fletcher factor, and high molecular weight kininogen.

Tests for fibrinolysis will be abnormal in greater than 75% of of patients with chronic liver disease and may be abnormal in patients with acute hepatic failure or cholestasis if DIC and secondary fibrinolysis are present.[6-8,62] Circulating plasmin and elevated FDP will be found in conjunction with decreased levels of plasminogen due to activation of the fibrinolytic system and plasminogen depletion. Good differential diagnostic tools in this respect for noting whether DIC is operative or whether low levels of clotting factors are present because of primary lysis are the B-beta 15-42 and related peptide determinations, in conjunction with fibronopeptide A, the platelet release proteins, platelet factor 4, and beta-thromboglobulin, and a positive or negative paracoagulation reaction.[6-8]

Tests of platelet function will likewise be abnormal for reasons discussed. Prolongation of the template bleeding time may be due to a combination of platelet function defects, as previously discussed, thrombocytopenia, or defects in the vasculature in patients with chronic liver disease or with acute hepatic failure or cholestasis. However, no characteristic aggregation or lumiaggregation patterns will be noted in these patients. In this regard it should be noted that a template bleeding time should not be performed in the presence of thrombocytopenia (platelet count less than 100,000/mm^3) because this may be associated with unnecessary bleeding and will give results that are meaningless. The degree of prolongation of the template bleeding time, as already noted, may be multifactorial, including simply that induced by heavy ethanol ingestion. However, it remains controversial as to whether the prolongation of the template bleeding time correlates with clinical propensity to hemorrhage. The use of a thrombin time or reptilase time will offer an indication of the degree of dysfibrinogenemia or hypofibrinogenemia present. However, the time in both of these laboratory modalities will also be prolonged with FDPs, rendering the results difficult to interpret with respect to precise reasons for the prolongation of these tests. It is clear that most test results of hemostasis will be markedly abnormal in patients with chronic or acute liver disease or cholestasis, and it is only with the use of a well-chosen hemostatic profile that each component of hemostasis can be assessed in conjunction with knowing what type of liver disease is present and the precise defect or combination of defects therefore delineated and a logical sequential approach to treatment of hemorrhage outlined (Table 7–15).

Management

All clinicians are well aware of the catastrophic hemorrhage that may occur in patients with chronic liver disease and the major challenge this disease presents for the laboratory, blood bank, pathologist, surgeon, hematologist, gastroenterologist, and internist. The mainstay of therapy in most patients is, unfortunately, still limited to infusions of fresh frozen plasma, Sengstaken-Blakemore tamponade, gastric lavage, and vasopressin infusion.[6,7,41] However, many patients fail to respond to these modalities of therapy. If the patient has significant fibrino(geno)lysis, the concomitant or subsequent use of antifibrinolytic

Table 7–15 Sequential Evaluation of Hemorrhage and Therapy in Patients with Liver Disease

Chronic liver disease
Coagulation factor defects
Primary fibrino(geno)lysis
Platelet function defects or thrombocytopenia
Vascular defects
Disseminated intravascular coagulation (rare)
Acute liver disease, hepatic failure, cholestasis
Coagulation factor defects
Disseminated intravascular coagulation (common)
Platelet function defects or thrombocytopenia
Liver transplantation rejection
Disseminated intravascular coagulation (common)

agents, usually episilon-aminocaproic acid may be indicated. This is used at a dose of 5 to 10 g slow intravenous push followed by 1 to 2 g/hour for 24 hours or until cessation of clinical hemorrhage is noted. If the patient is significantly thrombocytopenic, the liberal use of platelet concentrates should also be considered. Platelet concentrates will correct the thrombocytopenia and will usually alleviate bleeding from the platelet function defect which is almost always present in patients with acute or chronic liver failure. For patients failing to respond to the aforementioned modalities of therapy, the use of prothrombin complex concentrates, in conjunction with other components, such as platelet concentrates and other such indicated therapeutic modalities, may have to be resorted to.[16,68] An additional, although somewhat heroic approach, is to treat patients with exchange transfusions.[6,7]

The use of exchange transfusion or the infusion of prothrombin complex concentrate to control hemorrhage is probably not indicated in the patient with chronic liver disease and fulminant hemorrhage unless a surgically correctable bleeding point is demonstrated and the patient is thought to be a surgical candidate and the defect thought to be correctable, since these modalities will only achieve hemostasis for a short period of time.[6,7] In reality many patients with fulminant hemorrhage survive if they are approached in a logical and sequential manner, which must include a precise delineation of the exact type of liver disease, the exact hemostatic

defects present, and each defect defined and treated individually. The patient with cholestasis and abnormal synthesis of the prothrombin complex factors will usually respond to the immediate parenteral administration of vitamin K. The usual dose is 30 mg intramuscularly or 1 mg/minute intravenously. In addition, if brisk bleeding is present, the use of fresh frozen plasma or prothrombin complex concentrates may stop hemorrhage. However, it should be recalled that these patients may also develop a fulminant DIC-type syndrome and should be treated appropriately if this is present. In this regard patients with acute liver disease as well as cholestasis who develop DIC rarely develop intravascular microthrombi, and thus the advisability of using heparin in patients with cholestasis or acute liver failure with DIC is debatable. This general approach to the patient with acute or chronic liver disease of varied etiologies allows for successful blunting or arrest of hemorrhage to the point where the patient may become a reasonable candidate for surgical correction of the initiating event, which is most often peptic ulcer disease, a ruptured esophageal varix, or hemorrhagic gastritis in the patient with chronic liver disease. On the other hand, the patient with acute liver failure that is viral-, toxic-, or drug-induced is usually not a surgical candidate. The patient with cholestasis quite often is a surgical candidate and the infusions of fresh frozen plasma as well as the recognition of the presence or absence of DIC and the use of parenteral vitamin K may arrest hemorrhage. Therapeutic modalities available for the control of hemorrhage in liver disease are summarized in Table 7–16.

Summary

Hemorrhage in the patient with chronic liver disease can no longer be attributed to a simple decrease in the synthesis of Factors II, VII, IX, and X. Numerous defects may occur, and significant or life-threatening hemorrhage may be due to any one of or a combination of these defects. When approaching the patient with hemorrhage

Table 7–16 Available Therapeutic Modalities in Patients with Liver Disease

Coagulation faction defects
  Fresh frozen plasma
  Vitamin K (usually acute disease or cholestasis)
  Prothrombin complex concentrates (hazards)
  Plasma exchange (investigational)
Primary fibrino(geno)lysis
  Aminocaprioc acid
Platelet function defects or thrombocytopenia
  Platelet concentrates (8 to 10 U)
  Immunosuppressives (acute failure)
  Portacaval shunting (thrombocytopenia and
    hypersplenism)
Vascular defects
  No generally effective therapy
Disseminated intravascular coagulation
  Subcutaneous heparin (acute liver disease or failure)
  Heparin not indicated in chronic or terminal disease
  Platelet concentrates
  Washed packed red cells
  Antithrombin III concentrates
  Corticosteroids in selected cases (acute failure)
  Immunosuppressive therapy (transplantation
    rejection)

in chronic liver disease, it is a major clinical and clinical laboratory challenge to define precisely those defects that are most likely causing the hemorrhage, and then to deliver specific, logical, and effective therapy. If primary hyperfibrino-(geno)lysis is a major cause of hemorrhage, as it often is, antifibrinolytic therapy would be appropriate. Fresh frozen plasma may be used to correct hemorrhage associated with decreased or dysfunctional synthesis of Factors II, VII, IX, and X. If significant thrombocytopenia or platelet dysfunction is present, infusions of platelet concentrates are indicated. When the patient fails to respond to specific therapy directed at clearly defined defects, the use of prothrombin complex concentrates in combination with other components may have to be resorted to. However, this remains investigational and those choosing to use these therapeutic modalities should be aware of the potential for disseminated thromboses as well as hepatitis. The same arguments apply to the patient with acute liver failure or cholestasis; multifactorial defects may be present, including a fulminant DIC-type syndrome. Thus, one must consider all of the aforementioned defects and docu-

ment the presence or absence of DIC when designing effective and logical therapy for these patients.

Evaluating the patient with acute or chronic liver disease thus requires delineation of the type of disease present and to recall all of the types of defects that may occur in order to define precisely the defects present or absent and to treat each appropriately to stop the hemorrhage.

References

1. Abildgaard U, Fagerhol MK, Egeberg O: Comparison of progressive antithrombin activity and the concentrations of three thrombin inhibitors in human plasma. Scand J Clin Lab Invest 26:349, 1970.
2. Aledort LM: Clotting abnormalities in liver disease. Prog Liver Dis 5:350, 1976.
3. Amir-Ahmadi N, McGray RS, Marton F, Mitch W, Kantrowitz P, Zamcheck N: Reassessment of massive upper gastrointestinal hemorrhage on the wards of the Boston city hospital. Surg Clin North Am 49:715, 1980.
4. Aster RH: Pooling of platelets in the spleen. Role in the pathogenesis of "hypersplenic" thrombocytopenia. J Clin Invest 45:654, 1966.
5. Barnhart MI, Riddle JM: Cellular localization of profibrinolysin (plasminogen). Blood 21:306, 1963.
6. Bick RL, Murano G: Primary hyperfibrino-(geno)lytic syndromes. In Murano G, Bick RL (Eds): Basic Concepts of Hemostasis and Thrombosis. CRC Press, Boca Raton, FL, 1980, p 181.
7. Bick RL: Syndromes associated with hyperfibrino(geno)lysis. In Bick RL (Ed): Disseminated Intravascular Coagulation and Related Syndromes. CRC Press, Boca Raton, FL, 1983, p 105.
8. Bick RL: The clinical significance of fibrinogen degradation products. Semin Thromb Hemost 8:302, 1982.
9. Bick RL: Disseminated intravascular coagulation. In Bick RL (Ed): Disseminated Intravascular Coagulation and Related Syndromes. CRC Press, Boca Raton, FL, 1983, p 31.
10. Bick RL: Clinical relevance of antithrombin III. Semin Thromb Hemost 8:276, 1982.
11. Bick RL: Alterations of hemostasis associated with malignancy. In Murano G, Bick RL (Eds): Basic Concepts of Hemostasis and Thrombosis. CRC Press, Boca Raton, FL, 1980, p 213.
12. Bick RL: Clinical hemostasis practice: The major impact of laboratory automation. Semin

Thromb Hemost 9:139, 1983.

13. Bick RL: Clinical implications of molecular markers in hemostasis and thrombosis. Semin Thromb Hemost 10:290, 1984.

14. Bick RL, Fareed J, Squillaci G, Walenga J, Hermes EW, Messmore HL: Molecular markers of hemostatic processes. Implications in diagnostic and therapeutic management of thrombotic and hemorrhagic disorders. Fed Proc 42:4, 1983.

15. Bick RL: Vascular disorders associated with thrombohemorrhagic phenomena. Semin Thromb Hemost 5:167, 1979.

16. Bick RL, Schmalhorst WR, Shanbrom E: Prothrombin complex concentrate: Use in controlling the hemorrhagic diathesis of chronic liver disease. Am J Dig Dis 20:1, 1975.

17. Bick RL, Schmalhorst WR, Arbegast NR: Alterations of hemostasis associated with cardipulmonary bypass. Thromb Res 8:285, 1976.

18. Bick RL: Treatment of bleeding and thrombosis in the patient with cancer. In Nealon T (Ed): Care of the Cancer Patient. W.B. Saunders, Philadelphia, 1976, p 48.

19. Bick RL: Alterations of hemostasis associated with cardiopulmonary bypass: Etiology, pathophysiology, diagnosis and management. Semin Thromb Hemost 3:59, 1976.

20. Bick RL: Disseminated intravascular coagulation and related syndromes: Etiology, pathophysiology, diagnosis and management. Am J Hematol 5:265, 1978.

21. Bick RL: Alterations of hemostasis associated with malignancy: Etiology, pathophysiology, diagnosis and management. Semin Thromb Hemost 5:1, 1978.

22. Bick RL: Disseminated intravascular coagulation (DIC) and related syndromes. In Murano G, Bick RL, (Eds): Basic Concepts of Hemostasis and Thrombosis. CRC Press, Boca Raton, FL, 1980, p 163.

23. Bick RL: Disseminated intravascular coagulation and related syndromes. In Fareed J, Messmore H, Fenton J, Brinkhous KM (Eds): Perspectives in Hemostasis. Pergamon Press, New York, NY, 1981, p 122

24. Bohmig HJ: The coagulation disorders of orthotopic hepatic transplantation. Semin Thromb Hemost 4:57, 1977.

25. Braunstein KM, Evrenius K: Minimal heparin cofactor activity in disseminated intravascular coagulation and cirrhosis. Am J Clin Pathol 66:48, 1976.

26. Brinkhous KM, Smith HP, Warner Ed: Prothrombin deficiency and the bleeding tendency of obstructive jaundice and in biliary fistula. Effect of feeding bile and alfalfa (vitamin K). Am J Med Sci 196:50, 1938.

27. Brown JB: Platelet MAO and alcoholism. Am J Psychiatry 134:206, 1977.

28. Cederblad G, Korstan-Bengsten K, Olsen R: Observation of increased levels of blood coagulation factors and other plasma proteins in cholestatic liver disease. Scand J Gastroenterol 11:391, 1976.

29. Coccheri S, Palareti G, Dalmonte PR, Poggi M, Boggian O: Investigations on intravascular coagulation in liver disease: soluble fibrin monomer complexes in liver cirrhosis. Haemostasis 8:8, 1979.

30. Cowan DH: Effect of alcoholism on hemostasis. Semin Hematol 17:137, 1980.

31. Cowan DH: Thrombokinetic studies in alcohol-related thrombocytopenia. J Lab Clin Med 81:64, 1973.

32. Cowan DH, Graham Jr RC: Studies on the platelet defect in alcoholism. Thromb Diath Haemorrh 33:310, 1975.

33. Cowan DH, Hines JD: Thrombocytopenia of severe alcoholism. Ann Intern Med 74:37, 1971.

34. Cowan DH, Kikta M, Baunach D: Alteration of platelet cyclic AMP (cAMP) by ethanol. Thromb Haemost 38:270, 1977.

35. Cowan DH, Shook P: Effects of ethanol on platelet serotonin metabolism. Thromb Haemost 38:33, 1977.

36. Denson KWR: The levels of Factor II, VII, IX, and X by antibody neutralization techniques in the plasma of patients receiving phenindione therapy. Br J Haematol 20:643, 1971.

37. Donaldson GWK, Davies SR, Darg S, Richmond J: Coagulation factors in chronic liver disease. J Clin Pathol 22:109, 1969.

38. Dymock IW, Tucker JS, Woolf EL, Poller L, Thompson JM: Coagulation studies as a prognostic index in acute liver failure. Br J Haematol 29:385, 1975.

39. Eichner ER, Hillman RS: The evoluation of anemia in alcoholic patients. Am J Med 50:218, 1971.

40. Frick W: Thrombocytopenie und Lebercirrhose. Schweiz Med Wochenschr 97:407, 1967.

41. Gilberg DA, Silverstein FE, Auth DC, Rubin CE: Non surgical management of acute nonvariceal upper gastrointestinal bleeding. Prog Hemost Thromb 4:349, 1978.

42. Green G, Thompson JM, Poller L, Dymock IW: Abnormal fibrin monomer polymerization in liver disease. Gut 16:827, 1975.

43. Haselager EM, Vreeken J: Rebound thrombocytosis after alcohol abuse: A possible factor in the pathogenesis of thromboembolic disease. Lancet 1:774, 1977.

44. Haut MJ, Cowan DH: The effect of ethanol on hemostatic properties of human blood platelets. Am J Med 56:22, 1974.

45. Hillenbrand P, Parbhoo SP, Jedrychowski A, Sherlock S: Significance of intravascular coagulation and fibrinolysis in acute hepatic

failure. Gut 15:83, 1974.

46. Jandl JH, Lear AA: The metabolism of folic acid in cirhosis. Ann Intern Med 45:1027, 1956.

47. Karpatkin S, Strick N, Karpatkin MB, Siskind GW: Cumulative experience in the detection of antiplatelet antibody in 234 patients with idiopathic thrombocytopenic purpura, systemic lupus erythematosus, and other clinical disorders. Am J Med 52:776, 1972.

48. Kopec M, Wegrzynowicz Z, Budynski AZ, Latallo ZS, Lipinski B, Kowalski E: Interaction of fibrinogen degradation products (FDP) with platelets. Exp Biol Med 3:73, 1968.

49. Kowalski E, Kopec M, Niewiarowski S: An evaluation of the euglobulin method for the determination of fibrinolysis. J Clin Pathol 12:215, 1959.

50. Kowalski E: Fibrinogen derivatives and their biological activities. Semin Hematol 5:45, 1968.

51. Kumada T, Abiko Y: Enhancement of fibrinolytic and thrombolytic potential in the rat by treatment with an anabolic steroid, Furazabol. Thromb Haemost 36:451, 1976.

52. Lane PA, Scully MF, Thomas DP, Kakkar VV, Williams R: Acquired dysfibrinogenemia in acute and chronic liver disease. Br J Haematol 35:301, 1977.

53. Lechner K, Niesser H, Thaler E: Coagulation abnormalities in liver disease. Semin Thromb Hemost 4:40, 1977.

54. Lord JW, Andrus W: Differentiation of intrahepatic and extra hepatic jaundice. Response of the plasma prothrombin to intramuscular injection of menadione (2-methyl-1, 4-naphthoquinone) as a diagnostic aid. Arch Intern Med 68:199, 1941.

55. Major LF, Murphy DL: Platelet and plasma amine oxidase activity in alcoholic individuals. Br J Psychiatry 132:548, 1978.

56. Marder VJ, Budzynski AZ: The structure of fibrinogen degradation products. Prog Hemost Thromb 2:141, 1974.

57. Menon IS: A study of the possible correlation of euglobulin lysis time and dilute blood clot lysis time in the determination of fibrinolytic activity. Lab Pract 17:334, 1968.

58. Mossesson M: Fibrinogen catabolic pathways. Semin Thromb Hemost 1:63, 1974.

59. Murano G: Plasma protein function in hemostasis. In Murano G, Bick RL (Eds): Basic Concepts of Hemostasis and Thrombosis. CRC Press, Boca Raton, FL, 1980, p 43.

60. Murano G, Bick RL: Thrombolytic therapy. In Murano G, Bick RL (Eds): Basic Concepts of Hemostasis and Thrombosis. CRC Press, Boca Raton, FL, 1980, p 259.

61. Penny R, Rosenberg FC, Firkin BG: The splenic platelet pool. Blood 17:1, 1966.

62. Pises P, Bick RL, Siegal B: Hyperfibrinolysis in cirrhosis. Am J Gastroenterol 60:280, 1973.

63. Quick AJ, Stanley-Brown M, Bancroft FW: A study of the coagulation defect in hemophilia and in jaundice. Am J Med Sci 190:501, 1935.

64. Rake MO, Flute PT, Panell G, Williams R: Intravascular coagulation in acute hepatic necrosis. Lancet 1:533, 1970.

65. Ratnoff OD: Hemostatic defects in liver and biliary tract disease. In Ratnoff OD, Forbes CD (Eds): Disorders of Hemostasis. Grune & Stratton, New York, 1984, p 451.

66. Reeve EB, Franks JJ: Fibrinogen synthesis, distribution, and degradation. Semin Thromb Hemost 1:129, 1974.

67. Sahud MA: Platelet size and number in alcoholic thrombocytopenia. N Engl J Med 286:355, 1972.

68. Sandler SG, Rath CE, Ruder A: Prothrombin complex concentrate in acquired hypoprothrombinemia. Ann Intern Med 79:485, 1973.

69. Stenflo J: Vitamin K, prothrombin, and gamma-carboxyglutamic acid. N Engl J Med 296:624, 1977.

70. Straub PW: Diffuse intravascular coagulation in liver disease. Semin Thromb Hemost 4:29, 1977.

71. Straub PW: Intravascular coagulation in acute hepatic necrosis. Lancet 1:1339, 1970.

72. Sullivan LW, Herbert V: Suppression of hematopoiesis by ethanol. J Clin Invest 43:2048, 1964.

73. Thomas DP, Ream VJ, Stuart RK: Platelet aggregation in patients with cirrhosis of the liver. N Engl J Med 276:1344, 1967.

74. Tocantins LM: The hemorrhagic tendency in congestive splenomegaly (Banti's syndrome): Its mechanism and management. JAMA 136:616, 1948.

75. Walker ID, Davidson JF, Young P, Conkie JA: Plasma fibrinolytic activity following oral anabolic steroid therapy. Thromb Diath Haemorrh 34:236, 1975.

76. Wardle EN: Fibrinogen in liver disease. Arch Surg 109:741, 1974.

77. Workman EF, Lundblad RL: The role of the liver in biosynthesis of the non-vitamin K-dependent clotting factors. Semin Thromb Hemost 4:15, 1977.

8

Hemostasis Defects in General Surgery, Cardiac Surgery, Transplantation, and the Use of Prosthetic Devices

Surgery and cardiopulmonary bypass (CPB) are procedures associated with catastrophic intraoperative or postoperative hemorrhage. Surgical hemorrhage is of more than passing concern since it not only places severe demands on local blood bank facilities, but also may lead to prolonged hospitalization and significantly altered morbidity and mortality in patients. Many instances of surgical hemorrhage are clearly due to inadequate surgical technique, an "acquired silk deficiency." However, many other instances are due to alterations of hemostasis. Often, a defect in hemostasis is present before the surgical procedure and is simply not detected. However, severe alterations in hemostasis are also created by CPB procedures. When managing a postsurgical patient with hemorrhage, it is obvioulsy important to distinguish quickly between surgical and nonsurgical bleeding. This key question must be answered before a reasonable decision can be made regarding surgical versus medical control of hemostasis. Perhaps the most important function of the hematologist in this instance is to be able to inform the surgeon quickly if hemostasis is intact or potentially contributing to surgical hemorrhage. When surgical hemorrhage occurs, it is often fulminant and life-threatening; thus, effective managment of patients and reasonable decisions regarding reexploration versus medical management requires close teamwork between the hematologist, surgeon, and pathologist. Only with this approach can optimal care be given to critically ill patients who, in many instances, have undergone an elective procedure.

Prevention of Surgical Bleeding

Hemorrhage associated with surgery is often catastropic and life-threatening; overcautiousness must be emphasized in regard to prevention, differential diagnosis, and rapid effective therapy. Significant attention must be given to preventing surgical hemorrhage by uncovering hereditary, acquired, or drug-induced bleeding tendencies before subjecting a patient to general surgical procedures or CPB. An already existing bleeding diathesis, even though mild, when coupled with surgery or the alterations of hemostasis induced by cardiac surgery, can obviously lead to disastrous results.

History Taking

Many cases of surgical hemorrhage could be averted by simply obtaining an adequate hemostasis history. Ideally, this should be obtained before hospital admission in order to allow time for appropriate evaluation if a potential problem with hemostasis is uncovered. Most historical information needed for detecting overt or covert bleeding tendencies is well known and discussed in other chapters; however, for the surgeon or cardiovascular surgical reader who is not often confronted with this aspcct of medicine, the salient features of a bleeding history are outlined.[11] Key questions that often suggest a bleeding diathesis are: Does the patient have significant gingival bleeding with toothbrushing? Is there easy or spontaneous bruising? Has the patient experienced undue bleeding after dental extraction or prior surgical procedures? Is there a childhood history of epistaxis? Is menstrual flow normal or excessive? These simple questions certainly do not constitute a complete historical search for disorders of hemostasis, but a positive response is a good clue to the possibility of an underlying bleeding disorder. Obviously, all patients considered for surgery should also be questioned regarding epistaxis, hemoptysis, hematemesis, melena, hematochezia, and hematuria.

The family history should always include inquiries about bleeding tendencies in parents, siblings, and children; this may uncover a hereditary bleeding tendency that has remained silent because the hemostasis system has never been stressed by surgery or trauma. Of paramount importance and often neglected is a detailed drug history. In my experience many instances of surgical hemorrhage could be explained in retrospect by noting the ingestion of drugs known to interfere with hemostasis, primarily platelet or, less commonly, vascular function.[12] Many drugs interfere with hemostasis; often the bleeding is mild and classified as bothersome. However, when drug-induced defects are combined with surgery, hemorrhage may reach alarming proportions. Drugs may interfere with hemostasis by many mechanisms. Significant drugs will be covered in specific sections of this chapter. If the drug history is positive and surgery is elective rather than emergent, surgery should be postponed for 14 days, since most drugs interfering with platelet function are generally effective for as long as 10 to 14 days. If the drug history is positive for antiplatelet agents and the drug has been ingested within 14 days, and the surgery or cardiac procedure is emergent, the patient should be given an appropriate amount of platelet concentrates (6 to 8 U for an adult) just before surgery. In addition, for cardiac surgery the patient should receive a similar dose of platelet concentrates just before leaving the operating room and then each morning for 2 days postoperatively. This approach is somewhat vigorous but is important if lifethreatening hemorrhage is to be avoided.

For general surgical procedures, platelets are given preoperatively if the template bleeding time is greater than 15 minutes and given postoperatively only if bleeding occurs. If the template bleeding time is less than 15 minutes, platelets are not infused preoperatively, but used if bleeding occurs. Obviously, the presurgical patient should be questioned about the past use of warfarin or heparin anticoagulants. It is well known that patients previously on warfarin, even though the prothrombin time has returned to normal, have an increased bleeding risk with surgery.

Physical Findings

The less obvious physical findings that provide clues for potential bleeding problems will be presented, since the more overt physical findings of a potential bleeding diathesis, such as hemarthroses, hepatomegaly, and splenomegaly, are well known and covered in detail in appropriate chapters of this text. The patient's general appearance often provides hints of a bleeding tendency. All of the hereditary and acquired connective tissue disorders are often associated with a significant vascular defect and the potential for surgical hemorrhage. Additionally, most of the hereditary collagen vascular disorders are accompanied by poorly defined platelet function defects. Clinical clues heralding the presence of a collagen vascular disorder are well known to most clinicians and include the body habitus of Marfan's syndrome, blue sclerae, skeletal deformities, hyperextensible joints and skin, and nodular, spiderlike, or pinpoint telangiectasia. These suggestive signs should prompt a more complete investigation for the presence of a collagen vascular disorder before surgery is undertaken. The hereditary and acquired collagen vascular disorders that are most likely to be associated with general surgical bleeding will be discussed in appropriate sections. Other disorders that may be associated with a vascular defect and surgical bleeding include Cushing's syndrome, malignant paraprotein disorders, the allergic purpuras, and hereditary hemorrhagic telangiectasia.

Other subtle hints of an occult bleeding tendency are uncovered by careful observation of the integument and mucous membranes. Mucosal petechiae, purpura, or significant telangiectasia should be searched for and explained if present. Likewise, petechiae, significant ecchymoses (brusies greater than 2 cm in diameter), or telangiectasia of the skin, nailbeds, or sublingual areas must be looked for; these findings are often suggestive of a vascular or platelet function defect or significant thrombocytopenia. If any of these findings are present, they should be investigated and thoroughly explained before surgery is performed. The usual physical findings of the more common clinical disorders associated with a significant bleeding tendency, such as chronic liver disease, hypersplenism, chronic renal disease, rheumatoid arthritis, and systemic lupus erythematosus, are well known and will not be delineated here. In addition, prior laboratory screening will usually suggest the presence of any of these disorders if characteristic physical findings are absent. If the personal, family, or drug history or physical examination is suggestive of a potential or real bleeding tendency, surgery, especially cardiac, should be postponed until the defect is ruled out, or until it is fully delineated and a therapeutically sound approach to correcting hemostasis during surgery and during the postoperative period has been carefully designed. It should be emphasized that if such a procedure is followed, a bleeding disorder of any type is rarely, if ever, a contraindication to performing general or cardiac surgery.

Presurgical Laboratory Screening

Any preoperative laboratory and hemostasis screen should generally be simple and involve a minimum of expense to the patient, while providing adequate information. Usually, however, presurgical or precardiac bypass hemostasis screens are inadequate.[11,12,36] As with an adequate history and physical examination, one cannot be too cautious in screening for defects in hemostasis when a surgical procedure is contemplated. When preexisting hemostatic defects are combined with general surgical procedures (disruption of the vasculature) or the defects in hemostasis created by CPB the resultant hemorrhage is often catastrophic, but in many instances can be averted by wise screening of patients. The usually ordered SMA 12/60 biochemical screening survey, electrolytes, complete blood, and platelet count will detect the common acquired disorders often associated with a bleeding tendency, such as chronic liver disease, renal disease, and instances of "hypersplenism" or bone marrow failure of any etiology. Most commonly, a presurgical hemostasis screen consists only of a prothrombin time, activated partial thromboplastin time, and a platelet count. Although these simple tests will detect the majority of coagulation protein problems and thrombocytopenia, they provide absolutely no information about vascular or platelet function and ignore the possibility of pathologic fibrinolysis.

In my experience the vast majority of nontechnical hemorrhage associated with general surgical procedures or cardiac surgery hemorrhage are due to platelet function defects and less commonly to vascular defects; these are much more common causes of surgical bleeding than coagulation protein problems. Accordingly, we add one simple procedure to the routine preoperative surgical screen and would strongly advise all surgeons to consider the same. This test is the standardized template bleeding time, as described by Mielke and co-workers.[117] It provides a reasonable surgical screen for adequate vascular and platelet function.[13] It should be recalled that the template bleeding time should not be performed until adequate platelet numbers are documented by count or smear evaluation. We use the Simplate-II (General Diagnostics). For cardiac bypass surgery patients, in addition to the template bleeding time, we add a thrombin time or Fibrindex (Ortho Diagnostics) to the precardiac surgery screen.[14,37] In addition, the resultant clot is observed for 5 mintues after the test is performed. A normal thrombin time assures the absence of significant hypofibrinogenemia, dysfibrinogenemia, fibrinolysis, or fibrin(ogen) degradation product (FDP) elevation. The use of one or both of these tests in the presurgical screen adds only minimal cost and laboratory time, while providing valuable information not given by the routine tests. With respect to cardiac surgery, if hypothermic perfusion is to be done, cryoglobulins should also be measured before bypass.[37,52,87,117,135,136]

Hemorrhage Associated with General Surgery

Vascular Defects

Although most vascular defects are not strictly hematologic diseases, many are characterized or accompanied by a significant hemorrhagic diathesis and often present in this manner.[15] In addition, most, if not all, of these disorders can be accompanied by significant surgical hemorrhage; thus, the surgeon should be aware of the more common vascular disorders, especially those that may lead to vascular hemorrhage with surgery. Vascular disorders are characteristically manifested by petechiae, purpura, ecchymoses, or telangiectasia.[15,16] Although these are the most common manifestations, mucosal membrane bleeding (epistaxis, genitourinary, and gastrointestinal bleeding) may also occur. Commonly found in vascular disorders is a history of gingival bleeding with toothbrushing, bleeding after dental extraction, and a history of easy and spontaneous bruising.[15–17] The vast majority of vascular disorders and their propensity toward surgical hemorrhage will be detected by noting an abnormal template bleeding time and, usually, a normal platelet function test.

The vascular disorders that most commonly lead to hemorrhage in surgical patients are: hereditary hemorrhagic telangiectasia, collagen vascular disorders with a microvascular component, Cushing's syndrome, diabetes mellitus, multiple myeloma and other paraprotein disorders, amyloidosis, allergic purpuras, and aspirin ingestion.[17] In the patient with a known vascular disorder, little can be done to prevent hemorrhage other than the use of careful surgical technique. However, if the patient with a vascular

disorder and a propensity to surgical hemorrhage has not taken antiplatelet agents before surgery, and careful surgical hemostasis is strictly adhered to, significant intraoperative or postoperative hemorrhage rarely occurs. It should be emphasized, however, that the surgeon is well advised to know that one of these disorders, and the possibility of surgical hemorrhage, exists before subjecting a patient to a surgical procedure, especially if it is elective. It should be recalled that the template bleeding time is commonly normal in hereditary hemorrhagic telangiectasia and the allergic purpuras; thus, an adequate history and physical examination are imperative.

Platelet Defects

Thrombocytopenia is not uncommonly encountered in a general surgical practice and causes of thrombocytopenia most commonly seen by the surgeon are listed in Table 8–1. These are almost always, if not always, detected by the presurgical platelet count or careful evaluation of the peripheral blood smear. However, in the busy laboratory, even severe thrombocytopenia may be missed on a smear evaluation, and the presurgical patient should always have a quantitative platelet count. When thrombocytopenia is noted, the etiology should be delineated before surgery is undertaken.

The common drugs causing thrombocytopenia in surgical patients are also listed in Table 8–1 and the patient should be questioned about their use when encountering presurgical thrombocytopenia. This topic is also dealt with in more detail in Chapter 4. Surgical bleeding commonly does not occur with a platelet count greater than $100,000/mm^3$. However, if a patient has a lower platelet count and does not have immune thrombocytopenia, appropriate numbers of platelet concentrates are usually given before surgery and 6 to 8 U are kept available for the possibility of postsurgical hemorrhage. If the platelet count is greater than $100,000/mm^3$, but below normal, the patient is subjected to the surgical procedure with platelets being given only if significant

Table 8–1 Common Causes of Thrombocytopenia in Surgical Patient Populations

Aplastic anemia
Drug-induced
  Acetaminophen
  Aspirin
  Cephalosporins
  Chlorpropamide
  Digitalis preparations
  Meprobamate
  Penicillin compounds
  Phenobarbital
  Phenytoin
  Quinidine
  Streptomycin
  Thiazide diuretics
Hemolytic-uremic syndrome
Immune thrombocytopenia purpura
Infection
Liver disease
Low-grade DIC
Metastatic malignancy
Multiple blood transfusions
Myeloproliferative disorders
Severe iron deficiency
Splenomegaly or hypersplenism

Table 8–2 Common Platelet Function Defects in Surgical Patient Populations

Acquired storage pool disease
Circulating FDPs
Drug-induced
  Ampicillin
  Aspirin
  Carbenicillin
  Clofibrate
  Dyphenhydramine
  Dipyridamole
  Furosemide
  Gentamicin
  Glyceryl guaiacolate
  Ibuprofen
  Indomethacin
  Nitrofurantoin
  Papaverine
  Penicillin
  Phenothiazines
  Propanolol
  Sulfinpyrazone
  Tricyclic amines
Hereditary storage pool disease
Liver disease
Low-grade DIC
Multiple myeloma
Myeloproliferative disorders
Uremia

bleeding occurs intraoperatively or postoperatively. In our experience the most common causes of presurgical thrombocytopenia are malignancy and attendant chemotherapy, radiation therapy, marrow metastases, or drug-induced thrombocytopenia,[11,12,18,36] as delineated in detail in Chapter 4.

Platelet Function Defects

Platelet function defects clearly account for more than 50% of nontechnical surgical hemorrhage.[11,12,36] Platelet function defects that most commonly cause a surgical bleeding problem are given in Table 8–2. These are discussed in more detail in Chapter 4. Most of the hereditary platelet function defects are clinical oddities and extremely rare; the one most commonly seen and leading to surgical hemorrhage in our experience has been a hereditary storage pool defect, typically manifested by absent second wave aggregation to adenosine diphosphate (ADP) and epinephrine and totally absent aggregation to collagen in conjunction with normal ristocetin-induced platelet agglutination. In addition, the possibility of a storage pool defect should be considered when noting normal platelet numbers and a prolonged template bleeding time. Much more commonly, however, the surgeon will be confronted with acquired or drug-induced platelet function defects (Table 8–2). It should be emphasized that these are only the common drugs inducing postsurgical hemorrhage and for a more extensive list the reader is referred to Chapter 4 and several excellent reviews.[57,122,157,158] If presurgical template bleeding times are not performed, these disorders will not be detected by the routine presurgical screen. When surgical bleeding thought to be potentially due to a platelet function defect is suspected, a template bleeding time should be performed immediately; if it is prolonged, platelet aggregation should be measured.

Platelet function defects are treated in essentially the same manner as for thrombocytopenia. If a patient has a platelet function defect that has been uncovered preoperatively and has a template bleeding time of more than 15 minutes, the patient is infused with 6 to 8 U of platelet concentrates before the surgical procedure. If the template bleeding time is less than 15 minutes (normal, 4 to 9 minutes), then platelets are made available and infused only if significant intraoperative or postoperative hemorrhage occurs. Alternatively, if the defect is not uncovered before surgery and postsurgical bleeding occurs, if the template bleeding time is prolonged and platelet aggregation abnormalities are noted, appropriate numbers of platelet concentrates are given immediately to abort hemorrhage: usually 6 to 8 U in the adult, given twice a day or every morning, depending on the site and severity of hemorrhage. Our practice is to give platelets until significant hemorrhage stops.

Isolated Coagulation Factor Deficiencies

Isolated coagulation factor deficiencies are rarely a surgical problem, except in centers specializing in hemophilia and congenital coagulation protein problems, and are discussed in appropriate sections of this text (Chapter 5). However, far more commonly, the general and subspecialty surgeon will be faced with acquired multiple compartment defects. The most common of these are disseminated intravascular coagulation (DIC) and the hypoprothrombinemic problems, as seen with chronic liver disease, biliary obstruction, and other associated conditions. DIC is discussed in detail in Chapter 6 and the usual causes of hypoprothrombinemia in liver diseases are discussed in detail in Chapter 7 as are the bleeding diatheses associated with numerous liver diseases which are multifactorial. Chronic liver disease consists not only of coagulation factor problems, including deficiencies of the vitamin K dependent clotting factors, but also of vascular and platelet defects. The platelet defects may be quantitative or qualitative. Hypoprothrombinemic bleeding may be seen in the warfarin-treated patient, in the patient with acute liver insults, including hepatitis, and in those with hepatic cirrhosis. However, most of these defects will be detected by a careful his-

tory and adequate presurgical laboratory screening. It should be noted that even though a patient who has been on warfarin before surgery has a prothrombin time that has returned to normal, the patient still has an increased bleeding risk with a surgical procedure.[20,162] When vitamin K dependent clotting factor deficiency-type bleeding occurs, whether due to liver disease or to presurgical use of warfarin, it is best managed by the use of phytonadione, 20 mg intravenously (1 mg/minute) or intramuscularly, and the use of fresh frozen plasma, 2 to 4 U as necessary, as the site and severity of bleeding dictate. If bleeding is truly emergent and life-threatening, we have resorted, on occasion, to the use of prothrombin complex concentrates to correct the hemostatic defect quickly.[21] However, the use of these concentrates is not without hazard and they should be infused only by those experienced in management of thrombohemorrhagic phenomena.

Disseminated Intravascular Coagulation

DIC-type syndromes often lead to significant surgical hemorrhage. Typically, when a patient with a disorder associated with chronic low-grade underlying DIC is subjected to a surgical procedure, this precipitates an acute, fulminant DIC syndrome. Those conditions most commonly associated with chronic or subacute underlying DIC processes in patients who are surgical candidates are listed in Table 7–3.[22–24,38] A detailed description of the etiology, pathophysiology, diagnosis, and management of DIC, when fulminant, is given in detail in Chapter 6. It should be emphasized, however, that the surgeon should be aware of the disorders that may be associated with a low-grade DIC process that may not be detected by the use of routine presurgical screening. Primary fibrino(geno)lysis has been commonly blamed for many instances of post-transurethral prostatectomy (TURP) hemorrhage; however, in our experience even though primary fibrinogenolysis is occasionally seen and may account for massive post-TURP hematuria, far more common

Table 8–3 Disseminated Intravascular Coagulation Syndromes Commonly Seen in Surgical Patient Populations

Acidosis or shock
Biliary obstruction or cholestasis
Collagen vascular disorders
Crush injuries
Extensive burns
Hemolysis
Infection or sepsis
Metastatic malignancy
Obstetrical accidents
   Amniotic fluid embolism
   Placental abruptio
   Toxemia
   Retained fetus syndrome
Prosthetic devices
Transfusion reactions
Ulcerative colitis

causes are drug-induced platelet function defects and a chronic underlying DIC-type syndrome.[25] It has been suggested that a minimum DIC evaluation be performed on all patients undergoing TURP, since this may identify patients who are presdisposed to post-TURP hemorrhage.[116]

Alterations of Hemostasis Associated with Cardiopulmonary Bypass and Cardiac Surgery

Cardiac surgery using CPB is now a common procedure and, with popularization of coronary artery bypass grafting, is no longer limited to large centers, now being performed in most community hospitals. Widespread use of CPB has renewed awareness of the catastrophic intraoperative or postoperative hemorrhage that may be associated with this procedure. Hemorrhage during or after bypass is of more than passing concern, since it may lead to significant morbidity and mortality from an elective procedure, places significant demands on local blood banking facilities, and can lead to prolonged expensive hospitalizations.[8,36,37,59] The actual incidence of life-threatening hemorrhage associated with CPB appears to vary from 5 to 25%.[20,37,59,111,162]

Until recently, the pathophysiology of altered hemostasis created by CPB was poorly understood, and past failures to delineate it during CPB have, quite understandably, precluded the development of uniform concepts of successful prevention, adequate and rapid diagnosis, and effective control of hemorrage. Lack of understanding of CPB hemorrhagic syndromes has derived from several factors; since many past studies of hemostasis during CPB examined only isolated aspects of blood coagulation and ignored the complexities and interrelationships of the hemostasis system; failed to utilize coagulationists or hematologists, which in some instances led to the inappropriate choice of test systems and unclear or inappropriate interpretation of results, and despite available and sophisticated advances in modalities to assess the hemostatic system, utilized insensitive, inaccurate, or inappropriate test systems. For example, the euglobulin lysis time has been the most commonly utilized modality for studying CPB fibrinolysis, even though this test system has been questioned for the valid evaluation of clinically significant pathologic fibrinolysis.[39,40,77,115]

Various investigators have ascribed the hemorrhagic syndrome of CPB surgery to a wide variety of defects; each investigator has likewise placed varying degrees of importance on each defect, depending on which particular hemostatic parameters were monitored. In the past, the abnormalities most frequently cited to account for CPB hemorrhage have included inadequate heparin neutralization, protamine excess, heparin rebound, thrombocytopenia, hypofibrinogenemia, primary hyperfibrino-(geno)lysis, DIC, isolated coagulation factor deficiencies, transfusion reactions, and hypocalcemia. The suggestion that any or all of these defects may contribute to CPB hemorrhage clearly demonstrates that despite the finding of multiple defects in hemostasis, the basic pathophysiology of altered hemostasis during CPB remains confusing to many. It is equally clear that basic mechanisms of altered hemostasis associated with CPB must be completely understood and appreciated before an appropriate approach to rapid and effective therapy can be designed.

Thrombocytopenia

Early studies of hemostasis during CPB noted significant thrombocytopenia, about 50,000/mm^3 in patients undergoing bypass surgery; many investigators thought this responsible for bypass hemorrhage. In addition, Kevy and associates[94] noted that the degree of thromobocytopenia was related to the time on bypass and was much more pronounced with perfusions lasting greater than 60 minutes. A relationship between the degree of thrombocytopenia and time on bypass was also reported by Signore and co-workers.[146] Later studies noted similar findings,[134,155] and Porter and Silver[134] found that in the majority of patients undergoing CPB the platelet count fell to one third of the preoperative level. In addition, it was noted that thrombocytopenia did not abate until several days after CPB.[134] Earlier studies by Wright and co-workers[170] and von Kaulla and Swan[164] also recognized thrombocytopenia in association with CPB, but these investigators concluded that thrombocytopenia bore little, if any, relationship to actual bypass hemorrhage. Some studies finding thrombocytopenia during CPB concluded that this represented thrombocytopenia of DIC.[47,61,131,155] We,[26-29,36,37] as well as others,[55,63,120] have failed to find significant thrombocytopenia during CPB. This wide variability in experience most likely represents different surgical and pumping techniques, such as flow rates, normothermic or hypothermic perfusion, the oxygenation system used, time on bypass, and the priming solution. In our experience a flow rate of 40 ml/kg/min and a pump prime of 20 ml/kg of 5% dextrose and Ringer's lactate solution plus 5% dextrose and water in a ratio of 2:1 produces only minimal thrombocytopenia.[20,28,36] Figure 8–1 demonstrates changes in platelet number with this pumping technique. The dotted line represents the mean platelet counts in membrane oxygenation pumped system and the solid line represents the bubble oxygenation system[19] used in a total of 300 consecutive patients. In our experience the type of oxygenation mechanism used appears to play little role in causing thrombocytopenia, although with the bubble oxygenators it is slightly greater than that seen with mem-

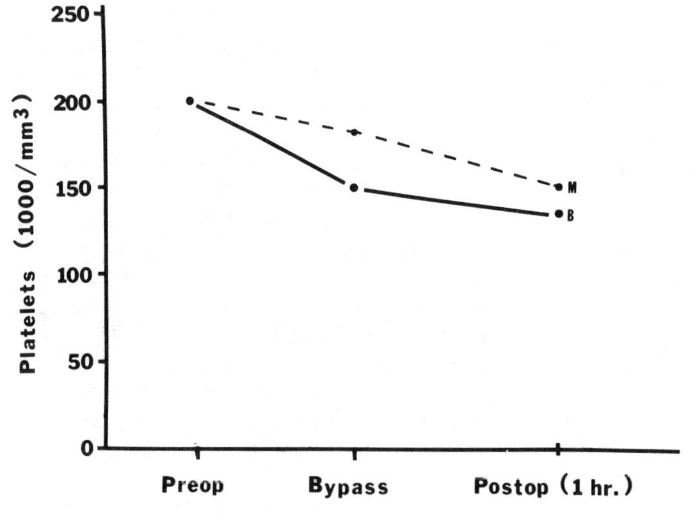

Fig. 8–1. Platelet function during CPB. Results from 300 patients.

brane oxygenators but this does not reach clinical significance. The most commonly cited mechanisms for the development of CPB thrombocytopenia are hemodilution, formation of intravascular platelet thrombi, platelet utilization in the pump or oxygenation system, and peripheral utilization due to DIC. We have failed to find a correlation between CPB hematocrit and platelet count, suggesting that hemodilution is not a major factor.[20,29,41] Indeed, the role, if any, of these mechanisms in producing CPB thrombocytopenia remains totally unclear.

Platelet Function Defects

In contrast to the numerous investigations regarding platelet number during CPB, there has been a surprising lack of interest in assessing platelet function during this procedure. Early investigators suspected that abnormalities of platelet function might occur because faulty clot retraction was noted.[146] These results were of unclear significance however, since other changes known to affect clot retraction, such as hypofibrinogenemia and thrombocytopenia, were also present. Another early study assessed platelet function before placing patients on CPB, but failed to evaluate platelet function during or after bypass.[86] In this study, abnormal preoperative platelet adhesion in glass bead columns was associated with increased postoperative bleeding. Salzman[139] studied platelet adhesion before, during, and after bypass and noted decreased adhesion to glass bead columns in all patients during bypass; however, the significance of this defect was difficult to evaluate, since all patients had marked thrombocytopenia, which is definitely known to alter adhesion studies[30,49,50] and in addition adhesion studies are generally thought to be without any clinical significance.[85,173] Further information from this particular study was that heparin, in doses used during CPB, did not alter platelet adhesion. This study concluded that a circulating anticoagulant might be responsible for the platelet function defect noted, since plasma from CPB patients altered adhesion when added to normal platelets. This circulating anticoagulant most likely represented FDPs.[36,37,40]

Salzman[139] also noted that perfusion temperature and the type of priming solution did not correlate with the development of abnormal platelet function. More recently, platelet adhesion studies have been performed in patients undergoing CPB without significant thrombocytopenia.[26,28,2941] In these studies platelet function, as measured by adhesion, decreased profoundly in all patients at the initiation of bypass; most patients demonstrated adhesion that decreased to 17% of preoperative levels. In one study little correlation was noted between hematocrit, fibrinogen level, or FDP titer and abnormal adhesions.[28] In addition, poor correlation was noted between chest tube blood loss and abnormal platelet function, as assessed by adhesion. Figure 8–2 depicts platelet adhesion changes during CPB. It must again be emphasized that recent studies have questioned the clinical significance of platelet adhesion by the glass bead column technique.[85,173] However, this degree of abnormal platelet function would certainly be expected to compromise hemostasis severely. Membrane oxygenation mechanisms are depicted by a dashed line and bubble oxygenation mechanisms are depicted by a solid line.[19] The platelet function defect is slightly more severe and tends to correct much more slowly when a membrane oxygenator is used compared with a bubble oxygenator. Platelet function, as assessed by template bleeding times or platelet aggregation or lumiaggregation, is abnormal in patients with platelet function defects,[50] von Willebrand's disease (ristocetin aggregation only),[49] and myeloproliferative disorders.[1] Many factors, some possibly altered by CPB, may affect platelet function; these include pH, absolute platelet count, hematocrit, drugs, and the presence of FDP.[1,31,37,40,84,99,100,122]

Although most studies do not clearly define the reasons for abnormal platelet function during CPB, they do suggest that several of the mechanisms first mentioned are most likely not involved. The finding of platelet counts greater than 100,000/mm^3 and hematocrit values greater than 30% in most patients with marked platelet dysfunction 1 hour after CPB suggests that the absolute platelet count and the

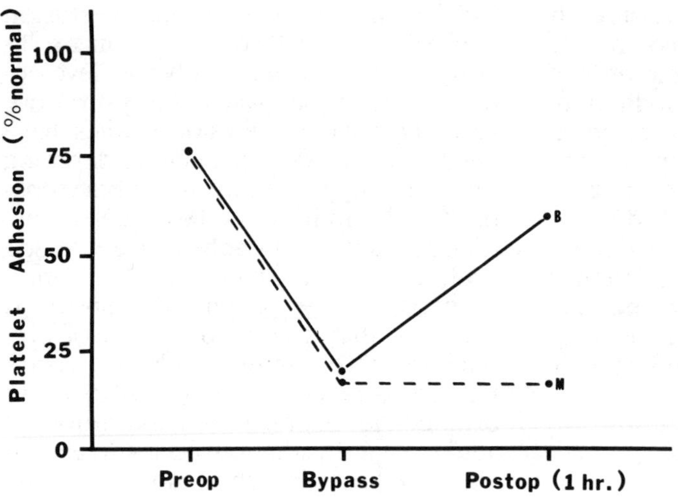

Fig. 8–2. Platelet numbers during CPB. Results from 300 patients.

hematocrit do not account for altered platelet function. In addition, most patients have a normal or near normal pH 1 hour after bypass surgery; thus, a change in pH is unlikely to account for abnormal platelet function during bypass surgery. Heparin, at levels higher than those attained in patients undergoing CPB, has not been shown to alter platelet function.[50,139] Circulating FDPs are known to interfere with platelet function, and these are present in approximately 85% of patients undergoing CPB.[37,40,99] However, there is poor correlation between levels of circulating FDP and the degree of abnormal platelet function during bypass surgery.[28,41] In addition, defective platelet function occurs in virtually 100% of patients undergoing CPB; thus, circulating FDP cannot account for altered platelet function in many instances.[20,28,36,37,41]

Other possible mechanisms of altered platelet function during CPB include platelet membrane damage by shearing force or contact with foreign material, resulting in a partial release of platelet contents, platelet membrane coating with nonspecific proteins or protein degradation products, or incomplete release reaction or nonspecific platelet damage induced by flow rates. Recent studies have shown selective platelet degranulation to occur during bypass surgery.[79] However, no studies reported thus far allow conclu-

sions to be drawn regarding the contribution of any of these mechanisms to alter platelet function during CPB. In one preliminary study of 29 patients, only 20% developed aggregation abnormalities during CPB; however, after heparin reversal with protamine sulfate 90% of patients developed aggregation abnormalities. These investigators ascribed this finding to a protamine and platelet interaction and not due to bypass itself.[152] We have recently completed platelet aggregation and lumiaggregation studies in 20 patients undergoing CPB surgery and in all 20 platelet aggregation and platelet release was markedly altered.[58,141] Typical preoperative, intraoperative and one hour postoperative lumiaggregation patterns are depicted in Figures 4–11 and 4–12. In addition, in all patients studied the aggregation and release reaction defect occurred within 10 to 15 minutes of starting bypass. Additionally, we have also noted that in all patients platelet factor 4 levels rise rapidly with the initiation of bypass. The aggregation defects appear to be similar with both membrane and bubble type oxygenators; however, the type of priming solution, albumin versus hydroxyethyl starch, does seem to alter the type of defects seen.[141] When studying platelet activation by scanning electron microscopy, we have noted that platelet activation appears to be more pronounced mid-bypass with membrane oxygenators than with bubble oxygenators.[58] Mid- and post-bypass platelet activation in patients after membrane oxygenation (Fig. 8–3) and after bubble oxygenation (Fig. 8–4) are typical of the 20 patients we have studied.

Regardless of the mechanisms involved, studies to date clearly reveal that a significant platelet function defect is induced in all patients undergoing CPB surgery. The magnitude of this defect would certainly be expected to have potential serious consequences for hemostasis during and after bypass. In addition, patients who have ingested drugs known to interfere with platelet function would be expected to have more blood loss than those not ingesting such agents, which would be expected to compound the defects already induced by CPB and potentiate the chance for hemorrhage. One small study has provided evidence for this conclusion.[31] Although diagnosis and management of hemorrhage associated with CPB will be discussed subsequently, it should be pointed out that this platelet function de-

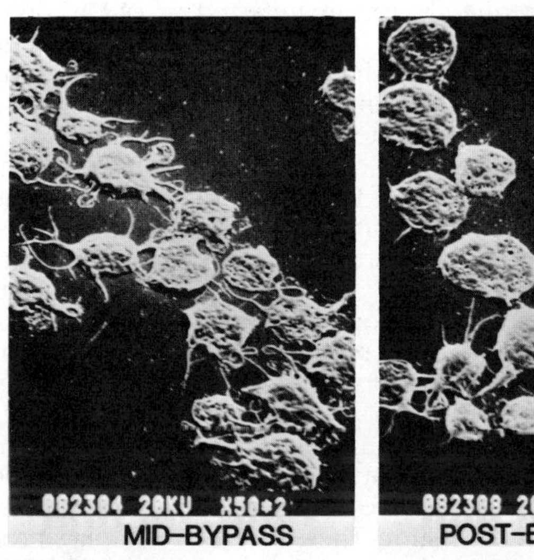

Fig. 8–3. Platelet activation with use of membrane oxygenator at mid-bypass and post-bypass.

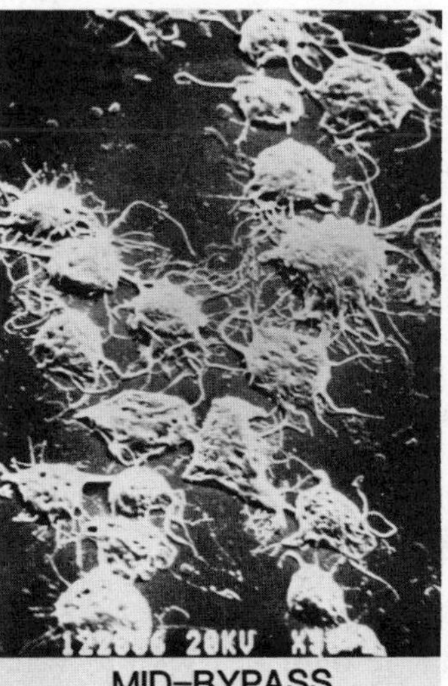

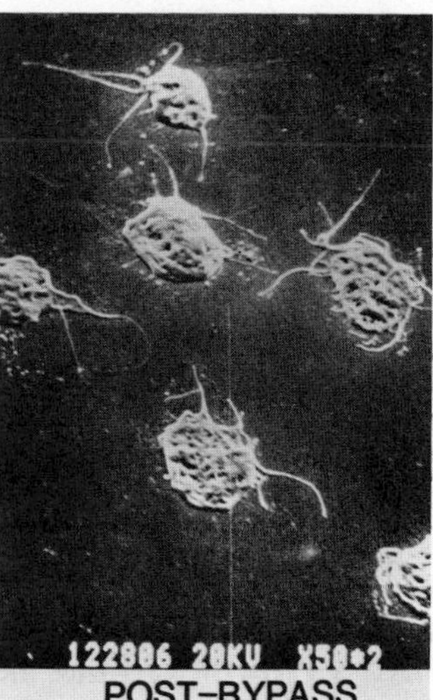

Fig. 8–4. Platelet activation with use of bubble oxygenator at mid-bypass and post-bypass.

fect is of major significance in hemorrhage occurring after CPB. In my experience, the use of platelet concentrates when there is a normal platelet count will usually promptly correct or significantly reduce most episodes of hemorrhage, during or after CPB.

Vascular Defects

Few studies of vascular defects during CPB have been reported. A syndrome of mild to moderate thrombocytopenic purpura accompanied by splenomegaly and atypical lymphocytosis after CPB has been reported by Behrendt and co-workers.[9] In this series the purpura was benign, self-limited, and frequently was manifested only after discharge from the hospital. Only one of seven patients had a complication after the development of this syndrome; this was glomerulonephritis of the type often seen in Henoch-Schönlein purpura. In addition, a case of fatal purpura fulminans was reported after extracorporeal circulation for coronary artery bypass grafting.[32] Massive purpura developed on the third postoperative day, followed by progressive renal failure. High doses of steroids and low molecular weight dextran provided no improvement and the patient died of renal failure on the 18th postoperative day. No abnormalities in hemostasis were detected by extensive laboratory testing. These two reports suggest that an inflammatory vasculitis may be associated with CPB; the most benign forms represented by purpura simplex and, rarely, purpura fulminans (without DIC) may be expected to occur.[20,36] Cardiac surgeons should be aware of this potential complication of bypass surgery. Aside from these two reports, no mention has been made in the literature of vascular defects associated with CPB surgery.

Isolated Coagulation Factor Defects

Numerous studies have examined and reported coagulation factor deficiencies during CPB. A wide variety of findings have been observed and, like the finding of thrombocytopenia, may only reflect differences in surgical or pumping techniques, such as flow rate and priming solution. Most studies have noted significant hypofibrinogenemia that does not seem to be correlated with perfusion time.[28,29,111,134,155,170] We,[28,29,40] and others,[111,155] have found fibrinogen levels to be closely correlated with the degree of CPB fibrinolysis; however, other investigators report little correlation between hypofibrinogenemia and degree of CPB fibrino(geno)lysis.[62,94] Figure 8–5 depicts correlations noted between fibrinogen, plasminogen, circulating plasmin, and FDP during CPB.[19,20,36] Some studies have concluded that hypofibrinogenemia occurs primarily as a consequence of DIC during pump surgery;[47,131,156] however, others have failed to find hypofibrinogenemia during CPB.[5,160] It seems reasonable to conclude from the studies reported that hypofibrinogenemia secondary to hyperfibrinolysis may be a frequent occurrence during CPB. This appears to be a rather consistent finding in the carefully studied series already noted and is most likely a major cause of hypofibrinogenemia associated with CPB.

Hyperfibrino(geno)lysis occurs in approximately 85% of patients undergoing bypass surgery. Most studies have also noted other coagulation factor deficiences in association with CPB; those most commonly found to be decreased and reported to play a role in CPB hemorrhage are Factors II, V, and VIII:C.[47,94,111,155,156,170] Some conclude that these changes are secondary to DIC,[47,120] whereas others describe these decreases to a primary fibrino(geno)lytic syndrome and plasmin-induced degradation of coagulation proteins.[20,28,29,37,40,111] Still others have failed to find a significant decrease in most coagulation factors during bypass surgery,[5,94,160] and two investigators have reported increased Factor VIII:C levels during perfusion.[5,168]

Disseminated Intravascular Coagulation

The pathophysiology of DIC was discussed in detail in Chapter 6. The question of whether DIC develops during bypass surgery has caused much confusion re-

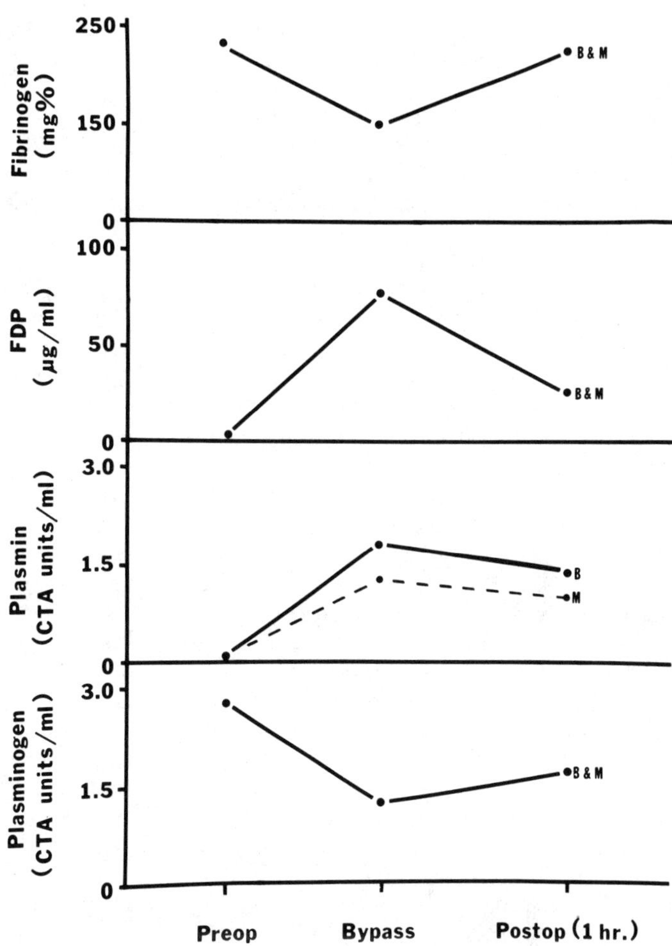

Fig. 8–5. Primary fibrino-(geno)lysis during CPB. Results from 300 patients.

garding altered hemostasis both during and after bypass. Numerous early studies of hemostasis during CPB concluded that DIC occurred.[47,73,129,131,156] However, many such studies monitored only isolated coagulation factors; the measured decreases were empirically described to presumed DIC, since no other explanation was evident. In particular, the findings of isolated fibrinogen, Factor VIII:C [131,170] or prothrombin complex factor deficiencies[63] were often assumed, usually erroneously, to be secondary to DIC, without appropriate confirmatory laboratory testing. In addition, two recent reports have concluded that DIC accounts for altered hemostasis during CPB.[96,120] In these reports of nine patients, the investigators concluded that DIC was present after noting that several

parameters of hemostasis worsened after heparin reversal with protamine. In particular, FDP elevation, hypofibrinogenemia, and hypoplasminogenemia appeared to become accentuated after the infusion of protamine. However, our experience,[20,28,29,36,37] as well as that of others,[76,111,134,146,160,164] has been the opposite; hypofibrinogenemia, hypoplasminogenemia, and FPD elevation are usually noted to be corrected rather rapidly and uniformly after the administration of protamine sulfate.

These findings would suggest that DIC is not associated with CPB surgery. DIC during cardiac surgery also seems unlikely in view of massive heparinization and the absence of significant or uniform thrombocytopenia reported in many studies in which hemostasis appears to be markedly abnormal.

Another finding that would certainly suggest that DIC is not present during CBP is the presence of normal or near normal antithrombin III levels.[20,41,111] Current evidence suggests that decreased antithrombin III levels are a reasonably good indicator of the development of acute or chronic DIC.[33,38,39] Only one study has shown decreased levels of antithrombin during CPB;[120] however, in the nine patients described, all had low levels of antithrombin III before bypass was initiated. In addition, the method used was quite old, and possibly influenced by the presence of FDP or heparin, rendering interpretation of these results unclear. Another consideration negating the probability that DIC occurs during CPB is the following: if DIC were present in patients undergoing CPB, the infusion of intravenous protamine sulfate would be expected to cause a massive precipitation of soluble fibrin monomer, with resultant extensive micro- and macrovascular occlusion. In my experience, only two of several thousand patients have had DIC in association with CPB.[20,36,37] Both patients developed DIC before CPB, one from cardiac arrest and the other from septicemia. In these two instances, bypass surgery was accomplished without incidence; however, when protamine sulfate was infused, massive vascular occlusion, including carotid and renal artery thrombosis, suddenly occurred.

To summarize, even though most early and several recent studies have detected primary fibrino(geno)lysis in association with CPB, only a few have concluded that DIC occurs. These conclusions most likely derive from the marked superficial similarities between primary fibrino(geno)lysis and DIC and the usual secondary fibrinolytic response and from the difficulty in making a clear-cut differential diagnosis between these two states in the absence of sophisticated and complete coagulation studies.

Primary Fibrino(geno)lysis

Fibrinolytic activity is generally decreased inhibited during and following most general surgical procedures.[102,159,171,172] However, most studies utilizing a variety of laboratory modalities have found increased fibrinolysis during and after CPB surgery.[20,28,29,34,36,37,40,55,62,76,94,111,134,141,146,160] Many earlier studies of hemostasis during CPB assessed fibrinolysis with the euglobulin lysis time; thus, the finding of fibrinolysis remained of unclear significance for a long period of time.[77,115] More recent studies of CPB hemostasis,[20,28,29,41,134] which have utilized more specific methods for assessing fibrinolysis, primarily synthetic substrate assays,[35,39,46,70,71,90] have confirmed earlier reports of a primary hyperfibrino(geno)lytic syndrome in the majority of patients undergoing CPB surgery. Figure 8–5 depicts changes in the fibrinolytic system in patients undergoing CPB. Because of early reports detecting primary hyperfibrino(geno)lysis during CPB, the emperical use of antifibrinolytics, usually epsilon-aminocaproic acid (EACA), has become commonplace. Despite the attendent hazards of this agent, which include hypokalemia, hypotension, ventricular arrhythmias, local or disseminated thromboses, and DIC syndromes,[123,137] many cardiovascular surgeons have frequently used this drug. Controlled studies with and without antifibrinolytics have failed to reveal any clear-cut differences in CPB hemorrhage,[62,111,155,162,163] and Gomes amd McGoon[76] and Tsuji and co-workers[160] have shown a definite increase in post-CPB hemorrage with the empirical use of antifibrinolytics. In our experience, the need to use EACA to control CPB hemorrhage is extremely rare;[20,35] this agent should only be used when concrete laboratory evidence of primary fibrino(geno)lysis is noted in the severely hemorrhaging CPB patient.

Several investigators finding primary fibrino(geno)lysis during CPB have concluded this to be inconsequential as a cause of post-perfusion hemorrhage,[146,155] whereas others have thought that this syndrome is triggered only by specific events, such as pyrogenicity of equipment, the use of low molecular weight dextran, or induction of anesthesia.[53,127,164] Since primary fibrino(geno)lysis occurs in the majority of patients subjected to CPB surgery, it seems more likely that activation of the fibrinolytic system may be occuring in the oxygenation mechanism or, alternatively, that pump-induced accelerated flow rates may activate the plasminogen-plasmin system or may alter endothelial plasminogen activator activity. We have recently noted marked activation of Factor XII in all patients undergoing CPB surgery, with approximately 70% of Factor XII being converted to Factor XIIa.[42] This is an additional potential activation pathway for the initiation of a primary fibrino(geno)lytic syndrome. However, the pathogenesis of fibrinolytic activation during CPB remains unclear. Although many investigators have noted enhanced fibrinolysis during CPB, a few studies have found only elevated fibrinolytic activator activity, with no systemically circulating plasmin.[62,73,94] Also, a few studies have failed to find any evidence of primary fibrino(geno)lysis in association with CPB[73,155,162,170]

The pathophysiology of primary hypofibrino(geno)lysis is familiar to many readers; a comprehensive review of primary lysis was presented in Chapter 7. However, the salient features of this syndrome will be outlined so that a complete understanding of the defects of hemostasis during CPB can be obtained. The pathophysiology of primary hyperfibrino(geno)lysis is depicted and summarized in Figure 7–2. Hemostasis is significantly altered when plasmin circulates systematically; the attendant systemic hypofibrinogenemia and plasmin-induced biodegradation of Factors V, VIII, and IX may severely compromise the hemostasis system.[37,40,130,144,145] In addition, the resultant FDP's futher derange hemostasis by intefering with thrombin activity, and with fibrin monomer polymerization and radically altering platelet function.[3,37,40,99,100,103,104]

These changes in hemostasis would certainly be expected to be associated with a significant hemorrhagic potential. In addition, it is easy to see how these alterations in hemostasis could be superficially confused with DIC and secondary fibrinolysis. Figure 8–6 compares the salient features of DIC and primary fibrinolysis. Table 8–4 defines a molecular marker profile that can be used to differentially diagnose primary fibrinolysis and DIC.[43]

Table 8–4 Molecular Marker Profiling in the Differential Diagnosis of Disseminated Intravascular Coagulation-Type Syndromes Versus Primary Fibrino(geno)lytic Syndromes

Marker	DIC	Primary Lysis
Fibrinopeptide A	Elevated	Normal
Fibrinopeptide B	Elevated	Normal
B-beta 15-42 peptide	Elevated	Normal
B-beta 1-42 peptide	Elevated	Elevated
B-beta 1-118 peptide	Elevated	Elevated
Platelet factor 4	Elevated	Normal
Beta-thromboglobulin	Elevated	Normal

Other Defects

Heparin "rebound" has received significant attention as a potential cause of CPB hemorrhage.[2,67,75,92,127] This was observed more often in earlier studies. With today's generally accepted doses of both heparin and protamine, both heparin rebound and inadequate heparinization are rarely, if ever, seen.[20,28,29,37,41,120] In fact, neither heparin rebound nor inadequate heparin neutralization have been documented as actual causes of hemorrhage during CPB.[20,61,156] Similarly, protamine excess has occasionally been incriminated as a source of hemorrhage during CPB; however, several carefully studied series have failed to note this phenomenon in a single patient undergoing CPB.[20,28,29,37,55,67,68] In addition, although protamine sulfate is a well known in vitro anticoagulant, it is unlikely that this agent is the cause of in vivo altered hemostasis or hemorrhage.[126]

Several investigators have reported that both coagulation defects and significant hemorrhage during CPB may be associated with hypothermic perfusion.[127,155,162,164] Our experience in comparing normothermic perfusions has led to the same conclusion.[34] Gomes and McGoon[76] and Porter and Silver,[134] have found no increased incidence of hemorrhage during CPB as a consequence of hypothermic perfusion. Many patients undergoing coronary artery bypass grafting for coronary occlusive disease have been on warfarin-type drugs.

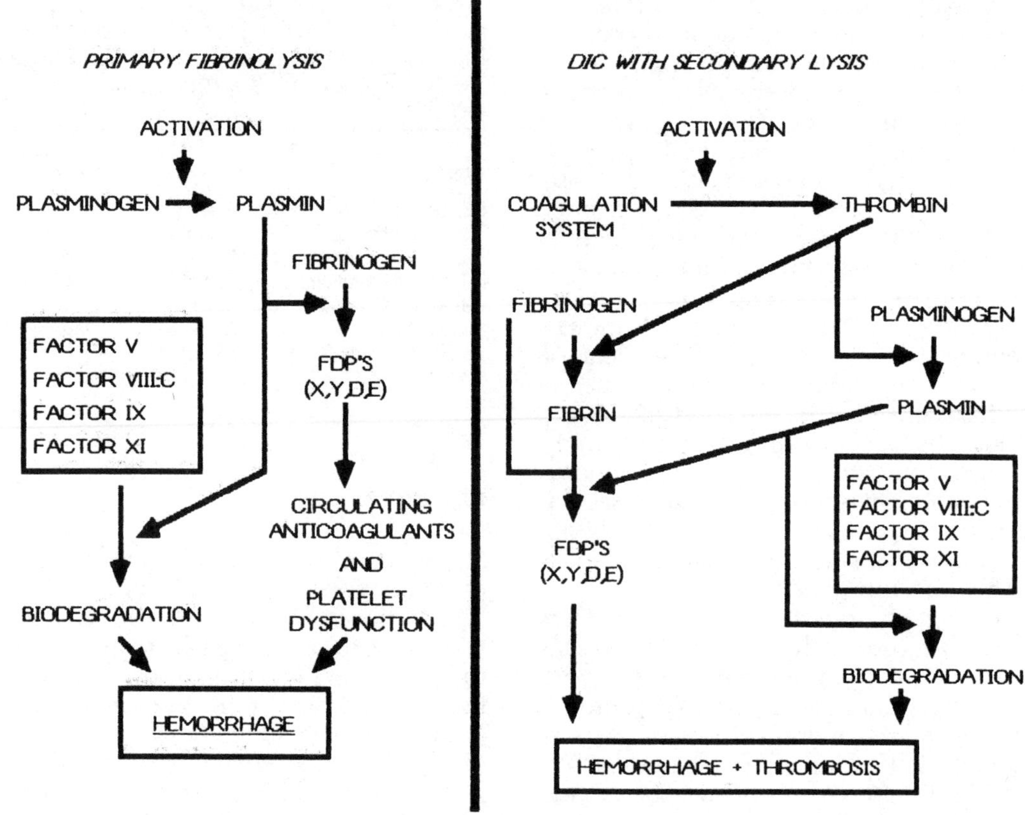

Fig. 8–6. A comparison of disseminated intravascular coagulation and primary fibrino(geno)lysis.

Verska and associates[162] have noted that even though the prothrombin time returns to normal before CPB, patients previously receiving warfarin-type therapy demonstrated more hemorrhage than those not previously on these agents. They also noted that increased hemorrhage was associated with a repeat bypass procedure; others, however, have noted no increased hemorrhage in association with a second procedure.[76,156] In addition, patients undergoing CPB for correction of cyanotic heart disease appear to have more severe derangements in hemostasis during perfusion, and thus a propensity to hemorrhage, than those operated on for noncyanotic heart disease.[76,146] Thus, increased hemorrhagic risk during CPB surgery appears to be associated with the prior use of warfarin drugs, hypothermic perfusion, and surgery for correction of cyanotic heart disease.

Summary of Hemostasis Pathophysiology During Cardiopulmonary Bypass

Many conclusions regarding altered hemostasis and resultant hemorrhage during CPB surgery are of questionable significance; for example, it appears that overheparinization, heparin rebound, inadequate protamine neutralization, and protamine excess, although receiving at least theoretical attention as potential sources of CPB hemorrhage, have not been documented as being responsible for bleeding associated with bypass surgery. Similarly, thrombocytopenia, almost certainly a potential source of hemorrhage, is an inconsistent finding during cardiac surgery. The finding of isolated coagulation defects during CPB has added little, except confusion, to an understanding of altered hemostasis during bypass surgery; most likely, these isolated findings simply represent isolated measurements of the results of hyperfibrino(geno)lysis and systemically circulating plasmin.

Although DIC has been thought by some to occur during CPB, most carefully performed studies have failed to document this. The significant doses of heparin used during CPB, the absence of thrombocytopenia, and the general correction of hypofibrinogenemia, hypoplasminogenemia, and elevated FDP after heparin neutralization all suggest that the presence of DIC during cardiac surgery is a very rare event. I have noted DIC in association with cardiac surgery only when another triggering event was provided, such as sepsis, shock, massive transfusions, or a frank hemolytic transfusion reaction.

Predisposing factors that do seem to be associated with enhanced cardiac surgery hemorrhage are long perfusion times, prior ingestion of warfarin-type drugs, cyanotic heart disease, hypothermic perfusions, and the preoperative ingestion of drugs known to interfere with platelet function. More importantly, evidence suggests that the majority of patients undergoing CPB surgery develop a primary hyperfibrino(geno)lytic syndrome, although the exact triggering mechanisms remain unclear, but may be due to Factor XII activation. However, the resultant secondary derangements in hemostasis will certainly create a potential for CPB hemorrhage. In addition, virtually all patients undergoing CPB procedures develop a severe platelet function defect. It is not clear if this defect is due to coating of platelet surfaces by FDP, membrane damage from the oxygenation mechanism, platelet damage from fast flow rates, or other unrecognized mechanisms. Whatever the triggering mechanisms, it is quite clear that the most significant alterations in hemostasis associated with CPB surgery are defective platelet function and primary fibrino(geno)lysis. These two defects alone or in combination certainly account for the majority of nonsurgical and nontechnical hemorrhage in patients undergoing CPB. Platelet function defects account for far more hemorrhagic episodes than primary hyperfibrino(geno)lysis.

Diagnosis of Hemorrhage During Cardiopulmonary Bypass

When bleeding occurs during or after bypass, it is obviously extremely important to define the defects as quickly as possible; only in this manner can specific and effective therapy be delivered.[20,37,150] As previously mentioned, many instances hemorrhage and CPB are clearly due to inadequate surgical technique, but alterations of hemostasis may also be responsible for accentuating hemorrhage. This discussion will be limited to nontechnical causes of CPB hemorrhage. The types of hemorrhage that occur during CPB are somewhat limited (Table 8–5).

The primary distinction to be made is between strictly surgical bleeding, defects in hemostasis, or a combination of the two. This distinction becomes more difficult and more important after the patient has left the operating room; during this period, a decision must be made regarding re-exploration and the adequacy of hemostasis for re-exploration. In distinguishing between surgical and nonsurgical bleeding, many physical findings are

Table 8–5 Hemorrhagic Syndromes Associated with Cardiopulmonary Bypass*

Platelet function defect
CPB-induced
Drug-induced
Primary fibrino(geno)lysis
Thrombocytopenia
Hyperheparinemia or rebound?
Disseminated intravascular coagulation (extremely rare)

* Listed in descending order of probability.

helpful: Is the bleeding localized or systemic? If the patient is already in the recovery room, the recognition of hematuria in association with petechiae and purpura, and oozing from intravenous sites in conjunction with increased chest tube blood loss and oozing from surgical sites, including the sternotomy wound and saphenous vein harvest site, mean a defect in hemostasis. On the other hand, increased chest tube blood loss alone often signifies a technical bleeding problem. When the patient is in the operating room, these same findings hold true; in addition, the surgeon will usually note bleeding or oozing throughout the surgical field in nontechnical bleeding. It is imperative therefore that communication between the surgeon and the hematologist or internist occur. Clinical suggestions of a systemic rather than local cause of hemorrhage are depicted in Table 8–6.

As soon as hemorrhage during CPB is seen or suspected, the following laboratory tests are ordered: prothrombin time, activated partial thromboplastin time, complete blood and platelet counts, examination of a peripheral smear, FDP level, heparin assay by synthetic substrate, thrombin or reptilase times, and plasminogen/plasmin levels by synthetic substrate methods.[20,37] Evaluation of the heparin level provides information on the potential effects heparin will have on other tests of hemostasis. The resultant clot from the thrombin and reptilase time tests is always observed for 5 minutes for evidence of lysis, thus providing rapid additional information regarding the presence or absence of a clinically significant primary hyperfibrino(geno)lytic syndrome. Additional evidence for or against primary lysis is ob-

tained by noting the FDP level.[108,140] A peripheral blood smear and platelet count are invaluable for rapidly evaluating the potential for thrombocytopenic bleeding. Plasminogen and plasmin levels obtained by synthetic substrate technique are not time-consuming, but are not used for an immediately diagnosis. However, they are invaluable in making decisions regarding antifibrinolytic therapy at a later time.[20,36,37] If significant primary fibrino(geno)lysis is present, FDPs will be significantly elevated and hypoplasminogenemia and circulating plasmin will be detected. If available, fibrinopeptide A levels will not be elevated but B-beta 15-42 and related peptides will be elevated. If, on the other hand, excess heparin is a potential problem, this will be noted by the heparin assay and in addition, the thrombin time will be markedly prolonged. If no significant clot lysis is observed in the clot formed during measurement of the thrombin time, and significant FDP elevation is not present, primary fibrino(geno)lysis should not dwelled upon.

All patients undergoing CPB display a platelet function defect; when bleeding occurs, I assume that this defect is always present and even though it might not be the primary reason for hemorrhage, platelet dysfunction can be assumed to be additive to any other defect, whether surgical or due to altered hemostasis. No tests of platelet function are done therefore, but platelets are immediately ordered for any patient who demonstrates hemorrhage during or after CPB.[20,36,37] The time period during which hemorrhage occurs, that is, interoperatively, after heparin neutralization, or in the recovery room, appears to bear little relationship to the etiology of the primary hemostatic defect responsible for hemorrhage. Exceptions to this are thrombocytopenic bleeding that usually occurs after the patient is in the recovery room and a significant drug-induced platelet function defect that is usually manifested as significant oozing as soon as the operative procedure is started. Tests ordered for the differential diagnosis of the causes of hemorrhage during CPB surgery are listed in Table 8–7.

Table 8–6 Clinical Evaluation of Hemorrhage in Cardiopulmonary Bypass Patients

Chest tube blood loss only? *or associated with*
Petechiae and purpura
Hematuria
Oozing from intra-arterial or intravenous lines
Bleeding from sternotomy or saphenous graft sites
Other systemic bleeding

Table 8–7 Laboratory Evaluation of Cardiopulmonary Bypass Hemorrhage

Platelet and complete blood count
Blood smear evaluation
  Prothrombin time
  Activated partial thromboplastin time
FDP titer
Heparin assay (synthetic substrate)
Thrombin time (observe for lysis)
Plasminogen assay (synthetic substrate)
Plasmin assay (synthetic substrate)

Management of CPB Hemorrhage

When one first sees a patient with hemorrhage from CPB, whether intraoperative or postoperative, it is of prime importance to note the type of bleeding (systemic versus local), to order a laboratory screen as outlined previously, and to administer 6 to 8 U of platelet concentrates as quickly as possible. Even though the use of platelet concentrates is somewhat empirical at this point, it is done for the sound reasons that virtually all patients have a significant platelet function defect that may be the primary reason for hemorrhage, and usually is if the bleeding is not related to the surgery, or this defect is likely to be accentuating bleeding from other causes, whether it be a surgical defect or defective hemostasis. In my experience, the quick administration of platelet concentrates, while awaiting the laboratory evaluation, will often stop or significantly reduce most instances of non-technical CPB hemorrhage.[20,36,37]

When bleeding begins immediately on initiation of surgery, a platelet function defect, usually drug-induced, can be assumed to be present until further laboratory investigation can be performed. In this instance, the patient should be given 6 to 8 u of platelet concentrates as quickly as possible, and the surgical wound should be closed if this is feasible. If a platelet function defect is found to be responsible for the hemorrhage (no laboratory evidence of significant fibrino(geno)lysis or

hyperheparinemia), 6 to 8 units of platelet concentrates should be repeated the evening after surgery and for 2 mornings postoperatively.

Thrombocytopenic hemorrhage should be controlled in the same manner, although greater numbers of platelet concentrates may be needed, as dictated by the initial platelet count, the site and severity of hemorrhage, and the response to platelet transfusions. Hyperheparinemia and heparin rebound, if thought to be a real clinical problem as documented by synthetic substrate assays, are managed by delivering 25% of the original calculated protamine sulfate dose; this is repeated every 30 to 60 minutes until bleeding ceases. It should again be emphasized hyperheparinemia and heparin rebound are not at all likely to be responsible for bleeding, and should be considered only if concrete laboratory evidence of hyperheparinemia is present and evidence of primary fibrino(geno)lysis is clearly absent. I have seen many instances of excessive heparinization due to mistakes in calculations and solution preparation; not one of these instances was associated with significant cardiac surgical hemorrhage. Similarly, protamine excess is rarely, if ever, a clinical probelm. This situation should never require therapy and should not be considered at the risk of ignoring other potential defects in hemostasis.

Primary hyperfibrino(geno)lysis is commonly present and may or may not be responsible for hemorrhage. This syndrome should not be treated empirically; antifibrinolytic therapy should be considered if the patient has failed to respond to platelet concentrates and there is documented laboratory evidence for this syndrome, as noted by the presence of hypoplasminogenemia, circulating plasmin, and elevated FDPs. In addition, for those having these testing systems available, the absence of elevated fibrinopeptide A and the presence of elevated B-beta 15-42 and related peptides offers further evidence for primary lysis. Primary hyperfibrino(geno)lytic bleeding is generally treated with EACA given as an initial dose of 5 to 10 g slow intravenous push followed by 1 to 2 g/hour until bleeding ceases or slows to a nonlife-threatening level. It should be recalled that EACA may be associated with ventricular arrhythmias, hypotension, hypokalemia, localized or diffuse thrombosis, and frank DIC. Thus, this agent should be injected slowly and patients should be monitored carefully with respect to renal output, blood pressure, and electrolytes.

Thrombohemorrhagic Complications of Prosthetic Devices and Transplantation

Exposure of the blood to foreign surfaces is often linked with thrombosis, which provides a major clinical obstacle to the use of prosthetic devices. The use of prosthetic devices have become commonplace in the management of patients with cardiovascular disease, renal disease, or chemotherapy, for long-term parenteral hyperalimentation, and for common angiographic studies.[36,72] The hemostatic complications following the insertion of prosthetic devices include consumption of coagulation factors, other plasma proteins, or platelets, the generation of microthrombi of little clinical consequences, and thrombosis or thromboembolism that may give rise to serious, life-threatening, or terminal vaso-occlusion. Under normal circumstances, the blood remains fluid because of numerous obvious factors, including a non-thrombogenic endothelial surface, endogenous fibrinolytic activity, natural protease inhibitors, such as antithrombin III and protein C, and the dilution and dispersion of procoagulant components of the blood.[44,45,69,143] All of these protective mechanisms are lost, to some degree, with the use of prosthetic devices.[36]

In general, slow flow rates are associated with local thrombotic events; however, fast flow rates are more commonly associated with a high shear force and embolization.[140] In addition, smooth prosthetic surfaces tend to favor little adhesiveness of a formed thrombus and thus embolization is more likely to occur than with a rough surface, which tends to favor firm fibrin clot formation and eventual neovascularization.[51] When blood is exposed to prosthetic devices or any foreign surface, plasma proteins are immediately absorbed, primarily fibrinogen, albumin, alpha- and beta globulins, gamma globulin, Factors VIII:C, XII, and XI, and thrombin.[6,89] Factors XII and XI may simply be absorbed or, alternatively, may become activated. Fibrinogen appears to be the major plasma protein absorbed and promotes subsequent platelet adhesion will be enhanced or induced not only by fibrinogen but also by gamma globulin, thrombin, and subsequent Factors XII and XI activation.[112] In addition, the activation of Factors XII or XI may induce intrinsic coagulation, with further fibrin formation generating a platelet-fibrin thrombus. As thrombotic surfaces form and embolize in the aforementioned manner, they may eventually overwhelm the ability of the reticuloendothelial system to clear them; subsequent thromboembolization with vascular occlusion and subsequent end organ infarction may occur.[97]

The most common defects that generally occur with prosthetic devices are as follows: (1) There may be a frank coagulation factor and platelet consumption with subsequent thrombocytopenia and resultant hemorrhage; (2) devices may cause partial platelet degranulation, with subsequent defective platelet function and resultant hemorrhage; (3) in cases of oxygenation or dialysis membranes, fibrin-platelet deposition will render the exchange ineffective and provide a focus for thromboembolus; and (4) micro- or macrothromboemboli of platelets or fibrin may give rise to serious clinical vaso-occlusive problems.[36,74] The use of anticoagulants, including warfarin-type drugs, heparin, and platelet suppressive agents, tends to normalize thrombotic and thromboembolic complications with prosthetic devices.[36] However, the problem still remains clinically significant, especially during CPB surgery, hemodialysis, angiographic studies, prosthetic heart valve placement, long-term intravenous catheterization, and the use of LeVeen shunts.[36] Additional problems are also associated with apheresis procedures, which will be discussed subsequently.

Intra-arterial or intravenous catheters are coated with fibrin or platelet aggregates when used for angiographic studies, long-term chemotherapy, infusions of fluids, and long-term parenteral hyperalimentation.[36,106] Thromboembolism occurs in approximately 2% of individuals catheterized for angiographic studies.[36,118] An additional complication is that an existing atherosclerotic plaque may be disrupted and embolize. The thromboembolic complications of short-term or long-term catheterization are usually minimized by the use of low-dose intravenous heparin.

Intra-aortic balloon assist is a widely utilized clinical procedure to control post-myocardial infarction, cardiogenic shock, and to stabilize selected patients after CPB surgery and other vascular surgical procedures.[48,125] The balloons in common use are made of polyurethane. Minimal to moderate fibrin formation and minimal platelet aggregation are noted with these assist balloons.[142] However, clinically significant problems may occur, including thrombosis, thromboembolism, vaso-occlusive ischemic changes in the lower extremities (the balloon is usually introduced via the left common femoral artery), and potential injury to the aortic wall. An additional hematologic complication with intra-aortic balloon assist is that of hemolysis, which occurs in up to 10% of patients. However, the use of heparin or heparin in conjunction with platelet suppressive therapy will minimize the thrombotic and thromboembolic risks associated with intra-aortic balloon assist. On rare instances, a frank DIC-type syndrome may also occur, especially if the balloon is in place for more than 5 days.

Renal hemodialysis is the mainstay of therapy for acute and chronic renal failure, as well as for the alleviation of acute poisoning. However, the formation of fibrin-platelet thrombi on the dialysis membrane greatly reduces its efficiency and provides a focus for embolization, with subsequent potential complications. In addition, renal hemodialysis is commonly associated with neutrophil adherence and complement activation on the dialysis membrane.[93] The complement activation may further add to clinical problems by the release of the anaphylatoxins C3a and C5a with subsequent leukoembolization as well. Since thrombosis and thromboembolism remain major clinical problems associated with renal hemodialysis, systemic or regional heparization is used. Regional heparinization consists of adding heparin to the arterial line as blood leaves the patient and neutralizing heparin with protamine in the venous line as blood returns to the patient. Some have considered heparin rebound to be a clinical problem with regional heparinization.[78]

Platelet-suppressive therapy has decreased platelet adhesion to dialysis membranes; however, antiplatelet agents must be used cautiously in the uremic patient with already compromised platelet function.[36,109,169] Access shunts in the form of surgically created arteriovenous (AV) shunts or prosthetic AV shunts are necessary for hemodialysis patients, frequently transfused patients, patients undergoing long-term parenteral hyperalimentation, long-term chemotherapy, and those committed to a long-term apheresis program.[5,167] Surgically created AV shunts tend to have fewer thrombotic complications than prosthetic shunts.[101] Although thrombosis of the shunt remains the major significant problem with these devices, infection is also of concern. Prosthetic shunts as well as surgically created shunts are usually "declotted" by the use of surgery or streptokinase with reasonably good success.[121] Anticoagulant therapy has not become commonplace for patients with AV shunts; however, it has been shown that dipyridamole will correct decreased platelet survival and increased platelet consumption in patients with these devices.[80] Aspirin alone will not decrease the incidence of shunt thrombosis. Prosthetic vascular grafts are primarily constructed of Dacron with sufficient porosity to allow for neovascularization, thrombus organization, and nutrient blood flow. Thrombotic occlusion of prosthetic grafts is not well controlled with heparin or warfarin-type drugs and is now most commonly treated with platelet suppressive therapy.[36]

Peritoneovenous shunting using a Le-

Veen valve has become a palliative procedure for the treatment of intractable ascites associated with severe liver disease.[107,138] A generalized hemorrhagic diathesis is frequently seen with the use of LeVeen shunts and appears to represent a straightforward DIC-type syndrome associated with accelerated fibrinogen and platelet destruction.[38,81,105,154] The removal of ascitic fluid at the time of valve implantation, as well as the use of anticoagulants, have been advocated to abort DIC in patients receiving LeVeen shunts[36,95] LeVeen shunts were also discussed in Chapters 6 and 7.

Alterations of Hemostasis Associated with Renal Disease and Renal Transplantation

The role of the hemostasis system as a mediator of renal vascular and glomerular damage remains unclear. Evidence suggesting participation of the hemostasis system in renal disease is based on morphologic, histochemical, serologic, and radioisotope studies as well as the noting of abnormal test results of hemostasis. It appears clear that renal diseases associated with a microangiopathic hemolytic anemia as a prominant feature are accompanied by activation of the hemostasis system with subsequent fibrin deposition, which appears responsible for progressive renal damage. However, the role of the hemostasis system in the pathogenesis of other glomerular diseases remains less clear and, in many instances, it is impossible to know if "activation" of the hemostasis system leads to renal damage or disease or alternatively if renal disease leads to activation of the hemostasis system with subsequent renal microvascular fibrin deposition. The mechanisms responsible for accelerating fibrin deposition in renal disease likewise remain unclear.[40] However, it does appear that fibrin deposition in glomeruli assumes an important pathogenetic role in crescent formation and eventual glomerular degeneration.[119] Fib-

rin appears not only deposited within capillaries, but also in Bowman's space, where it likely stimulates epithelial cell proliferation with subsequent crescent formation. In addition, fibrin leakage through capillary walls is thought to be due to focal membrane disruption. Crescent formation appears to pass through three well-defined stages: cellular, fibrocellular, and fibrotic. Crescent formation is a prominant feature of idiopathic extracapillary glomerulonephritis; however, in other glomerular diseases, including acute poststreptococcal nephritis, lupus nephritis, and anaphylactoid purpura, crescent formation appears to be less pronounced.

Immunoflourescent microscopy appears to be the best single technique for consistently detecting fibrinogen, fibrin, or FDPs in the kidney. These deposits have been consistently demonstrated by immunofluorescence even when histologic stains for fibrin or electron microscopy studies have been negative.[60] Fibrinogen, fibrin, and FDP deposits have been detected by immunochemical techniques either along the basement membrane within the mesangium or in the vascular walls in a variety of renal disease, including hemolytic-uremic syndrome, scleroderma, malignant hypertension, acute homograft rejection, postpartum renal failure, and rapidly progressive glomerulonephritis.[98,110,113] In addition, in hemolytic-uremic syndrome, postpartum renal failure, acute homograft rejection, scleroderma, and malignant hypertension, Factor VIII is present in the same areas as fibrinogen.[88] This finding suggests an active participation of the hemostasis system in leading to subsequent fibrin deposition in the aforementioned disorders. However, Factor VIII has not been found in epithelial cell cresents in proliferative nephritis or in the mesangium of patients with anaphylactoid purpura, all of which are areas of intense fibrinogen, fibrin, and FDP deposition. This finding suggests that differing mechanisms of fibrin deposition and hemostasis "activation" may exist in differing renal diseases.[148] It has been suggested that Factor VIII:C levels may be of prognostic significance in patients with glomerulonephritis, high levels being associated with a poor prognosis and a low probability of renal function returning to normal.[65] In addition, this increase is attributed to progressive vascular endothelial damage.

The clearance of deposited fibrin in the kidney may occur as a result of endothelial cell or mensangial cell phagocytosis or as a result of fibrino(geno)lysis by plasminogen activators in the associated vascular endothelium. It should be recalled that human kidney endothelial cells produce a potent plasminogen activator, urokinase. In the normal kidney, plasminogen activator activity may be demonstrated in glomeruli, arteries, arterioles, and veins.[91] However, there remains an unclear relationship between glomerular fibrin deposition and glomerular fibrinolysis in kidneys from patients with a wide variety of renal diseases. However, it has been observed that plasminogen activator activity is absent in the cortex of patients with acute renal homograft rejection, although the mechanisms responsible for loss of fibrinolytic activator activity are unknown.[10]

In general it has been suggested that serum FDPs are elevated in most of the aforementioned renal diseases and may be expected to vary with the activity and severity of the disease process.[153] However, it must be recalled that extrarenal sites of fibrino(geno)lysis will also result in elevated serum FDP levels, which, as will be discussed, are found in a number of renal diseases, including lupus nephritis, poststreptococcal progressive glomerulonephritis, anaphylactic purpura, hemolytic-uremic syndrome, nephrotic syndrome, focal sclerosis with hypertension, renal failure, and in membranous nephropathy. However, it has been demonstrated that urinary FDPs correlate much better with disease activity and fibrin deposition than do serum FDP levels.[82,83,133] It has been suggested that urinary FDP excretion may not correlate with disease activity, since variability may be noted with the degree of protein selectivity.[66] Others, however, have found that urinary FDP levels are indicative of renal fibrin deposition and not indicative of protein excretion selectivity.[114]

The role of platelets as mediators of renal disease remains unclear and confusing. However, abnormal platelet turnover, manifested by decreased platelet survival and increased platelet consumption as well as abnormal platelet aggregation patterns, has been noted in hemolytic-uremic syndrome, acute homograft rejection, membranoproliferative nephritis, glomerulosclerosis, diffuse proliferative nephritis, and diabetic nephropathy.[83] In addition, it has been noted that bilateral nephrectomy results in normalization of platelet survival in a variety of renal diseases, thus suggesting the presence of intrarenal platelet deposition.[83] Despite these findings, it remains unclear whether improvement in renal function will occur in patients treated with anticoagulant or platelet-suppressive therapy, even though such therapy tends to bring about normal platelet survival. Increased platelet aggregability has been documented in patients with Alport's syndrome, nephrotic syndrome, active glomerulonephritis, and in patients with diabetic nephropathy.[7] It must be appreciated that immune complex-induced endothelial injury and alterations of the renal basement membrane and other subendothelial surfaces may certainly result in primary platelet activation. This may provide procoagulant material for subsequent fibrin deposition in similar morphologic areas.[40]

In summary, the precise role of the hemostasis system as a modulator of renal diseases remains unclear.[40] The presence of decreased platelet survival and of fibrin(ogen), FDPs, and Factor VIII by immunoflourescent studies, and the noting of elevated urine and serum FDP levels in the majority of renal diseases present highly suggestive evidence of active participation of hemostasis in immune-mediated glomerular disease. Unfortunately, what remains unclear is whether activation of the hemostasis system may lead to renal microvascular fibrin deposition with subsequent renal disease or, alternatively, whether exposure of the hemostasis system to subendothelial collagen or other materials in the renal microenvironment will subsequently activate the hemostasis system.

Laboratory Findings of Hemostasis in Renal Disease

In patients with various renal disorders, the determination of serum and urinary FDP levels is useful for both aiding in diagnosis, assessing severity of disease, and in monitoring disease activity and potential efficacy of therapy. In general, the urinary FDP titer appears better correlated with severity and activity of disease. Urinary FDP titers of up to 50μg/dL have been noted in active renal disorders, including hydronephrosis, lupus nephritis, and proliferative glomerular nephritis; the levels generally correlate well with disease activity.[132] In contrast, patients with minimal renal disease or membranous lesions have FDP levels rarely exceeding 2μg/dL thus providing an important laboratory diagnostic tool.[40] However, in both types of lesions, including those associated with minimal nephrotic syndrome, serum FDP levels may be abnormally elevated. In addition, studies have shown that urinary FDP levels decrease when therapy for glomerular lesion appears to be effective.[4,132]

In pediatric renal disease, including chronic glomerular nephritis, Henoch-Schölein glomerulonephritis, and hemolytic-uremic syndrome, high serum FDP levels are often noted. In the presence of disease progression, urinary FDP levels may begin to increase and, when monitored in association with blood pressure, may provide evidence of effective therapy when a drop in titer and blood pressure are noted.[4]

Patients with upper urinary tract infections usually have elevated urinary FDP titers. Thus, the urinary FDP titer appears to be helpful in distinguishing the site of urinary tract infections.[166]

Patients with recent renal homograft transplant often show elevated levels of FDPs in serum and urine as the donor kidney begins to function. Although several investigators have reported that the determination of urinary FDP titers appears to be of little value in the diagnosis of early acute rejection,[54,56] other investigators have shown that the assay of FDPs in urine as well as serum do indeed provide a sensitive laboratory index of impending rejection.[124] In addition,it has been noted that the failure to note increasing levels of urinary FDPs to decrease after enhancing immunosuppressive therapy seems to correlate with rejection and may indicate the need for still more intensive therapy in attempting to salvage the graft.[56] Thus, sustained increased FDP titers appear to correlate with early graft rejection and herald the need for more aggressive therapy.

In summary, current evidence would suggest that serum and urine FDP titers may be a useful guide in the diagnosis, determination of severity and disease activity,and efficacy of therapy in numerous renal diseases. In addition, it appears that the determination of urinary FDP levels may aid in the differential diagnosis between membranous and glomerular lesions and in determining the site of urinary tract infection. In addition, current although incomplete evidence suggests that the determination of serum and urinary FDP levels may be useful in assessing the efficacy of successful steroid, immunosuppressive, anticoagulant, and platelet suppressive therapy in a wide variety of renal diseases. In addition, some evidence is beginning to accumulate to suggest that decreased platelet survival and increased platelet turnover may also be a diagnostic aid in assessing severity of renal disease and, more importantly, may be an effective way of monitoring efficacy of anticoagulant therapy or platelet suppressive therapy in a variety of renal diseases, including lupus nephritis and diabetic nephropathy. It appears that the pathophysiology of renal transplant rejection is a DIC-type syndrome probably induced by circulating immune complexes with the attendant triggering mechanisms, as delineated in detail in Chapter 6.

Aphresis

Aphresis (plasmapheresis, plasma exchange, leukopheresis, and plateletpheresis) has become a common procedure for the management of patients with a wide variety of hematologic and immunologic diseases, including thrombotic thrombocytopenic purpura, hemolytic-uremic syndrome, collagen vascular disorders, myasthenia gravis, hyperviscosity syndrome, and some instances of immune hemolytic anemias. Hemorrhage or thrombosis may occur with any of these apheresis procedures. Thrombosis and thromboembolism may occur in vivo or, alternatively, quite frequently occurs ex-vivo in the apheresis equipment and tubing.[161] Thrombocytopenia occurs in the majority of patients undergoing apheresis procedures and quite commonly the platelet count will drop to between 15 and 50% of the initial platelet count; the loss is less with discontinuous flow systems than with continuous flow systems. An additional problem that occurs during apheresis procedures is that of defective platelet function; this has been shown by using the Borchgrevink technique and has also been studied by use of the glass bead column adhesion method. By the Borchgrevink technique approximately 80% of patients undergoing apheresis procedures have decreases in platelet adhesion;[149] however, it should be noted that the glass bead column technique did not show this abnormality and this is in harmony with recent suggestions that the glass bead column test may not be of clinical significance.[85,173]

Other severe derangements in hemostasis also occur during apheresis procedures. The most pronounced changes in coagulation appear to be decreases in fibrinogen and Factor XI.[147] The fibrinogen level may drop to 50% of prepheresis levels and may remain depressed chronically for up to 72 hours. However, in most studies the fibrinogen level has not dropped below 50 mg/dL and thus thrombin times are only rarely prolonged.[64,147,161] It has also been noted that if there is greater than a 3.5 L exchange, the prothrombin time, activated partial thromboplastin times, and thrombin time commonly become prolonged.[128] It has also been noted that if there is a 2 to 5 L exchange, fibrinogen levels will decrease from 50 to 25% of normal and may not return to normal levels until approximately 3 days after pheresis.[128,161] How-

ever, this change in fibrinogen is commonly not associated with bleeding unless large amounts of heparin are also used during the pheresis procedure.[161] It has also been noted that Factor IX levels will decrease from 60 to 70% of normal if greater than a 4 L exchange occurs. Additional changes in coagulation are the noting of a 60 to 70% decrease in Factors II, V, VII, X, XI, and XIII.[161] In addition, Factor V and VII levels will usually become normal within 24 hours; however, Factors II, X, XI, and XIII levels will usually not become normal until approximately 48 hours after pheresis.[147,161]

An additional complication of apheresis is a significant decrease in antithrombin III that may lead to clotting in up to 25% of patients.[151,161] The thrombotic events and antithrombin III depletion associated with apheresis can be markedly blunted or eradicated by the use of heparin in the replacement fluid or by the infusion of fresh frozen plasma as a source of antithrombin III; this practice has, again, been noted to reduce or blunt markedly the in vivo and in vitro thrombotic and thromboembolic problems associated with apheresis.[151] It should also be noted that complement activation with the release of C3a and C5a and subsequent potential leukoembolization and endothelial damage may also occur with apheresis procedures.[165] In addition, if activation of the complement system proceeds to C8, 9 this may potentially also lead to or contribute to platelet and red cell release of procoagulant materials and subsequent thrombus formation.

Thus, apheresis is associated with significant changes in the hemostasis system, including thrombocytopenia, platelet dysfunction, and decreasing coagulation factor levels, with the most profound decreases being those of fibrinogen and Factor XI; most of these parameters return to normal in 24 to 48 hours after pheresis. Of additional significance is that antithrombin III levels tend to drop significantly during apheresis procedures, and unless heparin is used or antithrombin III is replaced by the use of fresh frozen plasma, thrombosis and thromboembolus can be a problem in up to 25% of patients undergoing apheresis procedures.

Summary

A review of the available literature regarding alterations of hemostasis associated with surgery, CPB surgery, transplantation, the use of prosthetic devices, and apheresis has been provided. The key to prevention of surgical hemorrhage is to obtain an adequate preoperative workup. Of extreme importance is an adequate history with respect to bleeding and thrombotic tendencies in both the patient and the family; of equal importance is a careful history regarding the use of drugs affecting hemostasis, especially drugs known to interfere with platelet function. A careful physical examination, searching for clues of a real or potential bleeding diathesis, may also prevent catastrophic cases of surgical hemorrhage. An adequate presurgical screen must be performed. In addition to the usual prothrombin time, partial thromboplastin time, and platelet count, a standardized template bleeding time (and thrombin time in patients subjected to CPB surgery) should be performed. The use of these simple testing modalities will guard against significant defects in vascular and platelet function. Most instances of non-technical surgical and cardiovascular surgical hemorrhage are due to several well-defined defects in hemostasis that should be readily controlled if approached in a logical manner as a team effort among all surgeons, pathologists, and hematologists.

References

1. Adams T, Schutz L, Goldberg L: Platelet function abnormalities in the myeloproliferative disorders. Scand J Haematol 13:215, 1975.
2. Akkerman JW, Runne WC, Sixma JJ, Zimmerman AE: Improved survival rates in dogs after extracorporeal circulation by improved control of heparin levels. J Thorac Cardiovasc Surg 68:59, 1974.
3. Alkjaersig N, Fletcher AP, Sherry S: Pathogenesis of the coagulation defect developing during pathological plasma proteolytic ("fibrinolytic") states. II. The significance, mechanism, and consequences of defective fibrin polymerization. J Clin Invest 41:917, 1962.
4. Ambrus JL, Baliah TR, Ambrus CM: Fibrin-fibrinogen degradation products in children with renal disease. NY State J Med 74:1396, 1974.
5. Bachmann F, McKenna R, Cole ER, Maiafi HJ: The hemostatic mechanisms after open-heart surgery. I. Studies on plasma coagulation factors and fibrinolysis in 512 patients after extracorporeal circulations. J Thorac Cardiovasc Surg 70:76, 1975.
6. Bagnall RD: Absorption of plasma proteins on hydrophobic surfaces. II. Fibrinogen and fibrinogen-containing protein mixtures. Biomed Biomater Res 12:203, 1978.
7. Bang NU, Trystad CW, Schroeder JE: Enhanced platelet function in glomerular renal disease. J Lab Clin Med 81:651, 1973.
8. Beall C, Yow EM, Blodwell RD, Hallman G, Cooley D: Open heart surgery without blood transfusion. Arch Surg 94:567, 1967.
9. Behrendt DM, Espstein SE, Morrow AG: Postperfusion nonthrombocytopenic purpura: An uncommon sequal of open heart surgery. Am J Cardiol 22:631, 1968.
10. Bergstein JM, Michael AF: Glomerular plasminogen activation activity in renal homograft rejection. Transplantation 17:443, 1974.
11. Bick RL, Shanbrom E: A systematic approach to the diagnosis of bleeding disorders. Med Counterpoint 6:27, 1972.
12. Bick RL: A systematic approach to the diagnosis of bleeding disorders. In Murano G, Bick RL (Eds): Basic Concepts of Hemostasis and Thrombosis. CRC Press, Boca Raton, FL, 1980, p 81.
13. Bick RL: Difficult Diagnostic Problems in Hemostasis and Thrombosis. American Society of Clinical Pathology Manual No 5549, Chicago, 1980.
14. Bick RL, Murano G: Primary hyperfibrino-(geno)lytic syndromes. In Murano G, Bick RL (Eds): Basic Concepts of Hemostasis and Thrombosis. CRC Press, Boca Raton, FL, 1980, p 181.
15. Bick RL: Vascular disorders associated with thrombohemorrhagic phenomena. Semin Thromb Hemost 5:167, 1979.
16. Bick RL: Current Concepts of Hemostasis and Thrombosis. Chicago, American Society of Clinical Pathology Manual No 5548, 1980.
17. Bick RL: Vascular disorders. In Murano G, Bick RL (Eds): Basic Concepts of Hemostasis and Thrombosis. CRC Press, Boca Raton, FL, 1980, p 89.
18. Bick RL: Alterations of hemostasis associated with malignancy: Etiology, pathophysiology, diagnosis, and management. Semin Thromb Hemost 5:1, 1978.
19. Bick RL: Alterations of hemostasis during car-

diopulmonary bypass: A comparison between membrane and bubble oxygenators. Am J Clin Path 73:300, 1980.

20. Bick RL: Alterations of hemostasis associated with cardiopulmonary bypass: Pathophysiology, prevention, diagnosis, and management. Semin Thromb Hemost 3:59, 1976.

21. Bick RL, Schmalhorst WR, Shanbrom E: Prothrombin complex concentrates: Use in controlling the hemorrhagic diathesis of chronic liver disease. Am J Dig Dis 20:741, 1975.

22. Bick RL: Disseminated intravascular coagulation (DIC) and related syndromes. In Murano G, Bick RL (Eds): Basic Concepts of Hemostasis and Thrombosis. Boca Raton, FL, 1980, p 163.

23. Bick RL: Disseminated intravascular coagulation and related syndromes: Etiology, pathophysiology, diagnosis and management. Am J Hematol 5:265, 1978.

24. Bick RL: Disseminated intravascular coagulation and related syndromes. In Fareed J, Messmore J, Fenton J, et al (Eds): Perspective in Hemostasis. Pergamon Press, New York, 1981, p 122.

25. Bick RL: Treatment of bleeding and thrombosis in the patient with cancer. In Nealon T (Ed): Management of the patient with Cancer. W. B. Saunders Co, Philadelphia, 1976, p 48.

26. Bick RL, Arbegast NR, Holtermann N, Crawford L, Schmalhorst WR: Platelet function abnormalities in cardiopulmonary bypass. Abstr. Circulation 50(Suppl):301, 1974.

27. Bick RL, Schmalhorst WR, Crawford L, Holterman M, Arbegast NR: The hemorrhagic diathesis created by cardiopulmonary bypass. Abstr. Am J Clin Pathol 63:588, 1975.

28. Bick RL, Arbegast NR, Crawford L, Holtermann L, Adams T, Schmalhorst WR: Hemostatic defects induced by cardiopulmonary bypass. Vasc Surg 9:28, 1975.

29. Bick RL, Schmalhorst WR, Arbegast NR: Alterations of hemostasis associated with cardiopulmonary bypass. Am J Clin Pathol 63:588, 1975.

30. Bick RL, Adams T, Schmalhorst WR: Bleeding times, platelet adhesion, and aspirin. Am J Clin Pathol 65:69, 1976.

31. Bick RL, Fekete LF: Cardiopulmonary bypass hemorrhage: Aggrevation by pre-op ingestion of antiplatelet agents. Vasc Surg 13:277, 1979.

32. Bick RL, Comer TP, Arbegast NR: Fatal purpura fulminans following total cardiopulmonary bypass. J Cardiovasc Surg (Torino) 14:569, 1973.

33. Bick RL, Kovacs I, Fekete LF: A new two stage functional assay for antithrombin III (heparin cofactor): Clinical and laboratory evaluation. Thromb Res 8:745, 1976

34. Bick RL, Bishop RC, Warren M, Stemmer E: Changes in fibrinolysis and fibrinolytic enzymes during extracorporeal circulation Abstr. Trans Am Soc Hematol 109, 1971.

35. Bick RL, Bishop RC, Shanbrom ES: Fibrinolytic activity in acute myocardial infarction. Am J Clin Path 57:359, 1972.

36. Bick RL: Alterations of hemostasis associated with surgery, cardiopulmonary bypass surgery, and prosthetic devices. In Ratnoff OD, Forbes CD (Eds): Disorders of Hemostasis. Grune & Stratton, New York, 1984, p 379.

37. Bick RL: Syndromes associated with hyperfibrino(geno)lysis. In Bick RL (Ed): Disseminated Intravascular Coagulation. CRC Press, Boca Raton, FL, 1983, p 105.

38. Bick RL: Disseminated intravascular coagulation. In (Bick RL (Ed): Disseminated Intravascular Coagulation. CRC Press, Boca Raton, FL, 1983, p 31.

39. Bick RL: Clinical hemostasis practice: The major impact of laboratory automation. Semin Thromb Hemost 9:139, 1983.

40. Bick RL: The clinical significance of fibrinogen degradation products. Semin Thromb Hemost 8:302, 1982.

41. Bick RL, Schmalhorst SW, Arbegast NR: Alterations of hemostasis associated with cardiopulmonary bypass. Thromb Res 8:285, 1976.

42. Bick RL: Factor XII activation during cardiopulmonary bypass. Blood 64:254, 1984.

43. Bick RL: Clinical implications of molecular markers in hemostasis and thrombosis. Semin Thromb Hemost 10:290, 1984.

44. Bick RL: Basic mechanisms of hemostasis pertaining to DIC. In (Bick RL (Ed): Disseminated Intravascular Coagulation. CRC Press, Boca Raton, FL, 1983, p 1.

45. Bick RL: Clinical relevance of antithrombin III. Semin Thromb Hemost 8:276, 1982.

46. Bishop RC, Ekert H, Gilchrist G, Shanbrom E, Fekete LF: The preparation and evaluation of a standardized fibrin plate for the assessment of fibrinolytic activity. Thromb Diath Haemorrh 23:202, 1970.

47. Blomback M, Noren I, Senning A: Coagulation disturbances during extracorporeal circulation and the postoperative period. Acta Chir Scand 127:433, 1964.

48. Bolooki N: Clinical Applications of Intra-aortic Balloon Pump. Futura Publishing, New York, 1977.

49. Bowie EJW, Owen CA, Thompson JH: Platelet adhesiveness in von Willebrand's disease. Am J Clin Pathol 52:69, 1969.

50. Bowie EJW, Owen CA: The value of measuring platelet adhesiveness in the diagnosis of bleeding diseases. Am J Clin Pathol 60:302, 1973.

51. Braunwald NS, Bonchek L: Prevention of thrombus formation on rigid prosthetic heart

valves by the ingrowth of autogenous tissue. J Thorac Cardiovasc Surg 54:630, 1967.

52. Brecker G, Cronkite EP: Morphology and enumeration of human blood platelets. J Appl Physiol 3:365, 1950.

53. Brooks DH, Bahnson HT: An outbreak of hemorrhage following cardiopulmonary bypass. J Thorac Cardiovasc Surg 63:449, 1972.

54. Case JD, Clarkson AR: Serum and urinary fibrin/fibrinogen degradation products in renal disease. Scand J Haematol (Suppl) 13:331, 1971.

55. Casteneda AR: Must heparin be neutralized following open heart operations? J Thorac Cardiovasc Surg 52:716, 1966.

56. Clarkson AR, Morton JB, Cash JD: Urinary fibrin/fibrinogen degradation products after renal homotransplantation. Lancet 2:1220, 1970.

57. Cohen LS: Clinical pharmacology of acetylsalicylic acid. Semin Thromb Hemost 2:146, 1976.

58. Coley B, Bick RL: Platelet activation during cardiopulmonary bypass: An electron microscopic comparison between membrane and bubble oxygenators. Am J Clin Pathol. In press.

59. Cordell AR: Hematological complications of extracorporeal circulation. In Cordell AR, Ellison RG (Eds): Complications of Intrathoracic Surgery. Little, Brown, Boston, 1979, p 27.

60. Davidson AM, Thomson D, MK MacDonald: Identification of intrarenal fibrin deposition. J Clin Pathol 26:102, 1973.

61. Deiter RA, Neville WE, Piffare R, Jasuja M: Preoperative coagulation profiles and post-hemodilution cardiopulmonary bypass hemorrhage. Am J Surg 121:689, 1971.

62. Derman UM, Rand PW, Barker N: Fibrinolysis after cardiopulmonary bypass and its relationship to fibrinogen. J Thorac Cardiovasc Surg 51:223, 1966.

63. deVries SI, von Creveld S, Groen P, Muller E, Wettermark M: Studies on the coagulation of the blood in patients treated with extracorporeal circulation. Thromb Diath Haemorrh 5:426, 1961.

64. Domen RE, Kennedy MS, Jones LL, Senhauser DA: Hemostatic imbalances produced by plasma exchange. Transfusion 24:336, 1984.

65. Ekgerg M, Nilsson IM: Factor VIII and glomerulonephritis. Lancet 2:1111, 1975.

66. Ekert H, Barratt TM, Chandler C: Immunologically reactive equivalents of fibrinogen in sera and urine of children with renal disease. NY State J Med 74:1396, 1974.

67. Ellison N, Betty CP, Blake DR, Wurzel H, Mac Vaugh H: Heparin rebound: Studies in patients and volunteers. J Thorac Cardiovasc Surg 67:723, 1974.

68. Ellison N, Ominsky AJ, Wollman H: Is pro-

tamine a clinically important anticoagulant? A negative answer. Anesthesiology 35:621, 1971.

69. Esmon CT: Protein-C: Biochemistry, physiology, and clinical implications. Blood 62:1155, 1983.

70. Fareed J: New methods in hemostatic testing. In Fareed J, Messmore H, Fenton J (Eds): Perspectives in Hemostasis. Pergamon Press, New York, 1981, p 310.

71. Fareed J, Messmore HL, Bermes EW: New perspectives in coagulation testing. Clin Chem 26:1380, 1980.

72. Forbes CD: Thrombosis and artificial surfaces. Clin Haematol 10:653, 1981.

73. Gans H, Subramanian V, John S, Casteneda AR, Lillehei CW: Theoretical and practical (clinical) considerations concerning proteolytic enzymes and their inhibitors with particular reference to changes in the plasminogen-plasmin system during assisted circulation in man. Ann NY Acad Sci 146:721, 1968.

74. George CRP, Slichter SJ, Quadracci LJ: A kinetic evaluation of hemostasis in renal disease. N Engl J Med 291:111, 1974.

75. Gollub S: Heparin rebound in open-heart surgery. Surg Gynecol Obstet 124:337, 1967.

76. Gomes MM, McGoon D: Bleeding patterns after open heart surgery. J Thorac Cardiovasc Surg 60:87, 1970.

77. Graeff H, Beller FK: Fibrinolytic activity in whole blood, dilute blood, and euglobulin lysis time tests. In Bang N, Beller FK, Deutsch E (Eds): Thrombosis and Bleeding Disorders, Theory and Methods. Academic Press, New York, 1970, p 328.

78. Hampers CL, Blanfox MD, Merrill JP: Anticoagulation rebound after hemodialysis. N Engl J Med 275:776, 1966.

79. Harker LA, Malpass, TW, Branson HE, Hessel EA, Slichter SJ: Mechanisms of abnormal bleeding in patients undergoing cardiopulmonary bypass: Acquired transient platelet dysfunction associated with selective α-granule release. Blood 56:824, 1980.

80. Harker LA, Slichter SJ: Platelet and fibrinogen survival in man. N Engl J Med 287:999, 1972.

81. Harmon DC, Demirjian Z, Ellman L, Fischer JE: Disseminated intravascular coagulation with the peritoneovenous shunt. Ann Intern Med 90:774, 1979.

82. Hedner U, Nilsson IM: Renal diseases and fibrinogen degradation products. In Hamburger J, Crosnier J, Maxwell MH (Eds): Advances in Nephrology. Year Book Publisher, Chicago, 1973, p 241.

83. Hedner U: Urinary fibrin/fibrinogen derivities. Thromb Diath Haemorrh 34:693, 1975.

84. Hellem AJ: The advances of human blood platelets in vitro. Scand J Clin Lab Invest (Suppl) 51:1, 1960.

85. Hirsh J: Laboratory diagnosis of thrombosis. In Coleman RW, Hirsh J, Marder VJ, Salzman EW (Eds): Basic Principles and Clinical Practice. J. B. Lippincott, Philadelphia, 1982, p 789.

86. Holswade GR, Nachman RL, Killip T: Thrombocytopathies in patients with open-heart surgery. Preoperative treatment with corticosteriods. Arch Surg 94:365, 1967.

87. Hougie C: Fundamentals of Blood Coagulation in Clinical Medicine. McGraw-Hill, New York, 1963. p 241.

88. Hoyer JR, Michael AF, Hower LW: Immunofluorescent localization of antihemophilic factor and fibrinogen in human renal diseases. J Clin Invest 53:1375, 1974.

89. Hubbard D, Lucas GL: Ionic changes of glass surfaces and other materials and their possible role in the coagulation of blood. J Appl Physiol 15:265, 1960.

90. Husby RM, Smith RE: Synthetic oligopeptide substrates: Their diagnostic application in blood coagulation, fibrinolysis, and other pathologic states. Semin Thromb Hemost 6:173, 1980.

91. Isacson S, Nilsson IM: The kidneys and the fibrinolytic activity of the blood. Thromb Diath Haemorrh 22:211, 1969.

92. Jaberi M, Bell WR, Benson DW: Control of heparin therapy in open-heart surgery. J Thorac Cardiovasc Surg 67:133, 1974.

93. Kapplow LS, Goffinet JA: Profound neutropenia during early phase of haemodialysis. JAMA 203:133, 1968.

94. Kevy SV, Glickman RM, Bernhard WF, Diamond L, Gross R: The pathogenesis and control of the hemorrhagic defect in open-heart surgery. Surg Gynecol Obstet 123:313, 1966.

95. Kitchens C: Personal communication.

96. Kladetsky RG, Popov-Cenic' S, Buttner W, Muller N, Egli H: Studies of fibrinolytic and coagulation factors during open-heart surgery with ECC. Thromb Res 7:579, 1975.

97. Knieriem HJ, Chandler AB: The effect of warfarin sodium on the duration of platelet aggregation. Thromb Diath Haemorrh 18:766, 1967.

98. Koffler N, Paronetto F: Immunofluorescent localization of immunoglobulins, complement and fibrinogen in human disease. J Clin Invest 44:1665, 1965.

99. Kowalski E, Kopec' M, Wegrzynowicz Z: Influence of fibrinogen degradation products (FDP) on platelet aggregation, adhesiveness, and viscous metamorphosis. Thromb Diath Haemorrh 10;406, 1963.

100. Kowalski E: Fibrinogen derivatives and their biologic activities. Semin Hematol 5:45, 1968.

101. Kuruvila KC, Beven EG: Arteriovenous shunts and fistulas for hemodialysis. Surg Clin North Am 51:1219, 1971.

102. Lackner H, Javid JP: The clinical significance of the plasminogen level. Am J Clin Pathol 60:175, 1973.

103. Larrieu MJ, Dray L, Ardaillou N: Biological effects of fibrinogen-fibrin degradation products. Thromb Diath Haemorrh 34:686, 1975.

104. Latallo ZS, Fletcher AP, Alkjersig N, Sherry S: Inhibition of fibrin polymerization by fibrinogen proteolysis products. Am J Physiol 202:681, 1962.

105. Lerner RG, Nelson JC, Corines P, del Guercio LRM: Disseminated intravascular coagulation: Complication of LeVeen peritoneovenous shunts. JAMA 240:240:2064, 1978.

106. Lessin LS, Jensen WH, Kelser GA: Scanning electron microscopy of thrombogenesis on vascular catheter surfaces. N Engl J Med 286:139, 1972.

107. LeVeen HH, Christoudias G, Ip M, Luft R, Falk G, Grosberg S: Peritoneovenous shunting for ascites. Ann Surg 180:580, 1974.

108. Lewis JH, Wilson HJ, Brandon JM: Counterelectrophoresis test for molecules immunologically similar to fibrinogen. Am J Clin Pathol 58:400, 1972.

109. Lindsay RM, Prentice CRM, Davidson JF: Hemostatic changes during dialysis, associated with thrombus formation on dialysis membranes. Br Med J 4:454, 1972.

110. MacDonald MK, Clarkson AR, Davidson AM: The role of coagulation in renal disease. In Kincaid-Smith P, Mathew TH, Becker EL (Eds): Glomerulonephritis. John Wiley & Sons, New York, 1973, p 923.

111. Mammen EF: Natural proteinase inhibitors in extracorporeal circulation. Ann NY Acad Sci 146:754, 1968.

112. Mason RG: The interaction of blood hemostatic elements with artificial surfaces. In Spaet TH (Ed): Progress in Hemostasis and Thrombosis. Grune & Stratton, New York, 1972, p 141.

113. McCluskey RT, Vassalli R, Gallo G: An immunofluorescent study of pathogenic mechanism in glomerular disease. N Engl Med 274:695, 1966.

114. McNicol GP, Prentice CRM, Briggs JD: Fibrinogen degradation products or FDP in renal disease: Estimation and significance of FDP in urine. Scand J Haematol (Suppl) 13:329, 1971.

115. Menon IS: A study of the possible correlation of euglobulin lysis time and dilute blood clot lysis time in the determination of fibrinolytic activity. Lab Pract 17:334, 1968.

116. Mertens BF, Greene LF, Bowie EJW, Elveback LR, Owen CA: Fibrinolytic split products and ethanol gelation test in preoperative evaluation of patients with prostatic disease. Mayo Clin Proc 49:642, 1974.

117. Mielke CH, Kaneshiro MM, Maher LA, Weiner

J, Rapaport SI: The standardized normal Ivy bleeding time and its prolongation by aspirin. Blood 34:204, 1969.

118. Moore CH, Wolma FJ, Brown RW, Derrick JR: Complications of cardiovascular radiology. A review of 1204 cases. Am J Surg 120:591, 1970.

119. Morita T, Susuki Y, Churg J: Structure and development of glomerular crescent. Am J Pathol 72:349, 1973.

120. Muller N, Popov-Cenic S, Buttner W, Kladetsky RG, Egli H: Studies of fibrinolytic and coagulation factors during open-heart surgery. II. Postoperative bleeding tendencies and changes in the coagulation system. Thromb Res 7:589, 1975.

121. Murano G, Bick RL: Thrombolytic therapy. In Murano G, Bick RL (Eds): Basic Concepts of Hemostasis and Thrombosis. CRC Press, Boca Raton, FL, 1980, p 259.

122. Mustard JF, Packham MA: Factors influencing platelet function: Adhesion, release, and aggregation. Pharmacol Rev 23:97, 1970.

123. Naeye RL: Thrombotic state after a hemorrhagic diathesis: A possible complication of therapy with epsilon aminocaproic acid. Blood 19:694, 1962.

124. Naish P, Peters DK, Shackman R: Increased urinary fibrinogen derivities after renal allotransplantation. Lancet 1:1280, 1973.

125. Okada M, Shiozawa T, Iizuka M, Kuno KO, Chen CC, Matsuda S, Yoneda K, Yano A, Kawai M, Asada S: Experimental and clinical studies on the effect of intra-aortic balloon pumping for cardiogenic shock following acute myocardial infarction. Artif Organs 3:271, 1979.

126. Ollendorff P: The nature of the anticoagulant effect of heparin, protamine, Polybrene, and toluidine blue. Scand J Clin Lab Invest 14:267, 162.

127. O'Neill JA, Ende N, Collins IS, Collins HA: A quantitative determination of perfusion fibrinolysis. Surgery 60:809, 1966.

128. Orlin JB, Berkman EM: Partial plasma exchange using albumin replacement. Removal and recovery of normal plasma constituents. Blood 56:1055, 1981.

129. Palester-Chlebowzyk M, Strzyzewska E, Sitowski W, Olender K: Detection of the intravascular coagulation of blood clotting. II. Results of the paracoagulation test in patients undergoing open-heart surgery, with extracorporeal circulation. Polish Med J 11:59, 1972.

130. Pechet L: Fibrinolysis. N Engl J Med 273:966, 1965.

131. Penick GD, Averette HE, Peters RM, Brinkhouse KM: The hemorrhagic syndrome complicating extracorporeal shunting of blood: An experimental study of its pathogenesis. Thromb Diath Haemorh 2:218, 1958.

132. Pitcher FM: Fibrinogen degradation products. Lab Equip Digest 11:109, 1973.

133. Portemont G, Vermylen J, Donati MB: Urinary excretion of fibrinogen/fibrin related antigen in glomerulonephritis. In Kincaid-Smith P, Mathew TH, Becker EL (Eds): Glomerulonephritis. John Wiley & Sons, New York, 1973. p 829.

134. Porter JM, Silver D: Alterations in fibrinolysis and coagulation associated with cardiopulmonary bypass. J Thorac Cardiovasc Surg 56:869, 1968.

135. Proctor RR, Rapaport SI: The partial thromboplastin time with kaolin. A simple screening test for first stage plasma clotting factor deficiencies. Am J Clin Pathol 36:212, 1961.

136. Quick AJ, Stanley-Brown M, Bancroft FW: A study of the coagulation defect in hemophilia and in jaundice. Am J Med Sci 190:501, 1935.

137. Ratnoff OD: Epsilon aminocaproic acid: A dangerous weapon. N Engl J Med 280:1124, 1969.

138. Reinhardt GF, Stanley MM: Peritoneovenous shunting for ascites. Surg Gynecol Obstet 145:419, 1977.

139. Salzman WE: Blood platelets and extracorporeal circulation. Transfusion 3:274, 1963.

140. Salzman EW: The events that led to thrombosis. Bull NY Acad Med 48:225, 1972.

141. Saunders CR, Carlisle L, Bick RL: Hydroxyethyl starch versus albumin cardiopulmonary bypass prime solutions. Ann Thorac Surg 35:532, 1983.

142. Schoen FJ, Delaria GA, Bernstein EF: Evaluation of intraaortic balloon surfaces by scanning electron microscopy. Surg Forum 23:167, 1972.

143. Seegers WH: Basic principles of blood coagulation. Semin Thromb Hemost 7:180, 1981.

144. Sharp AA: The significance of fibrinolysis. Proc R Soc Lond (Biol) 173:311, 1969.

145. Sherry S, Fletcher AP, Alkjaersig N: Fibrinolysis and fibrinolytic activity in man. Physiol Rev 39:343, 1959.

146. Signori EE, Penner JA, Kahn DR: Coagulation defects and bleeding in open heart surgery. Ann Thorac Surg 8:521, 1969.

147. Simon TL: Coagulation disorders with plasma exchange. Plasma Ter Transfusion Technol 3:147, 1982.

148. Sixma JJ, Kater L, Bouma BN: Immunofluorescent localization of Factor VIII-related antigen, fibrinogen, and several other plasma proteins in hemostatic plugs in humans. J Lab Clin Med 87:112, 1976.

149. Smith DA, Monaghan WP, Hann WD, Schumacher H: Evaluation of in vivo platelet adhesiveness during discontinuous-flow centrifugal thrombocytapheresis. Plasma Ther Transfusion Technol 4:37, 1983.

150. Soloway HB, Cornett BM, Donahoo JV, Cox SP: Differentiation of bleeding diathesis which occurs following protamine correction of heparin anticoagulation. Am J Clin Pathol 60:188, 1973.

151. Spiva DA, Robinson CS, Langley JW: Acute changes in antithrombin III levels during apheresis procedures. Plasma Ther Transfusion Technol 3:137, 1982.

152. Stass S, Bishop C, Fosberg R, Hartley M, Cramer M: Platelets as affected by cardiopulmonary bypass. Trans Am Soc Clin Pathol 35, 1976.

153. Steihm ER, Trugstad CW: Split products of fibrin in human renal disesase. Am J Med 46:774, 1969.

154. Strin SF, Fulenwider JT, Ansley JD, Evatt BL, Nordlinger B, Melemore P, Schwotzer L, Wideman CS: Accelerated fibrinogen and platelet destruction after peritoneovenous shunting. Arch Intern Med 141:1149, 1981.

155. Tice DA, Worth MH: Recognition and treatment of postoperative bleeding associated with open heart surgery. Ann NY Acad Sci 146:745, 1968.

156. Trimble AS, Herst R, Grady M, Crookston J: Blood loss in open heart surgery. Arch Surg 93:323, 1966.

157. Triplett DA: Quantitative or functional disorders of platelets. In Triplett DA (Ed): Platelet Function. American Society of Clinical Pathology, Chicago, 1978, p 123.

158. Triplett DA: Platelet disorders. In Murano G, Bick RL (Eds): Basic Concepts of Hemostasis and Thrombosis. CRC Press, Boca Raton, FL, 1980, p 95.

159. Tsitouris G, Bellet S, Eilberg R, Feinberg L, Sandberg H: Effects of major surgery on plasmin-plasminogen systems. Arch Intern Med 108:98, 1961.

160. Tsuji HK, Redington JV, Kay JH, Goesswald RK: The study of fibrinolytic and coagulation factors during open heart surgery. Ann NY Acad Sci 146:763, 1968.

161. Urbaniac SJ, Prowse CV: Hemostatic changes during plasma exchange. Plasma Ther Transfusion Technol 4:21, 1983.

162. Verska JJ, Lonser ER, Brewer LA: Predisposing factors and management of hemorrhage following open-heart surgery. J Cardiovasc Surg (Torino) 13:361, 1972.

163. Verska J: Letter to the editor. Ann Thorac Surg 13:87, 1972.

164. von Kaulla KN, Swan H: clotting deviations in man during cardiac bypass: Fibrinolysis and circulating anticoagulants. J Thorac Surg 36:519, 1958.

165. Wegmuller E, Kazatchkine MD, Nydegger UE: Complement activation during extracorporeal blood bypass. Plasma Ther Transfusion Technol 4:361, 1983.

166. Whitworth JA, Fairley KF, McIvor MA: Urinary fibrin-degradation products and the site of urinary infection. Lancet 1:234, 1973.

167. Williams BT, Blainey JD, Dawson-Edwards P, Hilton DD, Simpson KM: Use of the Quinton-Scribner arteriovenous shunt in the management of aplastic anemia. Br Med J 2:484, 1967.

168. Woods JE, Kirklin JW, Owen CA, Thompson JH, Taswell HF: The effect of bypass surgery on coagulation sensitive clotting factors. Mayo Clin Proc 42:724, 1967.

169. Woods JF, Ash G, Weston MJ: Sulfinpyrazone reduced deposition of fibrinon dialyser membranes. (Abstr.) Thromb Haemost 42:401, 1979.

170. Wright TA, Darte J, Mustard WT: Postoperative bleeding after extracorporeal circulation. Can J Surg 2:142, 1959.

171. Wuelfing D, Brandau KP: Fibrinolytic activity after surgery. Minn Med 51:1503, 1968.

172. Ygge J: Changes in blood coagulation and fibrinolysis during the postoperative period. Am J Surg 119:225, 1970.

173. Zimmerman TS, Meyer D: Factor VIII-von Willebrand factor and the molecular basis of von Willebrand's disease. In Coleman RW, Hirsh J, Marder VJ, Salzman EW (Eds): Hemostasis and Thrombosis: Basic Principles and Clinical Practice. J. B. Lippincott, Philadelphia. 1982, p 54.

9

Acquired Circulating Anticoagulants

Acquired circulating anticoagulants (inhibitors) directed against single factors or several factors are extremely rare causes of clinical hemorrhage. Acquired circulating anticoagulants are commonly associated with reasonably well-defined disease entities, drugs, or other clinical situations and may occur in otherwise normal individuals. Any coagulation factor may be effected. Circulating anticoagulants as complications in transfused patients with congenital coagulation factor defects will not be discussed.

Clearly the most common circulating anticoagulants of clinical significance are fibrin(ogen) degradation products (FDPs); the mechanisms of action of FDPs in interfering with hemostasis has been well defined in Chapters 6 and 7 and include impairment of fibrin monomer polymerization and interference with platelet function.[6,7] The next most common circulating anticoagulant of clinical relevance is that of malignant paraprotein, and mechanisms of action of paraprotein with respect to impeding hemostasis and thrombosis are discussed in detail in Chapter 10.[8,56] In addition, when suspecting circulating anticoagulants, the Munchausen's syndrome, the deliberate self-administration of warfarin-type drugs must be considered,[2,80] and in hospitalized patients one must consider the potentially unrecorded yet very real use of heparin to keep intravenous lines open, etc. Several early excellent reviews have recognized the importance of circulating anticoagulants and have paved the way for a more thorough understanding of circulating anticoagulants and the clinical situations in which they arise. The first early large review of circulating anticoagulants was presented by Margolius and co-workers, followed by excellent reviews by Deutsch and Lechner,[23] and Feinstein and Rapaport.[27]

Acquired inhibitors occurring in noncongenitally deficient patients may be divided into two types. The first includes inhibitors that inactivate individual coagulation factors, commonly in a progressive, usually irreversible time-dependent manner.[8,27,70] The vast majority of these are immunoglobulins (specific antifactor antibodies). Subtyping of these reveal that most of the immunoglobulins are IgG, generally IgG_4. Kappa light chains are more common than lambda light chains in circulating IgG anticoagulants.[8] The second type of circulating inhibitor is characterized by being reversible (or partially reversible), immediate in action, representing a strictly protein-protein interaction (complex formation) with either a specific factor or group of coagulation factors.[8,56] These types of anticoagulants often do not destroy the coagulation factor attacked and the biologic activity of the coagulation factor may be recovered if the complex can be dissociated. These types of anticoagulants are most commonly seen in malignant or benign paraprotein disorders, with the interaction being between paraprotein and a specific or group of clotting factors. Circulating anticoagulants should be strongly suspected when an otherwise healthy individual begins to develop unexplained bleeding or when coagulation testing gives contradictory or confusing results.[8]

Acquired Inhibitors to Specific Coagulation Factors

Less than ten cases of acquired inhibitors to fibrinogen have been reported; of these, two have occurred in transfused afibrinogenemic patients.[24,74] In noncongenital deficient patients, the anticoagulant has been associated with autoimmune disorders (two cases of systemic lupus), chronic inflammatory disorders (chronic active hepatitis),[38,51] and Down's syndrome (one case)[69] In addition, one case was reported in a multiple transfused patient who most likely had disseminated intravascular coagulation.[66] In the cases so studied the antibody was identified as an IgG, and in one case the antibody was found to interfere with the release of fibrinopeptide A. In some patients a mild hemorrhage tendency has been present, but in others no abnormal clinical hemostasis defects were encountered.

Antiprothrombin (Factor II) antibodies in cases of noncongenital Factor II deficiency are extremely rare and have been seen exclusively in patients with systemic lupus erythematosus.[88,89,95] In this instance a clear-cut distinction from a specific anti-II antibody versus a lupus anticoagulant has remained unclear.

Acquired antibody to Factor V has occurred in at least 16 patients, and in almost 70% the development of the antibody was preceded by a surgical procedure.[10,16,17,21,27–31,48,63,65,78,94,100] To complicate etiologic mechanisms further, 50% of the surgical patients thus far reported had ingested streptomycin as part of their operative course. An anti-Factor V antibody has also been associated with the use of streptomycin in several nonsurgical patients. Most patients have had a mild bleeding problem, but bleeding has been severe or fatal in a few isolated cases.[16,17,94,100] Both IgG and IgM have been incriminated. Therapy, when necessary, is generally limited to fresh frozen plasma; however, one patient was treated successfully with platelet concentrates.[16] Anti-Factor VII antibodies have only been reported once, and this was in association with a case of probable carcinoma of the lung.[13] In this case, the antibody was found to be IgG. Surgery was not performed because of abnormal hemostasis studies; thus, the diagnosis was not confirmed, and the cell type remains unknown.

Anti-VIII antibodies occur in 8 to 10% of patients with hemophilia A; these were discussed in Chapter 5. Anti-VIII antibodies are one of the more common circulating anticoagulants occurring in otherwise healthy individuals and in selected clinical situations; thus, they should be suspected in healthy individuals who suddenly develop an unexplained hemorrhagic diathesis.[8,23,27,58,70,90] In addition, an anti-VIII antibody is the most likely circulating anticoagulant to be present in the patient without lupus who develops a circulating anticoagulant in the absence of malignant paraprotein or elevated FDPs.[8,58,90] An excellent recent review has summarized a survey of 215 nonhemophiliac patients with inhibitors to Factor VIII and has provided significant insight into the clinical manifestations of anti-VIII antibodies in such patients.[45] In this survey it was found that greater than 46% of patients had no underlying disease condition, 8% had developed an anti-VIII antibody in association with rheumatoid arthritis, more than 7% developed an anti-VIII antibody in the course of a normal postpartum state, almost 7% were associated with a disseminated malignancy, slightly more than 5% were associated with drug ingestion, an equal number were associated with systemic lupus, more than 4% were associated with other, less common, autoimmune disorders, 4.5% were associated with dermatologic disorders, and approximately 10% were thought to be due to other rare isolated clinical disorders. The peak incidence was in patients between 50 and 80 years of age, who constituted greater than 65% of those in the survey. It was also found that the clinical outcome in postpartum patients was relatively good, with 85% of patients surviving, and the anti-Factor VIII antibody eventually disappared. Of the survivors, 36% were not treated and the remainder received some type of immunosuppressive therapy. However, this survey also indicated that patients developing a circulating anticoagulant in association with an autoimmune disorder fared rather poorly and persistence of the antibody or death occurred in 36% of patients; the remainder survived with the use of some type of immunosuppressive therapy. When evaluating the total cases in this large survey, 56% of patients survived the development of an antiplatelet antibody and 44% died from a hemorrhagic complication of the circulating anti-

VIII antibody. Of those surviving, the majority received some type of immunosuppressive therapy, whereas the majority of those who died (62%) received no immunosuppressive therapy. This large survey thus confirms the suggestions of others[82] that the use of immunosuppressive therapy in nonhemophilic patients who develop an anti-VIII antibody is clearly warranted. Interestingly, nonhemophilic patients who develop an acquired anti-VIII antibody do not commonly have the types of bleeding usually associated with hemophilia A and, thus, rarely have intra-articular bleeding, deep intramuscular bleeding, or intracranial bleeding, but more commonly have large subcutaneous ecchymoses.

Acquired von Willebrand's disease, or the development of an acquired anticoagulant to the von Willebrand portion of the Factor VIII macromolecular complex has been reported in more than 20 patients.[1,12,23,27,39,44,47,52–54,58,68,70,73,79,83,90,91,93,104] The vast majority of these patients have had some type of autoimmune disorder, lymphoma, or a malignant paraprotein disorder. The interaction between malignant or benign paraprotein in coagulation factors is discussed in Chapter 10. One patient developed an anti-von Willebrand factor antibody after pesticide exposure,[97] and one was noted to develop in a patient with Wilms' tumor[79] in whom the antibody decreased with surgical resection of the malignancy. In most instances, the bleeding has not been severe and has been compatible with a mild acquired von Willebrand's-type disease. Therapy has been that of immunosuppression, cryoprecipitate, and other appropriate measures to control the underlying disease process, whether it be myeloma, other paraprotein disorders, or autoimmunity.

Anti-IX antibodies only rarely occur in nonhemophilia B patients[3] and the most common clinical situation in which they occur are postpartum females, patients with systemic lupus, and in rare individuals with rheumatic fever.[23,27,57,70,75,90,96] Like anti-VIII antibody in the nonhemophilic patient, the anti-IX antibody often abates with the use of immunosuppressive therapy in the form of prednisone, azathioprine, or cyclophosphamide.

Only two cases of an anti-X antibody have been reported, both occurring in patients with leprosy.[77] One patient was ingesting dapsone; however, this was after developing the antibody, and thus leprosy, rather than drug ingestion, appeared to be the common occurrence. Neither patient had a clinically significant bleeding diathesis. Of more clinical relevance is the association of a selective Factor X deficiency associated with systemic amyloidosis; although an anti-X antibody has not clearly been found in the circulation, it is thought that amyloid fibrils may selectively bind with Factor X and remove it from the circulation.[36,37,46,92] Thus, although a "circulating anticoagulant" cannot be demonstrated in the circulation, it appears that amyloid may, in fact, represent an extracirculatory Factor X inhibitor via the interaction of Factor X and amyloid fibrils. In vivo recovery studies, as discussed in Chapter 5, support this mechanism.[36,37]

Anti-XI antibodies in noncongenital patients have occurred in only 11 individuals, ten having an autoimmune disorder[1,15,20,25,33,55,70,90,95,99] and one having pneumonia thought to be due to an adenovirus.[4] Anti-Factor XII antibody has thus far been reported only in systemic lupus, in Waldenströms macroglubulinemia, and in a patient with glomerulonephritis.[3,40,85] A severe deficiency of Factor XII has been found in association with angioimmunoblastic lymphadenopathy, but a circulating anticoagulant could not be demonstrated.[61]

Acquired anti-XIII antibody has occurred in at least eight otherwise hemostatically normal individuals.[23,27,34,42,60,62,64,70–72,86,90] Most of these patients had received isoniazid therapy, and one patient developed an anti-XIII antibody with a drug-induced systemic lupus-type syndrome.[102] It is thought that the inhibitor either reacts with the thrombin activation site on the alpha chain of Factor XIII or, alternatively, prevents fibrin cross-linking by reacting with sites on fibrinogen.[27,90] Some patients developing an anti-XIII antibody have had profuse bleeding in association with this inhibitor.

Lupus Anticoagulants

The lupus anticoagulant has long been described and several early reviews[9,11,23,27,43,70] as well as numerous recent reviews[18,59,87,89,98] have begun to provide data on the nature of this elusive "anticoagulant." Lupus anticoagulants have been defined as immunoglobulins interfering with phospholipid-dependent tests of coagulation.[89,98] Unlike the other factors previously discussed, the lupus anticoagulants do not inhibit the activity of specific coagulation factors and may occur in up to 10% of patients with systemic lupus erythematosus.[35,59] The frequency of bleeding due to the lupus anticoagulant is clearly less than 1% of patients developing this anticoagulant.[18,59,89,98] Of interest, almost a quarter of the patients with systemic lupus plus the lupus anticoagulant will have a concomitant significant prothrombin deficiency and more than 40% and will have significant associated thrombocytopenia.[89] In this regard, bleeding in association with the lupus anticoagulant almost always occurs in patients with associated hypoprothrombinemia or thrombocytopenia, and there is no reported increase in surgical hemorrhage in patients with the lupus anticoagulant alone.[89] An additional unclear feature is that isolated prothrombin deficiency may occur in patients with systemic lupus who do not have the lupus anticoagulant; in this instance the mechanism remain unknown.[27,58,89] It has been noted that infusions of plasma have failed to correct adequately the isolated Factor II deficiency in lupus patients, suggesting the presence of an anti-Factor II antibody, as previously discussed.[19,84]

A laboratory characteristic of lupus anticoagulants are that all phospholipid-dependent coagulation tests are prolonged, including the prothrombin time, the activated partial thromboplastin time, and the Russell's vipor venom time.[27,89,90] Of these tests, the activated partial thromboplastin time appears to be the most sensitive.[27,89] When studying patients with lupus, it is important to recognize that if the prothrombin time is significantly prolonged (defined as a prothrombin ratio of greater than 2.0) hypoprothrombinemia rather than the lupus anticoagulant should be suspected.[89] It has also been clearly shown that the sensitivity of the activated partial thromboplastin time to the presence or absence of the lupus anticoagulant is highly dependent on the reagents used; this has been reviewed by Mannucci and co-workers.[67] It has been noted that the use of platelet-poor plasma enhances the sensitivity of all of the phospholipid-dependent tests to the presence of the lupus anticoagulant[26,70] and that the use of platelet-rich plasma may diminish the sensitivity of these tests to the presence of lupus anticoagulants and may actually mask the presence of a lupus anticoagulant.[32]

Two lupus anticoagulant assays are popular. The first consists of a prothrombin time in which the thromboplastin is diluted[87] to give a "normal time" of 60 seconds and when noting a time of 65 seconds or longer, a lupus anticoagulant is considered to be present.[87,89] A problem with this test is that it may miss IgM lupus anticoagulants. It has been suggested[89] that a superior test to detect both IgG and IgM is a "modified" Russell's vipor venom time in which the venom is diluted to give a "normal" time of 23 to 27 seconds and the phospholipid is then diluted to a minimal level that will continue to support this range; a prolongation of this system will not correct with a mixture of patient and normal plasma. Of interest, biologic false-positive tests for syphilis are seen in up to 40% of patients with systemic lupus;[49,89] however, biologic false tests for syphilis are seen in 50 to 90% of patients with systemic lupus plus the lupus anticoagulant.[58,87,89] in addition, it should be recognized that almost 40% of patients with biologic false-positive tests for syphilis will have a lupus anticoagulant and in this clinical setting the lupus anticoagulant should be searched for. Thromboembolism occurs in approximately 10% of patients with systemic lupus; however, if a patient with systemic lupus also has the lupus anticoagulant, thromboembolism is a complication in 25 to 50% of cases.[41,50,76,81,89] Lupus anticoagulants may occur in normal individuals and in other disease states besides lupus and may occur in association with drug ingestion; the most commonly cited drugs are chlorpromazine or procainamide.[5,14,22,103,105]

Summary

Those rare clinical instances of acquired circulating anticoagulants in noncongenitally deficient patients have been discussed. Although these circulating anticoagulants are extremely interesting and may, on rare occasion, give rise to clinically significant or, indeed, fatal hemorrhage, it should be emphasized these anticoagulants are, in fact, extremely rare. Circulating FDPs and malignant paraprotein acting as circulating anticoagulants are far more common causes of clinically significant hemorrhage than are the specific antifactor antibodies discussed. When finding circulating anticoagulants in the absence of circulating FDPs or paraprotein, the most likely to be found in clinical practice are an anti-Factor VIII antibody or the lupus anticoagulant.

References

1. Aberg H, Nilsson IM: Recurrent thrombosis in a young woman with a circulating anticoagulant directed against Factors XI and XII. Acta Med Scand 192:419, 1972.
2. Agle DP, Ratnoff OD, Spring GK: The anticoagulant malingerer. Psychiatric studies in three patients. Ann Intern Med 73:67, 1970.
3. Bateman D, Gokal R, Prescott R, Hamilton PJ, Kerr DNS: Minimal-change glomerulonephritis associated with circulating anticoagulant to Factor XII. Br Med J 281:358, 1980.
4. Beck DW, Strauss RGH, Kisker CT, Henrisksen RA: An intrinsic coagulation pathway inhibitor in a 3-year-old child. Am J Clin Pathol 71:470, 1979.
5. Bell WR, Boss GR, Wolfson JS: Circulating anticoagulant in the procainamide-induced lupus syndrome. Arch Intern Med 137:1471, 1977.
6. Bick RL: The clinical significance of fibrinogen degradation products. Semin Thromb Hemost 8:302, 1982.
7. Bick RL: Disseminated intravascular coagulation. In Bick RL (Ed): Disseminated Intravascular Coagulation and Related Syndromes. CRC Press, Boca Raton, FL, 1983, p 31.
8. Bick RL: Acquired circulating anticoagulants and defective hemostasis in malignant paraprotein disorders. In Murano G, Bick RL (Eds): Basic Concepts of Hemostasis and Thrombosis. CRC Press, Boca Raton, FL, 1980, p 205.
9. Biggs R, Denson KWE: The mode of action of a coagulation inhibitor in the blood of two patients with disseminated lupus erythematosus. (DLE). Br J Haematol 10:198, 1964.
10. Blecker SM, Williams AC: Post extraction bleeding in a patient with an acquired circulating anticoagulant against Factor V. Oral Surg 32:533, 1971.
11. Breckenridge RT, Ratnoff OD: Studies on the site of action of a circulating anticoagulant in disseminated lupus erythematosus. Am J Med 35:813, 1963.
12. Brody J, Haider M, Rossman RE: A haemorrhagic syndrome in Waldenstrom's macroglobulinemia, secondary to immune absorption to Factor VIII. N Engl J Med 300:408, 1979.
13. Campbell E, Sanal S, Mattson J, Walker L, Estry S, Mueller L, Schwarz M, Hamptom S: Factor VII inhibitor. Am J Med 68:962, 1980.
14. Canoso RT, Hutton RA, Deykin D: A chlorpromazine-induced inhibitor of blood coagulation. Am J Hematol 2:183, 1977.
15. Castro O, Farber LR, Clyne LP: Circulating anticoagulants against Factors IX and XI in systemic lupus erythematosus. Ann Intern Med 77:543, 1972.
16. Chediak J, Ashenhurst JB, Garlick I, Desser RK: Successful management of bleeding in a patient with Factor V inhibitor by platelet transfusions. Blood 56:835, 1980.
17. Coots MC, Muhleman AF, Glueck HI: Hemorrhagic death associated with a high titer Factor V inhibitor. Am J Hematol 4:193, 1978.
18. Coots MC, Miller MA, Glucck HI: The lupus inhibitor: A study of its heterogeneity. Thromb Haemost 46:734, 1981.
19. Corrigan JJ, Patterson JH, May NE: Incoagulability of the blood in systemic lupus erythematosus. A case due to hypoprothrombinemia and a circulating anticoagulant. Am J Dis Child 119:365, 1970.
20. Cronberg S, Nilsson IM: Circulating anticoagulant against Factors XI and XII together with massive spontaneous platelet aggregation. Scand J Haematol 10:309, 1973.
21. Crowell EB: A spontaneous Factor V inhibitor in an elderly man. Clin Res 19:664, 1971.
22. Davis S, Furie BC, Griffin JH, Furie B: Circulating inhibitors of blood coagulation associated with procainamide-induced lupus erythematosus. Am J Hematol 4:401, 1978.
23. Deutsch E, Lechner K: Circulating anticoagulants. In Bang NU, Beller FK, Deutsch E, Mammen EF (Eds): Thrombosis and Bleeding Disorders. Georg Thieme Verlag, Stuttgart, 1971, p 286.
24. DeVries A, Rosenberg T, Kochwa S, Boss JH: Precipitating antifibrinogen antibody appearing after fibrinogen infusions in a patient with congenital afibrinogenemia. Am J Med 30:486, 1961.
25. DiSabatino CA, Clyne LP, Malawista SE: A circulating anticoagulant directed against Factor XI_a in systemic lupus erythematosus. Arthritis Rheumatol 22:1135, 1979.
26. Exner T, Rickard A, Kronenberg H: A sensitive

test demonstrating lupus anticoagulant and its behavioural patterns. Br J Haematol 40:143, 1978.

27. Feinstein DI, Rapaport SI: Acquired inhibitors of blood coagulation. Prog Hemost Thromb 1:39, 1972.

28. Feinstein DI, Rapaport SI, McGehee WG, Patch JM: Factor V anticoagulants: Clinical, biochemical, and immunogic observation. J Clin Invest 49:1578, 1970.

29. Feinstein DI, Rapaport SI, Chong MMY: Factor V inhibitor: Report of a case, with comments on a possible effect of streptomycin. Ann Intern Med 78:385, 1973.

30. Feinstein DI: Acquired inhibitors of Factor V. Thromb Haemost 39:663, 1978.

31. Ferguson JH, Johnston CL, Howell DA: A circulating inhibitor (anti-AcG) specific for the labile factor V of the blood-clotting mechanism. Blood 13:382, 1958.

32. Firkin BG, Booth P, Hendrix L, Howard MA: Demonstration of a platelet bypass mechanism in the clotting system using an acquired anticoagulant. Am J Hematol 5:81, 1978.

33. Fischer DS, Clyne LP: Circulating Factor XI and disseminated intravascular coagulation. Arch Intern Med 141:515, 1981.

34. Flore PA, Ellis LD, Dameshek HL, Lewis JH: XIII inhibitor and antituberculous therapy. Clin Res 19:418, 1971.

35. Frick PG: Acquired circulating anticoagulants in systemic "collagen disease." Autoimmune thromboplastin deficiency. Blood 10:691, 1955.

36. Furie B, Greene E, Furie BC: Syndrome of acquired Factor X deficiency and systemic amyloidosis. In vivo studies of the metabolic fate of Factor X. N Engl J Med 297:81, 1975.

37. Furie B, Voo L, McAdam PWG, Furie BC: Mechanism of Factor X deficiency in systemic amyloidosis. N Engl J Med 304:827, 1981.

38. Galankis DK, Ginzler EM, Fikrio SM: Monoclonal IgG anticoagulants delaying fibrin aggregation in two patients with systemic lupus erythematosus (SLE). Blood 52:1037, 1978.

39. Gan TE, Sawers RJ, Koutts J: Pathogenesis of antibody-induced acquired von Willebrand syndrome. Am J Hematol 9:363, 1980.

40. Gandolfo GM, Afeltra A, Amoroso A, Biancolella F, Ferri GM: Circulating anticoagulant against Factor XII and platelet antibodies in systemic lupus erythematosus. Acta Haematol 57:135, 1977.

41. Gladman DD, Urowitz MB: Venous syndromes and pulmonary emobolism in systemic lupus erythematosus. Ann Rheum Dis 39:340, 1980.

42. Godal HC: An inhibitor to fibrin stabilizing factor (FSF, Factor XIII). Scand Haematol 7:43, 1970.

43. Gonyea L, Herdman R, Bridges RA: The coagulation abnormalities in systemic lupus erythematosus. Thromb Diath Haemorrh 20:457, 1968.

44. Govault-Heilmann M, Dumond MD, Intrator L, Chenal C, Lejone JL: Acquired von Willebrand syndrome with IgM inhibitor against von Willebrand's factor. J Clin Pathol 32:1030, 1979.

45. Green D, Lechner K: A survey of 215 non-hempholic patients with inhibitors to Factor VIII. Thromb Haemost 45:200, 1981.

46. Greipp PR, Kyle RA, Bowie EJW: Factor-X deficiency in amyloidosis: A critical review. Am J Hematol 11:443, 1981.

47. Handin RI, Martin V, Moloney WL: Antibody-induced von Willebrand's disease: A newly defined inhibitor syndrome. Blood 48:393, 1976.

48. Handley DA, Duncan BM: A circulating anticoagulant specific for Factor V. Pathology 1:265, 1969.

49. Harvey AM, Shulman LE, Tumulty PA: Systemic lupus erythematosus. Review of the literature and clinical analysis of 138 cases. Medicine (Baltimore) 33:291, 1954.

50. Harvey AM, Shulman LE: Systemic lupus erythematosus and biologic false positive test for syphilis. In Dubois EL (Ed): Lupus Erythematosus. University of Southern California Press, Los Angeles, 1974, p 196.

51. Hoots WK, Carrell NA, Wagner RH, Cooper HA, McDonagh J: A naturally occurring antibody that inhibits fibrin polymerization. N Engl J Med 304:857, 1981.

52. Ingram GI, Kingston PG, Leslie J, Bowie EJ: Four cases of acquired von Willebrand's syndrome. Br J Haematol 21:189, 1979.

53. Ingram GI, Prentice CR, Forbes CD, Leslie J: Low Factor-VIII-like antigen in acquired von Willebrand's syndrome and response to treatment. Br J Haematol 25:137, 1973.

54. Joist HH, Cowan JF, Zimmerman TS: Acquired von Willebrand's disease: Evidence for a quantitative and qualitative Factor VIII disorder. N Engl J Med 298:988, 1978.

55. Krieger H, Breckenridge RT: Circulating anticoagulant interfering with the action of Factor XI_a in lupus. Blood 42:1002, 1974.

56. Lackner H: Hemostatic abnormalities associated with dysproteinemias. Semin Hematol 10:125, 1973.

57. Largo R, Sigg P, von Felton A, Straub PW: Acquired Factor IX inhibitor in a nonhemophilic patient with autoimmune disease. Br J Haematol 26:129, 1974.

58. Lechner K: Acquired inhibitors in non-hemophilic patients. Haemostasis 3:65, 1974.

59. Lee SL: Miotti AB: Disorders of hemostatic function in patients with systemic lupus erythematosus. Semin Arthritis Rheum 4:241, 1975.

60. Lewis JH, Szeto ILF, Ellis LD, Bayer WL: An acquired inhibitor to coagulation Factor XIII. Johns Hopkins Med J 120:401, 1967.

61. Londino AV, Luparello FJ: Factor XII deficiency in a man with gout and angioimmunoblastic lymphadenopathy. Arch Intern Med 144:1497, 1984.

62. Lopaciuk S, Bykowska K, McDonagh JM, McDonagh RP, Yount WJ, Fuller CR, Cooperstein L, Gray A, Lorand L: Differences between Type I autoimmune inhibitors of fibrin stabilization in two patients with severe hemorrhagic disorder. J Clin Invest 61:1196, 1978.

63. Lopez VA, Pfugshaupt R, Butler R: A specific inhibitor of human clotting factor V. Acta Haematol 40:275, 1968.

64. Lorand L, Maldonado N, Fradera J, Atencio AC, Robertson, B, Urayama T: Haemorrhagic syndrome of autoimmune origin with a specific inhibitor against fibrin stabilizing factor (Factor XIII). Br J Haematol 23:17, 1972.

65. Lust A, Bellon A: A circulating anticoagulant against Factor V. Acta Clin Belt 33:62, 1978.

64. Mammen EF, Schmidt KP, Barnhart MI: Thrombopiebitis migrans associated with circulating antibodies against fibrinogen. Thromb Diath Haemorrh 18:605, 1967.

67. Mannucci PM, Caciani MT, Mari D, Meucci P: The varied sensitivity of partial thromboplastin and prothrombin time reagents in the demonstration of lupus-like anticoagulants. Scand J Haematol 22:423, 1979.

68. Mant MJ, Hirst J, Gauldie J, Bienenstock J, Pineo GF, Luke KH: von Willebrand's syndrome presenting as an acquired bleeding disorder in association with a monoclonal gammopathy. Blood 42:429, 1973.

69. Marceniac E, Greenwood MF: Acquired coagulation inhibitor delaying fibrinopeptide release. Blood 53:81, 1979.

70. Margolius A, Jackson DP, Ratnoff OD: Circulating anticoagulants: A study of 40 cases and a review of the literature. Medicine (Baltimore) 40:145, 1961.

71. McDevitt NB, McDonagh J, Taylor HL, Roberts HR: An acquired inhibitor to Factor XIII. Arch Intern Med 130:772, 1972.

72. McGehee WG, Feinstein DI, Carpenter G, Rapaport SI: Factor XIII inhibitor in a patient receiving INH. Arch Intern Med 130:772, 1972.

73. McGrath KM, Johnson CA, Stuart JJ: Acquired von Willebrand disease associated with an inhibitor to factor VIII antigen and gastrointestinal telangiectasia. Am J Med 67:693, 1979.

74. Menache D: Abnormal fibrinogens. Thromb Diath Haemorrh 29:525, 1973.

75. Miller K, Neeley JE, Krivit W, Edson JR: Spontaneously acquired Factor IX inhibitor in a nonhemophilic child. J Pediatr 93:232, 1978.

76. Mueh JR, Herbst KD, Rapaport SI: Thrombosis in patients with the lupus anticoagulant. Ann Intern Med 92:156, 1980.

77. Nes PM, Hymas PG, Gesme D, Perkins HA: An unusual Factor-X inhibitor in leprosy. Am J Hematol 8:397, 1980.

78. Nilsson IM, Hedner U, Ekberg M, Denneberg T: A circulating anticoagulant against Factor V. Acta Med Scand 195:73, 1974.

79. Noronha PA, Kruby HA, Maurer HS: Acquired von Willebrand disease in a patient with Wilms tumor. J Pediatr 95:997, 1979.

80. O'Reilly RA, Aggeler PM: Covert anticoagulant ingestion: Study of 25 patients and review of world literature. Medicine (Baltimore) 55:389, 1976.

81. Peck B, Hoffman GS, Franck WA: Thrombophlebitis is systemic lupus erythematosus. JAMA 240:1728, 1978.

82. Penner JA, Kelly PA: Management of patients with Factor VIII or IX inhibitors. Semin Thromb Hemost 1:386, 1975.

83. Pool-Wilson PA: Acquired von Willebrand's syndrome and systemic lupus erythematosus. Proc R Soc Med 65:561, 1972.

84. Rapaport SI, Ames SB, Duvall BJ: A plasma coagulation defect in systemic lupus erythematosus arising from hypoprothrombinemia combined with antiprothrombinase activity. Blood 15:212, 1960.

85. Raz I, Ramon A, Lahav M: Inhibition of blood coagulation Factor XI-XII by monoclonal IgM. Isr J Med Sci 11:1392, 1975.

86. Rosenberg RD, Colman RW, Lorand L: A new haemorrhagic disorder with defective fibrin stabilization and cryofibrinogenaemia. Br J Haematol 26:269, 1974.

87. Schleinder MA, Nachman RL, Jaffe EAS, Coleman M: A clinical study of the lupus anticoagulant. Blood 48:499, 1976.

88. Scully MF, Ellis V, Kakkar VV, Savidge GF, Williams YF, Sterndale H: An acquired coagulation inhibitor to Factor II. Br J Haematol 50:655, 1982.

89. Shapiro SS, Thagarajan P: Lupus anticoagulants. Prog Hemost Thromb 6:263, 1982.

90. Shapiro SS, Hultin M: Acquired inhibitors to the blood coagulation factors. Semin Thromb Hemost 1:336, 1975.

91. Simone JV, Cornet JA, Abildgaard CF: Acquired von Willebrand's syndrome in systemic lupus erythematosus. Blood 31:806, 1968.

92. Spero JA, Lewis JH, Hasiba U, Ellis LD: Treatment of amyloidosis associated with Factor X deficiency. Thromb Haemost 35:377, 1976.

93. Stabelforth P, Tamagnini GC, Dormandy KM: Acquired von Willebrand syndrome with inhibitors both to Factor VIII clotting activity and ristocetin-induced platelet aggregation. Br J Haematol 33:565, 1976.

94. Stirling ML, Parker AC, Keller AJ, Urbaniak SJ:

Factor V inhibitor and bullous pemphigoid. Br Med J 2:677, 1977.

95. Struzik T, Haricki Z, Hawiger R, Biernacka B: Cryocoagulopathy with presence of immuno antithrombin in the course of lupus erythematosus disseminatus. Acta Med Pol 5:61, 1964.

96. Torres A, Lucia JF, Oliveros A, Vazquez C, Torres M: Anti-Factor IX circulating anticoagulant and immune thrombocytopenia in a case of Takayasu's arteritis. Acta Haematol 64:338, 1980.

97. Veltkamp JJ, Stevens P, Pla's MVD, Loeliger EA: Production site of bleeding factor (acquired morbus von Willebrand). Thromb Diath Haemorrh 23:412, 1970.

98. Veltkamp JJ, Kerkhoven P, Loeliger EA: Circulating anticoagulant in disseminated lupus erythematosus. Haemostasis 2:253, 1974.

99. Vercellotti GM, Mosher DF: Acquired Factor XI deficiency in systemic lupus erythematosus. Thromb Haemost 48:250, 1982.

100. Wajima T, Schenk DA, Maloney TR: Severe bleeding associated with circulating anticoagulant to Factor V. Blood 54:308, 1979.

101. Wautier JL, Levy-Toledano S, Caen JP: Acquired von Willebrand's syndrome and thrombopathy in a patient with chronic lymphocytic leukemia. Scand J Haematol 16:128, 1976.

102. Wilner GR, Holt PJL, Bottomley J, Maciver JE: Practolol therapy associated with a systemic lupus erythematosus-like syndrome and inhibitor to Factor XIII. J Clin Pathol 30:770, 1977.

103. Zarrabi MH, Zucker S, Miller F, Derman RM, Romano GS, Hartnett JA, Varma AP: Immunologic and coagulation disorders in chlorpromazine-treated patients. Ann Intern Med 91:914, 1979.

104. Zettervall O, Nilsson IM: Acquired von Willebrand's disease caused by a monoclonal antibody. Acta Med Scand 204:521, 1978.

105. Zucker S, Zarrabi MH, Romano GS, Miller F: IgM

10
Alterations of Hemostasis in Malignancy

Alterations of hemostasis in malignancy have long been recognized; Trousseau[150] in 1865 was the first to note this strong association, and Morrison[113] initiated a major study of changes of altered hemostasis in patients with malignancy as early as 1932. Alterations of hemostasis in patients with malignancy are extremely complex and present major clinical challenges and problems, and many instances of bleeding or thrombosis in patients with malignancy remain unexplained.[15] However, often the mechanisms are known and will be discussed.

Alterations of hemostasis secondary to malignancy are certainly multifaceted and the development of clinically significant hemorrhage or thrombosis in these patients often represents the total clinical expression of numerous changes in the hemostatic system.[16] The major alterations of hemostasis that occur in malignancy, with particular emphasis on those thought to be most clinically significant with respect to morbidity and mortality, and, in addition, an approach to diagnostic problems and management are discussed.

Hypercoagulability and Thrombosis

Pathophysiology

The first described abnormality of hemostasis in malignancy was that of "hypercoagulability" and thrombosis, and the first large study in blood changes in cancer patients revealed "accelerated bleeding times" in more than 60% of patients studied.[113,150] Since these classic descriptions, many investigators have reported hypercoagulability and thrombosis in association with virtually all types of malignancy.[3,48,52,57,79,86,109,125,144] Many have found elevated clotting factors in pa-

tients with malignancy and the factors most commonly elevated, and thus in the past implicated in causing hypercoagulability, have been Factors I, V, VIII:C, IX, and XI.[3,48,62,109,128] Additionally, many patients with malignancy are noted to have shortened activated or nonactivated partial thromboplastin times, accelerated prothrombin times, and accelerated clotting times.[109,128] Although these parameters have often been assumed to be indicative of hypercoagulability, there is, in fact, no proof of this,[106] and none of the aforementioned laboratory parameters actually correlate with the development of a clinical thrombotic event in an individual patient.[15,16]

Increased fibrinogen and platelet catabolism (increased turnover and decreased survival) occurs in many patients with disseminated malignancy.[142] In addition, increased titers of fibrin(ogen) degradation products (FDP), fibrinopeptide A, cryofibrinogens, fibrin monomer, B-beta 15-42 and related peptides, platelet factor 4, beta-thromboglobulin, and altered fibronectin and antithrombin levels are seen in many patients with disseminated malignancy.[4,32,43,48,51,56,127,134,142,155–157] These findings strongly suggest that many patients with cancer have a low-grade disseminated intravascular coagulation (DIC) process. The shortened survival of fibrinogen, platelets, and other coagulation proteins is often followed by an over-compensatory increase in coagulation factors and fibrinolytic enzymes, although these latter proteins may be decreased in selected myeloproliferative disorders.[9] In addition, these changes are frequently accompanied by a significant decrease in major coagulation inhibitors, including antithrombin III and protein C, although the exact mechanisms of decreases in antithrombin III and protein C remain controversial and may be due to consumption or may be due to defective hepatic synthesis.[17,79,109,135] However, this sequence of changes alters the balance between coagulation, fibrinolysis, and inhibition of the clotting and fibrinolytic system and may render patients highly susceptable to a significant clinical event secondary to only minor changes in the overall hemostatic system. This may then predispose the patient to a localized intravascular coagulation (thrombosis or thromboembolism) or a classic DIC-type syndrome associated with hemorrhage or thrombosis. Thrombus formation is the more common of the two expressions of intravascular coagulation in the patient with solid tumors and may approach 40 to 50% in selected cancer patient populations.[44] In some instances, the degree of alteration in coagulation factors has been correlated with the amount of tumor present and overall patient survival.

Some coagulation abnormalities tend to normalize quite readily after initiation of therapy for the particular malignancy; this phenomena may be noted after surgery, radiation therapy, chemotherapy, or hormonal manipulation.[3,48,142] In this respect, however, it has recently been noted that hormonal therapy may also lead to decreases in antithrombin III and make the patient more susceptable to a thrombotic event.[54] Alterations of hemostasis induced by chemotherapeutic and hormonal agents will be discussed in appropriate sections of this chapter.

The mechanisms by which malignant tissue initiates localized or DIC is highly complex; however, many malignant tissues are capable of releasing procoagulant materials and, in some instances, fibrinolytic materials as well into the systemic circulation. Regardless of the mechanisms, when compared with normal tissue, most malignant tissue is capable of initiating the clotting process via numerous multifaceted processes and many pathologic tumor specimens are commonly noted to be associated with surrounding fibrin formation. Many malignant tissues have the ability to initiate fibrin formation without apparent subsequent activation of the fibrinolytic system.[31,121] Many types of malignant tissue are also capable of releasing a "thromboplastin-like" activity and may provide this activity either systemically or locally to initiate a clotting process; the amount released will most likely dictate whether a localized intravascular coagulation event (thrombus) or a systemic DIC-type syndrome occurs. Low levels of antithrombin III, regardless of its cause, will allow this process to start more easily and to proceed without normal inhibition once it has begun,[109] for example, in the patient with significant liver metastases and subsequent decreased or defective antithrombin III synthesis.[17] The process of DIC in malignancy is discussed in subsequent sections.

Mucinous adenocarcinomas are tumors that are commonly associated with thrombus formation; in these malignancies it has been demonstrated that the sialic acid moiety of secreted mucin is capable of initiating coagulation by the nonenzymatic activation of Factor X to Factor Xa.[52,128,129] In pancreatic carcinoma the release of systemic trypsin is thought to trigger the intravascular coagulation event. Also, it has been shown that the amount of trypsin released can be correlated with the degree of disseminated thrombi; patients with carcinoma of the body or tail of the pancreas have minimal ductal obstruction, and thus large amounts of trypsin release and far more thrombotic and thromboembolic episodes than patients with carcinoma of the head of the pancreas, with maximal ductal obstruction and minimal trypsin release.

DIC represents the "coagulopathy" of adenocarcinoma of the prostate;[122,133] however, malignant prostatic tissue has the ability not only to activate the procoagulant system, but also to activate the fibrinolytic system independently. In this instance, both a DIC and secondary fibrinolysis in association with inordinantly excessive fibrino(geno)lysis from both primary activation and activation secondary to DIC occurs. Thus, this coagulopathy will more often be manifested as hemorrhage rather than thrombosis, demonstrating the wide variability of clinical expression in DIC, depending on the balance between activation of the procoagulant system versus the fibrino(geno)lytic system. Therapy of prostatic carcinoma is often followed by a correction of general hemostasis parameters, including alterations of the procoagulant and fibrinolytic system. This is noted particularly with administration of estrogens, whereas testosterone has been noted to enhance coagulation abnormalities in many patients.[37,120,127]

Hypercoagulability in cancer patients may also arise from platelet abnormalities. The role of platelets in contributing to thrombosis in malignancy was suspected many years ago, and the first large study of this phenomena was initiated by Moolten and associates[112] in 1949. These studies revealed abnormal increases in platelet numbers as well as abnormal morphology, platelet lysis, and defective adhesion to glass wool. In addition, a correlation was noted between platelet adhesiveness and the development of thrombosis; the increased platelet adhesion was better correlated with thrombosis than was thrombocytosis in malignancy. Increased platelet adhesion, as measured by shortened bleeding times, accelerated thromboplastin generation, shortened prothrombin consumption, and increased adhesion to glass has been studied in numerous cancer patient populations and appears to be a uniform abnormality in a wide variety of solid tumors.[3,48,94,109,113] However, it is not clear whether these alterations are primary disturbances caused by the malignancy or whether they are due to initial earlier changes in the coagulation system that activate platelets and render them hyperaggregable.

Thrombocytosis is a well-recognized accompaniment of malignancy and most commonly is associated with carcinoma of the pancreas, lung, gastrointestinal tract, ovary, breast, and myeloproliferative syndromes. Those patients undergoing bone marrow suppressive therapy will have less thrombocytosis than patients not being so treated.[48,94,109,113] The most pronounced instances of thrombocytosis are usually noted in the myeloproliferative syndromes.[1] As with coagulation protein abnormalities and hypercoagulability, thrombocytosis and increased platelet aggregability generally correlate very poorly with the actual development of a clinical thrombotic event in an indivdidual patient. Thus, the actual significance of these in vitro laboratory findings remains unclear.

As already outlined, there are various mechanisms enabling malignant tissue to induce changes in coagulation factors and platelets to create a hypercoagulable state, i.e., an increased predisposition to thrombosis, as an expression of an underlying intravascular clotting process, which may be systemic or may remain localized. This intravascular coagulation may be mild and manifested only by abnormal tests of hemostasis, such as elevated levels of fibrinogen degradation products (FDP), B-beta 15-42 and related peptides, fibrinopeptide A, circulating fibrin monomer, and other such tests that are generally interpreted as representing hypercoagulability. However, this intravascular coagulation may proceed to more than a laboratory phenomenon and be expressed clinically as localized thrombosis or thromboembolus, or in more extreme cases may be manifested as a systemic DIC-type event associated with hemorrhage or thrombosis. The malignancies most associated with thrombosis are listed in Table 10–1. The overall incidence of thrombosis in malignancy is approximately 15%, but may be higher in specific tumors, such as in pancreatic carcinoma in which this phenomenon may be seen in more than 50% of patients.[15,16,79,144] The patient with malignancy is much more likely to develop postoperative thrombophlebitis than is the patient without cancer. In cancer of the gastrointestinal tract the incidence of postoperative thrombosis and thromboembolus may approach 40%.[15,16,52,82,128,129]

Management of Thrombosis and Thromboembolus in the Patient with Malignancy

Antitumor therapy is associated with some correction of abnormal hemostasis, and this has especially been appreciated in prostatic carcinoma. Because of this, treated patients are less susceptible to thrombosis and thromboembolus, and when thrombotic episodes develop in the untreated patient, consideration should be given to antineoplastic therapy. The use of anticoagulants, both warfarin and heparin, as well as antiplatelet agents, usually in the form of aspirin plus di-

Table 10–1 Malignancies Commonly Associated with Thrombosis

Colon
Gallbladder
Gastric
Lung
Myeloproliferative syndromes
Ovary
Pancreas
Paraprotein disorders

Table 10–2 Liver Metastases and Antithrombin Levels

Malignancy	Antithrombin	Liver
Breast	33	Involved
Hodgkin's disease	75	Involved
Breast	80	Involved
Breast	58	Involved
Ovary	76	Involved
Colon	83	Involved
Breast	71	Involved
Colon	92	Involved
Carcinoid	160	Involved
Colon	160	Involved
Hodgkin's disease	120	Clear
Breast	92	Clear
Lung	121	Clear
Lung	117	Clear
Breast	112	Clear
Ovary	92	Clear
Pancreas	104	Clear
Breast	140	Clear
Breast	104	Clear
Breast	150	Clear

pyridamole, have been associated with some correction of altered coagulation factors and normalization of both fibrinogen and platelet consumption (increased turnover and decreased survival).[15,16,37,48,142] Despite these findings, however, cancer patients are notoriously resistant to anticoagulant therapy, and thrombotic events are often noted to continue after the initiation of anticoagulant therapy.[10,15,16]

In my experience, warfarin and less commonly intravenous heparin are not only usually ineffective but may also be associated with significant bleeding problems in patients with malignancy, probably due to large areas of necrotic tumor surface.[10,15,16] This has also been experienced by others, who have noted a high incidence of fatal hemorrhage associated with the use of intravenous heparin in patients with malignancy.[142] In addition, many patients with malignancy have decreased antithrombin III levels,[17] and the response to heparin will be less than optimal. This is especially common in patients with liver metastases, as is demonstrated in Table 10–2. On the other hand, experience with antiplatelet agents in patients with malignancy has been quite good. I commonly use aspirin, 600 mg twice daily, to be taken with 30 mL of liquid antacid in combination with dipyridamole at a dose of 50 mg four times a day in patients with cancer and thrombosis.[10,15,16] This is usually found effective for the immediate prophylaxis of extension of thrombi as well as for long-term prophylactic therapy in cancer patients with recurrent thrombosis. In this regard it should be noted that warfarin or heparin are generally contraindicated in patients with malignancy and thrombosis or

thromboembolus if metastases to the central nervous system are present.[10,15,16] The use of aspirin and dipyridamole preoperatively or immediately postoperatively seems effective for prophylaxis in those patients with tumors known to be associated with a high rate of post-operative thrombosis. Usually, bleeding complications are not noted in association with antiplatelet therapy, even in the patient with recent gastrointestinal surgery. However, the importance of using concomitant liquid antacids and enteric-coated aspirin cannot be overstressed. Alternatively, low-dose subcutaneous heparin can be safely used in most preoperative patients with malignancy as prophylaxis for postoperative thrombosis or pulmonary embolus. However, intravenous or high-dose heparin therapy should not be used in this instance.

For those using antiplatelet agents, it should be emphasized that the antiplatelet effect of these agents may last for 4 to 10 days after the last dose, and this should be considered in the event of bleeding or planned nonemergent surgery or other invasive procedures. However, bleeding from antiplatelet therapy can easily be controlled by the use of appropriate numbers of platelet concentrates, as outlined in Chapter 4. When the patient with malignancy has life-threatening thrombosis and has adequate levels of antithrombin III, low-dose heparin is highly useful and appears to be equally effective as large doses of heparin and is not often associated with bleeding from tumor surfaces, which may potentially occur with intravenous doses of heparin.

Hemorrhage

Leukemias

Hemorrhage may precede the overt clinical diagnosis of leukemia by several months; this is commonly noted in acute leukemias.[87,95,96] Petechiae, purpura, and ecchymoses are the most common prediagnostic manifestations and they, or other less commonly noted types of hemorrhage, are present in 40 to 70% of patients with acute leukemia at the time of diagnosis.[30,55,114] The most common sites of hemorrhage in patients with acute leukemia are the skin, eye, and mucosal membranes, including epistaxis, gingival bleeding, and gastrointestinal bleeding.[95,96] However, it should be recalled that retinal bleeding can occur in up to 15% of patients at the time of presentation and in up to 50% of patients with acute leukemia as the disease progresses.[30,76] In acute leukemia, hemorrhage is a common cause of death, accounting for deaths in up to 40% of patients[30,74] (second only to infection in the past two decades). This is probably due to the more intensive chemotherapy and attendant immunosuppression, as well as the major impact of the development of platelet concentrate therapy to help control thrombocytopenia, the most common cause of fatal hemorrhage in acute leukemia patients.[69,95,96] Clinical bleeding manifestations in acute leukemia are summarized in Table 10–3.

Hemorrhage is less commonly a problem in the chronic myeloid or lymphoid leukemias.[15,16,95,96,115] However, in both chronic myelogenous leukemia or chronic lymphocytic leukemia local or diffuse thromboses or thromboembolism may frequently occur.[10,15,16,88] Many pa-

Table 10–3 Hemorrhagic Manifestations in Acute Leukemias

Hemorrhage may preceed diagnosis by months; petechiae, purpura, and ecchymoses most common
Up to 70% have petechiae and purpura at diagnosis
Retinal hemorrhage in 15% at diagnosis
Retinal hemorrhage in 50% during course of disease
Most patients will have hemorrhage of skin or mucosal membranes during course
Hemorrhage is the cause of death in 40%

tients with chronic leukemia commonly have bothersome bleeding, usually manifest as petechiae, purpura, ecchymoses, or oozing from mucosal membranes, including the gastrointestinal and genitourinary tracts. Only rarely do these patients have retinal bleeding or other serious life-threatening bleeding unless severe thrombocytopenia (usually drug-induced) or thrombocytosis or thrombocythemia develops. Alterations of hemostasis associated with malignant thrombocytosis and thrombocythemia are discussed in detail in Chapter 4. As with chronic myelogenous leukemias, chronic lymphocytic leukemias also more commonly are associated with thrombosis or thromboembolus in the early course of the disease.[15,16,88] Hemorrhage, however, becomes a problem later in the course of the disease as thrombocytopenia from chemotherapy or marrow infiltration, liver infiltration, or other hemostasis defects, including DIC secondary to the leukemia itself, sepsis, transfusions, or other causes may begin to become manifest.[10,15,16,18]

Hemorrhage may occur in any of the leukemias, but is most commonly noted in acute promyelocytic leukemia, acute myelomonocytic leukemia, and acute granulocytic leukemia. Life-threatening or severe hemorrhage is less commonly seen in chronic myelogenous leukemia, chronic lymphocytic leukemia, and pure monocytic leukemia.[16,95–98]

There are numerous mechanisms for the development of significant or life-threatening hemorrhage in all types of leukemia, and these will be discussed as categories of defects, including platelets, the coagulation proteins, mechanisms for the development of DIC, abnormalities of the vasculature, and the leukemia cell as a source of various clot-promoting materials, fibrino(geno)lytic materials, and other materials that may alter or disrupt the hemostasis system.

Platelets

The most common single cause of serious or life-threatening hemorrhage in acute or chronic leukemias is thrombocytopenia.[15,16,95,96] Thrombocytopenia is most commonly due to chemotherapy or marrow infiltration; grades of thrombocytopenia, and the chemotherapeutic agents most likely to cause thrombocytopenia are outlined in detail in Chapter 4. However, less common causes of thrombocytopenia in patients with leukemia are the development of DIC with consumption of platelets, infection-induced immune or nonimmune thrombocytopenia, or splenomegaly and associated hypersplenism with increased platelet sequestration. A more detailed discussion of these mechanisms is given in Chapter 4.

In clinical practice when seeing severe thrombocytopenia in patients with leukemia, all of these mechanisms must be considered because even though the most common cause of thrombocytopenia is chemotherapy, drug-induced, or from marrow infiltration, any combinations of several or even almost all of the aforementioned mechanisms may be operative and must be corrected if life-threatening hemorrhage is to be successfully treated. Mechanisms of thrombocytopenia in leukemia are summarized in Table 10–4.

In patients with acute myelogenous leukemia the platelet count commonly

Table 10–4 Mechanisms of Thrombocytopenia in Leukemia

Bone marrow infiltration (myelophthisis)
Chemotherapy
Radiation therapy
Bacteremia
Disseminated intravascular coagulation
Infection-induced (immune and nonimmune)
Splenomegaly and hypersplenism
Immune thrombocytopenia purpura
Myelofibrosis
Richter's syndrome (chronic lymphocytic leukemia)

drops below 10,000/mm^3 during remission induction therapy;[137,158] bleeding is uncommon when the platelet count is greater than 10,000/mm^3 in patients undergoing remission induction. However, when the platelet count drops below 5000/mm^3, severe hemorrhage is frequently a problem. During remission induction, a daily urine examination for red cells and a daily stool guiaic should be obtained as soon as the platelet count drops below 50,000/mm^3. A positive result in either of these tests gives a reasonable indication that serious hemorrhage may be impending. If the urine and stool samples remain negative, prophylactic platelet concentrate therapy should not be empirically given unless the platelet count is less than 5000/mm^3. At this point the daily infusion of 6 to 8 U of platelet concentrates each day is warranted to avoid irreversible life-threatening hemorrhage and should be continued until the platelet count is consistently greater than 10,000/mm^3 and significant bleeding or early signs of bleeding, as manifested by positive quiaics or blood in the urine, are negative.

Chronic myelogenous leukemia is only rarely associated with platelet counts of less than 10,000/mm^3;[15,16,95,96] however, as in acute leukemias when the platelet count is less than 50,000/mm^3, the same principles of management as previously outlined also apply. More commonly, chronic myeloid leukemias are associated with hemorrhage or thrombosis secondary to a severe thrombocytosis/thrombocythemia. The general characteristics of this complication as well as the diagnostic problems and therapeutic approach to essential thrombocythemia or secondary thrombocythemia in patients with leukemias are discussed in Chapter 4.

Like chronic myelogenous leukemia, chronic lymphocytic leukemia is rarely, at least in the early course of the disease, associated with platelet counts of less than 50,000/mm^3. As previously discussed, when the platelet count is less than 50,000/mm^3 the previously outlined approach should be followed. However, as chronic lymphatic leukemia begins to enter a terminal phase, thrombocytopenia may become a very significant problem. This can come about from the institution of more vigorous chemotherapeutic attempts, severe marrow replacement, infections, or the development of various immune-mediated thrombocytopenic problems, including Richter's syndrome or an immune thrombocytopenic purpura-type syndrome. Severe thrombocytopenia may also occur after the development of significant hypersplenism or a frank DIC-type syndrome. The same management principles as outlined previously should be instituted, depending on the mechanisms or combination of mechanisms involved.

Platelet Dysfunction

Significant platelet function defects even with normal or elevated platelet counts are almost uniformly noted in chronic myelogenous leukemia, essential thrombocythemia, and other myeloproliferative syndromes.[1,15,16,95] The characteristics of platelet dysfunction in essential thrombocythemia were discussed in Chapter 4. Almost uniformly platelet function defects are noted in chronic myelogenous leukemia and these defects commonly lead to or contribute to significant hemorrhage. Although many types of defects are seen, the most common and uniform are impaired aggregation to adenosine diphosphate (ADP) and epinephrine as well as defective platelet factor 3 release.[40,41,146] In addition, a deficiency or absence of alpha granules has been noted in patients with myeloproliferative syndromes and platelet function defects.[110] It should be emphasized that the platelet function defect associated with chronic myelogenous leukemia or essential thrombocythemia commonly leads to or contributes to significant clinical hemorrhage, especially if coupled with other defects in the hemostasis system.[15,16,19,97] If the platelet count is decreased or normal, the defect can be overcome by the use of appropriate numbers of platelet concentrates. Platelet dysfunction associated with hemorrhage and an elevated platelet count (greater than 700,000/mm^3) is usually rapidly corrected by plateletpheresis.

Platelet dysfunction is less commonly a problem in acute leukemias; some have reported normal platelet response to most usual aggregating agents,[136] whereas others have noted impaired platelet function as assessed by platelet aggregation to thrombin, ADP, epinephrine, and collagen in patients with acute leukemias.[47] The abnormal release of platelet factor 3 has also been noted in patients with acute leukemia.[95] Although platelet function defects in chronic myelogenous leukemia are well known to contribute to significant hemorrhage, the role of abnormal platelet function as a significant cause of hemorrhage in acute leukemias remains less clearly defined. Platelet dysfunction is much less commonly seen in chronic lymphocytic leukemia and in monocytic leukemia than in the myelogenous leukemias or other myeloproliferative syndromes.[95]

Coagulation Protein Abnormalities

Liver infiltration with subsequent defective or decreased synthesis of the prothrombin complex factors is commonly a problem in acute leukemias; in addition, impaired synthesis of other factors may also occur.[95,99] Thus, if the patient with acute leukemia develops significant liver infiltration, there may be defective synthesis of any combination of not only Factors II, VII, IX, and X, but also fibrinogen, Factors V, VIII:C, XI, XII, and XIII, prekallikrein, high molecular weight kininogen, plasminogen, or antithrombin III, and protein C.[15,16,95,96,135] In addition, fibronectin levels are commonly decreased in acute leukemia; this may be due to decreased synthesis or to consumption after the development of a DIC-type syndrome. This phenomenon has been reported to correlate reasonably well with infectious episodes, and thus DIC rather than defective synthesis would appear to be incriminated as the mechanism for decreased levels of fibronectin in patients with acute leukemia.[135] Cholestasis occurs in a significant number of patients with acute leukemia, and this often leads to defective synthesis of the vitamin K dependent clotting factors and on occasion to a frank DIC syndrome.[50,95,96] However, as will be discussed subsequently, there are also other more significant mechanisms for the development of DIC in patients with acute leukemia.

Chronic lymphocytic leukemia may also be associated with significant liver infiltration, especially as the disease progresses and approaches its terminal stages.[95,98,99] This may, as in the acute leukemias, lead to impaired or decreased synthesis of the prothrombin complex factors as well as any other combination of factors synthesized by the liver. Thus, many patients with chronic lymphocytic leukemia will demonstrate prolonged prothrombin times, which may be noted to correct with more intensive appropriate chemotherapeutic agents. Factors V, VIII:C, and fibrinogen may behave as acute phase reactants and may therefore be high, low, or normal in patients with chronic lymphocytic leukemia. Thus, the activated partial thromboplastin time may be highly variable because of the highly variable levels of Factors V and VIII:C and fibrinogen. Defective hepatic synthesis of coagulation factors due to hepatic infiltration in chronic lymphocytic leukemia is an uncommmon cause of life-threatening hemorrhage. Chronic myelogenous leukemias may also be associated with significant hepatic infiltration; however, this is much less commonly a problem than in acute leukemias or chronic lymphocytic leukemia.[95,97] Patients with chronic myelogenous leukemia who do not have DIC will usually have normal or near normal global tests of hemostasis, and defective hepatic synthesis due to leukemic infiltrates is rarely a singular problem accounting for hemorrhage in patients with chronic myelogenous leukemia.

Fibrinolysis

Numerous alterations in the fibrinolytic system of patients with acute leukemia have been reported; however, the findings have been notoriously inconsistent, with increased fibrinolytic activity reported by some[136] and decreased fibrinolytic activity noted by others.[33] One study found a correlation between leukocytosis, subsequent leukostasis, and enhanced fibrinolytic activity; however, this is an isolated report that has not been confirmed.[100] In general, significant changes in the fibrinolytic system components have not been noted in patients with chronic myelogenous leukemia or chronic lymphocytic leukemia.[95,97,98] High plasminogen activator activity has been reported in association with chronic myeloid leukemias,[84,149] but not lymphocytic leukemias.[95,98] One study demonstrated that 30% of patients with acute leukemias have high fibrinolytic activity; these patients also demonstrated low antiplasmin levels, as well as the presence of circulating plasmin-antiplasmin complexes. These findings did not appear to correlate with findings suggestive of procoagulant activity or of DIC, and thus these fibrinolytic alterations appeared to be independent of intravascular procoagulant activity.[154]

Disseminated Intravascular Coagulation in Leukemia

Myeloblasts, promyelocytes, monocytes, and lymphoblasts all contain and are capable of releasing procoagulant materials or enzymes in patients with acute leukemia.[15,16,53,63,65,67,95,96,105,131] Thus, DIC may complicate the course of acute leukemia in up to 50% of patients.[77,147] In addition, blast cells may possess fibrinolytic activity or fibrinolytic system activator activity.[46,58,65,95,96,100,130,153] Granulocytes of chronic granulocytic leukemia are also capable of releasing procoagulant enzymes and activity, as well as antithrombin-type materials.[95,97] Granulocytes of chronic myelogenous leukemia release an antiheparin-like activity that appears to be derived from myeloperoxidase.[95,148] Mature lymphocytes of chronic lymphocytic leukemia also release procoagulant materials that appear to be phospholipoprotein or "thromboplastin-like" in composition.[88,95,98] Due to this capability of releasing procoagulant materials into the systemic circulation and thus activating (triggering) the coagulation system, virtually any leukemia can be associated with acute or chronic DIC.[15,16,18,20,21]

Acute promyelocytic leukemia is the most common followed by acute myelomonocytic leukemia, acute myeloblastic leukemia, and acute lymphoblastic leukemia, in descending order of probability.[18,20] Acute DIC is seen much less commonly in chronic leukemias than in acute leukemias and is more likely to be seen with chronic myelogenous leukemia than in chronic lymphocytic leukemia. The development of DIC is of major significance with respect to survival in the acute leukemias and is a frequent complication of acute promyelocytic leukemia. The survival of patients with acute promyelocytic leukemia can be significantly improved if development of DIC is blocked or an existing DIC is blunted by the early use of low-dose (subcutaneous) heparin.[5,18,20,68] A detailed discussion is presented in Chapter 6.

Vascular Defects

Significant vascular defects may also develop in patients with acute leukemia; these defects are often neglected or forgotten, but may be responsible for or contribute to significant hemorrhage.[95,96] Although vascular defects are of clinical significance in the acute leukemias, they are not likely to be a clinical problem in patients with chronic leukemias. Patients with acute leukemias commonly demonstrate increased vascular permeability due to infiltration of the vasculature by leukemic cells, hyperviscosity or leukostasis of the vasa vasorum, or foci of extramedullary hematopoiesis in the vessel wall.[141,151,152]

In summary, it must be recalled that numerous defects of hemostasis may be associated with acute and chronic leukemias, and when significant hemorrhage occurs, the defects may be multifactorial and consist of a combination of any one, several, or all of the previously described defects. Only by carefully evaluating the patient from both the clinical and laboratory standpoints and carefully delineating the presence or absence of each of these defects can rational and effective therapy be delivered. Hemorrhagic syndromes associated with leukemia are summarized in Table 10–5.

Table 10–5 Hemorrhagic Syndromes in Leukemias

Thrombocytopenia
Platelet dysfunction
Disseminated intravascular coagulation
   Leukemia cell procoagulant activity
   Bacteremia
   Massive transfusions
   Shock
Coagulation protein defects
   Liver infiltration
   Cholestasis
   Drug-induced
Primary fibrinolysis
   Leukemia cell proteolytic activity
   Drug-induced
Vascular defects
   Infiltration
   Hyperviscosity or leukostasis
   Extramedullary hematopoiesis

Hemorrhage and Solid Tumors

Although thrombosis is more commonly the abnormality of hemostasis manifested with solid tumors, and hemorrhage is more commonly associated with acute leukemias, hemorrhage may also be a significant clinical problem in patients with solid tumors as well.[15,16] As discussed previously, intravascular coagulation is present in many patients with malignancy and manifests varying clinical expressions, the most extreme form being acute fulminant DIC and catastrophic hemorrhage. DIC in cancer patients may be acute or chronic.[10,18,20,21] The chronic form is slightly more common and is manifested clinically by mild to moderate bleeding, usually of the integument or mucous membranes.[18] Easy and spontaneous bruising, petachiae and purpura, echymoses, gingival bleeding, and minor gastrointestinal bleeding are usual manifestations. In contrast, acute DIC, as discussed in detail in Chapter 6, is characterized by an explosive catastrophic hemorrhage, with bleeding usually being from at least three unrelated sites at the same time. The most commonly noted abnormalities are petechiae, purpura, and ecchymoses, seen in conjunction with significant gastrointestinal, pulmonary, or genitourinary hemorrhage. In addition, most patients with acute DIC will have oozing from intravenous sites or sites of other invasive procedures, such as intra-arterial lines, subclavian catheters, and hepatic artery catheters.[15,16,18,20,21] Although these are the most common bleeding manifestations, more life-threatening bleeding, such as intracranial and intrapulmonary hemorrhage with massive hemoptysis may also occur. This form of DIC has been noted in association with almost all types of solid tumors and is most commonly seen in carcinoma of the lung, gallbladder, stomach, colon, breast, ovary, malignant melanoma[8,49,66,109,128,129,143] and is especially common in carcinoma of the prostate.[60,122,127,133] Table 6–2 lists malignancies most commonly associated with DIC. In these latter disorders, initiation of chemotherapy has occasionally been associated with triggering or acceleration of DIC.[18,48,66,67,92] The initiation or enhancement of DIC in association with initiation of antineoplastic therapy is presumably due to release of thromboplastin-like or other clot-promoting materials or enyzmes from necrotic tumor cells. In acute promyelocytic leukemia, low-dose heparin therapy given before starting cytotoxic drugs may protect against this development, as previously discussed.[5,18,68,73] Most patients with disseminated solid malignancy have some laboratory or clinical evidence of DIC; many patients with malignancy never develop clinical manifestations of DIC, but if one looks for laboratory findings of DIC, these are almost always present. The patient with disseminated malignancy represents a special problem, in that DIC may be manifested as an acute, subacute, or chronic form, and as local thrombosis, diffuse thrombosis, thromboembolism, minor hemorrhage, diffuse hemorrhage, or any combination thereof.[15,16,18,20,21]

There are numerous potential mechanisms by which malignancy may provide triggers for DIC. The hemorrhagic syndrome associated with prostatic carcinoma remained poorly understood for a long time. Many consider this to represent DIC with secondary fibrinolysis, whereas others believe the hemorrhage associated with prostatic carcinoma to be a primary hyperfibrinolytic syndrome.[34,133]

It is now clearly recognized that both processes occur in malignant prostatic disease and may occur to a smaller extent in benign prostatic disease as well. Malignant prostatic tissue contains procoagulant materials that may be released into the circulation, triggering a DIC process with the usual secondary fibrinolytic response. In addition, malignant prostatic tissue may independently either directly or indirectly activate the fibrinolytic system, leading to a primary hyperfibrino(geno)lytic syndrome. Thus, prostatic carcinoma is commonly associated with DIC and the usual secondary fibrinolytic response plus a primary hyperfibrino(geno)lytic syndrome. This explains why, from the clinical and laboratory standpoint, patients with prostatic carcinoma more often present with an overwhelming fibrino(geno)lytic syndrome, a minimal procoagulant problem, and the clinical manifestations of this are, of course, hemorrhage rather than diffuse thrombosis. A recent study has shown that evidence for DIC, as defined by the presence of elevated FDPs or soluble fibrin monomer, is noted in many patients before surgery for malignant prostatic disease.[107] In addition, after transurethral resection of the prostate (TURP), blood loss appears to be correlated with preoperative evidence of DIC. These findings suggest that it is necessary to look for laboratory manifestations of DIC before attempting TURP in patients with prostatic disease because these parameters may be predictive with respect to postoperative bleeding, blood loss, and necessity of blood replacement.[18,107]

DIC may commonly be associated with pancreatic carcinoma. In this incidence, DIC is more commonly manifested as diffuse thrombosis rather than diffuse hemorrhage, because the prcoagulant activity appears to dominate and secondary fibrinolysis is minimal. DIC, manifested as acute disseminated thrombosis, is more commonly seen in carcinoma of the body and tail of the pancreas because there is little ductal obstruction and a large amount of trypsin release, the trypsin having thrombin-like activity. In carcinoma of the head of the pancreas there is more ductal obstruction and less trypsin release into the systemic circulation and thus there is less commonly an associated disseminated intravascular thrombosis (DIC) type syndrome.

In patients with adenocarcinoma of numerous primary sites, the mechanism for DIC may be multifaceted. However, as previously mentioned, it is known that the sialic acid moiety of secreted mucin from adenocarcinomatous tissue is capable of causing the nonenzymatic activation of Factor X to Factor Xa.[128,129] This can easily provide a trigger for systemic thrombin generation and a subsequent course of acute or subacute DIC.[18,22] In addition, this sequence could lead to thrombosis alone.[18,20,21] It is likely that less clearly defined additional mechanisms exist for initiating DIC in malignancy. The systemic release of necrotic tumor tissue or enzymes with procoagulant or phospholipoprotein-like activity may activate the early phases of coagulation or platelet release. In addition, many tumors undergo neovascularization; this process could potentially produce abnormal endothelial cell lining that may either cause a platelet release or generation of Factor XIIa or XIa with subsequent procoagulant activation and the development of an acute, subacute, or chronic DIC-type process.[18,20,21,38,59] Table 10–6 lists the usual laboratory features found in most patients with disseminated malignancy and disorders of hemostasis. These findings are often associated with and are interpreted as a hypercoagulable state or a predisposition to thrombus formation; however, these findings most likely simply represent complicated changes of a subacute or chronic DIC process that may or may not become clinically manifested.

Another common trigger for DIC in the patient with malignancy is the use of LeVeen shunts for malignant ascites. Patients with malignant ascites must be carefully selected for this procedure; if ascitic fluid is positive for malignant cells, the placement of a LeVeen shunt is usually not successful,[42] does not lead to significant prolongation of good quality life, and is commonly associated with the development of an acute DIC-type process.[23,72,93,145]

Table 10–6 Typical Abnormal Hemostasis Findings in Patients with Disseminated Malignancy

Elevated fibrinogen (with decreased survival)
Elevated fibrin(ogen) degradation products
Circulating soluble fibrin monomer
Elevated fibrinopeptide A
Elevated fibrinopeptide B
Cryofibrinogenemia
Decreased plasminogen
Elevated plasmin
Elevated B-beta 15-42 related peptides
Decreased fibronectin
Decreased antithrombin III
Decreased protein C
Elevated Factor VIII:C
Thrombocytosis (with decreased survival)
Thrombocytopenia (with decreased survival)
Elevated platelet factor 4
Elevated beta-thromboglobulin

DIC may be aborted by removal of ascitic fluid at the time of shunt placement.[132] In this clinical setting a less common although significant complication of LeVeen shunting in the patient with malignant ascites is that of thromboembolism.[42]

A significant amount of discussion has concerned the association of malignancy and DIC; this is one of the most common clinical settings in which clinicians will have to contend with acute, subacute, or chronic DIC. In addition, especially in malignancy DIC may display highly varied clinical manifestations. For example, the patient with malignancy may demonstrate accelerated procoagulant activity with minimal fibrinolytic response and diffuse thrombosis or may have a moderate procoagulant drive with overwhelming secondary fibrinolytic activation and subsequent purely hemorrhagic manifestations.[15,16,18,20,21] Also, any combination between these two extremes may be seen in patients with disseminated solid tumor.[15,16] The patient with malignancy and associated DIC presents a major problem in management and thus a clear understanding and definition of possible triggering events is desirable and often necessary for efficacious control of the intravascular clotting process.

Diagnosis of Disseminated Intravascular Coagulation

Clinical

The clinical diagnosis of DIC need not be difficult; the key to a high index of suspicion is to simply note the appropriate type of bleeding in the patient with malignancy.[15,16,18] The type of bleeding manifested by most patients with acute or subacute DIC is suggestive of multiple hemostatic compartment-type defects. For example, most patients with acute DIC will bleed from at least three unrelated sites at one time.[15,16,18] This may be expressed in a wide variety of ways and commonly is seen as melena and hematochezia, epistaxis, hemoptysis in association with oozing from intra-arterial or intravenous invasion sites, hematuria, and associated findings of petechiae and purpura.[18,20,21] This type of bleeding or these combinations of bleeding should immediately suggest that multiple hemostatic compartments are involved. When noting this type of bleeding presentation in cancer patients, one can be almost assured of a diagnosis of DIC. Also, most cancer patients with acute DIC display shock and associated end organ hypoxia or ischemic changes.[18] This may be manifested in a wide variety of ways, depending on end organ involvement and degree of occlusive changes. Renal failure, due to fibrin thrombi deposited in the renal microvasculature is a frequent manifestation, as is pulmonary failure or central nervous system symptoms. Additionally, one must recall the interplay between coagulation proteins and other protein systems. Specifically kinin generation and complement activation often account for many of the attendant signs and symptoms in these bleeding or thrombosing patients, including pain and shock. Many patients with malignancy and subacute or chronic DIC will not display fulminant and multiple site type bleeding, which is more typically seen in those with acute DIC;

chronic DIC patients more commonly complain of minor mucosal membrane bleeding, often manifested as excessive gingival bleeding with toothbrushing, minor hemoptysis, bothersome epistaxis, and at times hematuria.[10,18,20,21] Patients with malignancy will often complain of easy and spontaneous bruising and petechiae and purpura, which may not be noticed by the patient and may only represent minimal findings found by the clinician after careful examination. When the patient with malignancy presents with diffuse thrombosis, this may only be a manifestation of the opposite clinical spectrum of DIC. In this setting, DIC should be strongly considered and the patient appropriately studied for confirmatory evidence and appropriate therapy started if the diagnosis is confirmed.[10,18,20,21,24]

Laboratory Diagnosis

The laboratory diagnosis of DIC is discussed in detail in Chapter 6; however, the salient features with regard to oncology will be discussed. Although noting the type of bleeding in the appropriate clinical setting can virtually assure a diagnosis of DIC, laboratory confirmation is desirable, if not mandatory, before committing a cancer patient to heparin, low-dose heparin, or other antiprocoagulant type therapy. Understanding the pathophysiology of DIC makes it clear that these patients will have numerous abnormal laboratory tests of hemostasis. Most laboratory data are abnormal in the acute form of DIC only, and in subacute or chronic DIC associated with malignancy many laboratory parameters of hemostasis may be difficult to interpret or may be within normal limits.[18,20,21,24] Table 10–7 lists the laboratory tests that are typically abnormal in acute and chronic DIC in the patient with malignancy. It must be recalled that in addition to malignancy itself, other common complications seen in cancer patients may act as triggers for DIC, including sepsis, initiation of radiation therapy,

Table 10–7 Typical Laboratory Findings of Acute and Chronic DIC in Disseminated Malignancy

Acute and chronic
Microangiopathic hemolytic anemia
Schistocytosis
Reticulocytosis
Leukocytosis
Elevated fibrin(ogen) degradation products
Circulating soluble fibrin monomer
Elevated fibrinopeptide A
Elevated B-beta 15-42 related peptides
Circulating plasmin
Decreased platelet survival
Large "young" platelets
Elevated platelet factor 4
Elevated beta-thromboglobulin
Acute only
Decreased antithrombin III
Decreased protein C
Decreased fibronectin
Clotting factors: Normal, up, or down
Hypoplasminogenemia
Decreased antiplasmin
Thrombocytopenia
Chronic only
Fibrinogen borderline or normal
Clotting factors borderline or normal
Antithrombin III normal or decreased
Protein C normal or decreased
Plasminogen normal or decreased
Platelets normal or borderline low

microangiopathic hemolytic anemia, hemolytic anemia of any etiology, hemolytic transfusion reactions, and transfusions of large amounts of banked whole blood.[18,20]

Therapy

Therapy of DIC in the cancer patient represents a major clinical challenge; my approach is outlined in Table 6–26. Efficacious therapy is multiphasic and must be approached in a sequential manner.[18] The first and most important modality is to treat the malignancy, since this is providing the triggering procoagulant material for intravascular coagulation to occur. Therapy may be surgical, radiotherapy, chemotherapy, or endocrine manipulation as the clinical situation warrants. Treatment of the trigger (tumor) is often associated with cessation or significant improvement

of DIC. Until attempts at antineoplastic therapy are initiated, subsequent therapy of bleeding or thrombosis is often unsuccessful. This is especially true if the manifestation of DIC and malignancy is that of thrombosis; unless the malignancy is well controlled, cancer patients are notoriously resistant to anticoagulant therapy.[10,15,16,18] If significant bleeding continues after reasonable attempts to control the malignancy, anticoagulant therapy must be considered. For the patient with malignancy and acute DIC, low-dose heparin therapy at 80 to 100 U/kg is given subcutaneously three to four times a day as the site and severity of hemorrhage dictates.[18] Patients with chronic DIC and bothersome but not life-threatening hemorrhage are started on antiplatelet agents in the form of aspirin and dipyridamole, as previously discussed. These are usually successful at stopping the chronic intravascular clotting process. It should be noted that the use of antiplatelet agents in chronic DIC will usually require 24 to 36 hours to stop the intravascular clotting process; however, the use of low-dose heparin will usually stop the process within 4 to 8 hours.

Other Defects

Cancer patients may also develop bleeding from other coagulation factor abnormalities; these other defects are less common, however, and are usually associated with less serious hemorrhage than that associated with DIC. Patients with malignancy, especially those with liver metastases, may acquire deficiencies of the prothrombin complex factors.[60,109] When this results in significant or life-threatening bleeding, vitamin K is usually ineffective and the hemorrhage must be controlled with fresh frozen plasma, or prothrombin complex concentrates.[25] However, before using these modalities as primary modes of therapy, DIC must be excluded. Extrahepatic or intrahepatic biliary obstruction and cholestasis, due to tumor at any site in the biliary tree in the patient with malignancy, is often associated with malabsorption of vitamin K and defective synthesis of the vitamin K dependent factors. In this setting, DIC may also occur, although this is less commonly a complication than simple decreased synthesis of the prothrombin complex factors.

Factor XIII deficiency or dysfunction is common in malignancy and is most pronounced in patients with liver metastases.[102,143] This may be due to decreased Factor XIII activators or impaired removal of Factor XIII inhibitors by the invaded liver. Also, Factor XIII is associated with albumin, and cancer patients with hypoalbuminemia may be Factor XIII deficient, although usually not to a clinically significant degree. In cancer patients, acquired Factor XIII deficiency may or may not cause hemorrhage; more commonly, impaired clot formation and poor wound healing will be noted. When Factor XIII deficiency is thought to cause or contribute to hemorrhage, it can be managed by transfusions with fresh frozen plasma given at a dose of 5 mL/kg every 7 to 10 days.[78]

Patients with liver metastases will often have low levels of other clotting factors synthesized in the liver, including fibrinogen, Factors V, VIII:C, XI, and XII, prekallikrein, high molecular weight kininogen, plasminogen, antithrombin III, and fibronectin. However, the decreased synthesis of all of these are of unclear clinical significance. Of particular concern in malignancy is the development of a dysfibrinogenemia with either primary hepatoma or liver metastases. Abnormalities in fibrin monomer polymerization are manifestations of this dysfibrinogenemia and may lead to significant hemorrhage in the patient with disseminated malignancy and liver metastases or the patient with primary hepatoma.[15,16]

Acquired circulating anticoagulants may occur in a wide variety of tumors; however, these have been isolated findings and have an unclear relationship to actual hemorrhage in many instances. Many are heparinoid in nature and are found in association with carcinoma of the lung and myeloma.[10,15,16,26,39,83,117,123] Some appear to inhibit the activation phase of coagulation or act as antithrombins, and these have been most commonly noted in association with carcinoma of the breast.[102] Of more clinical significance,

circulating anticoagulant in the form of FDPs may assume paramount clinical importance in cancer patients with low-grade covert intravascular coagulation; the mechanism by which FDPs interfere with hemostasis has been previously discussed in Chapters 6 and 7. Circulating anticoagulants may assume major importance in the paraprotein disorders, as will be discussed subsequently.

Primary Fibrino(geno)lysis

Primary fibrino(geno)lysis has been repeatedly noted in patients with disseminated malignancy.[44,120,127,143] In this disorder, hemorrhage, as discussed in detail in Chapter 7, is caused by plasmin-induced biodegradation of numerous clotting factors, including fibrinogen, Factors V and VIII:C, as well as the impairment of hemostasis by circulating FDPs that interfere with fibrin monomer polymerization, thrombin generation, and platelet function.[27,28] Although primary hyperfibrinolysis occurs in malignancy, DIC is a much more common cause of hemorrhage in the cancer patient. Many malignant tissues are capable of spontaneous fibrinolytic activity and activation of the fibrinolytic system. This has been noted in patients with carcinoma of the breast, thyroid, colon, and stomach; however, the greatest activity is seen in patients with disseminated sarcoma.[15,16,44] If patients with carcinoma of the breast, thyroid, colon, or stomach develop a systemic hemorrhagic syndrome, the cause is most likely DIC, and only rarely is it due to primary activation of the fibrinolytic system and a primary hyperfibrino(geno)lytic syndrome. However, the opposite is true in patients with disseminated sarcoma. If these patients develop a systemic hemorrhage syndrome, the most common cause is primary hyperfibrino(geno)lysis and only rarely is it due to DIC.[15,16,55] Kwaan and McFadzean[89] noted a decrease in tumor fibrinolytic activity in patients with liver metastases and ascribed this phenomena to increased levels of fibrinolytic inhibitors that appear with liver involvement. Primary hyperfibrino(geno)lytic hemorrhage is treated with agents that inhibit the fibrinolytic system. My approach is to give epsilon-aminocaproic acid as an initial 5 to 10 g by slow intravenous push followed by 1 to 2 g/hour for 24 hours or until bleeding ceases.[28] At the end of 24 hours, the patient may be placed on oral therapy if necessary. Those using this agent should be aware of the hypotension, hypokalemia, and ventricular arrhythmias that may develop. Of course, the use of epsilon-aminocaproic acid is contraindicated in the patient with DIC.[18]

Platelets and Bleeding

Thrombocytopenia

Thrombocytopenia is clearly the most common cause of hemorrhage in patients with both solid tumors and hematologic malignancies.[142] In addition, thrombocytopenia is commonly the result of bone marrow suppression by radiation therapy, or chemotherapy; in this regard alkylating agents are clearly the worst offenders.[101,138] Drugs causing thrombocytopenia may be classified as mild, moderate, and severe. Thrombocytopenia also commonly results from bone marrow invasion by tumor and in general correlates well with the degree of marrow invasion.[48,109,142] Marrow metastases should be suspected and carefully searched for when unexplained thrombocytopenia develops in the patient with malignancy. This is accomplished by examination of the bone marrow aspirate or biopsy, although biopsy is much more reliable than a simple aspirate in detecting and evaluating bone marrow involvement by a carcinoma.[6,70,80,81,91]

In addition to bone marrow suppressive therapy and marrow metastases, cancer patients may develop other types of thrombocytopenia. When splenomegaly develops as a part of the malignant process, hypersplenism and subsequent thrombocytopenia may ensue.[71] Development of splenic metastases is more common than generally recognized, especially in carcinoma of the lung, breast, prostate, colon, and stomach.[104,108] This may lead to reactive hypersplenism and thrombocytopenia.[142] If clinically feasible, splenectomy may be of benefit in these situations. If splenectomy is considered, in an attempt to control thrombocytopenia secondary to hypersplenism, a preoperative infusion of epinephrine may be helpful in predicting the response to this rather heroic procedure in patients with disseminated malignancy.[15,16,20] When thrombocytopenia from decreased bone marrow production or increased splenic sequestration becomes significant, platelet concentrates provide the mainstay of management. Platelet counts below 10,000/mm^3 are commonly associated with spontaneous and serious hemorrhage, whereas platelet counts greater than 30,000/mm^3 are usually not associated with this complication unless the patient is challenged with trauma or surgical stress.[64] My general approach is to infuse platelet concentrates in most situations if the platelet count is less than 10,000/mm^3, unless the patient develops signs of bleeding above this level or when surgery or other invasive procedures are contemplated. Platelet concentrates are now readily available and provide the most efficient modality of platelet replacement therapy. An ideal platelet concentrate contains approximately 1.2×10^{11} platelets and in general 1 U of platelet concentrate will elevate the platelet count by about 5000 to 7000/mm^3 in an adult and by about 10,000 to 12,000/mm^3 in an infant. In practice, 6 to 8 U of platelet packs are usually administered to the severely thrombocytopenic adult every time the platelet count falls below 10,000/mm^3. Appropriately reduced numbers are used for children and infants.[75] If long-term platelet transfusions are anticipated and appropriate facilities are available HLA compatible platelets should be used if possible, especially in leukemia patients who may be candidates for bone marrow transplantation.[15,16]

ITP occasionally occurs in patients with solid tumors, but is more commonly noted in patients with lymphoreticular malignancies.[45] When ITP occurs in association with malignancy, the approach to management should be that generally used for this disorder, using steroids and possibly splenectomy if indicated and as outlined in Chapter 4. In cases of ITP that remain refractory to the usual forms of therapy, the use of intravenous vincristine or intravenous gamma globulin may be potentially useful.[2,103] Another type of increased platelet destruction that may be rarely associated with malignancy is thrombotic thrombocytopenia purpura.[36,116] This rare syndrome is commonly fatal when it develops in the cancer patient, but may respond to vigorous plasmapheresis, plasma exchange, or the use of intravenous prostacyclins,[116] as discussed in Chapter 4.

Platelet Function Defects

Abnormalities of platelet function are commonly found in association with both solid and hematologic malignancies. Because of relatively frequent episodes of intravascular coagulation and resulting elevated FDPs noted in cancer patients, the coating of platelet surfaces by these fragments probably constitutes the most common cause of platelet dysfunction in patients with malignancy.[15,16,27] However, additional platelet abnormalities are also noted in cancer patients. Platelet factor 3 is commonly decreased in patients with cancer.[61] Other platelet function defects have also been consistently noted in cancer patients and include defective platelet aggregation to ADP and other presumptive evidence of platelet dysfunction as manifested by a prolonged thromboplastin generation test, prolonged template bleeding times, positive tourniquet tests, and poor clot retraction.[48,61,126,139] It remains unclear whether these defects develop secondary to the malignancy itself, whether they come about from partial release of platelet contents after contact with malignant tissue, or whether they develop in response to activated clotting factors. The malignant paraprotein disorders are commonly associated with platelet function abnormalities that develop from coating of platelet surfaces by circulating immunoglobulins.[29,90] Consistent platelet aggregation abnormalities

are found in the myeloproliferative syndromes[1] and in preleukemia.[61] The exact significance of these numerous platelet function defects in contributing to hemorrhage in patients with solid tumors remains unclear. However, these platelet function defects may correlate better with the development of hemorrhage in cancer patients than does the actual platelet count.[61,126] At the very least, these defects must be presumed to be active in aggravating bleeding in cancer patients who have an already severely compromised hemostasis system or attendant thrombocytopenia.

Clinical clues to the existence of a platelet function defect include the noting of easy or spontaneous bruising, gingival bleeding, petechiae and purpura, and other minor forms of mucosal membrane bleeding when there is a normal platelet count. Also, a prolonged template bleeding time is a good screening test for the possibility of platelet dysfunction in patients with malignancy, and when noting a prolonged template bleeding time, platelet aggregation or lumiaggregation should be performed to delineate the type of defect, if it is present.[11] Unless secondary to intravascular coagulation, bleeding due to or aggravated by a platelet function defect requires platelet concentrate replacement therapy. This should be approached in essentially the same manner as that outlined for thrombocytopenia and is discussed in Chapter 4. In addition, the patient with malignancy and a documented associated platelet function defect should be strongly cautioned regarding the use of common drugs known to interfere with platelet function; for a complete list of these drugs the reader is referred to Chapter 4. Mechanisms of hemorrhage in disseminated malignancy are summarized in Table 10–8.

Defective Hemostasis in Malignant Paraprotein Disorders

Defects in hemostasis associated with malignant paraprotein disorders are well

Table 10–8 Hemorrhagic Syndromes in Disseminated Malignancy*

Thrombocytopenia
Disseminated intravascular coagulation
Decreased clotting factors
Primary fibrino(geno)lysis
Platelet dysfunction
Vascular defects
Circulating anticoagulants

* Listed in descending order of probability.

known, since these commonly lead to significant clinical hemorrhage and subsequent major management difficulties. Alterations of hemostasis in malignant paraprotein disorders are expressed as either hemorrhage, thrombosis, or a combination of the two; however, hemorrhage is much more common than thrombosis.[15,29]

The actual incidence of hemorrhage in malignant paraprotein disorders varies somewhat, depending on the particular disease present. Approximately 15% of patients with IgG myeloma experience hemorrhage, whereas those with IgA myeloma have a 40% incidence of hemorrhage.[15,29] In addition, patients with Waldenström's macroglobulinemia or IgM myeloma have a greater than 60% incidence of significant hemorrhage.[3,29,124]

There are numerous reasons for hemorrhage in patients with malignant paraprotein disorders, and some of these are not simply due to alterations of the hemostasis system. The most common reasons for hemorrhage are due to abnormalities in hemostasis, which are manifestations of circulating paraprotein and the mechanisms by which these paraproteins alter hemostasis will be subsequently discussed. In addition, uremia and attendant abnormal platelet function accounts for significant hemorrhage in many of these patients; also, liver failure or hypersplenism may be associated with defects in hemostasis in patients with malignant paraprotein disorders.[10,15,29] Hypersplenism is a frequent accompaniment of malignant paraprotein disorders, and significant thrombocytopenia due to splenic sequestration of platelets may reach alarming proportions. Many patients with malignant para-

protein disorders develop liver disease with resultant decreased synthesis of the prothrombin complex factors, abnormal fibrinogen (dysfibrinogenemia), abnormal fibrinolytic activity, and other coagulation protein defects associated with diffuse myelomatous involvement of the liver. DIC has been reported in myeloma and may account for significant hemorrhage in selected patients. Thrombocytopenia due to chemotherapy or radiation therapy may also lead to hemorrhage in patients with malignant paraprotein disorders. In addition, significant thrombocytopenia obviously may occur from bone marrow replacement and multiple myeloma, light chain disease, and Waldenström's macroglobulinemia.

Thrombocytopenia

Thrombocytopenia is commonly seen in malignant paraprotein disorders, but is often not pronounced enough to account for clinically significant bleeding. Thrombocytopenia can occur via several mechanisms in myeloma, primarily by the development of hypersplenism and increased platelet sequestration, liver disease, radiation therapy, chemotherapy, or bone marrow replacement, as previously discussed.

Platelet Function Defects

Platelet function defects are much more common causes of hemorrhage in malignant paraprotein disorders than is thrombocytopenia.[29] Many patients with multiple myeloma demonstrate a prolonged template bleeding time that correlates reasonably well with clinical bleeding; however, many patients will have normal or shortened bleeding times even with marked defects in platelet function. Platelet aggregation or lumiaggregation studies are usually markedly abnormal in most patients with circulating paraprotein, and these studies correlate reasonably well with predisposition to clinical hemorrhage.[15,29] Platelet aggregation abnormalities in a patient with multiple myeloma both pretherapy and after plasmapheresis are shown in Figures 10–1 and 10–2. Abnormalities of platelet func-

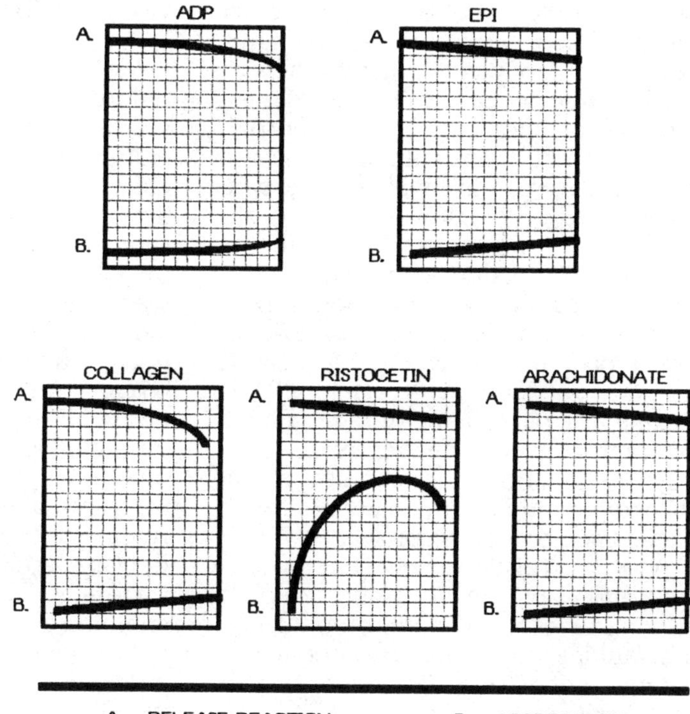

Fig. 10-1. Platelet function in myeloma before plasmapheresis. A: Release reaction; ADP: adenosine diphosphate; B: aggregation; EPI: epinephrine.

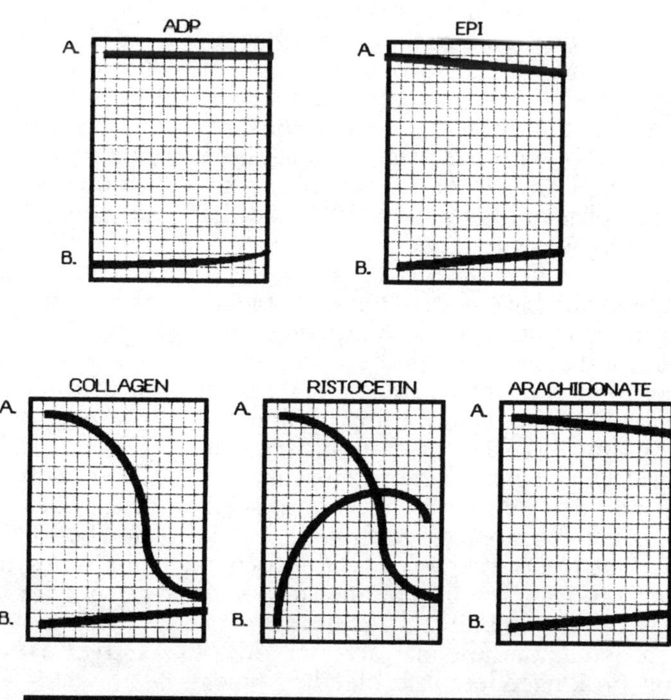

Fig. 10-2. Platelet function in myeloma after plasmapheresis. See Figure 10-1 for meaning of acronyms.

tion in multiple myeloma have not been clearly defined, but are most commonly due to coating of platelet membrane surfaces by paraprotein.[15,29] Platelet aggregation abnormalities are seen in approximately 80% of patients with myeloma and do not tend to correlate well with the type of paraprotein.[15,29] However, there appears to be some correlation with the quantity of paraprotein circulating. Platelet factor 3 release has been normal more often than abnormal in my patient population with myeloma and associated abnormal platelet lumiaggregation.[10] It is thought that platelet membrane coating by paraprotein is not a strict antigen-antibody reaction, but rather simply a chemical paraprotein-protein interaction with platelet membrane receptor sites. There is poor correlation between platelet aggregation abnormalities and template bleeding times in my patient population with multiple myeloma or other malignant paraprotein disorders. Up to 80% of patients with malignant paraprotein disorders have markedly abnormal aggregation and release; epinephrine-induced aggregation is abnormal in approximately 90% of patients, ADP-induced aggregation and release is abnormal in approximately 60% of patients, and collagen-induced aggregation is abnormal in approximately 60% of patients with malignant paraprotein disorders.[12] It appears that the most sensitive indicator of abnormal platelet aggregation in multiple myeloma is epinephrine-induced platelet aggregation.[15,29] It is of interest that some patients demonstrate markedly abnormal platelet lumiaggregation but will have normal template bleeding times and absence of clinical bleeding.

In addition to these there are other causes of abnormal platelet function. in multiple myeloma, including uremia, the development of liver disease, and circulating FDPs. Malignant paraproteins may coat the vasculature, interfere with normal endothelial function, or precipitate in the vasa vasorum, interfering with vascular function. Paraprotein may interfere with in vivo collagen-induced platelet aggregation, and all of these may account for not only prolonged template bleeding times, but also interference with the normal platelet-endothelial cell interaction.

Coagulation Proteins

Malignant paraprotein is known to interfere with a number of coagulation proteins. Probably the most publicized alteration of the coagulation system in malignant paraprotein disorders is the inhibition of a single specific clotting factor, such as Factor VIII:C. However, in reality, this phenomena is relatively rare and the least common cause of hemorrhage by paraprotein-coagulation protein interactions. When specific inhibition of blood coagulation factors by paraprotein does occur, it is usually somewhat selective; for example, IgG paraprotein is commonly directed against Factors II, VII, and X, or thrombin; alternatively IgA and IgM paraprotein is more commonly directed against the larger coagulation proteins, primarily Factors V and VIII:C activity. The most common coagulation protein interaction appears to be inhibition of fibrin monomer polymerization. It appears that paraprotein selectively attacks fibrin monomer and impedes polymerization into a stable fibrin clot. It is unclear if paraprotein coats the intact fibrinogen molecule and impedes the generation of fibrin monomer after exposure to thrombin, or, alternatively, if paraprotein attacks fibrin monomer only after its generation from fibrinogen.[29,90] It has been proposed, but not proved, that the Fab segment is the primary site of attachment to fibrin monomer by paraprotein. The noting of an abnormal thrombin time or reptilase time, which occurs in greater than 50% of patients, is a good indication of inhibition of fibrin monomer polymerization in paraprotein disorders and correlates reasonably well with clinical hemorrhage as a result of this phenomenon.[15,29] The presence of an abnormal thrombin time or reptilase time appears to be well correlated with clinical bleeding. However, there does not appear to be good correlation between abnormal prolonged thrombin times and reptilase times and the quantity or type of paraprotein present.

Other Defects

Chronic low-grade DIC is present in some patients with malignant paraprotein disorders, although this is relatively uncommon.[15,29] Also, enhanced fibrinolytic activity is present in a number of patients with malignant paraprotein disorders. This is manifested by the noting of circulating elevated FDPs, the presence of circulating plasmin, and the absence of soluble fibrin monomer complexes. The mechanism by which this occurs is unclear. To complicate these defects further, rare patients develop circulating heparinoids that have, on occasion, been responsible for severe terminal hemorrhage.[26,83,123]

Treatment of Hemorrhage in Malignant Paraprotein Disorders

Therapy of hemorrhage in patients with malignant paraprotein disorders presents difficult management problems. The exact alterations of hemostasis associated with hypersplenism, uremia, liver infiltration, and bone marrow infiltration are usually best controlled by appropriate management of the paraprotein disorder itself. This also applies to paraprotein inhibition of platelet function, coagulation protein defects, or interference by paraprotein of fibrin monomer polymerization. Often, these defects will correct somewhat, if not completely, with decreases in the myeloma cell population induced by chemotherapy or radiation therapy. When bleeding becomes of marked significance and rapid control of hemorrhage is desired, vigorous plasmapheresis is usually effective as a means for rapidly lowering the paraprotein concentration and restoring normal or near normal hemostasis.[140]

Effects of Chemotherapy on the Hemostasis System

Chemotherapeutic agents may alter hemostasis by a variety of mechanisms.[15] The most common and significant of these have been previously discussed and include the thrombocytopenia so commonly associated with bone marrow suppressive cytotoxic drugs as well, as the initiation of DIC or enhancement of DIC by cytotoxic drugs or hormones in both solid tumors and acute promyelocytic or myelomonocytic leukemia. Antineoplastic agents that may significantly interfere with hemostasis, along with their mechanisms, are listed in Table 10–9.

L-asparaginase therapy is commonly associated with significant hypofibrinogenemia, which is an almost universal complication of this drug. Although earlier investigators attributed this phenomena to decreased fibrinogen synthesis,[7] more recent studies have shown this to come about from the synthesis of functionally abnormal fibrinogen. This phenomena is thought probably to arise from reactions from L-asparaginase and asparagine residues of the fibrinogen molecule.[35] In addition, L-asparaginase may induce a DIC-type syndrome. Mithramycin therapy is also associated with hemorrhage in greater than 50% of patients receiving this drug; although this agent causes thrombocytopenia, hemorrhage is more likely thought to be the result of impaired platelet function, hyperfibrino(geno)lysis, and decreased levels of Factors II, V, VIII:C, and X.[15,111] When these findings are present, the triggering of DIC by Mithramycin seems a reasonable probability. Actinomycin D has also been associated with significant hemorrhage; this occurs because it is a potent vitamin K antagonist and the result of this, of course, is defective synthesis of Factors II, VII, IX, and X.[119] Use of doxorubicin[13] and Daunorubicin[14] has

Table 10–9 Antineoplastic Drugs Altering Hemostatis

Drug:	Mechanism:
Actinomycin-D	Vitamin K Antagonist
L-Asparaginase	Dysfibrinogenemia
	Hypofibrinogenemia
Melphalan	Platelet Dysfunction
	Hypofibrinogenemia
Mithramycin	Thrombocytopenia
	DIC Syndrome
Adriamycin	Primary Fibrinolysis
Daunomycin	Primary Fibrinolysis

also been associated with primary activation of the fibrinolytic system and subsequent clinical hemorrhage. Melphalan, cytosine arabinoside, daunorubicin, vincristine, and vinblastine induce platelet function defects; however, the clinical significance of these defects remains unclear at present with respect to clinically significant hemorrhage.[15,85]

Summary

As outlined, the patient with disseminated malignancy has many alterations of hemostasis. These are multifaceted and all of these defects must be taken into account when trying to control hemorrhage or thrombosis in cancer patients. In addition, hemorrhage or thrombosis is often the final clinical event in many patients with disseminated solid tumor or hematologic malignancies. Patients with malignancy present a major clinical challenge in this new era of oncologic awareness. More aggressive care has led to prolonged survival for patients and thus a longer time frame in which these complications may develop. Thus, these complications are occurring more commonly. It is important to realize that these alterations of hemostasis do exist and that they must be approached in a sequential and logical manner with respect to diagnosis. Only in this way can responsible, efficacious, and rational therapy be delivered to patients. By far the most common alteration of hemostasis in malignancy is that of hemorrhage associated with thrombocytopenia, either drug-induced, radiation-induced, or from bone marrow invasion. However, hemorrhage due to DIC is also quite common and may present as hemorrhage, thrombosis, thromboembolus, or any combination thereof. Many antineoplastic drugs as well as radiation therapy may lead to or significantly enhance hemorrhage in patients with malignancy. Thrombosis, which is also commonly seen in the patient with malignancy, is usually a low-grade DIC manifested as an intravascular thrombotic or thromboembolic event rather than an intravascular proteolytic

(hemorrhagic) event. When suspecting this, confirmatory laboratory evidence must be sought and the patient treated appropriately. When approaching the patient with malignancy and either hemorrhage or thrombosis, all of the potential defects in hemostasis must be taken into account, defined from the laboratory standpoint, and treated in as precise and logical manner as possible.

References

1. Adams T, Schultz L, Goldberg L: Platelet function abnormalities in the myeloproliferative disorders. Scand J Haematol 13:215, 1974.
2. Ahn YS, Harrington WJ, Seelman RC: Vincristine therapy of idiopathic and secondary thrombocytopenias. N Engl J Med 291:376, 1974.
3. Amundsen MA, Spitell JA, Thompson JH: Hypercoagulability associated with malignant disease and with the postoperative state. Ann Intern Med 58:608, 1963.
4. Astedt B, Svanberg L, Nilsson IM: Cancer, FDP, and radiotherapy. Br Med J 2:47, 1972.
5. Bennett RM: Acute leukemia. In: Rappaport H (Ed): Proc Tutorial in Hematopathology. University of Chicago Press, Chicago, 1980.
6. Berkheiser SW: The incidence of malignant cells in routine bone marrow examination. Cancer 8:958, 1955.
7. Bettigole RF, Himelstein ES, Oettgen HF: Hypofibrinogenemia due to L-asparaginase: Studies of fibrinogen survival using autologous ^{131}I-fibrinogen. Blood 35:195, 1970.
8. Biben RL, Tyan ML: Hemorrhagic diathesis in carcinoma of the stomach: A case report. Ann Intern Med 17:917, 1958.
9. Bick RL, Adams T: Fibrinolytic activity in myeloproliferative disorders. Clin Res 21:264, 1963.
10. Bick RL: Treatment of bleeding and thrombosis in the patient with cancer. In Nealon T (Ed): Management of the Patient with Cancer. W.B. Saunders, Philadelphia, 1976, p 48.
11. Bick RL, Adams T, Schmalhorst WR: Bleeding times, platelet adhesion, and aspirin. Am J Clin Pathol 65:69, 1976.
12. Bick RL, Klein CA, Fekete LF: Alterations of hemostasis associated with malignant paraprotein disorders. Trans Am Soc Hematol 1976, p 163.
13. Bick RL, Fekete LF, Wilson WL: Adriamycin and fibrinolysis. Thromb Res 8:467, 1976.

14. Bick RL, Fekete L, Murano G: Daunomycin and fibrinolysis. Thromb Res 9:201, 1976.

15. Bick, RL: Alterations of hemostasis associated with malignancy: Etiology, pathophysiology, diagnosis and management. Semin Thromb Hemost 5:1, 1978.

16. Bick RL: Alterations of hemostasis associated with malignancy. In Murano G, Bick RL (Eds): Basic Concepts of Hemostasis and Thrombosis. CRC Press, Boca Raton, FL, 1980, p 213.

17. Bick RL: Clinical relevance of antithrombin III. Semin Thromb Hemost 8:276, 1982.

18. Bick RL: Disseminated intravascular coagulation. In Bick RL (Ed): Disseminated Intravascular Coagulation and Related Syndromes. CRC Press, Boca Raton, FL, 1983, p 31.

19. Bick RL, Wilson WL: Essential (hemorrhagic) thrombocythemia: A clinical and laboratory study of 14 patients. Am J Clin Pathol 81:799, 1984.

20. Bick RL: Disseminated intravascular coagulation and related syndromes. In Murano G, Bick RL (Eds): Basic Concepts of Hemostasis and Thrombosis. CRC Press, Boca Raton, FL, 1980, p 163.

21. Bick RL: Disseminated intravascular coagulation and related syndromes. A review. Am J Hematol 5:265, 1978.

22. Bick RL: Basic mechanisms of hemostasis pertaining to DIC. In Bick RL (ed): Disseminated Intravascular Coagulation and Related Syndromes. CRC Press, Boca Raton, FL, 1983, p 1.

23. Bick RL: Alterations of hemostasis associated with surgery, cardiopulmonary bypass surgery, and prosthetic devices. In Ratnoff OD, Forbes CD (Eds): Disorders of Hemostasis. Grune & Stratton, New York, 1984, p 379.

24. Bick RL: Disseminated intravascular coagulation: A clinical/laboratory study of 48 patients. Ann NY Acad Sci 370:843, 1981.

25. Bick RL, Schmalhorst WR, Shanbrom E: Prothrombin complex concentrates: Use in controlling the hemorrhagic diathesis of chronic liver disease. Am J Dig Dis 20:741, 1975.

26. Bick RL: Circulating heparin activity in multiple myeloma. Blood 64:924, 1984.

27. Bick RL: The clinical significance of fibrinogen degradation products. Semin Thromb Hemost 8:302, 1982.

28. Bick RL: Syndromes associated with hyperfibrino(geno)lysis. In Bick RL (ed): Disseminated Intravascular Coagulation and Related Syndromes. CRC Press, Boca Raton, FL, 1983, p 105.

29. Bick RL: Acquired circulating anticoagulants and defective hemostasis in malignant paraprotein disorders. In Murano G, Bick RL (Eds): Basic Concepts of Hemostasis and Thrombosis. CRC Press, Boca Raton, FL, 1980, p 205.

30. Boggs DR, Wintrobe MM, Cartwright CE: Acute leukemias: Analysis of 322 cases and review of the literature. Medicine (Baltimore) 41:163, 1962.

31. Boggust WA, O'Brien DJ, O'Meara RA: The coagulative factors of normal human and human cancer tissue. Ir J Med Sci 6:131, 1963.

32. Boughton BJ, Simpson A: Plasma fibronectin in acute leukemia. Br J Haematol 51:487, 1982.

33. Brakman P, Snyder J, Henderson ES, Astrup T: Blood coagulation and fibrinolysis in acute leukemia. Br J Haematol 18:135, 1970.

34. Brassinne C, Coone A, Jijs M, Tagnon HJ: Characterization of two direct fibrinogenolytic activities and one proteolytic inhibitor activity in the human prostate. Thromb Res 8:803, 1976.

35. Brodsky I, Conroy JF: The effects of chemotherapy on hemostasis. Cancer Chemother 2: 85, 1972.

36. Brook J, Konwaler BE: Thrombotic thrombocytopenic purpura: Association with metastatic gastric carcinoma and a possible auto-immune disorder. Calif Med 102:222, 1965.

37. Brown RC, Campbell DC, Thompson JH: Increased fibrinolysin with malignant disease. Arch Intern Med 109:129, 1962.

38. Bull B, Rubenberg M, Dacie J, Brain MC: Microangiopathic hemolytic anemia: Mechanisms of red-cell fragmentation. Br J Haematol 14:643, 1968.

39. Bussel JB, Steinherz PG, Miller DR, Hilgartner MW: A heparin-like anticoagulant in an 8-month-old boy with acute monoblastic leukemia. Am J Hematol 16:83, 1984.

40. Caen J, Sinakoz Z, Sultan V, Uainer H, Bernard J: Les troubles du functionnement des plaquettes dans les leukemies myeloides chroniques. Nouv Rev Fr Hematol 6:719, 1966.

41. Cardamone JM, Edson J, McArthur JK, Jacob HS: Abnormalities of platelet function in the myeloproliferative disorders. JAMA 221:270, 1972.

42. Cheung DK, Raaf JH: Selection of patients with malignant ascites for a peritoneovenous shunt. Cancer 50: 1204, 1982.

43. Choate JJ, Mosher DF: Fibronectin concentration in plasma of patients with breast cancer, colon cancer, and acute leukemia. Cancer 51:1142, 1983.

44. Cliffton EE, Grossi CE: Fibrinolytic activity of human tumors as measured by the fibrinplate method. Cancer 8:1146, 1955.

45. Cocking JB: Thrombocytopenic purpura with bronchogenic carcinoma. Postgrad Med J 42:521, 1966.

46. Cooperberg AA, Neiman GMA: Fibrinogenopenia and fibrinolysis in acute myelogenous leukemia. Ann Intern Med 42:706,

1955.

47. Cowan DM, Haut MJ: Platelet function in acute leukemia. J Lab Clin Med 79:893, 1972.

48. Davis RB, Theologides A, Kennedy BJ: Comparative studies of blood coagulation and platelet aggregation in patients with cancer and non-malignant disease. Ann Intern Med 71:67, 1969.

49. Didisheim P, Bowie EJW, Owen CA: Intravascular coagulation fibrinolysis (ICF) syndrome and malignancy: Historical review and report of two cases with metastatic carcinoid and with acute myelomonocytic leukemia. Thromb Diath Haemorrh 36:215, 1969.

50. Diebold J, Camilieri TP, Delarue J: Les lesions hepatiques au cours des leucoses. Etude histopathologique. Ann Anat Pathol 14:41, 1969.

51. Douglas JT, Lowe GDO, Forbes CD, Prentice CRM: Beta-thromboglobulin and platelet counts: Effect of malignancy, infection, age, and obesity. Thromb Res 25:459, 1982.

52. Edwards EA: Migrating thrombophlebitis associated with carcinoma. N Engl J Med 240:1031, 1949.

53. Eiseman G, Stefanini M: Thromboplastic activity of leukemic white cells. Proc Soc Exp Biol Med 86:763, 1954.

54. Enck RE, Rios CN: Tamoxifen treatment of metastatic breast cancer and antithrombin III levels. Cancer 53:2607, 1984.

55. Evans HE, Wolman IJ: Problems in the diagnosis and management of acute leukemia in childhood. Clin Pediatr 10:571, 1971.

56. Fareed J, Walenga JM, Bick RL, Bermes EJ, Messmore HL: Impact of automation on the quantitation of low molecular weight markers of hemostatic defects. Semin Thromb Hemost 9:355, 1983.

57. Fisch C, Jones AW, Gambill WD: Acute thrombophlebitis associated with carcinoma of the stomach. Gastroenterology 18:290, 1951.

58. Fisher S, Ramot B, Kreisler B: Fibrinolysis in acute leukemia. Isr Med J 19:195, 1960.

59. Folkman J: Tumor angiogenesis: Therapeutic implications. N Engl J Med 285:1182, 1971.

60. Frick PG: Acute hemorrhagic syndrome with hypofibrinogenemia in metastatic cancer. Acta Haematol (Basel) 16:11, 1956.

61. Friedman IA, Schwartz SO, Leifhold SL: Platelet function defects with bleeding. Arch Intern Med 113:177, 1964.

62. Fumarola D, del Bono G: The blood coagulation patterns in malignancy. Prog Med Napoli 14:327, 1958.

63. Galloway MJ, Mackie MJ, McVerry BA: Combinations of increased thrombin, plasmin, and non-specific protease activity in patients with acute leukemia. Haemostasis 13:322, 1983.

64. Garner GF: Platelet transfusion. In Baldini MG, Elbe S (Eds): Platelets: Production, Function and Storage. Grune & Stratton, New York, 1974, p 393.

65. Girolami A, Cliffton EE: Fibrinolytic and proteolytic activity in acute and chronic leukemia. Am J Med Sci 51:638, 1966.

66. Goodnight SH: Bleeding and intravascular clotting in malignancy: A review. Ann NY Acad Sci 230:271, 1974.

67. Gralnick HR, Tan HK: Acute promyelocytic leukemia. A model for understanding the role of the malignant cells in hemostasis. Hum Pathol 5:661, 1974.

68. Gralnick HR, Bagley J, Abrell E: Heparin treatment for the hemorrhagic diathesis of acute promyelocytic leukemia. Am J Med 52:167, 1974.

69. Han T, Stutzman L, Cohen E, Kim U: Effect of platelet transfusion on hemorrhage in patients with acute leukemia. Cancer 19;1937, 1966.

70. Hansen HH, Muggia FM, Selawry OS: Bone marrow examination in 100 consecutive patients with bronchogenic carcinoma. Lancet 1:443, 1971.

71. Harker LA, Finch CA: Thrombokinetics in man. J Clin Invest 48:963, 1969.

72. Harmon DC, Demirjian Z, Ellman L, Fischer J: Disseminated intravascular coagulation with the peritoneovenous shunt. Ann Intern Med 90:714, 1979.

73. Henderson ES: Acute myelogenous leukemia. In Williams WJ, Beutler E, Erslev AJ, Rundles RW (Eds): Hematology. McGraw Hill, New York, 1977, p 830.

74. Hersh EM, Bodey GP, Nies BA, Freireich EJ: Causes of death in acute leukemia: A ten year study of 414 patients from 1954-1963. JAMA 193:105, 1965.

75. Heustis DW, Bove JR, Busch S: Practical blood transfusion. Little, Brown, Boston, 1969.

76. Holt JM, Gordon-Smith EG: Retinal abnormalities in diseases of the blood. Br J Opthalmol 53:145, 1969.

77. Huth K, Loffler H, Lechlemayer U: Verbrauchskoagulopathie bei unreifzelligen Keukosen. Verh Dtsch Ges Inn Med 74:147, 1968.

78. Ikkala E: Transfusion therapy in congenital deficiencies of plasma factor XIII. Ann NY Acad Sci 202:200, 1972.

79. Innerfield I, Anrist A, Benjamin JW: Plasma antithrombin patterns in disturbances of the pancreas. Gastroenterology 19:843, 1951.

80. Jamshidi K, Swaim WR: Bone marrow biopsy with unaltered architecture: A new biopsy device. J Lab Clin Med 77:335, 1971.

81. Jonsson U, Rundles RW: Tumor metastases in bone marrow. Blood 6:16, 1951.

82. Kakkar VV, Howie CT, Nicolaides AN: Deep

vein thrombosis of the leg: Is there a "high risk" group. Am J Surg 120:527, 1970.

83. Khooray MS, Nesheim ME, Bowie EJW, Mann KG: Circulating heparan sulfate proteoglycan anticoagulant from a patient with a plasma cell disorder. J Clin Invest 65:666, 1980.

84. Kirchmayer S, Stalowa I, Biernacka B, Slizowska H: Measurements of proteolytic activity of leukoblasts—a new diagnostic method. Pol Arch Med Wewn 44:365, 1970.

85. Klener P, Kubisz P, Suranova J: Influence of cytotoxic drugs on platelet functions and coagulation. Thromb Hemost 37:53, 1977.

86. Kremer WB, Laszlo J: Hematologic effects of cancer. In Holland JF, Frei E (Eds): Cancer Medicine. Lea & Febiger, Philadelphia, 1973, p 1965.

87. Kumar S, Monorama B: Pre-leukemic acute myelogenous leukemia. Acta Haematol (Basel) 3:21, 1970.

88. Kuznik BI, Kuzmiehco EL, Alnikov GP: On the role of leukocytes in the process of blood coagulation in chronic lymphocytic leukemia. Probl Gematol Pereliv Krovi 14:3, 1969.

89. Kwaan HC, Lo R, McFadzean AJS: Antifibrinolytic activity in primary carcinoma of the liver. Clin Sci 18:251, 1959.

90. Lachner H: Hemostatic abnormalities associated with dysproteinemias. Semin Hematol 10:125, 1973.

91. Lanier PF: Sternal marrow in patients with metastatic cancer. Arch Intern Med 84:891, 1949.

92. Leavy RA, Kahn SD, Brodsky I: Disseminated intravascular coagulation: A complication of chemotherapy in acute promyelocytic leukemia. Cancer 26:142, 1970.

93. Lerner RG, Nelson JC, Corines P, del Guercio LRM: Disseminated intravascular coagulation: Complication of LeVeen peritoneovenous shunts. JAMA 240:2064, 1984.

94. Levin J, Conley CL: Thrombocytosis associated with malignant disease. Arch Intern Med 114:487, 1964.

95. Lisiewicz J: Mechanisms of hemorrhage in leukemias. Semin Thromb Hemost 4:241, 1978.

96. Lisiewicz J: Acute leukemias. In Hemorrhage in Leukemias. Polish Medical Publishers, Warsaw, 1976, p 51.

97. Lisiewicz J: Chronic granulocytic leukemia. In Hemorrhage in Leukemias. Polish Med Publishers, Warsaw, 1976, p 82.

98. Lisiewicz J: Chronic lymphocytic leukemia. In Hemorrhage in Leukemias. Polish Med Publishers, Warsaw, 1976, p 104.

99. Lisiewicz J, Moszcynski P: Disturbances of hemostasis in patients with various leukemia types in the light of results of basic tests of

blood coagulation and fibrinolysis. Przegl Lek 29:389, 1972.

100. Lisiewicz J, Moszcynski P: Leukocytois and fibrinolytic activity of the blood in the leukemic patients. Rev Med Interna 1:37, 1975.

101. Livingston RB, Carter SK: Single agents in cancer chemotherapy. Plenum Press, New York, 1970.

102. Marguliusa A, Jackson DP, Ratnoff OD: Circulating anticoagulants: A study of 40 cases and review of the literature. Medicine (Baltimore) 40:145, 1961.

103. Marmont AM, Damasio EE, Gori E: Vinblastine sulfate in idiopathic thrombocytopenic purpura. Lancet 2:94, 1971.

104. Marymount JH, Gross S: Patterns of metastatic cancer in the spleen. Am J Clin Pathol 40:58, 1963.

105. Matsuoka M, Onishi Y: Pathologic cells as procoagulant substances of disseminated intravascular coagulation syndrome in acute promyelocytic leukemia. Thromb Res 8:263, 1976.

106. Mersky C: Altered blood coagulability in patients with malignant tumors. Ann NY Acad Sci 230:289, 1974.

107. Mertins BF, Green LF, Bowie EJW, Elveback LR, Owen CA: Fibrinolytic split products and ethanol gelation test in pre-operative evaluation of patients with prostatic disease. Mayo Clin Proc 49:642, 1974.

108. Miale JB: Laboratory medicine hematology. C.V. Mosby, St. Louis, 1972, p 53.

109. Miller SP, Sanchez-Avalos J, Stefanski T: Coagulation disorders in cancer I Clinical and laboratory studies. Cancer 20:1452, 1967.

110. Miyagawa K, Kawakita Y: Ultrastructure of blood platelets in various hematologie disorders. Acta Haematol Jpn 32:64, 1969.

111. Monto RW, Talley RW, Caldwell MJ: Observation on the mechanisms of hemorrhagic toxicity in mithramycin therapy. Cancer Res 29:697, 1969.

112. Moolton SE, Vroman L, Broman GMS: Role of blood platelets in thromboembolism. Arch Intern Med 84:667, 1949.

113. Morrison M: An analysis of the blood picture in 100 cases of malignancy. J Lab Clin Med 17:1071, 1932.

114. Moszczynski P, Lisiewicz J: The liver function in leukemic patients in the light of enzymatic studies. Pol Tyg Lek 29:1925, 1974.

115. Moszczynski P, Lisiewicz J: Early symptoms of acute and chronic leukemias in 300 patients. Med Wiejska 8:249, 1973.

116. Nalbandian RM, Henry RL, Bick RL: Thrombotic thrombocytopenic purpura. Semin Thromb Hemost 5:216, 1979.

117. Nenci GG, Berrettini M, Parise P, Agnelli G: Persistent spontaneous heparinemia in sys-

temic mastocytosis. Folia Haematol (Leipz) 109:453, 1982.

118. Nussbaum M, Morse BS: Plasma fibrin stabilizing factor activity in various diseases. Blood 23:669, 1964.

119. Olson RE: Vitamin K-induced prothrombin formation antagonism by actinomycin-D. Science 145:926, 1964.

120. Omar JB, Saxena HS, Mitel HS: Fibrinolytic activity in malignant diseases. J Assoc Physicians India 19:293, 1971.

121. O'Meara RAQ: Coagulation properties of cancers. Ir J Med Sci 394:474, 1958.

122. Owen CA, Oels HC, Bowie EJW: Chronic intravascular coagulation syndrome. Thromb Diath Haemorrh 36:197, 1969.

123. Palmer RN, Rick ME, Rick PD, Zeller JA, Gralnick HR: Circulating heparan sulfate anticoagulant in a patient with a fatal bleeding disorder. N Engl J Med 310:1696, 1984.

124. Perkins HA, Mackenzie MR, Fudenberg HH: Hemostatic defects in dysproteinemias. Blood 35:695, 1970.

125. Perlow S, Daniels JL: Venous thrombosis and obscure abdominal malignancy. Arch Intern Med 97:184, 1956.

126. Perry S: Coagulation defects in leukemia. J Lab Clin Med 50:229, 1957.

127. Phillips LL, Skrodelis V, Furey CA: The fibrinolytic enzyme system in prostatic cancer. Cancer 12:721, 1959.

128. Pineo GF, Brain MC, Gallus AS: Tumors, mucus production, and hypercoagulability. Ann NY Acad Sci 230:262, 1974.

129. Pineo GF, Regorczi F, Hatton MWC: The activation of coagulation by extracts of mucin: A possible pathway of intravascular coagulation accompanying adenocarcinomas. J Lab Clin Med 82:255, 1973.

130. Pisciotta AV, Schulz EJ: Fibrinolytic purpura in acute leukemia. Am J Med 19:824, 1955.

131. Polliack A: Acute promyelocytic leukemia with disseminated intravascular coagulation. Am J Clin Pathol 56:155, 1971.

132. Qazi R, Savlov ED: Peritoneovenous shunt for palliation of malignant ascites. Cancer 49:600, 1982.

133. Rapaport SI, Chapman CG: Coexist hypercoagulability and acute hypofibrinogenemia in a patient with prostatic carcinoma. Am J Med 27:144, 1959.

134. Rickles FR, Edwards RL, Barb C, Cronlund M: Abnormalities of blood coagulation in patients with cancer. Fibrinopeptide A generation and tumor growth. Cancer 51:301, 1983.

135. Rodeghiero F, Mannucci PM, Vigano S, Barbui T, Gugliotta L, Cortellaro M, Dini E: Liver dysfunction rather than intravascular coagulation as the main cause of low Protein C and anti-

136. Rosner F, Dobbs JV, Ritz DN, Lee SL: Disturbances of hemostasis in acute myeloblastic leukemia. Acta Haematol (Basel) 43:65, 1970.

137. Rosove MH: Hematologic complications of cancer and its treatment. In Haskell CM (Ed): Cancer Treatment. W.B. Saunders, Philadelphia, 1985, p 864.

138. Rubin P, Casareh GW: Clinical radiation pathology. W.B. Saunders, Philadelphia, 1968, p 778.

139. Sanchez-Avalos J, Soong BCF, Miller SP: Coagulation disorders in cancer. II. Multiple myeloma. Cancer 23:1388, 1969.

140. Schwab PJ, Fahey JL: Treatment of Waldenstroms macroglobulinemia by plasmapheresis. N Engl J Med 263:574, 1960.

141. Shustrova NM: On the permeability of vascular walls in some disorders of the blood system. Doctoral Dissertation Alma-Ata, Russia, 1965.

142. Slickter SJ, Harker LA: Hemostasis in malignancy. Ann NY Acad Sci 230:252, 1974.

143. Soong BCF, Miller SP: Coagulation disorders in cancer: Fibrinolysis and inhibitors. Cancer 25:867, 1970.

144. Sproul EF: Carcinoma and venous thrombosis: The frequency of association of carcinoma in the body or tail of the pancreas with multiple venous thrombosis. Am J Cancer 34:566, 1938.

145. Stein SF, Fulenwider JT, Ansley JD, Evatt BL, Nordlinger B, McLemore P, Scwotzer L, Wideman CS: Accelerated fibrinogen and platelet destruction after peritoneovenous shunting. Arch Intern Med 141:1149, 1981.

146. Sultan Y, Delobel J, Caen J: Anomalies de l'hemostase primaire au cours de leucemies myeloides chroniques et des autres syndromes myeloproliferatifs. Actual hematol 3:95, 1969.

147. Sultan C, Gounault M, Varet B: Relationship between the cell morphology of acute myeloblastic leukemia and occurrence of a syndrome of disseminated intravascular coagulation. Proceedings of the XIV International Congress of Hematology, Sau Paulo, (Abstr.), 1972, p 603.

148. Sznajd J, Naskalski J, Liciewicz J: Antiheparin activity of myeloperoxidase and ribonuclease of chronic granulocytic leukemia leukocytes. Pol Arch Med Wewn 42:207, 1969.

149. Tatarsky J, Sinakos Z, Larrieu MJ, Bernard J: Leukocytes et fibrinolyse. II. Etudes des leukocytes pathologiques. Nouv Rev Fr Hematol 7:95, 1967.

150. Trousseau A: Phlegmasia alba dolens. Clinique Medicale de L'Hotel Dieu de Paris 3. Edition 2, Balliere, Paris, 1865.

151. Trunova LE: The pathogenesis of the hemor-

rhagic system in acute leukemia. Vrach Delo 11:41, 1965.

152. Valkov J: Histologic studies of extramedullary hemopoiesis in leukemias and its relationship to the blood vessels. Med Fizkult 42:35, 1963.

153. van Creveld J, Mochtar JA: Fibrinolysis in acute leukemia. Pediatr Ann 194:65, 1960.

154. Wado H, Nagano T, Tomeoku M, Kuto M, Karitani Y, Deguchi K, Shirakawa S: Coagulant and fibrinolytic activities in the leukemic cell lysates. Thromb Res 30:315, 1982.

155. Walenga JM, Fareed J, Mariani G, Messmore HL, Bick RS, Emanuele RM: Diagnostic efficacy of a simple radioimmunoassay test for fibrinogen/fibrin fragments containing the B-beta 15-42 sequence. Semin Thromb Hemost 10:252, 1984.

156. Yip ML, Lee S, Sacks HJ: Nonspecificity of the protamine test for intravascular coagulation. Am J Clin Pathol 57:487, 1972.

157. Yodo Y, Abe T: Fibrinopeptide A (FPA) level and fibrinogen kinetics in patients with malignant disease. Thromb Haemost 46:706, 1981.

158. Zighelboim J, Foon KA, Gale RP, Haskell CM: Acute myelogenous leukemia. In Haskell CM (Ed): Cancer Treatment. W.B. Saunders, Philadelphia, 1985, p 694.

11
Clinical Approach to the Patient with Thrombosis, Thromboembolus, and Pulmonary Embolus

Thrombosis, thromboembolus, and pulmonary embolus are major clinical problems seen in a wide variety of clinical practices. Pulmonary embolus remains a major cause of death in the United States, and thus it is extremely important to diagnose quickly those individuals who are predisposed to or who have thrombosis and thromboembolus and to institute treatment. As in all areas of medicine, a thorough clinical evaluation of the patient remains the mainstay of diagnosis and only after this should laboratory, radiographic, nuclear imaging and invasive techniques, including angiography, be performed. Only in the appropriate clinical setting can the results of these ancillary tests be correctly interpreted and a specific diagnosis made, resulting in specific, efficacious, and rapid therapy.

History Taking

When evaluating the patient with a predisposition to thrombus formation or a suspected thrombotic event, it is important to first elicit a chief complaint, including an in-detail inquiry about symptoms and how long the symptoms have been present. Following this, one must carefully question the patient about associated disease conditions, with particular emphasis on those known to be associated with an increased predisposition to venous or arterial thrombotic events. Of particular importance with respect to increased risk of venous thrombotic events are oral contraceptive use, obesity, sustained hypertension, a history of malignancy, a history of abdominal, thoracic, obstetrical, or orthopedic surgery, pregnancy, the pre-

sence or absence of heart disease, a past history of venous thrombosis, chronic venous insufficiency, varicosities, and the possibility of stigmata of other rarer predisposing disorders, such as Behçet's syndrome and cystathionine beta-synthase deficiency. If suspecting a predisposition to arterial thrombotic events, the patient should be carefully questioned about the presence or absence of ischemic heart disease, hypertension, hypercholesterolemia, hyperlipidemia, obesity, smoking history, hyperglycemia, peripheral vascular vaso-occlusive disease, a history of myocardial infarction, angina, high dietary fat intake, lack of exercise, and the use of oral contraceptives, both estrogenic and progestational. In addition, the sex of the patient may be relevant.

After this careful inquiry about associated disease conditions that are known to be associated with an increased predisposition to venous or arterial thrombotic events, the patient must be carefully questioned about any regular drug intake, with particular attention to the use of contraceptive agents. In addition, a history should be elicited regarding the use of aspirin, aspirin-containing compounds, antihypertensives, cough medications, digitalis, hormones, cortisone, diabetic medications, thyroid medications, analgesics, weight reducing pills, anticoagulants, phenytoin, diuretics, antibiotics, barbiturates, tranquilizers, or antidepressants.

The presence or absence of a medical history of angina, coronary artery disease, heart disease, diabetes, emphysema, recurrent bronchitis, recurrent pneumonia, asthma, tuberculosis, herpes zoster, measles, mumps, chickenpox, rheumatic fever, scarlet fever, hepatitis, peptic ulcer disease, liver disease, jaundice, renal disease, hives, venereal disease, anemia, seizures, or mental disease, as well as a history of chronic venous insufficiency, any type of arterial or venous thrombotic event, or of varicosities should be elicited and recorded. A very thorough surgical history should also be obtained, especially of the immediate past, for abdominal, thoracic, gynecologic, or orthopedic surgery. The patient should also be carefully questioned about any recent injuries or accidents, especially those involving the extremities or chest. The patient should be asked about any known allergy to medications or any other agents

Following this, a very careful review of systems should be taken, as discussed in Chapter 2.

In the female patient the date of the last Papanicolaou smear should be obtained. Following this, a pregnancy history should be taken including the number of pregnancies, miscarriages, premature births, children born alive and stillborns, abortions, number and nature of cesarean sections, and any potential complications of pregnancy, including any suggestion of preeclampsia or eclampsia, the nature of the blood pressure during these episodes, and any thrombotic problems.

The details of a personal and family history are given in Chapter 2.

Physical Examination

The physical examination should begin with a careful evaluation of the body habitus and general health, the noting of the presence or absence of obesity, muscle wasting, skin complexion, skin turgor, and the presence or absence of good hygiene. The vital signs should be recorded, including the height, weight, body surface area, temperature, sitting, standing, and supine blood pressure, and careful recording of the pulse and the noting of the character and regularity of the pulse. Next, the head is examined carefully, searching for any subcutaneous nodules in the scalp and an evaluation of occipital, cervical, submental, or supraclavicular lymphadenopathy. The pupils

should be evaluated for reactivity to light and accommodation and the conjunctivae carefully evaluated. The equality of the pupils should be recorded. A careful funduscopic examination should be performed; if suspecting a pulmonary embolus, the noting of retinal venous dilation is indicative of pulmonary artery pressure of greater than 30 mm Hg. Hearing should be carefully checked with both Weber and Rinne testing; Weber testing may lateralize in the presence of transient ischemic attacks, small stroke syndromes, or a frank cerebral vascular thrombotic event. The oral mucosa should be carefully examined, including the sublingual area for vascular anamolies. Additionally, the carotid pulses should be evaluated and auscultated for the presence or absence of bruits. The noting of jugular venous distention is suggestive of a pulmonary artery pressure of greater than 30 to 35 mm Hg and is suggestive of a large pulmonary embolus in the appropriate clinical setting. Next the patient should be evaluated for sternal, rib, cervical, thoracic, and lumbosacral spine tenderness. The chest should be carefully aus cultated and percussed and diaphragmatic excursion should be documented. The usual physical findings of a patient with a pulmonary embolus may be normal, or one may note findings compatible with pleural effusion, and there may be tachypnea, localized inspiratory wheezing, rhonchi, rales, pleural friction rub, or findings of consolidation. There may be increased tactile fremitus, dullness to percussion, or tubular breathing sounds.

A careful evaluation of the heart should be performed with careful recording of the heart sounds, the presence or absence of murmurs, and the presence or absence of findings suggestive of acute cor pulmonale, including a right ventricular heave, a right-sided gallop, accentuated second heart sound, or a murmur of tricuspid insufficiency. Again, the presence or absence of distended jugular veins and a positive hepatojugular reflex should be recorded when suspecting a pulmonary embolus. The finding of these is strongly suggestive of pulmonary artery pressure that is increased. Following evaluation of the heart and heart sounds, one should evaluate the peripheral pulses, including the brachial, radial, ulnar, and femoral. Both the femoral arteries and the aorta should also be auscultated for the presence or absence of murmurs. The popliteal, posterior tibial, and dorsalis pedis pulses are usually evaluated at the same time as the extremities.

Following the cardiorespiratory evaluation the abdomen should be evaluated for the presence or absence of tenderness, normal bowel sounds, hepatomegaly, hepatic tenderness, splenomegaly, splenic tenderness, costovertebral angle tenderness or bruits, or any abdominal masses. A careful rectal examination is performed unless there is a contraindication to this. In this regard it is important to record the presence or absence of prostatic enlargement and localized tenderness. The genitalia are thoroughly examined.

Evaluation of the extremities is very important in a patient with suspected venous thrombosis, since the physical findings of deep vein thrombosis are somewhat unreliable; however, their reliability is markedly enhanced by careful and specific evaluation. The presence or absence of findings of chronic venous insufficiency, including varicosities, ankle edema, and chronic hemosiderin deposits should be carefully searched for and noted if found. Additionally, the popliteal, dorsalis pedis, and posterior tibial pulses should be evaluated for their presence and character. The toes should be carefully inspected for evidence of pallor, cyanosis, chronic ulcerative changes, or chronic atrophic changes suggestive of chronic vascular insufficiency. The inguinal areas, anterior medial thighs, popliteal fossae, and calfs should be carefully evaluated for evidence of erythema, tenderness, swelling, hyperpyrexia, or the demonstration of a frank venous cord. In this regard the palpation of a distinct cord is the more reliable physical finding of a venous thrombus; however, the findings of a demonstrable increase in diameter of the calf, popliteal area, or thigh and associated edema are also reliable findings. Alternatively, the presence or absence of Homans sign is not highly reliable. It must be remembered that with significant venous thrombosis there may be a compartmental compression syndrome either anterior tibial,

posterior tibial, or of the thigh, which results in arterial compromise, as well as in the sharp pain, cyanosis, redness, swelling, tenderness of a cord noted in association with venous disease and interference with arterial vascular flow leading to more cyanosis, pallor, exaggerated swelling, and a dull persistent ache in conjunction with decreased or absent pulses by palpation. These pulses, however, are usually demonstrable by Doppler.

Examination of the integument and the neurologic examination are described in Chapter 2.

Ancillary studies are often necessary when dealing with patients who are hypercoagulable or are suspected of having venous or arterial thrombotic or thromboembolic events or pulmonary embolus. With respect to pulmonary embolus, diagnostic aids are readily available, which need to be interpreted in the appropriate clinical setting. Usually one will note elevated enzymes, including lactate dehydrogenase, SGOT, and creatine phosphokinase; however, these are nonspecific findings, although nearly 90% of patients with a pulmonary embolus will have a partial oxygen pressure of less than 80 mm Hg. Other laboratory tests that are often positive are elevated fibrin(ogen) degradation products and soluble fibrin monomer, and elevated fibrinopeptide A levels and platelet factor 4 levels are commonly noted in patients with pulmonary embolus or extensive deep vein thrombosis. A baseline electrocardiogram should always be performed in a patient with venous thrombosis or suspected pulmonary embolus. This may be normal; however, more commonly it will demonstrate findings of acute cor pulmonale and right ventricular failure. Almost always, a sinus tachycardia will be present; however, transient atrial premature systoles, atrial flutter, or atrial fibrillation may also be present in the presence of a significant pulmonary embolus. The extremity leads commonly show an S-1 Q-3 pattern consisting of a deep S wave in lead 1, a prominent Q wave, and an inverted T wave in lead 3 and depression of ST segments in leads 2 and 1. The precordial leads will often show T-wave inversions in right precordial leads, a complete or incomplete right bundle branch block, and a QR pattern in leads V-3, V-1, and V-2 in association with negative T waves. As a result of generalized myocardial ischemia, the precordial leads may show ST segment depressions or T-wave inversions. Thus, the following patterns are strongly suggestive of an acute pulmonary embolus and acute right heart failure: S-1, Q-3, T-3 pattern associated with T-wave inversion in lead 3 and the right precordial leads, and an S-1, Q-3, T-3 pattern in association with a complete or incomplete right bundle branch block.

As with a baseline electrocardiogram, a baseline chest radiograph should always be obtained in a patient with suspected thrombus or pulmonary embolus. The vast majority of patients with a pulmonary embolus will have an abnormal chest radiograph, even though many of the findings are not characteristic. The most common defect found is that of a patchy infiltrate; however, characteristic humped-shaped infarcts at the lung base or in other areas of the pulmonary parenchyma may also be found. Less commonly, a pleural effusion will be noted; there may be local constriction of pulmonary vessels and fullness of pulmonary arteries at the hilum. There may be an area of oligemia (Westermark's sign). These findings should be correlated with ventilation perfusion lung scans using technetium-99 labeled macroaggregated albumin. Often one will note perfusion defects in the same areas as pulmonary infiltrates; if the pulmonary infiltrate is smaller than the perfusion defect, a pulmonary embolus is likely. Alternatively, if the infiltrative defect on a chest radiograph is larger than a perfusion defect, the probability of pulmonary embolus is unlikely. Ventilation scans that are of low probability for a pulmonary embolus are those demonstrating single or multiple defects that are less than 3 to 4 cm in diameter or, as mentioned, a perfusion defect that is smaller than a radiographic infiltrate. However, the presence of a perfusion defect that is larger than a radiographic infiltrate or than a segment in size may be considered positive. Perfusion defects equal to or smaller than chest radiographic infiltrates fall into an intermediate probability category, and in this instance the patient should be treated for

a pulmonary embolus or should be subjected to pulmonary angiography if this will change the therapy being contemplated. The noting of a normal perfusion lung scan is strong evidence that the patient does not have a pulmonary embolus. However, the finding of a normal chest radiograph is not strong evidence of the absence of a pulmonary embolus, and when appropriate clinical suspicion is present, a perfusion scan should always be performed.

Approximately 95% of pulmonary emboli arise from deep vein thrombi of the lower extremities which are most commonly proximal to the popliteal vein and are less commonly noted to be present in the calf veins. When a patient has a documented pulmonary embolus, a search for presence or absence of venous thrombi should be performed. Alternatively, in the patient without a pulmonary embolus but with only clinically suspected deep vein thrombosis, confirmatory procedures should be performed. There is much debate as to the relative efficacy and safety of ascending venography versus radioactive fibrinogen scans versus ascending thromboscintigraphy using technetium-99 labeled macroaggregated albumin. I prefer ascending thromboscintigraphy, because a simultaneous perfusion ventilation scan can be performed at the same setting. There are associated difficulties with other invasive procedures; the radioactive fibrinogen scan is associated with a high incidence of false-negative and false-positive results and is insensitive to thrombi above the lower thigh because of increased radioactive background activity in the pelvic vessels and bladder. In addition, positive results will be found if there is perivascular hemorrhage or inflammation, and radioactive fibrinogen scanning cannot distinguish between old and new thrombi. Doppler ultrasonography is of high reliability except for lesions below the knee; however, the results may be influenced by collateral circulation and venous recannalization. Venography is, of course, the most reliable way to demonstrate venous thrombi of the lower extremities; however it is extremely painful and time-consuming and associated with allergic reactions. My main reason for not using the procedure is the associated 10% incidence of post-venogram venous thrombosis. Thromboscintigraphy is of high reliability and an experienced radiologist or nuclear medicine specialist can distinguish the difference between old and new thrombi. An additional advantage is that a simultaneous pulmonary perfusion ventilation scan for pulmonary embolus can be performed and the procedure is virtually unassociated with side effects, thrombosis, or allergic reactions. Figure 11–1 demonstrates a positive thromboscintigram and Figure 11–2 is a perfusion scan from the same patient. Figures 11–3 and 11–4 demonstrate a positive venogram and pulmonary angiogram in another patient.

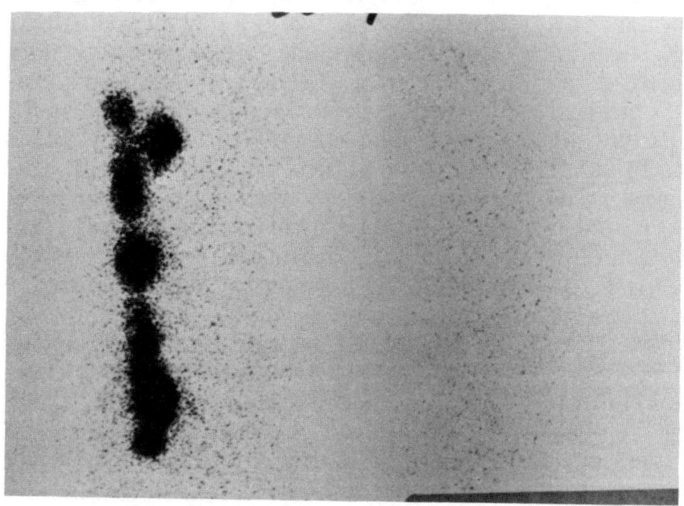

Fig. 11–1. Right leg thromboscintigram. There are diffuse multiple areas of thrombi below the knee and at the calf compatible with thrombosis in the calf and near the ankle.

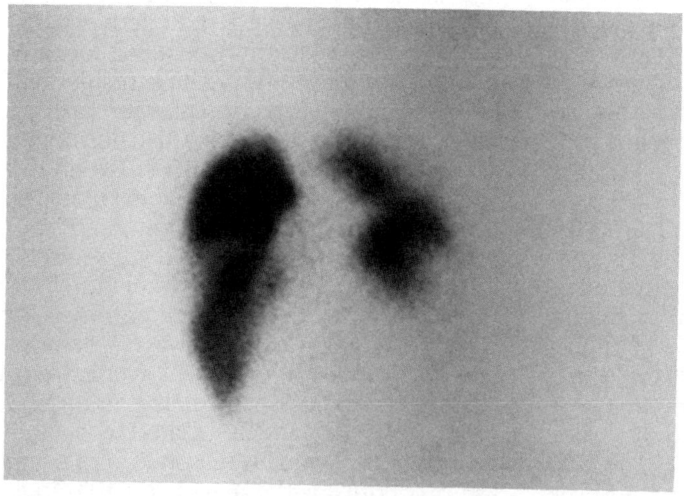

Fig. 11–2. Lung scan. There are multiple segmental perfusion defects without corresponding ventilation defects, more marked in the right middle lobe, right upper lobe, left lingula, and left base, representing multiple pulmonary emboli.

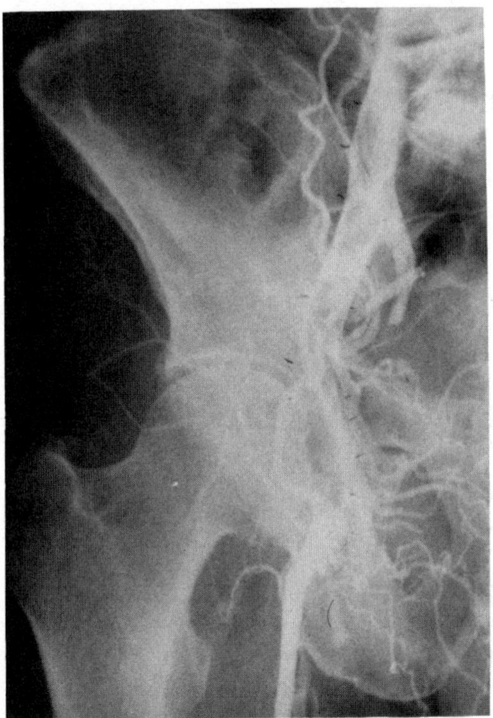

Fig. 11–3. Right leg venogram. Thrombosis of the right common femoral, external iliac, and common iliac veins with nonpacification of the right superficial femoral, popliteal, and deep veins occluded with thrombi.

Summary

Since thrombotic or thromboembolic events are often irreversible and can lead to a high degree of morbidity and, indeed, mortality, it is of obvious extreme importance to evaluate carefully these patients from the clinical standpoint as well as with the use of ancillary testing procedures. This applies to patients who are hypercoagulable or to patients recently having a thrombotic event. Only in this way can prophylactic therapy or therapy in treating the underlying event be instituted before the patient has sustained an unalterable and often catastrophic insult that will lead to prolonged morbidity or mortality.

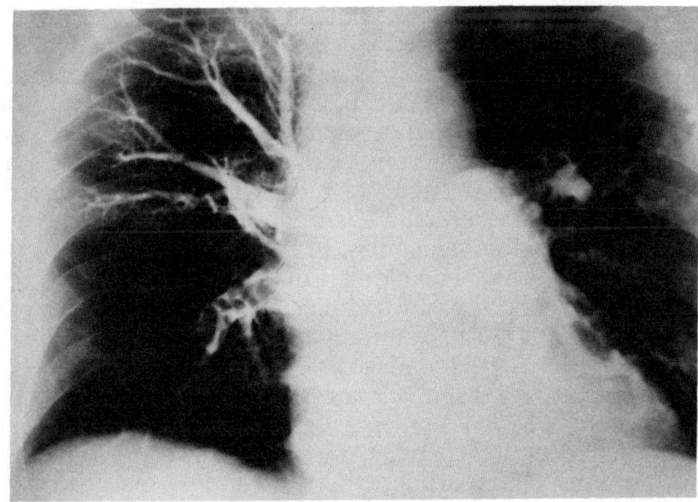

Fig. 11–4. Pulmonary angiogram. Multiple defects are noted in the branch to the right upper and lower lung zones secondary to pulmonary embolism.

12
Hypercoagulability and Thrombosis

Hypercoagulability and thrombosis are poorly understood phenomena. In clearly at least 50% of patients undergoing thrombotic or thromboembolic events a definitive etiologic reason is not identifiable. Despite "sophistication" in blood coagulation laboratories and in clinical hemostasis practice, the etiology of hypercoagulability and thrombosis often remains a mystery. However, the advent of new molecular marker profiling may change this trend and allow for the prediction of those patients who are at increased risk for thrombosis; the discovery of new inhibitor systems and new congenital deficiencies may now allow for defining the etiology in many patients experiencing arterial or venous thrombotic events, as these newer assays become more generally available.[15-17] In the past, modalities of hemostasis testing in the laboratory have not allowed for significant conclusions to be made regarding the etiology of thrombotic events. Many changes in the hemostasis system that have been reported to occur in association with hypercoagulability and thrombosis may not be of etiologic significance but may simply be the consequence of an already occurring thrombotic event, even though the event may, at the time of measuring hemostasis parameters, be subclinical. Therapy for hypercoagulability and thrombosis, likewise, has been largely empirical; this is to be expected, since clinicians and investigators are just beginning to understand etiologic aspects and to develop reasonably accurate diagnostic tools for the assessment of hypercoagulable and thrombotic disorders. In general, as was described more than 100 years ago, there are still only three primary factors in thrombus formation: changes in the blood flow, changes in the circulating blood, and changes in the vessel wall.[18]

Changes in Blood Flow

With respect to changes in the blood flow, very little is known regarding venous thrombosis and the initiation of thrombus formation. Several theories exist, and the most popular of these, with respect to why altered blood flow leads to thrombus formation, was advanced by Hume and co-workers,[99] who proposed that during periods of stasis, especially in venous valve pockets, there is activation of Factors XII, XI, and IX. Because of activation of these early "contact activation" factors, there is generation of Factor X_a, which in turn generates thrombin activity, which then propagates thrombus formation via two mechanisms: fibrin formation and the induction of platelet aggregation with subsequent availability of platelet factor 3 and adenosine diphosphate. This then cascades into more platelet aggregation and more blood coagulation. An additional theory is that during stasis there is a significant amount of endothelial sloughing with exposure of subendothelial collagen and the subsequent activation of platelets, Factor XII to Factor XIIa, and Factor XI to Factor XIa; any one of these three events could then lead to thrombin generation and thrombus formation.[19] However, it is quite possible that these hypotheses are only several of many potential alterations in coagulation and platelet function that may lead to thrombus formation when systemic stasis is present. These theories are depicted in Figures 12–1 and 12–2.

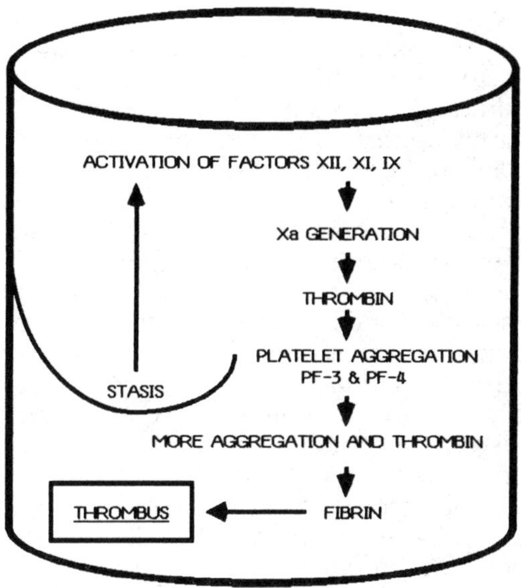

Fig. 12-1. Stasis in venous valve pockets.

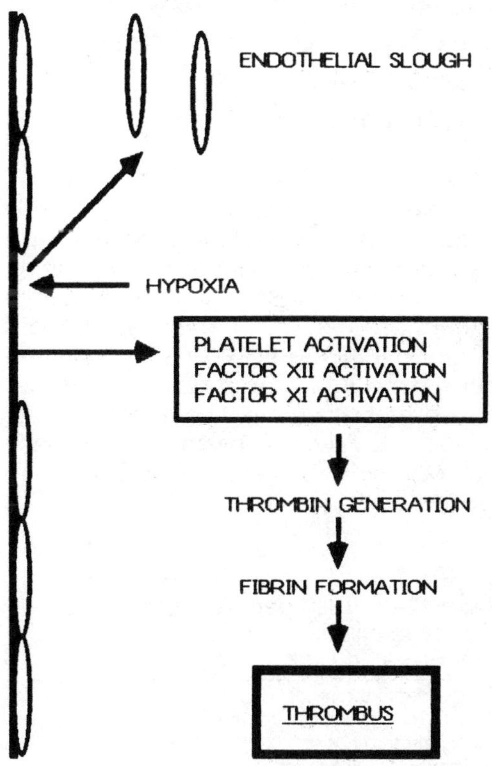

Fig. 12-2. Stasis and the endothelium.

Changes in the Circulating Blood

Changes in the circulating blood, both before and after thrombosis, are well defined; however, the meaning of many of these hemostasis laboratory changes remains unclear. Some of these changes are difficult to assess because they have been measured after the fact (thrombosis). In addition, even though many are thought to be measured before the fact, some changes may have been measured when subclinical thrombus formation and fibrin deposition was already occurring. Table 12-1 depicts changes in circulating blood that could, theoretically, lead to hypercoagulability, thrombosis, or both.

Increased platelet reactivity as measured by a variety of techniques has been noted in association with various thrombotic and thrombohemorrhagic disorders associated with hypercoagulability.[93,100] In general, increased platelet reactivity is noted in patients with acute thrombosis.[44] However, this has usually been assessed after the fact. It is significant that platelet hyperactivity is most often normal in patients with aged arterial thrombi, suggesting that platelet hyperreactivity plays an unclear role in the etiology of arterial thrombotic and thromboembolic problems. It has been well documented that increased platelet reactivity is seen in many patients with recurrent deep vein thrombosis.[104] However, again, this has usually been assessed after thrombosis has been clinically detected. The postoperative state is known to be associated with an increased incidence of thrombosis, and in a general surgical postoperative population, increased platelet reactivity can usually be measured.[66] Likewise, in postpartum women, the risk of thrombosis is increased and in many postpartum patients increased platelet reactivity can be demonstrated. Additionally, increased platelet reactivity has been found in many patients with disseminated malignancy; this is discussed in detail in Chapter 10.

Table 12–1 Alterations in Circulating Blood Leading to Thrombosis

Increased platelet reactivity
Increased coagulation factors
Decreased coagulation inhibitors
Decreased fibrinolytic activity
Increased fibrinolytic inhibitors
Increased lipids?

Interestingly, studies have also demonstrated increased platelet reactivity in patients with diabetes mellitus, a disorder commonly associated with hypercoagulability and increased predisposition to thrombus formation.[94] Additionally, increased platelet reactivity is noted in many individuals with generalized atherosclerosis. It remains controversial, however, as to whether any correlation exists between increased platelet reactivity, as measured by a variety of available techniques, and the incidence of an actual clinical thrombotic event. The only conclusion that can be drawn at present is that measurements of increased platelet reactivity are probably important predisposing factors in thrombus formation, especially when coupled with other changes in the hemostasis system. However, evidence that increased platelet reactivity, as measured by a variety of laboratory techniques, actually leads to clinical thrombosis is lacking.[12,18]

Changes in circulating coagulation factors have also been well documented in both thrombosis and its situations leading to thrombus formation (hypercoagulability). Increased coagulation factors are often noted postoperatively in general surgical patients in the postoperative period, in patients with fractures or trauma, in patients with chronic inflammatory disorders, such as ulcerative colitis, in disseminated malignancy, in acute thrombosis, and in patients with recurrent deep vein thrombosis with or without pulmonary emboli.[18,57,153,154] Like the finding of increased platelet reactivity, however, many increases in coagulation factors described have been measured after the fact and the significance of these findings remains unclear with respect to these changes being of etiologic significance or simply being a result of subclinical fibrin deposition. The coagulation factors most commonly increased in the aforementioned disorders are fibrinogen, Factors V, and VII, VIII:C, and VIII:RAg.[58] In addition, many investigators have measured "increased thromboplastin generation" in these same disorders. It must be emphasized, however, that there is a poor correlation between any individual increased clotting factor and the development of a clinical thrombotic event.[18] Factor VIII and fibrinogen are the coagulation factors most often noted to be increased and are found to be increased in pregnancy, chronic inflammatory disorders, disseminated malignancy, in the postoperative state, and in intravascular hemolytic disorders.[18] All of these situations are associated with an increased risk of thrombosis. Disorders associated with hypercoagulability, thrombosis, and elevated clotting factors are summarized in Table 12–2.

Coagulation Inhibitors and Hypercoagulability, Thrombosis, and Thromboembolus

It has been postulated and generally accepted that coagulation occurs in a cybernetic manner with fibrin deposition and subsequent lysis occurring as a continuous process.[5,103,177] The manifestations of normal hemostasis versus increased fibrin deposition (thrombosis) or increased fibrino(geno)lysis (hemorrhage) depends on the delicate balance between the procoagulant system and its associated in-

Table 12–2 Disorders Associated with Hypercoagulability and Thrombosis with Elevated Clotting Factors

Acute arterial thrombosis
Chronic inflammatory disorders
Deep vein thrombosis
Disseminated malignancy
Fractures
Hemolysis
Postoperative state
Pregnancy
Trauma

hibitors.[88,129,176] Primary inhibitors of the procoagulant and fibrino(geno)lytic system are comprised of antithrombin III (AT III), protein C, alpha-2-macroglobulin, alpha-1-antitrypsin, C1 esterase inhibitor, and alpha-2-antiplasmin.[20] Antithrombins were first described in 1939 by Brinkhous and co-workers.[47] The first large survey of antithrombins was reported by Seegers and associates in 1952.[173]

The most important of the antithrombins appears to be AT III-heparin cofactor. An additional important and more recently described inhibitor, to be discussed subsequently, is protein C. Early work considered heparin cofactor (antithrombin II) to be distinct from AT III; however, it now appears that antithrombin II-heparin cofactor activity and AT III are the same.[3,159] AT III has activity not only against thrombin, but also other serine proteases generated during coagulation, including Factors X_a, IX_a, XI_a, XII_a, plasmin, and kallikrein.[174,175,199] In addition, AT III has inhibitory activity against protein C. In most instances, especially with respect to activity against thrombin and Factor X_a, this activity is thought to be markedly accelerated by heparin.[167,206] Differing molecular weights of heparin appear to have differing inhibitory effects on antithrombin III, with higher molecular weight forms of heparin accelerating inhibitory activity against Factor II_a and descending molecular weight of fractions and fragments having concomitantly decreased anti-II_a activity and concomitantly increased anti-X_a activity. The kinetics of these reactions have been described and are listed in Table 12–3 with respect to USP heterogenous heparin.[109,213] When the hemostasis system is driven in the procoagulant direction with attendant generation of serine proteases and eventual fibrin formation, AT III consumption would be expected to occur, since it is thought to combine irreversibly with activated clotting factors.[166] From at least a theoretical standpoint one would expect to see pathologic consumption of antithrombin III in conditions associated with the pathologic acceleration of procoagulant activity and the pathologic generation of thrombin and other serine proteases, such as occurs in

Table 12–3   Kinetics of the Antithrombin III and Heparin Interaction

Heparin absence
2 μg AT III inhibit 1 U Factor Xa
Heparin presence
1 μg AT III inhibits 15 U Factor Xa (30-fold acceleratory activity with heparin)
Therefore
1 U Factor Xa generates 50 U Thrombin (Factor IIa)
1 μg AT III inhibits 15 U Factor Xa (in the presence of heparin at 0.01 U/mL)
Thus, 1 μg AT III, in the presence of heparin is able to inhibit the generation of 750 U of Factor IIa (thrombin)

many disorders, including deep vein thrombosis, pulmonary embolism, and disseminated intravascular coagulation (DIC); to a large extent this same consumption is seen with respect to protein C. Alternatively, since AT III, a very important serine protease inhibitor, is thought to be highly important in protection against thrombus formation one would likewise expect an increased predisposition to thrombus formation and an inadequate response to subsequent heparinization in situations associated with significant decreases in AT III. Additionally, decreases in protein C, to be discussed subsequently, are also associated with increased thrombotic tendencies.

AT III is an alpha-2-globulin with a molecular weight of approximately 65,000 daltons.[1,142] Its specific characteristics have been recently described in detail.[70,141] AT III is purified by chromatography with heparin Sepharose.[145,190] In the absence of heparin, AT III appears to inactivate thrombin and other serine proteases in a progressive, irreversible manner following second order kinetics.[1] In addition, AT III inactivates other serine proteases, including Factors X_a, IX_a, XI_a, XII_a, and kallikrein, although with less efficiency than with respect to its inhibition of thrombin.[119,120,174,175,184,199] It has been thought that approximately 70% of the total inhibition of the serine protease procoagulant system may be ascribed to antithrombin III and approximately 25 to 30% attributed to alpha-2-macroglobulin and other inhibitors.[1,170] However, other more recent evidence has suggested that greater than 90% of the total inhibition of the procoagulant system may be ascribed to AT III and perhaps only 5 to 7% to alpha-2-macroglobulin and other inhibitors.[147,180] In fact, the relative general contributions of AT III, protein C, and alpha-2-macroglobulin in inhibiting the procoagulant system are still unclear and remain to be defined. In the presence of heparin, the inactivation of thrombin and Factor X_a by AT III is markedly accelerated and is almost instantaneous. Rosenberg and Damus [166] have demonstrated that heparin interacts with AT III by binding to lysine residues of the AT III molecule and thus presumably markedly enhancing its inhibitory activity. However, heparin also combines with thrombin and Factor X_a, and thus it is still a matter of controversy whether the neutralization of thrombin and Factor X_a by AT III is due to the interaction of heparin with AT III or, alternatively, the interaction of heparin with the particular serine protease involved.[97,124,205,212]

Another proposed mechanism is that a molecule of heparin may bind to AT III and thrombin.[165] In the presence of heparin, the preferential target of AT III is thrombin, followed by Factor X_a. Proposed mechanisms of action of AT III are summarized in Figures 12–3 and 12–4. It has recently been clearly demonstrated that differing molecular weight subspecies of heparin have different activities with respect to the interaction of AT III and Factor X_a or interaction with the vasculature (vascular proteoglycans).[11,156,195,208] As mentioned previously, anti-II_a (thrombin) activity of heparin appears to be greatest with higher molecular weight forms and as the molecular weight is decreased the anti-II_a activity decreases and the anti-X_a activity increases, respectively. During the aforementioned processes, heparin appears not to be consumed.[50] After the formation of AT III and a serine protease complex, heparin dissociates from the complex and thus acts as a catalyst. The kinetics of the heparin and serine protease interaction have been well elucidated, providing evidence that only a minute amount of heparin needs to be present to accelerate the inhibitory activity of AT III (See Table 12–3).[2,13,109] Endogenous

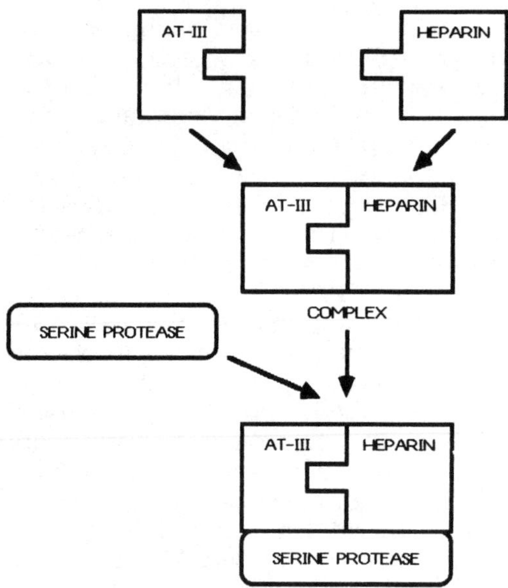

Fig. 12–3. Antithrombin III activity, model I.

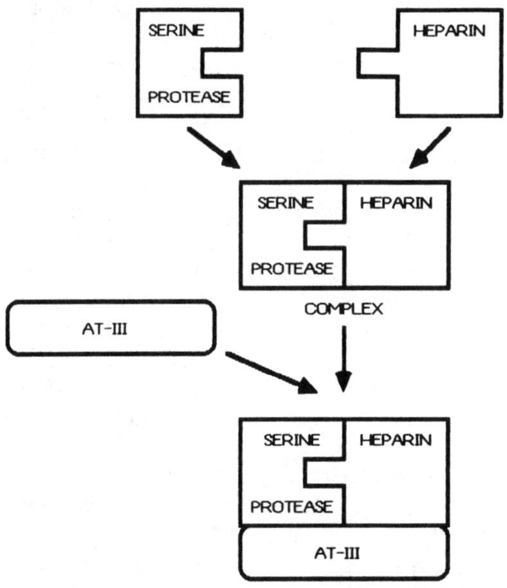

Fig. 12–4. Antithrombin III activity, model II.

heparin is rarely, if ever, detected in the blood in significant amounts, except in selected pathologic conditions, such as certain malignancies. When exogenous heparin is delivered to the blood compartment, it is rapidly absorbed by the surface of endothelial cells; this endothelial-bound heparin may be far more important physiologically than circulating heparin with respect to thrombus formation in man.[105,106,125,126] In this regard, it should be recognized that some of the vascular proteoglycans, other than heparin, are also able to absorb AT III and enhance the rate of inhibition of thrombin and Factor X_a, and possibly other serine proteases, by AT III.[90,208] The obvious major physiologic significance of this activity is implied but not yet conclusively proved.

Most studies reveal that the physiologic range of AT III in normal human blood is quite narrow.[20,39,158] In addition, only moderate decreases of AT III are often of significant clinical relevance with respect to thrombus formation or thromboembolus.[20,194] Infants have approximately 50% of normal adult AT III levels; however, the adult level is reached at an early age.[189] The mechanisms by which a potential deficiency of AT III may occur are as follows: (1) a defect in synthesis that may occur in the congenital form as well as in several acquired forms, such as liver disease; (2) increased consumption of AT III resulting from the generation of pathologic levels of serine proteases, such as might be expected to occur in DIC-type syndromes, extensive deep vein thrombosis, massive pulmonary embolization, and diffuse small and large venous and arterial thrombo-occlusive events; (3) loss of AT III from the intracellular compartment, such as may occur with selected renal diseases; and (4) increased protein catabolism.[20,194] These mechanisms are listed in Table 12-4.

Table 12-4 Mechanisms of Antithrombim III Deficiency

Decreased synthesis
  Congenital form
  Acquired form
Dysfunctional synthesis
  Congenital form
  Acquired form
Increased consumption
  Disseminated intravascular coagulation
  Deep venous thrombosis
  Pulmonary embolus
  Diffuse vaso-occlusive diseases
Proteinuria and nonselective loss of AT III
Increased nonselective protein catabolism

Pathologic Decreases in Antithrombin III

Hereditary Deficiency

Hereditary Thrombophilia

Hereditary thrombophilia, or congenital deficiency of AT III, is usually inherited as an autosomal dominant disease, although variant inheritance has also been described.[171] In the majority of patients with classic hereditary deficiency of AT III there appears to be a reduced synthesis of a biologically normal AT III molecule,[171] but this may also be associated with a dysfunctional AT III molecule.[171,211] Thus, the absent and the dysfunctional forms exist. In addition, one variant has been described that is not associated with a thrombotic tendency.[161] The prevalence of hereditary deficiency of AT III is not known for certain in view of only recent screening and the more widespread use of quantitative AT III assays. At the present time, however, the incidence appears to be between 1 in 2,000 and 1 in 5,000.[160,168] However, this incidence may change with more widespread use of AT III assays in patients with hypercoagulability and thrombosis because of the development of easy automated synthetic substrate techniques for the assay. Perhaps of more clinical relevance, is the question of how many patients with deep vein thrombosis or pulmonary embolus seen in a general population have actually had these events because of hereditary AT III deficiency. The answer to this question will have to await large population studies; however, at this time it appears that the prevalence of hereditary antithrombin deficiency in a general patient population with thrombotic or thromboembolic events is approximately 3 to 4%.[20,22,121]

Patients with classic hereditary deficiency of AT III have a marked increased risk of venous thrombotic events and pulmonary embolism.[20,54,127,194,197,198,203] These events typically appear in the mid to late teenage years. The most common sites of thrombosis are the deep vein structures of the lower extremities. However, an additional characteristic site of thrombosis is the mesenteric veins.[59] The classic presentation is that of recurrent deep vein thrombosis with or without pulmonary embolization.[20,127,194] From the family studies reported, it appears that the deficiency of AT III need not be especially severe for thrombotic events to occur; some individuals have deep vein thrombosis and pulmonary emboli at between 50 and 70% biologic activity, whereas others with low AT III levels may not have thrombosis at all.[20,54,127,197,198,203] Thus, heterozygotes are certainly also at an increased risk for severe venous thrombotic and thromboembolic events. Many patients with hereditary thrombophilia treated with oral anticoagulants have an increase in AT III levels after the initiation of therapy.[20,65,134,148] However, there have also certainly been patients reported to be unresponsive to oral anticoagulant therapy and demonstrate no significant increases in AT III levels.[20,107,123,150] A typical family with congenital deficiency of AT III is presented in Table 12–5. One in this family was treated with oral anticoagulants and two were treated with combination platelet suppressive therapy (aspirin and dipyridamole); the increases in AT III levels were identical, which presumably occur due to "blunting" of low levels of intravascular procoagulant drive (and presumed fibrin deposition), thus decreasing intravascular concentrations of the serine protease and increasing AT III biologic activity. The results of anticoagulant and antiplatelet therapy in this family are depicted in Figure 12–5. These results suggest that hereditary thrombophilia patients not demonstrating the desired AT III response to oral anticoagulant therapy may be given a trial of combination platelet suppressive therapy to see if this modality will enhance their AT III levels. In addition, the AT III biochemical characteristics of this family and two similar families have been published.[209]

Recently available for treating hereditary AT III deficiency are very potent AT III concentrates, the use of which will be discussed in subsequent sections. However, Figure 12–6 depicts the increase in AT III and subsequent prolongation of the partial thromboplastin time (PTT) in a congenital AT III-deficient patient receiving AT III concentrate therapy and heparin. Table 12–6 summarizes the characteristics of congenital AT III deficiency.

Table 12–5 Congenital Antithrombin III Deficiency: A Typical Family

Mother
A 52-year-old Caucasian female with life-long history of recurrent deep vein thrombosis and two episodes of pulmonary embolus. AT III level at presentation was 79% biologic and immunologic assay (patient was in warfarin therapy at time of these determinations)

Son
An 18-year-old Caucasian male with a 5-year history of deep vein thrombosis; he had experienced three episodes of pulmonary emboli, the first at age 13 years. AT III level at presentation was 59% biologic and immunologic assay

Daughter
A 16-year-old Caucasian female with seven episodes of deep vein thrombosis, but no pulmonary emboli. The first episode of deep vein thrombosis was at age 12 years. AT III level at presentation was 52% by biologic and immunologic assay

Father
Not available for study.

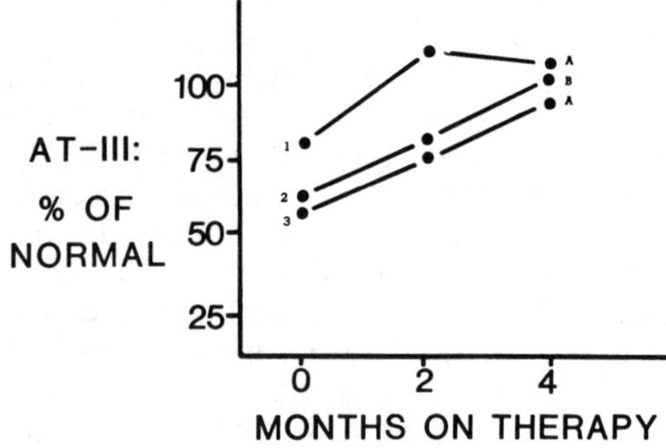

Fig. 12–5. The effect of different treatment modalities on three members of a family with antithrombin III deficiency. A: aspirin and dipyridamole; B: sodium warfarin; 1: mother; 2: son; 3: daughter.

Deep Vein Thrombosis and Pulmonary Embolism

Many risk factors are known to be associated with the development of deep vein thrombosis and pulmonary embolism, including age, blood group, obes-

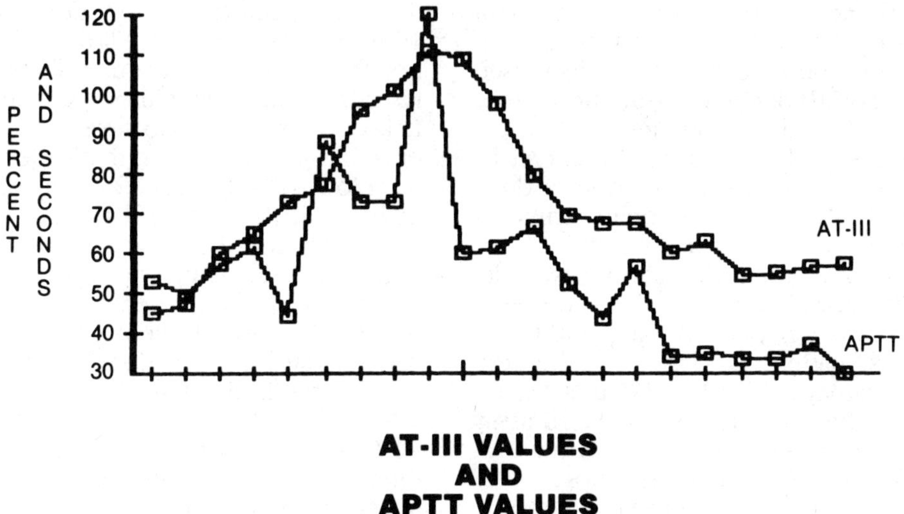

Fig. 12–6. Correlation of the activated partial thromboplastin time (APTT) with increasing antithrombin III (AT-III) concentrate infusion in a patient with congenital thrombophilia.

Table 12–6 Characteristics of Congenital Antithrombin III Deficiency

Clinical features
  Autosomal dominant trait
  Absence form and dysfunctional forms exist
  Venous thrombosis begins in mid to late teens
  Pulmonary emboli are common
  Mesenteric vessels particularly susceptible
  Thrombosis occurs commonly in heterozygotes
  Thrombosis may occur at AT III levels below 75%
Laboratory features
  Low AT III levels by biologic activity
  Low immunologic AT III levels in absence form
  Normal immunologic levels in dysfunctional form
  Global tests of coagulation are normal
  Tests of fibrinolysis are normal
  Template bleeding time is normal
  Platelet aggregation is normal
  Activated PTT may not be prolonged adequately or at
    all during intravenous heparin therapy
Therapy
  Oral anticoagulants
  Antiplatelet agents (aspirin plus dipyridamole)
  AT III concentrates
  Heparin usually ineffective

ity, the use of oral contraceptives, and numerous specific clinical events, such as malignancy, the postoperative or postpartum state, cardiovascular disease, and a past history of deep vein thrombosis, and varicose veins.[140] Interestingly, there is an inverse correlation between smoking and venous thrombotic disease, although a positive correlation between arterial thrombosis and smoking exists. Approximately 70% of individuals with deep vein thrombosis or pulmonary embolization have decreased levels of AT III before the initiation of anticoagulation therapy. However, the greatest majority of these individuals have decreased AT III levels because of consumption when the thrombus developed and only 3 to 4% have had a thrombotic event because of a deficiency of AT III. There appears to be a rough correlation between the severity of the intravascular thrombotic event (such as deep vein thrombosis and pulmonary emboli) and the degree of decrease in AT III levels in the majority of acquired cases. In general, the degree of decrease correlates generally with DIC, iliofemoral thrombosis, pulmonary embolization, bilateral calf thrombosis, and single calf thrombosis in descending order of decrease of AT III.[24,90] Table 12–7 presents data on pretherapy and post-therapy antithrombin III levels in 40 patients with deep vein thrombosis with and without pulmonary embolism.[17,20,43] Table 12–8 gives the correlations noted in our laboratories between the degree of decrease in AT III and the site and severity of the thrombotic event.

It should again be emphasized that more than 90% of patients with a deep vein thrombotic event have decreased levels of AT III due to consumption rather than to a hereditary deficiency. My usual practice is to obtain a pretreatment AT III level in any individual in whom a deep vein thrombosis or pulmonary embolus is present or strongly suspected.[17,20] The purpose of this determination is twofold: to gain information regarding the potential efficacy of heparin therapy and to detect those patients who may have hereditary deficiency of AT III.[17,20] In this regard, it should be noted that some AT III assay systems may render erroneously high results, leading to a missed diagnosis of AT III deficiency.[23-25] If the AT III level is significantly decreased, the patient is again measured 1 to 2 months later in the "steady state" when no detectable intravascular thrombosis is occurring to ascertain whether the initial decrease was due to increased consumption or a hereditary deficiency.[20]

With respect to post-treatment AT III levels, it should be noted that decreases in AT III have been noted after heparin therapy. Specifically, in several studies a 10 to 15% decrease in AT III levels have been associated with the use of intravascular heparin; this is without any apparent risk of thrombosis. However, my experience has generally been that patients who have low AT III levels before the initiation of heparin therapy tend to have normal levels within 24 hours after the institution of therapy. Subcutaneous heparin therapy aiming for a plasma heparin level of between 0.01 and 0.1 U/L is usually used in my hematology practice.[18,20,22,40] However, in the individuals depicted in Table 12–7 25% still have abnormally decreased AT III levels after the initiation of heparin therapy, but only 2 individuals of 40 patients had a subsequent decrease of pretreatment AT III levels after the initiation of heparin therapy.[20]

Oral Contraceptives and Antithrombin III

Numerous reports have appeared in the literature concerning AT III levels in patients taking oral contraceptives.[45,53,55,108,163,215] Numerous conflicting reports are found and have recently been summarized in a review article rendering rational perspective to the issue of oral contraceptives, thromboembolism, and the hemostasis system.[30] Many investigators have found decreased levels of AT III and many others have found unchanged levels of AT III in women ingesting oral contraceptives.[130] These marked discrepancies are most likely due to differences in testing techniques.[20] AT III measurements in serum instead of plasma have yielded more consis-

Table 12–7 Antithrombin III Levels in Deep Vein Thrombosis

	Antithrombin (% NHP)	Percent of Patients Abnormal
Pretreatment	77.0	67
Post-treatment*	105.3	25
Normal range	89 to 125	

* Subcutaneous calcium heparin: 80 to 100 U/kg. three times a day.

Table 12–8 Antithrombin III Level and Severity of Thrombotic Event

Severity	Event	Antithrombin III Level (% NHP)	SD
I	Single calf thrombus	109.0	18.3
II	Bilateral calf thrombi	104.8	25.3
III	Isolated pulmonary embolus	83.2	20.2
IV	Iliofemoral thrombus	81.5	6.4
V	Deep vein thrombosis plus pulmonary embolus	66.5	9.9
VI	Acute DIC	62.6	18.5
	Normal values	89–125	

tent decreases in oral contraceptive pill users; however, these serum systems are not adequate to quantitate the ability of the patient to inactivate thrombin and other serine proteases, since they measure the amount of AT III left after clotting.[139,188] Additional discrepancies have been found in studies measuring AT III levels in oral contraceptive users by both immunologic and biologic techniques. In one such study, the biologic activity was found to be decreased in 55% of women, whereas the immunologic level was abnormal in only 12%.[1162] It has been reported that estrogens may reduce AT III levels by approximately 15% and the greater reductions appear to be correlated with higher doses of estrogens.[69,98] In addition, recent studies have shown specific binding between estrogens as well as other steroids and AT III.[149] Thus, one might deduce a potential relationship between decreases in AT III levels and thrombotic tendencies in women on oral contraceptives. However, at the present time, the data are too conflicting to come to any firm conclusions regarding the clinical relevance of decreased AT III levels in women taking oral contraceptive agents.

It is to be hoped that careful studies using reliable plasma AT III determinations, preferably by synthetic substrate assays, will become more commonly used and this issue more carefully understood. It should be noted also that the use of serum AT III levels is to be condemned because these determinations are without clinical relevance.[20,130,139,188]

Antithrombins and Coronary Artery Disease

The role of thrombosis and coronary artery ischemia and coronary artery disease remains controversial,[115,146] but the role of AT III with respect to atherogenesis and myocardial infarction remains even less clear. However, it has been reported that AT III levels are decreased in many patients with coronary artery disease and in those at high risk for coronary artery disease. Yue and co-workers[214] examined a large population of patients and found excellent correlation between AT III levels and those at low risk for ischemia, those at high risk for ischemia, those with chronic ischemic heart disease on heparin, those with chronic ischemic disease without heparin, and those with acute myocardial infarction. In this study AT III levels decreased concomitantly in each of these groups of patients. Another study reported a significant decrease in AT III levels in patients with postmyocardial infarction and with generalized atherosclerotic vaso-occlusive peripheral vascular disease.[157] Banarjee and co-workers[10] have reported decreased AT III levels in women and men with generalized atherosclerosis. Innerfield and co-workers[102] reported decreased AT III levels in patients with coronary artery occlusion. However, Hedner and Nilsson[92] have reported normal AT III levels in patients with myocardial infarction. All of these studies, except that of Innerfield and associates have relied solely on clinical diagnosis, and angiographic evidence of coronary artery disease has been lacking. Bick and Faulstick[26] have also recently studied 102 individuals with angiographically documented coronary artery disease. In these plasma levels of biologic AT III activity were determined at the time of coronary artery catheterization and at the time of catheter removal. These results are given in Table 12–9. In these patients undergoing coronary artery angiography only 10 patients (9.8%) had decreased AT levels. However, 17% of patients had decreased AT III levels after catheterization. This further supports the suggestion of others that angiographic dyes in general may alter AT III levels.[117] In this study an attempt to correlate AT III levels with the type of intracoronary lesion was made.

Table 12–9 Antithrombin III and Coronary Artery Disease

	Antithrombin III Level (% NHP)	SD
During catheterization	119.5	26.9
After catheter removal	108.2	21.2
p value	0.009	
Normal range	89 to 125	

However, no significant differences were found when patients were segregated into those with specific coronary artery involvement (lesions of the left anterior descending coronary artery, circumflex artery, or right coronary artery; Table 12–10), nor were there any correlations when compared with class of coronary artery disease (class I through IV; Table 12–11). Thus, the role of antithrombins in coronary artery disease is conflicting and unclear at the present time; however, it appears that the majority of patients with documented coronary artery disease, proved by angiographic studies, have normal AT III levels, and it would thus appear that the determination of AT III levels in patients with coronary artery disease is without clinical relevance.[20,26]

Renal Disease, Liver Disease, and Antithrombin III

Patients with proteinuria lose AT III in the urine along with other plasma proteins,[191] and, urinary AT III levels can be correlated with urinary proteinuria as well as with urinary albumin.[192] Concomitant with this, plasma AT III levels correlate inversely with urinary proteinuria.[112]

Table 12–10   Antithrombin III and Coronary Artery Involvement*

	Antithrombin III Level (% NHP)	SD
Left anterior descending	116.6	29.3
Right coronary artery	115.0	24.3
Circumflex artery	166.6	34.5

* Involvement equals greater than 50% occlusion.

Table 12–11   Antithrombin III and Class of Coronary Artery Disease

Class	No. Patients	Antithrombin III (%)	Increased	Decreased
0	35	124	12	3
I	12	109	2	2
II	26	118	4	3
III	18	127	7	1
IV	11	104	2	1

There is a well-recognized risk of deep vein thrombosis and pulmonary embolism in patients with nephrotic syndrome.[114] However, these individuals have many other conditions that may also constitute high-risk factors for this complication, including high concentrations of various clotting factors and prolonged bed rest and subsequent stasis.[111,196] Thus, it is not clear whether there exists a causal relationship between decreases of AT III in patients with nephrotic syndrome and the increased risk of thrombosis and thromboembolic disease seen in these patients. It has been noted that glucocorticoid therapy may enhance AT III levels in patients who are deficient secondary to urinary proteinuria. This may be due to steroid-induced stimulation of AT III synthesis or, alternatively, may be due to a direct effect of steroids on renal protein loss.[116]

AT III levels are often noted to be decreased in patients with chronic liver disease[20,39] and normal in patients with acute hepatitis,[86,96] unless the patient with acute fulminant hepatitis develops severe fulminant DIC.[27–29] However, the significance of this finding remains unclear, since patients with chronic liver disease and hepatic failure have no apparent increased risk of thrombosis. The decrease in AT III may be counterbalanced by the severe defects in hemostasis and subsequent "hypocoagulability" often associated with acute and chronic liver disease[30,41,122] However, if the patient with chronic liver disease has a catastrophic event, such as being provided with a trigger for DIC (for example, sepsis or massive transfusions), then this low-level procoagulant inhibitor balance may be quite readily disrupted and subsequent catastrophic thrombohemorrhagic disease results.

Disseminated Intravascular Coagulation Syndromes and Antithrombin III

DIC and related syndromes were discussed in detail in Chapter 6; these syndromes are intermediary mechanisms of disease commonly recognized throughout all medical disciplines.[27–29,31] DIC syndromes are almost always associated with a triggering disease process state and are only rarely isolated events. There are many recognized triggers, most of which have been shown to be associated with low AT III levels, including severe burns complicated by infection, malignancy, acute promyelocytic leukemia, septicemia, and obstetrical accidents.[27–29,31,56,81,143] This is to be expected; AT III has activity against thrombin and other serine proteases generated during blood coagulation. Thus, in a situation such as DIC in which the hemostasis system is driven in the procoagulant direction with attendant (massive?) generation of serine proteases, including thrombin and Factor X_a, AT III consumption would be expected to occur due to irreversible binding with these activated clotting factors. Indeed it has been shown that radioactive AT III represents a useful probe for the study of in vivo thrombin formation and subsequent fibrin deposition.[51] Thus, from at least a theoretical standpoint, one would expect a pathologic consumption of AT III in conditions associated with pathologic acceleration of procoagulant activity and the pathologic generation of thrombin and other serine proteases, such as commonly occurs in DIC.[4,27–29,31–33,183] Several studies have, in fact, shown significant decreases in AT III levels in patients with DIC. This was discussed in detail in Chapter 6.

Our work has clearly revealed significant and early decreases in AT III in the majority of patients with DIC, and these decreases are noted before the onset of anticoagulant (usually heparin) therapy.[19,27,31–33] These studies suggest that AT III determinations may be of significant aid in diagnosing a DIC process. Also of significant importance are data and experience suggesting that the monitoring of AT III levels, following the use of heparin therapy (usually given subcutaneously) in DIC may represent an effective means of establishing efficacy of therapy in DIC with respect to blunting or stopping the intravascular clotting process. AT III levels pretreatment and post-treatment in 50 individuals with DIC are depicted in Table 12–12. In addition, Table 6–14

Table 12–12 Antithrombin III Levels in Disseminated Intravascular Coagulation

	Antithrombin III Level (% NHP)	SD	Percent Patients Abnormal
Pretherapy	63.1	25	92
Post-therapy*	106.7	32	18
p value	<0.001		
Normal range	89 to 125		

* Subcutaneous heparin.

demonstrates the reliability of laboratory tests in patients with DIC.[33] This same reliability has been found by other investigators as well.[183] Thus, I have come to rely heavily on AT III levels in conjunction with the noting of elevated FDPs, the presence of circulating soluble fibrin monomer, the presence of thrombocytopenia, the presence of hypofibrinogenemia, and the elevation of fibrinopeptide A in conjunction with elevated B-beta 15-42 related peptides in aiding in a reliable diagnosis of DIC.[15,17,19,27] In addition, the noting of a return to normal or near normal post-treatment AT III and fibrinopeptide A levels and platelet markers (either platelet factor 4 or beta-thromboglobulin) and a decrease in B-beta 15-42 and related peptides provide useful indices in assessing the efficacy of heparin or other types of anticoagulant therapy in patients with DIC.[15,17,19]

Therapeutic Antithrombin III Concentrates

AT III concentrates have been used investigationally and may become generally available in the near future. These may be of potential value in therapy for the patient with DIC, "consumption" associated with acute or chronic liver disease, the control of hereditary deficiency of AT III deficiency, and in eradicating thrombogenicity of prothrombin complex concentrates. Most investigational clinical experience with AT III concentrates has been directed toward therapy for control of "consumption" or frank DIC in association with acute liver failure. Vogel and co-workers[201] treated 22 patients with acute liver disease with

AT III concentrates when patient AT III levels decreased below 80%. They found antithrombin therapy to be highly successful in stopping "intravascular consumption" at a dose of 250 U delivered over 3 hours. These investigators also concluded AT III concentrates to be useful for improving the prognosis in patients with acute liver failure. In addition, Egbring and co-workers[64] and Braude and co-workers[46] treated six patients with acute hepatic failure, and both groups concluded that AT III concentrates are effective in prolonging survival in these patients.

Kakkar[110] reported on the therapeutic use of AT III concentrates for treating four postoperative patients who had AT III levels of less than 50% of normal; none of these patients had a postoperative thromboembolic event. In addition, Kakkar studied 50 patients who were randomized between AT III concentrate or placebo plus low-dose heparin; treatment was delivered preoperative for total hip replacement. The results appear promising.[110] Egbring and associates[63] treated ten patients with hereditary and acquired AT III deficiency and reported these concentrates to be of benefit in treating thromboembolic disease in all patients. It was their experience that patients with AT III levels of less than 75% of normal would not respond adequately to heparin therapy. Bick and co-workers[32] treated five patients with acute DIC with an AT III concentrate; all five patients survived and the use of AT III was therefore an effective therapy and a potential alternative to heparin or miniheparin therapy.[19,32] Schipper and co-workers[172] and Thaler and co-workers[193] in two independent studies each treated five patients with DIC-type syndromes with AT III concentrates. Schipper and associates concluded that the concentrate was effective, as determined by noting decreased fibrinopeptide A levels and increased fibrinogen levels but uncorrectable fibrinogen survival, for a period of 48 hours after the infusion. However, Thaler and colleagues terminated their study without clear-cut conclusions regarding efficacy. Dunn and co-workers[62] have shown that endotoxin-induced DIC in dogs can be successfully aborted with the use of AT III concen-

trates. The conclusion from this study was that AT III appeared to be as effective as heparin in controlling DIC and may have distinct advantages over heparin with respect to overall survival and bleeding risk. Also, it has been demonstrated that potential thrombogenicity of prothrombin complex concentrates may be controlled by the addition of AT III to this therapeutic fraction before its infusion into patients.[207]

It is my opinion and that of others that AT III concentrates are most likely the specific antiprocoagulant therapy of choice for patients with acute DIC.[19,20,27,95] It is hoped that prospective randomized clinical trials using AT III concentrates in patients with acute DIC and patients with "consumption" due to acute hepatic failure can be initiated in the near future to determine if, in fact, efficacy is present and equal to or even better than current modalities of therapy.

Clinical Indications for Antithrombin Determinations

With the development and ready availability of simple and reproducible AT III determinations by synthetic substrate assay (fluorogenic or chromogenic assay), this laboratory testing modality is generally available at a minimum expense for virtually all clinical laboratories and should certainly be available to those institutions dealing with patients with thrombohemorrhagic disorders.[17,20] In this regard, synthetic substrate methods for the determination of AT III are clearly the methods of choice; clot-based methods should no longer be used in the clinical laboratory.[17,43,70–72,194] I have adopted the following indications for determining AT III levels: (1) Identification of patients who may be at high risk for thrombotic or thromboembolic disease. In general, if the level of AT III is less than 75% of normal activity, the individual should be assumed to have an increased risk of thrombotic or thromboembolic disease and appropriate prophylactic therapy should be considered. (2) To determine the potential responsiveness to heparin therapy. Patients with lower AT III levels may respond less than ideally, or not at all, to heparin therapy. Patients who have an AT III level of less than 40% biologic activity will usually not respond to heparin therapy at any dose and another form of therapy should be considered when appropriate. Alternatively, if the biologic AT III level is greater than 60% of normal activity, patients will usually respond to heparin. (3) When a patient's AT III deficiency is identified, all family members should also be studied in order to find other affected individuals. Prophylactic therapy with oral anticoagulants should be considered. For those patients not responding to oral anticoagulants, a combination of aspirin and dipyridamole appears to be effective. Of course, to determine efficacy of therapy in individuals with hereditary AT III deficiency requires additional subsequent antithrombin III determinations. (4) To determine the efficacy of therapy in DIC. It has been clearly shown that post-treatment AT III determinations are a reliable index to determine if control of the intravascular clotting process in DIC has been established after delivery of subcutaneous or intravenous heparin. In addition, the determination of AT III has also proved to be a highly useful diagnostic tool for DIC patients.

Thus, AT III determinations are an important part of the battery of tests used to establish a diagnosis of DIC. This was discussed in detail in Chapter 6. After the institution of appropriate therapy, AT III determinations are used to establish whether or not the intravascular coagulation process has been blunted or stopped. The role of AT III determinations in rendering information regarding efficacy of therapy in other thrombotic or thromboembolic disorders has not yet been clearly established.

Many unrelated clinical conditions that are associated with significant decreases in AT III have been summarized. In addition, prospects for future therapy with AT III concentrates have been discussed. The clinical indications for AT III determinations, including the reasons for performing the assay and those specific patient populations subjected to AT III assays in my clinical practice, have been outlined. It is to be anticipated that with the new general availability of simple reliable AT III assay systems using synthetic substrates that more and more patient populations will be studied and clinical indications for the use of AT III determinations as well as AT III concentrates may become more firm or may, indeed, change (Table 12–13).

Protein C

Protein C is a newly rediscovered vitamin K dependent protein that also appears to be a major inhibitor of the procoagulant system and may actually equal or exceed the importance of AT III.[68,185] Protein C was first discovered in 1960 by Mammen and associates,[131] who also noted the inhibitory nature of protein C. Protein C was rediscovered in 1976 by Stenflo.[186] Seegers and co-workers,[178] in 1976, quickly demonstrated that their initial protein C, originally referred to as autoprothrombin II-A, and Stenflo's rediscovered protein C were the same inhibitory protein.[67] Since the rediscovery of protein C, great interest has centered around its modes of inhibitory action as well as its role in disease states.

Protein C is a vitamin K dependent protein synthesized in the hepatocyte and has

Table 12–13 Clinical Indications for Antithrombin III Determinations

Patients with a history of deep vein thrombosis or pulmonary embolus
Patients with active deep vein thrombosis or pulmonary embolus
Patients developing a recurrent thrombotic event during heparin therapy
Preoperative patients with a personal or family history of deep vein thrombosis or pulmonary embolus
Patients with disseminated intravascular coagulation or a related syndrome
Patients with a family history of deep vein thrombosis or pulmonary embolus
Patients demonstrating inadequate prolongation of the activated PTT or other global clotting test while on heparin therapy
Possibly patients considering taking oral contraceptives; indications in this instance are not clearly established

a molecular weight of approximately 56,000 daltons.[185,186] Protein C exerts its primary inhibitory activity by inactivating Factors V and VIII:C.[185] To perform this inactivation, protein C must first be activated by thrombin.[67,68,185] Thrombin, which activates protein C to protein Ca (activated form) must first be bound to endothelial thrombomodulin after which thrombin acquires its ability to activate protein C.[67,185] In addition, thrombomodulin-bound thrombin loses its ability to convert fibrinogen to fibrin and also loses its ability to activate platelets.[67] Protein Ca is a serine protease and its activity is inhibited by AT III;[67] in addition, its inhibitory activity in degrading Factors V and VIII:C is markedly enhanced by protein S, another vitamin K dependent factor.[204] This factor was discovered in 1977 by DiSchipio and co-workers[60] in Seattle, hence the designation S. The exact mechanisms by which protein S accentuate the activity of activated protein C in degrading Factors V and VIII:C, which must occur in the presence of phospholipid, remains unclear.[160] Mechanisms of action of protein C are summarized in Figure 12-7.

Congenital Deficiency of Protein C

Congenital deficiency of protein C is inherited as an autosomal dominant trait, and the clinical characteristics are amazingly similar to congenital AT III deficiency.[13,49,68,82,83,127,135,179] Recurrent deep vein thrombosis and pulmonary embolus begins to occur typically in the late teenage years.[13,49,68,82,83,127,135,179] Two forms of the disease exist; patients may have an absence of the protein (CRM−form) or may have a dysfunctional protein (CRM+form); absence of the protein, thus far, appears to be more common than the presence of a dysfunctional protein.[14,52,85,127] In addition, like AT III deficiency, venous thrombi and thromboemboli, especially pulmonary emboli, commonly occur in heterozygous as well as homozygous patients.[82,127] Most homozygous patients have succumbed to thrombi and thromboemboli during early infancy.[82,136,179,181] One homozygous infant is thus far surviving with the prophylactic use of a protein C-containing prothrombin complex concentrate.[136,181] Thus, when seeing such patients, the presence of con-

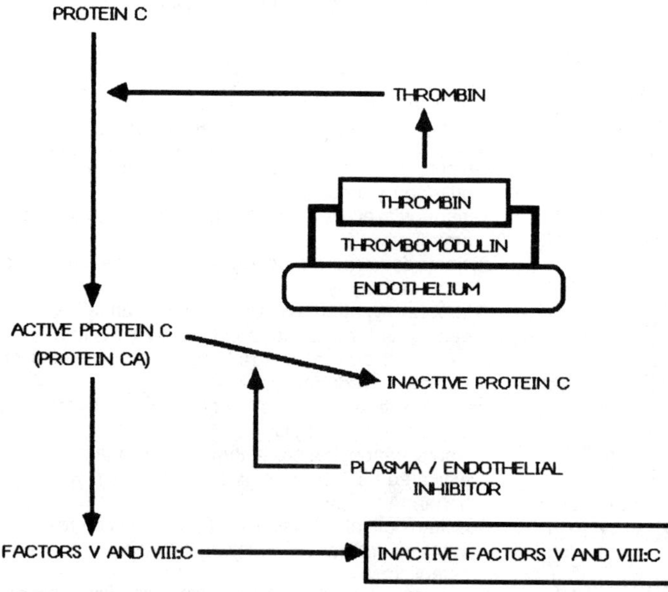

Fig. 12-7. Protein C activity.

genital protein C deficiency should strongly be considered, and a protein C assay performed.

Preliminary evidence would suggest that congenital protein C deficiency may actually be a more common cause of thrombosis or thromboembolus than AT III deficiency. The actual incidence of congenital protein C deficiency will only become known when assays become more widely available. It should be noted, however, that numerous protein C assays, some fully automated, are currently available for the clinical laboratory.[7,52,79,169] At the present time it is known that congenital AT III deficiency accounts for approximately 3 to 4% of all patients presenting with deep vein thrombosis or pulmonary embolus; however, preliminary estimations suggest that congenital protein C deficiency may account for 6 to 10% of these patients. Clinical characteristics of congenital protein C deficiency are summarized in Table 12–14.

Acquired Protein C Deficiency

Acquired protein C deficiency is commonly seen in patients with acute DIC, extensive deep vein thrombosis, and severe liver disease.[82,84,132] In addition, protein C levels may be decreased in postopera-

tive patients, but the role of this decrease in contributing to or causing postoperative deep vein thrombosis remains unclear.[132] Assays for protein C biologic and immunologic activity are now readily available and in most instances can be automated by synthetic substrate technique for biologic reactivity or immunologic activity and hemostasis laboratories should be encouraged to use this assay in all patients who develop deep vein thrombosis or pulmonary embolus and who present without other identifiable or obvious causes for these events.

Altered Fibrinolytic Activity in Hypercoagulability and Thrombosis

Decreased fibrinolytic activity and decreased fibrinolytic activator activity, at least in theory, should predispose to thrombus formation. It should be recalled that plasminogen, a precursor of plasmin, is synthesized in the liver or eosinophils; however, it appears that the majority of physiologically important plasminogen activator activity is from vascular endothelium or via indirect activation by activated Hageman factor.[200] Activation pathways were discussed in detail in Chapter 1. Hypoactivity of the fibrinolytic system and predisposition to thrombus formation can arise from either decreased plasminogen levels, decreased plasminogen activator activity, or increased fibrinolytic inhibitor activity. Mechanisms of hypoactivity of fibrinolysis are summarized in Table 12–15.

Table 12–14 Characteristics of Congenital Protein C Deficiency

Clinical features
  Autosomal dominant trait
  Absence form and dysfunctional forms exist
  Homozygous patients often die of thrombosis in early
    infancy
  Deep vein thrombosis and pulmonary embolus begin
    in mid to late teenage years
  Warfarin-induced skin necrosis often seen
  Clotting is common in heterozygotes
  Congenital deficiency may account for 5% to 10% of
    all patients with early clotting problems
Laboratory features
  Low biological protein C levels
  Low immunologic protein C levels in absence form
  Normal immunologic protein C levels in dysfunctional
    form
Therapy
  Warfarins?
  Prothrombin complex concentrates?
  Heparin for acute thrombotic events

Table 12–15 Mechanisms Leading to Hypoactivity of the Fibrinolytic System

Decreased plasminogen levels
Decreased plasminogen activators
  Plasma activators
  Endothelial activators
  Abnormal Factor XII activation pathway
Increased fibrinolytic system inhibitors
  Alpha-2-antiplasmin
  Alpha-2-macroglobulin
Inhibition of plasminogen activators

Decreased fibrinolytic activity has been noted in acute myocardial infarction as well as in patients with generalized atherosclerosis,[21,151] and in patients with scleroderma and thrombotic thrombocytopenic purpura.[6,152] In patients with generalized atherosclerosis the decrease in fibrinolytic activity may be due to vascular intimal damage and the loss of fibrinolytic plasminogen activator activity.[9,137,185,208]

Decreased fibrinolytic activity is present in acute pulmonary embolism, but whether this is of etiologic significance or simply due to consumption remains unclear.[6] In general, decreased fibrinolytic activity is also noted in patients with recurrent deep vein thrombosis, patients on oral contraceptives, and in most patients in the postoperative state.[34,133] The observations of decreased plasminogen levels in patients with deep vein thrombosis, recurrent thrombotic disease, and pulmonary emboli assumes major importance if the patient is considered a candidate for thrombolytic therapy.[144] If plasminogen levels are decreased significantly, thrombolytic therapy with streptokinase or urokinase may not be efficacious.[144] Diseases with decreased fibrinolytic activity are summarized in Table 12–16.

Increased inhibitors of the fibrinolytic system are noted in numerous disorders; the primary inhibitors being alpha-2-antiplasmin and alpha-2-macroglobulin. Their mechanisms of inhibitory activity were discussed in Chapter 1. These two inhibitors are found to be increased in pulmonary fibrosis, malignancy, infections, acute myocardial infarction, and thromboembolic disease.[80] Also, alpha-2-macroglobulin and alpha-1-antitrypsin (another inhibitor of the fibrinolytic system) are increased in the post-operative state as well as in pregnancy, diabetes, and in users of oral contraceptives.[18] Diseases with increased fibrinolytic system inhibitors are listed in Table 12–17.

Inhibitors of the fibrinolytic system are normal in most individuals with recurrent deep vein thrombosis. As with other changes in the circulating blood, increased inhibitors of fibrinolytic activity (alpha-1-antitrypsin and alpha-2-antiplasmin) have usually been noted after the fact and it remains speculative as to whether these increases may actually be of etiologic significance or whether they are due to an "acute phase reaction" secondary to an already present thrombotic event.[76]

There is inhibition of fibrinolytic activitor activity in the postoperative state, in infections, and in general inflammatory disorders as well as in such selected disorders as scleroderma and thrombotic thrombocytopenic purpura.[91,152] However, there is no detectable inhibition against fibrinolytic activator activity in patients with acute thrombosis or thromboembolus. It can only be concluded that, in general, reactive processes are associated with thrombosis and hypofibrinolysis, the latter coming about through several potential mechanisms: decreased plasminogen, decreased plasminogen activator activity, increased fibrinolytic inhibitors, and increased plasminogen activator inhibition. The significance of these findings remains

Table 12–16 Disorders with Decreased Fibrinolytic Activity

Acute myocardial infarction
Atherosclerosis
Congenital plasminogen defects
Deep vein thrombosis
Diabetes mellitus
Disseminated intravascular coagulation
Liver disease
Malignancy
Oral contraceptive use
Postoperative patients
Pregnancy
Pulmonary fibrosis
Scleroderma
Septicemia
Thrombotic thrombocytopenic purpura

Table 12–17 Disorders with Increased Inhibitors to the Fibrinolytic System

Acute myocardial infarction
Deep vein thrombosis
Diabetes mellitus
Infections
Malignancy
Oral contraceptive use
Postoperative patients
Pregnancy
Pulmonary embolus
Pulmonary fibrosis

unclear since it is not known whether many of these changes were present before subclinical thrombus formation and thus potentially of etiologic significance or whether they simply developed as a consequence of thrombosis. Mechanisms for decreased fibrinolytic activity are summarized in Table 12–15, and assays currently available for components of the fibrinolytic system are listed in Table 12–18.

Congenital Plasminogen Deficiency

Congenital plasminogen deficiency is thus far considered rare,[128] although it may be found to be much more common than previously suspected with the now ready availability of reliable and simple plasminogen assays by synthetic substrate methods.[16,71,72,101] The disorder is inherited as an autosomal recessive trait.[8] Both the absence form (CRM−) and the dysfunctional form (CRM+) have been described, although thus far the dysfunctional form appears to be the more common type.[8,89,128] Clinically, patients demonstrate similarities to congenital AT III deficiency and congenital protein C deficiency. Congenital deficient plasminogen patients begin to experience thrombotic events in their late teenage years.[8,89,113,128] The most common thrombotic events are deep vein thrombosis and pulmonary embolization.[8,89,113,128] Arterial thrombotic and thromboembolic events are not a prominent characteristic disease. Venous thrombotic and thromboembolic events occur when the plasminogen level is less than 40% of normal biologic activity.[128] Both homozygous and heterozygous patients

can be identified by the use of synthetic substrate assays for biologic activity of plasminogen; additionally, a comparison of biologic activity with immunologic levels may be used to identify those patients who have dysfunctional plasminogen versus those with quantitative hypoplasminogenemia (heterozygotes) or aplasminogenemia (homozygotes). All usual global tests of coagulation, including the platelet count, prothrombin time, partial thromboplastin time, thrombin time, and bleeding time are normal and the diagnosis depends on specific plasminogen assay for biologic activity performed by synthetic substrate methods.[17,128] Successful therapy has included the use of heparin, warfarin-type drugs, antiplatelet agents, and, interestingly, urokinase.[113,128] The clinical characteristics of congenital plasminogen deficiency are summarized in Table 12–19.

Changes in the Vessel Wall

Changes in the vessel wall are probably the most common etiologic factors in arterial thrombus formation.[182,187] These changes can come about via numerous mechanisms. Collagen can be exposed by

Table 12–18 Assays Available for Components of the Fibrinolytic System*

Plasminogen assay
Plasmin assay
Endothelial plasminogen activator
Alpha-2-antiplasmin
Alpha-2-macroglobulin

* All are automated by synthetic substrate, ELISA, or laser nephelometry.

Table 12–19 Characteristics of Congenital Plasminogen Deficiency

Clinical features
Autosomal recessive trait
Absence form and dysfunctional form exist
Thrombotic events begin in mid to late teens
Deep vein thrombosis is common
Pulmonary embolization is common
Arterial thrombotic events are rare
Thrombosis occurs when plasminogen is less than 40%
Laboratory features
Low biologic plasminogen activity
Low immunologic plasminogen in absence form
Normal immunologic plasminogen in dysfunctional form
Therapy
Warfarin
Heparin
Antiplatelet drugs
Urokinase

local injury to the vessel, as well as by inflammatory vascular changes. In addition, stasis, hypoxia, acidosis, and shock may also give rise to endothelial sloughing with exposure to subendothelial collagen and activation of coagulation. Exposed collagen has a capacity to initiate platelet aggregation and release as well as to activate the blood coagulation system by the activation of Factor XII to XII_a and the activation of Factor XI to XI_a.[18,19,27,210] In addition, endothelial plasminogen activator activity may be decreased and is, indeed, usually decreased in many vascular disorders, including scleroderma and thrombotic thrombocytopenic purpura. It is significant that there is much less endothelial plasminogen activator activity in the lower extremities compared with the upper extremities, and this may account for, or at least contribute to, the higher incidence of thrombosis in the lower extremities.[155] Decreased fibrinolytic activator activity is found in approximately 75% of patients with recurrent deep vein thrombosis, and this is often ascribed to primary vascular damage. The significance of this, however, remains unclear. In addition, it has recently been shown that the distribution and amount of various vascular proteoglycans may be correlated with arterial thrombotic and thromboembolic disease. Recent excellent summaries of this rapidly evolving topic are available.[187,208]

Laboratory Evaluation and Diagnosis of Hypercoagulability and Thrombosis

Older techniques for assessing platelet hyperactivity have primarily been measurements of altered platelet aggregability as measured by the standard platelet aggregometer and noting enhanced slopes of aggregation, although these data have not generally proved of clinical usefulness. However, newer molecular markers of platelet reactivity, such as platelet factor 4 and beta-thromboglobulin as well as various numerous platelet or endothelial prostaglandin derivatives, including thromboxane B_2, prostacyclin, and cyclo-oxygenase assays, are fully automated procedures by radioimmunoassay technique, and may soon be available by ELISA. These are proving to be potentially highly useful in assessing platelet reactivity in hypercoagulable conditions as well as in subclinical and clinical thrombotic disorders, including patients with deep vein thrombosis, thromboembolus, unstable angina, alterations of hemostasis associated with malignancy, and with numerous arterial thrombotic and thromboembolic events and other general microvascular disorders.[15–17,73,74] These new molecular markers of platelet reactivity are proving to be useful tools for both the diagnosis and monitoring of antithrombotic and antiplatelet therapy in patients with these types of problems. Many persons with hypercoagulability or thrombotic disorders are noted to have elevated platelet factor 4, beta-thromboglobulin, and thromboxane B_2 levels, which quite commonly decrease after the institution of effective antithrombotic therapy.[15–17,73,74]

Thus, molecular markers of platelet reactivity that are readily available to the clinical laboratory by fully automated procedures are the platelet factor 4 level, beta-thromboglobulin level, and various prostaglandin derivatives, including the immediate breakdown products of thromboxane A_2 (thromboxane B_2, and prostacyclin (6-keto-PGF_{-1}alpha). Recent evidence would suggest that several or all of these markers may be of benefit in aiding in a diagnosis as well as monitoring efficacy of therapy in patients with a wide variety of hypercoagulable disorders and thrombosis. This is especially true of the platelet factor 4 and beta-thromboglobulin measurement. Platelet survival by a variety of techniques has been noted to be altered in patients with hypercoagulability and with clinical thrombus formation.[82] A new fully automated method for the assessment of platelet survival by platelet size distribution profiling is readily available to the clinical laboratory and may be performed on either Baker, Coulter, or similar instruments.[17,35,61] Platelet indices as markets of both acute thrombosis and response to antithrombotic therapy have recently been studied, including mean platelet volume (MPV), platelet crit (PCT), and platelet distribution width (PDW).[17,35,36] In addition, platelet population distribution graphics generated by the Baker or Coulter devices readily allow for the automated calculation of average platelet size (APS), MPV, and the percentage of large, normal, and small platelets (LP, NP, and SP) circulating in the patient.[17,35,36,61]

These platelet indices have recently been performed on 113 normal volunteers to establish normal values, and on 52 patients with acute thrombosis.[17,37] Values were obtained at the time of diagnosis and repeated 24 hours after the initiation of antithrombotic therapy delivered as aspirin, 600 mg orally twice a day, plus dipyridamole, 50 mg orally four times a day. Studies have been done in parallel on the Coulter S-Plus II, the Coulter ZBI and Channelyzer, and the Baker 810. Acute thrombosis is associated with an increase in MPV, PCT, APS, and percentage of LP and a decrease in PDW and percentage of SP. All changes were noted to be statistically significant when compared with normal controls. In addition, the initiation of antithrombotic therapy was associated with a decrease toward normal of the MPV, PCT, APS, and percentage of NP and LP and an increase toward normal of the PDW and percentage of SP. Both Coulter and Baker instruments gave remarkably similar results; however, more significant changes between most of these indices were noted on the Baker 810 instrument when comparing normal volunteers versus patients with thrombosis. In addition, platelet size distribution profiling (percentage of SP, NP, and LP) appears slightly more reliable on the Baker instrument; however, the "downtime" on this instrument detracts from its desirability and reliability.

The results of these studies would suggest that platelet indices and platelet size distribution profiling may provide a simple, rapid, and readily available fully automated method for detecting enhanced platelet consumption and decreased platelet survival, thus aiding in a diagnosis of acute thrombosis and assessing response to antithrombotic or antiplatelet therapy.[17,35–37,61] Changes in platelet size distribution profiles and platelet indices in thrombosis

before and after therapy are summarized in Table 12–20 and changes in platelet size distribution profiling in normal subjects and patients with thrombosis are depicted in Figure 4–31. Changes in MPV and PCT during thrombosis and after therapy are shown in Figures 4–30 and 4–32 and changes in platelet factor 4 levels before and after therapy in patients with deep vein thrombosis are depicted in Figure 12–8. The Baker 810 and S Plus II are depicted in Figures 12–9 and 12–10.

As mentioned previously, numerous coagulation factors are found to be elevated in patients with hypercoagulability and thrombosis; however, in general, the measurements of these factors, including fibrinogen, Factors VIII:C and IX, and other related factors do not appear to be useful with respect to either diagnosis or monitoring of efficacy of therapy. Decreases in coagulation inhibitors, both AT III and protein C, do appear to be of significant diagnostic and therapeutic monitoring efficacy in patients with hypercoagulability and undergoing subclinical and clinical thrombotic and thromboembolic events.[17,20,82,127,185] Automated methods for assessing AT III as well as protein C are readily available and are of paramount diagnostic efficacy, especially if a congenital deficiency is found.[17,20,52,127,185] However, the monitoring efficacy of protein C remains to be established.

The clinical indications for AT III determinations were discussed previously. Another recent advance in the diagnosis of hypercoagulability and thrombosis has been the development of fibrinogen chromatography.[5,77] Much useful data has

Table 12–20 Changes in Platelet Distribution Profiles and Platelet Indices in Acute Thrombosis

Parameter	Thrombosis	Post-therapy
Mean platelet volume	Increase	Decrease
Average platelet size	Increase	Decrease
Platelet crit	Increase	Decrease
% large platelets	Increase	Decrease
% normal platelets	No change	No change
% small platelets	Decrease	Increase
Platelet distribution width	Decrease	Increase

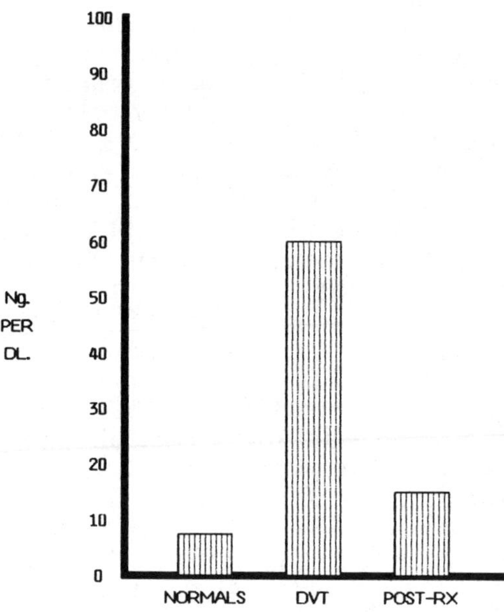

Fig. 12–8. Changes in platelet factor 4 in patients with deep vein thrombosis.

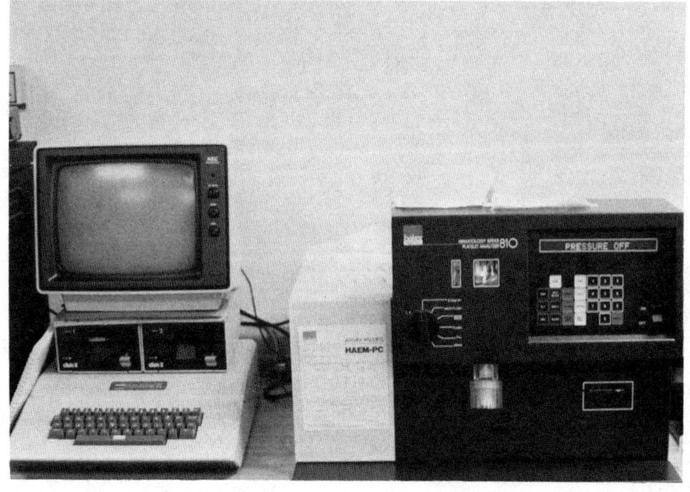

Fig. 12–9. The Baker 810 used for platelet size distribution profiling and platelet indicies in acute thrombosis.

come from this modality, and it is likely that this may be a highly applicable and available clinical tool in the near future. The procedure is now automated to the point where it can be performed in several hours; however, the equipment and time required is still formidable for the routine clinical hemostasis laboratory. Fibrinogen chromatography when used clinically is able to detect several fibrinogen sub-

species: (1) fibrin monomer (molecular weight of approximately 320,000 daltons) is fibrinogen minus fibrinopeptide A and fibrinopeptide B; (2) fibrinogen dimer has molecular weight of approximately 650,000 daltons and represents one intact fibrinogen molecule complexed with one fibrin monomer; (3) fibrinogen polymer (molecular weight of approximately 400,000 to 1,000,000 daltons), which is fib-

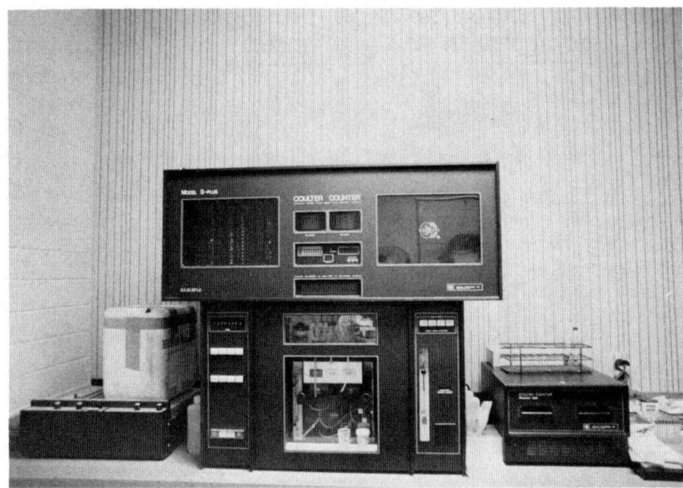

Fig. 12–10. The Coulter S-PLUS II used for platelet size distribution profiling and platelet indicies in acute thrombosis.

rinogen complexed with various fibrin(ogen) fragments; (4) fibrinogen first derivative (molecular weight of 267,000 daltons), which represents fibrinogen that has been cleaved at the carboxyterminal end of the A-alpha chain by plasmin; (5) the X, Y, D, and E fibrin(ogen) fragments. The applicability of fibrinogen chromatography becomes evident when looking at disorders characterized by the presence of fibrinogen dimer and fibrinogen polymer. In general, thrombosis is characterized by an increase in fibrin(ogen) complexes of molecular weight of 450,000 daltons or greater, and when these fragments are found one may presume that increased fibrin deposition is occurring. As a thrombus resolves, due to fibrinolysis, the following is noted: (1) a decrease in fibrin-(ogen) complexes, (2) an increase in FDP, and (3) an increase in fibrinogen first derivative.[78] In addition, there will be a decrease in fibrinopeptide A and fibrinopeptide B levels. The new techniques to detect thrombin generation rapidly by the use of fibrinopeptide A titers are readily available; fibrinopeptide A is noted to be elevated in numerous hypercoagulable and thrombotic disorders and is commonly noted to decrease with the institution of successful antithrombotic therapy.[15–17,73]

Another modality that may prove useful in hypercoagulability, and subclinical and clinical thrombosis is the simultaneous determination of B-beta 15-42 and related peptides.[75,164] As plasmin begins to circulate, B-beta peptides 1 through 118 and 1 through 42 begin to circulate; however, if thrombin has been present, to remove fibrinopeptide B (the first 14 amino acids on the B-beta chain) B-beta 15-42 levels will also be increased. Thus, patients with circulating thrombin will have elevated fibrinopeptide A and fibrinopeptide A levels, and B-beta 1 through 118 and 1 through 42 peptides. However, as plasmin begins to circulate one will also note the elevation of B-beta 15-42 and related peptides, thus allowing for the conclusion that thrombus resolution is beginning. The molecular profiling of hypercoagulable patients as well as patients with subclinical and clinical thrombosis is now becoming available; molecular profiling for the detection of hypercoagulability and thrombosis is given in Table 12–21.

Newer assays for components of the fibrinolytic system are also now readily available and may aid greatly in a diagnosis of hypercoagulability and thrombosis, and these synthetic substrate assays are for plasminogen, plasmin, endothelial plasminogen activator activity, and alpha-2-antiplasmin.[17,71,72,101] One can also perform alpha-2-macroglobulin levels by automated techniques, including ELISA and radioimmunoassays and other immunologic procedures[17] (Table 12–18).

The traditional older methods for assessing hypercoagulability and thrombosis,

Table 12–21 Molecular Marker Profiling for Hypercoagulability and Thrombosis*

Fibrinopeptide A
Fibrinopeptide B
B-beta 15–42 related peptides
Platelet factor 4
Beta-thromboglobulin
Thromboxanes
Prostacyclins (6-keto-PGF-I-alpha)
Soluble fibrin monomer
Fibrinogen degradation products
Antithrombin III
Protein C
Plasminogen
Alpha-2-antiplasmin
Endothelial plasminogen activator

* All may be fully automated by synthetic substrates, ELISA, radioimmunoassay or laser nephelometry.

such as the activated PTT, nonactivated PTT (Kingdon assay), the fibrinogen level, and the noting of elevated coagulation factors have contributed very little to the understanding of hypercoagulability and thrombosis and have likewise, in general, not been associated with useful information regarding diagnosis or efficacy of therapy. However, newer assays are becoming available by automated techniques, including the synthetic substrate equivalent of the activated PTT, the so-called intrinsic pathway generated thrombin test, the synthetic substrate equivalent of the prothrombin time, the so-called extrinsic pathway generated thrombin test, the AT III level by synthetic substrate assay, protein C levels by synthetic substrate assays as well as synthetic substrate assays for fibrinolytic system components.[17,71] In addition, radioimmunoassays and potentially ELISA procedures for fibrinopeptide A, fibrinopeptide B, platelet reactive products, including platelet factor 4 and beta-thromboglobulin, thromboxane B_2, and 6-keto-PGF$_1$-alpha are also available for molecular profiling by automated techniques.[15–17,71–73] Of additional interest are assays of B-beta 15-42 and related peptides. Platelet indices and platelet survival as assessed by platelet size distribution profiling by automated techniques, as previously discussed, in conjunction with automated procedures for the aforementioned molecular markers of platelet reactivity are proving to be useful for both diag-

nosing and monitoring the efficacy of therapy in hypercoagulable patients as well as patients with subclinical and clinical thrombotic and thromboemolic events. Older and newer laboratory tests for the evaluation of hypercoagulability and thrombosis are given in Table 12–22.

Additionally, when assessing patients with hypercoagulability and thrombosis, nonhemostasis testing methods are also usually applicable and at times must be considered. These include such procedures as complete blood count, platelet count, and evaluation of platelet morphology, reticulocyte count, general biochemical screening surveys, autoimmune evaluations, paraprotein evaluations, an evaluation for occult malignancy, as well as consideration for angiography, thromboscintigraphy, ventilation perfusion scan, pulmonary angiography, peripheral vascular angiography, and vascular biopsies for morphology and special staining techniques.[17,18] Nonhemostasis techniques often needed for assessing hypercoagulability and thrombosis are summarized in Table 11–23.

Selected hemostasis laboratory values in 118 consecutive patients with deep vein

Table 12–22 Testing Modalities for Assessing Hypercoagulability and Thrombosis

Older Methods (Manual)*	Newer Methods (Automated)†
Prothrombin time	Extrinsic pathway generated thrombin
Activated PTT	
Nonactivated PTT	Intrinsic pathway generated thrombin
FDP elevation	
Protamine sulfate	Antithrombin III
Aggregation?	Protein C
Platelet aggregates?	Plasminogen
Clotting factor levels?	Plasmin
	Plasminogen activator
	Alpha-2-antiplasmin
	Alpha-2-macroglobulin
	Fibrinopeptide A
	FDP elevation
	Protamine sulfate
	Platelet factor 4
	Beta-thromboglobulin
	Protaglandins
	Thromboxanes
	Platelet survival

* Clot-based methods.
† Synthetic substrates, radioimmunoassay, ELISA.

Table 12–23 Nonhemostasis Modalities for Assessing Hypercoagulability and Thrombosis

Complete blood count
Platelet count
Sedimentation rate
Biochemical screening survey
Lipid profile
Orotic acid crystals
Angiography
Thromboscintigraphy
Ascending venography
Ventilation perfusion scan
Vascular biopsy
Immunofluorescent stains
Hyperviscosity

thrombosis with or without pulmonary embolus have recently been examined.[17,37] All patients except three with hereditary thrombophilia were treated similarly: heparin subcutaneously, 80 to 100 U/kg every 6 hours for 4 days, followed by aspirin and dipyridamole. Studies were obtained at the time of diagnosis and repeated in 24 hours; the selected studies on these 118 patients were AT III, platelet factor 4, alpha-2-macroglobulin, alpha-1-antitrypsin, alpha-2-antiplasmin, plasminogen, platelet indices, and platelet size distribution profiling. It was found that the average pretherapy AT III level was 91% (normal, 89 to 129%) and the post-therapy level was 95%. Forty-eight percent of all patients had significantly decreased AT III levels before the initiation of therapy and 9% had elevated AT III levels. Of those with elevated levels, 50% had disseminated malignancy. After the initiation of therapy, 36% of patients still had decreased AT III levels. Platelet factor 4 levels were elevated in 82% of patients before the initiation of therapy with an average level of 57 µg/dL. After the initiation of therapy, only 11% of patients had persistent elevated levels, 89% being normal after initiation of antithrombotic therapy. Platelet factor 4 levels before and after therapy in this group of patients with deep vein thrombosis are depicted in Figure 12–8. Only 3% of patients had low plasminogen levels before the initiation of therapy; however, it could be anticipated that these patients would potentially not respond ideally to thrombolytic therapy. Alpha-2-macroglobu-

lin levels and alpha-1-antitrypsin levels remained normal and unchanged both before and after therapy. Twenty percent of patients were found to have low alpha-2-antiplasmin levels before the initiation of therapy. The pretherapy MPV was 8.35 µm^3 with 55% of patients having elevated MPVs. All but one patient with a pulmonary embolus had markedly elevated MPVs with the average being 9.1 (normal, 5.4 to 7.4 µm^3, Coulter ZBI Channelyzer). The average post-therapy MPV was 7.5, with 27% of patients still remaining abnormal. These MPV results are summarized in Figure 4–32.

In assessing the results of this study the platelet factor 4 level appears to be quite reliable in aiding in a diagnosis of deep vein thrombosis and in monitoring efficacy of therapy. The AT III levels, of less reliability diagnostically, appear to be highly useful for predicting a potential response to heparin or other anticoagulant therapy and for detecting congenital AT III deficiency (3% in this series of 118 patients) and for monitoring efficacy of therapy. Plasminogen levels were found to be useful, since 3% of patients had significant hypoplasminogenemia and would, presumably, not respond ideally to thrombolytic therapy. Twenty percent of individuals had low alpha-2-antiplasmin levels. This was presumably due to activation of the fibrinolytic system and partial inhibition of circulating plasmin. Platelet size distribution profiling, as discussed previously, appeared to be useful in both the diagnosis and in monitoring of antithrombotic therapy. Thrombosis was associated with an increase in the MPV and in the percentage of large platelets, whereas therapy was associated with a decrease in these parameters and an increase in the percentage of small platelets. In addition, the finding of an MPV greater than 8.5 µm^3 in patients with deep vein thrombosis suggests the development of concurrent pulmonary embolization.

In summary, the laboratory diagnosis of hypercoagulability and thrombosis is in its infancy, despite recent advances in the coagulation laboratory. However, with newer automated modalities being applied to large populations of patients, it is expected that molecular markers of platelet reactivity and altered blood protein function (coagulation, fibrinolysis, and inhibitors) may become highly useful in diagnosing and monitoring therapy in patients who are hypercoagulable or who have subclinical or clinical thrombosis. It is further anticipated that with the widespread use of automated molecular marker profiling, we will be able to detect and treat those patients who are hypercoagulable before they have a life-threatening thrombotic event or before a serious thrombohemorrhagic event leads to irreversible and lifelong morbidity.

Therapy

Therapy of hypercoagulability and frank thrombosis will differ markedly, depending on the condition being treated; specific therapy has been covered in relevant sections of this chapter and other chapters of this text. In patients who are hypercoagulable, those patients with a predisposition to thrombus formation, prophylaxis may be in the form of platelet suppressive therapy, as will be discussed in Chapter 13, oral anticoagulant therapy, or low-dose heparin therapy, also discussed in Chapter 13, or fibrinolytic enhancement therapy, as outlined in Chapter 14. Specific antithrombotic therapy in DIC is discussed in Chapter 6, and anticoagulant therapy for both hypercoagulability, thrombosis, and thromboembolus in malignancy is discussed in detail in Chapter 10.

My general approach to prophylactic therapy in hypercoagulable patients is to use a combination platelet suppressive therapy in the form of enteric coated aspirin, 600 mg twice a day, each dose to be taken with 30 mL of liquid antacid for gastric mucosal protection, and dipyridamole, 50 mg orally four times a day. If headaches develop with this dose of dipyridamole, the dose is decreased to 50 mg three times a day or to 25 mg four times a day. If a patient is intolerant to aspirin or there exists a contraindication to aspirin therapy, sulfinpyrizone, 200 mg three times a day, each dose also to be taken with 30 mL of liquid antacid for gastric mucosal protection, is substituted. An alternative approach to prophylaxis is to use subcutaneous heparin at 2500 U every 8 to 12 hours in the patient who is willing to give self injections, or to use intrapulmonary heparin at 10,000 to 20,000 U/week by ultrasonic nebulizer.[17,18,38] The use of intrapulmonary heparin for prophylaxis is still investigational, but the results thus far are encouraging, and this approach is certainly convenient to patients.[38] Approaches to prophylactic therapy in the patient with hypercoagulability and an increased predisposition to thrombus formation are summarized in Table 12–24.

My approach to treating active thrombotic disease, including arterial thrombi and thromboemboli, deep vein thrombosis, and pulmonary embolus, are as follows. Deep vein thrombosis of the lower extremities is treated by starting the patient on subcutaneous calcium heparin at a dose of 80 to 100 U/kg three times a day, assuming the AT III level is greater than 40% biologic activity.[17,20,40] In addition, both legs are elevated 15° above the hip joints, patients are kept at bed rest for 24 hours, and are immediately taught antiembolic leg exercises that are to be performed at least six times a day, starting on the first day. These antiembolic exercises consist simply of alternate dorsiflexion and plantor flexion of each foot until the calf of that particular leg is fatigued; the patient is instructed to do only one leg at a time. Also, at the time of admission, medium compression pantyhose are ordered. These will take several days to ob-

Table 12–24 An Approach to the Prophylaxis of Hypercoagulability and Thrombosis

---

Platelet suppressive therapy
    Aspirin, 600 mg twice a day, each dose with 30 mL
        of liquid antacid
    Dipyridamole, 50 mg four times a day
    Sulfinpyrazone, 200 mg twice a day, each dose with
        30 mL of liquid antacid
    A combination of aspirin and dipyridamole or sulfin-
        pyrazone and dipyridamole is needed
Low-dose heparin therapy
    Intrapulmonary calcium heparin by ultrasonic
        nebulizer, 10,000 to 20,000 U/week, or
    Outpatient self-administration of subcutaneous
        heparin at 80 U/kg two to three times a day

---

tain and are not put on the patient until at least the third day after the thrombotic event. The patient is encouraged to begin ambulation after the first 24 hours and to continue to do so until discharge. On the third day, or occasionally the fourth day, depending on the clinical situation, the patient is taken off subcutaneous calcium heparin and started on aspirin plus dipyridamole in the previously discussed doses. Twenty-four hours after starting aspirin and dipyridamole, the patient is discharged. As an outpatient, the patient is instructed to continue with the aforementioned antiembolic leg exercises at least six times a day, is told not to indulge in any activities that involve bending the knee or thigh for greater than 20 minutes at a time, and is told to wear the medium compression pantyhose during waking hours. If the patient remains thrombosis-free for 6 months, the pantyhose and dipyridamole are discontinued, and the patient is instructed to continue aspirin and antiembolic leg exercises indefinitely.

Using this approach, my experience has been that in 118 patients so treated, there has been a rethrombosis rate of 14% in 16,992 patient follow-up days, or a rethrombosis rate of 0.3% per year.[17,22] If the patient with deep vein thrombosis has a concurrent pulmonary embolus, the same approach is taken unless there is presence of unstable hemodynamics, in which case streptokinase, as outlined in Chapter 14, is used.[144] If a patient has a recurrent thrombosis on the just defined outpatient regimen, streptokinase may then be considered for the acute recurrent thrombotic event, and outpatient prophylaxis in these patients is often in the form of weekly intrapulmonary heparin[38] for a minimum period of 6 months. This approach to treating deep vein thrombosis and pulmonary embolus is outlined in Table 12–25.

Arterial thrombi and thromboemboli are usually treated with subcutaneous calcium heparin at the same dose described previously in conjunction with papaverine hydrochloride. After the acute episode has resolved, the patient is taken off calcium heparin and is placed on aspirin and dipyridamole at the doses previously defined and continued on papaverine hydrochloride 150 mg orally twice a day. If the

Table 12–25 An Approach to the Patient with Deep Vein Thrombosis with or without Pulmonary Embolus*

Subcutaneous calcium heparin: 80 to 100 U/kg three times a day
Elevate legs 15° on admission
Antiembolic leg exercises on admission
Fit for medium compression panty hose (not put on until day 3)
Ambulation after 24 hours
Platelet suppressive therapy at day 3 (concurrently stop heparin)
Discharge at day 3 or day 4, on aspirin plus dipyridamole or sulfinpyrazone plus dipyridamole
Stop dipyridamole and antiembolic stockings at 6 months if no recurrence
Continue with exercises and aspirin or sulfinpyrazone indefinitely

* Thrombolytic therapy if indicated: pulmonary embolus with unstable hemodynamics or recurrent deep vein thrombosis on heparin.

patient remains thrombosis-free for 6 months, the dipyridamole is stopped. Depending on the site, severity, and type of the arterial thrombotic or thromboembolic event, thrombolytic therapy, rather than subcutaneous calcium heparin, may be used.[144]

Summary

Known alterations of hemostasis in the hypercoagulable patient and in the patient undergoing subclinical and clinical thrombus formation have been discussed. It remains unclear as to whether many of these alterations are of etiologic significance or manifestations (consequences) of already present and perhaps clinically undetectable thrombus formation. At present, many common laboratory modalities do not allow for a differentiation between "cause and effect." It is hopeful that in the near future, practical techniques, such as those previously outlined, and primarily consisting of fully automated synthetic substrate assays as well as molecular marker techniques that detect subclinical changes in the coagulation system, will become more generally available for diagnosing prethrombotic events and for monitoring the patient who has had a thrombotic event and for detecting a patient who is potentially predisposed to thrombosis so that the patient can be treated prophylactically before unalterable morbidity or, in fact, mortality occurs.

References

1. Abildgaard U: Purification of two progressive antithrombins of human plasma. Scand J Clin Lab Invest 19:190, 1967,
2. Abildgaard U: Binding of thrombin to antithrombin III. Scand J Clin Lab Invest 24:23, 1969.
3. Abildgaard U, Graven K, Godal HC: Assay of progressive antithrombin in plasma. Thromb Diath Haemorrh 24:224, 1970.
4. Abildgaard U, Fagerhol M, Egeberg O: Comparison of progressive antithrombin activity and the concentration of three thrombin inhibitors in human plasma. Scand J Clin Lab Invest 26:349, 1970.
5. Alkjaersig N, Roy L, Fletcher AP: Analysis of gel exclusion chromatography data by chromatographic plate theory analysis: Application to plasma fibrinogen chromatography. Thromb Res 3:525, 1973.
6. Almer LD, Pandolfi M, Osterlin S: The fibrinolytic system in patients with diabetes mellitus with special reference to diabetic retinopathy. Opthalmologica 170:353, 1975.
7. American Diagnostica, Activated Protein C assay, American Diagnostic Newsletter, Greenwich, CT, 1984.
8. Aoki N, Moroi M, Sakata Y, Yoshida N, Matsuda M: Abnormal plasminogen. A hereditary molecular abnormality found in a patient with recurrent thrombosis. J Clin Invest 61:1186, 1978.
9. Astrup T: Tissue activators of plasminogen. Fed Proc 25:42, 1966.
10. Banerjee R, Sahni A, Kumar V, Arya M: Antithrombin III deficiency in maturity onset diabetes mellitus and atherosclerosis. Thromb Diath Haemorrh 31:339, 1974.
11. Barrowcliffe T, Johnson E, Eggleton C, Thomas DP: Anticoagulant activities of lung and mucous heparins. Thromb Res 12:27, 1978.
12. Becker J: The relation of platelet adhesiveness of postoperative venous thrombosis of the legs. Acta Chir Scand 138:781, 1972.
13. Bertina RM, Broekmans AW, van der Linden IK, Mertens K: Protein C deficiency in a Dutch family with thrombotic disease. Thromb Haemost 48:1, 1982.
14. Bertina RM, Broekmans AW, van Es-Krommenhoek T, van Wijngaarde A: The use of a functional assay for plasma protein C in the diagnosis of protein C deficiency. (Abstr.) Thromb Haemost 50:350, 1983.
15. Bick RL: Clinical implications of molecular markers in hemostasis and thrombosis. Semin Thromb Hemost 10:290, 1984.
16. Bick RL, Fareed J, Squillaci G, Walanga J, Bermes EW, Messmore HL: Molecular markers of hemostatic processes. Implications in diagnostic and therapeutic management of thrombotic and hemorrhagic disorders. Fed Proc 42:4, 1983.
17. Bick RL: Clinical hemostasis practice: The major impact of laboratory automation. Semin Thromb Hemost 9:139, 1983.
18. Bick RL: Hypercoagulability and thrombosis. In Murano G, Bick RL (Eds): Basic Concepts of Hemostasis and Thrombosis. CRC Press, Boca Raton, FL, 1980, p 237.
19. Bick RL: Disseminated intravascular coagulation. In Bick RL (Ed): Disseminated Intravascular Coagulation and Related Syndromes. CRC Press, Boca Raton, FL, 1983, p 31.
20. Bick RL: Clinical relevance of antithrombin III. Semin Thromb Hemost 8:276, 1982.
21. Bick RL, Bishop RC, Shanbrom E: Fibrinolytic activity in acute myocardial infarction. Am J Clin Pathol 57:359, 1972.
22. Bick RL: Deep venous thrombosis: Clinical evaluation of 118 consecutive patients. Thromb Haemost 50(1):305, 1983.
23. Bick RL: Discrepant AT-III and fibrinogen levels on the DuPont ACA system. Am J Clin Pathol 80:891, 1983.
24. Bick RL, McClain BJ: A comparison of the Protopath and DuPont ACA antithrombin III assays in 149 patients with DIC, deep venous thrombosis, and hereditary thrombophilia. Am J Clin Pathol 82:371, 1984.
25. Bick RL, Wheeler A, Camposano, N: A comparative study of the DuPont antithrombin III and fibrinogen assay systems. Am J Clin Pathol 83:541, 1985.
26. Bick RL, Faulstick D: Antithrombins and coronary artery disease. Am J Clin Pathol 81:773, 1984.
27. Bick RL: Disseminated intravascular coagulation and related syndromes. In Murano G, Bick RL (Eds): Basic Concepts of Hemostasis and Thrombosis. CRC Press, Boca Raton, FL, 1980, p 163.
28. Bick RL: Disseminated intravascular coagulation. Pract Cardiol 7:147,245, 1981.
29. Bick RL: Disseminated intravascular coagulation and related syndromes. In Fareed J, Messmore HL, Fenton JW, Brinkhous KM (Eds): Perspectives in Hemostasis. Pergamon Press, New York, 1981, p 122.
30. Bick RL: Syndromes associated with hyperfibrino(geno)lysis. In Bick RL (Ed): Disseminated Intravascular Coagulation and Related Syn-

dromes. CRC Press, Boca Raton, FL, 1983, p 105.

31. Bick RL: Disseminated intravascular coagulation and related syndromes. A review. Am J Hematol 5:265, 1978.

32. Bick RL, Oukes ML, Wilson WL, Fekete LF: Antithrombin III (AT-III) as a diagnostic aid in disseminated intravascular coagulation. Thromb Res 10:721, 1977.

33. Bick RL, Bick MD, Fekete LF: Antithrombin III patterns in disseminated intravascular coagulation. Am J Clin Pathol 73:577, 1980.

34. Bick RL, Thompson WB: Fibrinolytic activity: Changes induced with oral contraceptives. Obstet Gynecol 39:213, 1972.

35. Bick RL, McClain BJ: Platelet indicies as markers of acute thrombosis and response to antithrombotic therapy. Am J Clin Pathol 81:798, 1984.

36. Bick RL, McClain BJ: Platelet indicies as markers of acute thrombosis and response to antithrombotic therapy. Thromb Haemost 50:153, 1983.

37. Bick RL, McClain BJ: Deep venous thrombosis: A laboratory evaluation of 118 consecutive patients. Thromb Hemost 50:237, 1983.

38. Bick RL, Ross ES: The clinical use of intrapulmonary heparin. Semin Thromb Hemost 11:213, 1985.

39. Bick RL, Kovac I, Fekete L: A new two-stage functional assay for antithrombin III (heparin co-factor): Clinical and laboratory evaluation. Thromb Res 8:745, 1976.

40. Bick RL: Monitoring heparin therapy. Diag Dialog 1:1, 1979.

41. Bick RL, Murano G: Primary hyperfibrino-(geno)lytic syndromes. In Murano G, Bick R (Eds): Basic Concepts of Hemostasis and Thrombosis. CRC Press, Boca Raton, FL, 1980, p 181.

42. Bick R: Disseminated intravascular coagulation: A clinical/laboratory study of 48 patients. Ann NY Acad Sci 370:843, 1981.

43. Bick RL, McClain B: A clinical comparison of chromogenic, fluorometric and natural (fibrinogen) substrate assays for determination of antithrombin III. Am J Clin Pathol 77:238, 1982.

44. Bobek K, Kepelak V: Laboratory diagnosis of venous thrombosis. Acta Med Scand 160:121, 1958.

45. Bounameaux N, Duckert F, Walter M, Bounameaux Y: The determination of antithrombin III. Comparison of six methods. Effect of oral contraceptive therapy. Thromb Haemost 39:607, 1978.

46. Braude S, Arias J, Houghes R, Canalese J, Gimson A, Williams R, Scully M, Kakkar V: Antithrombin III infusion during fulminant hepatic failure. Thromb Haemsot 46:369, 1981.

47. Brinkhous KM, Smith HP, Warner ED, Seegers WH: Inhibition of blood clotting and unidentified substances which act in conjunction with heparin to prevent the conversion of prothrombin to thrombin. Am J Physiol 125:683, 1939.

48. Broekmans AW, Bertina MR, Loelinger EA, Hofmann V, Klingemann HG: Protein C and the development of skin necrosis during anticoagulant therapy. (Letter.) Thromb Haemost 49:255, 1983.

49. Broekmans AW, Veltkamp JJ, Bertina R: Congenital protein C deficiency and venous thromboembolism. N Engl J Med 309:340, 1983.

50. Carlstrom A, Lieden K, Bjork I: Decreased binding of heparin to antithrombins following the interaction between antithrombin and thrombin. Thromb Res 11:785, 1977.

51. Chandra S, Bang N, Marks C: Radiolabeled AT-III as a probe for the detection of activation of blood coagulation in vivo. Thromb Res 9:9, 1976.

52. Comp PC, Nixon R, Esmon CT: Determination of functional levels of protein C, an antithrombotic protein, using thrombin/thrombomodulin complex. Blood 63:15, 1984.

53. Conard J, Samama M, Salomon Y: Antithrombin III and the oestrogen content of combined oestro-progesterone contraceptives. Lancet 2:1148, 1972.

54. Conard J, Samama M, Norellou M, Casenave B, Griguer P, Barsotti J, Merreman G, Godeau P: Congenital antithrombin III deficiency in 3 families (7 affected members). (Abstr.) Thromb Haemost 42:128, 1979.

55. Conard J, Casenave B, Samama M, Horellou M, Zorn J, Neau C: AT-III content and antithrombin activity in oestrogen-progesterone and progesterone-only treated women. Thromb Res 18:675, 1980.

56. Corrigan J: Changes in the blood coagulation system associated with septicemia. N Engl J Med 279:851, 1968.

57. Davidson E, Tomlin S: The levels of plasma coagulation factors after trauma and childbirth. J Clin Pathol 16:112, 1963.

58. Davis RB, Theologides A, Kennedy BJ: Comparative studies of blood coagulation and platelet aggregation in patients with cancer and non-malignant disease. Ann Intern Med 71:67, 1969.

59. Dayan L, Donadio D, David E, Huguet M: Maladie thromboembolique familiale recidivante par deficit congenital en anti-thrombine III. Etude preliminaire de 3 observations. Nouv Presse Med 7:3229, 1978.

60. DiScipio RG, Hermodson MA, Yates SG, Davie EW: A comparison of human prothrombin, factor IX (Christmas factor), factor X (Stuart factor), and protein S. Biochemistry 16:698,

322Disorders of Hemostasis and Thrombosis

1977.

61. Dumoulin-OLagrange M, Capelle C: Evaluation of automated platelet counters for the enumeration and sizing of platelets in the diagnosis and management of hemostatic problems. Semin Thromb Hemos 9:235, 1983.

62. Dunn E, Prager R, Penner J: The effect of heparin and antithrombin III on endotoxin induced disseminated intravascular coagulation (DIC). Trans Am Soc Hematol, 1976, p 9.

63. Egbring R, Meneche B, Fuchs F, Jacobi J, Heimburger N, Havemann K: Antithrombin III determination of an amidolytic method before and after AT-III substitution. (Abstr.) Thromb Haemost 42:225, 1979.

64. Egbring R, Klingemann H, Heimburger N, Karges H, Beule J, Seitz R, Havemann K: Antithrombin III substitution in acute hepatic failure due to CCl_4 intoxication. (Abstr.) Thromb Haemost 46:373, 1981.

65. Egeberg O: Inherited antithrombin III deficiency and thrombo-embolism. V Congress of International Society of Thrombosis and Haemostasis. (Abstr.) 1975, p 170.

66. Emmons PR, Mitchell JRA: Post-operative changes in platelet clumping activity. Lancet 1:71, 1965.

67. Esmon CT, Esmon NL: Protein C activation. Semin Thromb Hemost 10:122, 1984.

68. Esmon CT: Protein C: Biochemistry, physiology and clinical implications. Blood 62:1155, 1983.

69. Fagerhol M, Abildgaard U: Immunologic studies in human antithrombin III. Influence of age, sex, and use of oral contraceptives on serum concentration. Scand J Haematol 7:10, 170.

70. Fareed J, Messmore HL, Walgena JM, Bermes EW, Bick RL: Laboratory evaluation of antithrombin III: A critical overview of currently available methods for antithrombin III measurements. Semin Thromb Hemost 8:288, 1982.

71. Fareed J, Messmore HL, Bermes EW: New perspectives in coagulation testing. Clin Chem 26:1380, 1980.

72. Fareed J, Messmore HL, Walenga J, Bermes EW: Diagnostic efficacy of newer synthetic substrate methods for assessing coagulation variables: A critical overview. Clin Chem 28:2025, 1983.

73. Fareed J, Walenga JM, Bick RL, Bermes EW, Messmore HL: Impact of automation on the quantitation of low molecular weight markers of hemostatic defects. Semin Thromb Hemost 9:355, 1983.

74. Fareed J, Walenga JM: Current trends in hemostasis testing. Semin Thromb Hemost 9:380, 1983.

75. Fareed J, Bick RL, Squallaci C, Walenga J, Messmore HL, Bermes EW: Clinical and experimental studies using a modified radioimmunoassay for B-beta 15-42 related peptides. Thromb Haemost 50:300, 1983.

76. Fischer CL, Gill LW: Acute phase proteins. In Ritzmann SE, Daniels JC (Eds): Serum Protein Abnormalities. Little, Brown, Boston, 1975, p 331.

77. Fletcher AP, Alkjaersig N: Blood hypercoagulability, intravascular coagulation, and thrombosis: New diagnostic concepts. Thromb Diath Haemorrh 45:389, 1971.

78. Fletcher AP, Alkjaersig N: Laboratory diagnosis of intravascular coagulation. In Poller L (Ed): Recent Advances in Thrombosis. Churchill Livingstone, London, 1973, p 87.

79. Francis RB, Patch MJ: A functional assay for Protein C in human plasma. Thromb Res 32:605, 1983.

80. Ganrot PO: Studies on serum protease inhibitors with special reference to α-2 macroglobulin. Acta Univ Lund Sect 2:2, 1967.

81. Gralnick H, Tan H: Acute promyelocytic leukemia: A model for understanding the role of the malignant cell in hemostasis. Hum Pathol 5:661, 1974.

82. Griffin JH: Clinical studies on protein C. Semin Thromb Hemost 10:162, 1984.

83. Griffin JH, Evatt B, Zimmerman TS, Kleiss AJ, Wideman C: Deficiency of Protein C in congenital thrombotic disease. J Clin Invest 68:1370, 1981.

84. Griffin JH, Mosher DF, Zimmerman TS, Kleiss AJ: Protein C, an antithrombotic protein, is reduced in hospitalized patients with intravascular coagulation. Blood 60:261, 1982.

85. Griffin JH, Bezeaud A, Evatt B, Mosher D: Functional and immunologic studies of protein C in thromboembolic disease. (Abstr.) Blood 62:301a, 1983.

86. Hallen A, Nilsson I: Coagulaton studies in liver disease. Thromb Diath Haemorrh 11:51, 1964.

87. Harker L: Platelet survival time: Its measurement and use. Prog Hemost Thromb 4:321, 1978.

88. Harpel PC, Rosenberg RD: Alpha-2-macroglobulin and antithrombin-heparin cofactor: Modulators of hemostasis and inflammatory reactions. Prog Hemost Thromb 3:145, 1976.

89. Hasegawa DK, Tyler BJ, Edson JR: Thrombotic disease in three families with inherited plasminogen deficiency. Blood 60:213, 1982.

90. Hatton M, Berry L, Regoeczi E: INhibition of thrombin by antithrombin III in the presence of certain glycosaminoglycans found in the mammalian aorta. Thromb Res 13:655, 1978.

91. Hedner U, Nilsson IM: Urokinase inhibitors in serum in a clinical series. Acta Med Scand 189:185, 1971.

92. Hedner U, Nilsson I: Antithrombin III in clin-

ical material. Thromb Res 3:631, 1973.

93. Hellem AJ: Platelet adhesiveness. Ser Haematol 1:99, 1968

94. Hellem AJ: Adenosine diphosphate induced platelet adhesiveness in diabetes mellitus with complications. Acta Med Scand 190:291, 1971.

95. Hellgren M, Javelin L, Hagnevik K, Blomback M: Antithrombin III concentrate as adjuvant in DIC treatment. A pilot study in 9 severely ill patients. Thromb Res 35:459, 1984.

96. Hensen A, Loeliger E: Antithrombin III. Its metabolism and function. Thromb Diath Haemorrh (Suppl) 9:1, 1973.

97. Hook M, Bjork I, Hopwood J, Lindahl U: Anticoagulant action of heparin: Separation of high-activity ad low-activity heparin species by affinity chromatography on immobilized antithrombin. FEBS Lett 66:90, 1976.

98. Howie P, Mallinson A, Prentice C, Horn C, McNicol G: Effect of combined oestrogen-progesterone oral contraceptives, oestrogen, and progesterone on antiplasmin and antithrombin activity. Lancet 2:1329, 1970.

99. Hume M, Sevitt S, Thomas DP: Venous thrombosis and pulmonary embolism. Harvard University Press, Cambridge, MA, 1970.

100. Hume M, Chan YK: Examination of the blood in the presence of venous thrombosis. JAMA 200:747, 1967.

101. Husby RM, Smith RE: Synthetic oligopeptide substrates: Their diagnostic application in blood coagulation, fibrinolysis, and other pathological states. Semin Thromb Hemost 6:173, 1980.

102. Innerfield I, Goldfsicher J, Reichter-Reiss H, Greenberg J: Serum antithrombins in coronary artery disease. Am J Clin Pathol 65:64, 1976.

103. Irwin JF, Seegers WH, Andary TJ, Fekete LF, Novoa E: Blood coagulation as a cybernetic system: Control of autoprothrombin-C (X_a) formation. Thromb Res 6:431, 1975.

104. Isacson S, Nilsson IM: Coagulation and platelet adhesiveness in recurrent "idiopathic" venous thrombosis and thrombophlebitis. Acta Chir Scand 138:263, 1972.

105. L Jaques, Mahadoo J: Pharmacodynamics and clinical effectiveness of heparin. Semin Thromb Hemost 4:298, 1978.

106. Jaques L: The chemical and anticoagulant nature of heparin. Semin Thromb Hemos 4:277, 1978.

107. Johansson L, Hedner UY, Nilsson I: Familial antithrombin III deficiency as pathogenesis of deep venous thrombosis. Acta Med Scand 204:491, 1978.

108. Kakkar S, Bentley P, Chan P, MacGregor I, Ward V, Docksey S, Kakkar V: Oral contraceptives, AT-III, and deep vein thrombosis. (Abstr.) Thromb haemost 42:26, 1979.

109. Kakkar V, Low dose heparin in the prevention of venous thromboembolism—rationale and results. Thromb Diath Haemorrh 33:87, 1974.

110. Kakkar V: The clinical use of anti-thrombin III. (Abstr.) Thromb Haemost 42:265, 1979.

111. Kanfer A, Kleinknecht D, Boyer M, Josso F: Coagulation studies in 45 cases of the nephrotic syndrome without uremia. Thromb Diath Haemorrh 24:562, 1970.

112. Kauffmann R, Veltkamp J, van Tilburg N, van Es L: Acquired antithrombin III deficiency and thrombisis in the nephrotic syndrome. Am J Med 65:607, 1978.

113. Kazama M, Tahara C, Suzki Z, Gohchi K, Abe T: Abnormal plasminogen; a case of recurrent thrombosis. Thromb Res 21:517, 1981.

114. Kendall A, Lohmann R, Dossetor J: Nephrotic syndrome. A hypercoagulable state. Arch Intern Med 127:1021, 1971.

115. Knudsen J, Gormsen J, Skagen K, Amtorp O: Changes in platelet function, coagulation, and fibrinolysis in uncomplicated cases of acute myocardial infarction. Thromb Haemost 42:1513, 1979.

116. Kobayashi N, Takeda Y: Studies of the effects of estradiol, progesterone, cortisol, thrombophlebitis, and typhoid vaccine on synthesis and catabolism of antithrombin-III in the dog. Thromb Haemost 37:111, 1977.

117. Krause W, Lang A: Effect of angiography of blood coagulation. (Abstr.) Thromb Haemost 38:73, 1977.

118. Kudryk B, Robinson D, Netre' C, Hessel B, Blomback M, Blomback B: Measurement in human blood fibrinogen/fibrin fragments containing the B-beta 15-42 sequence. Thromb Res 25:277, 1982.

119. Kurachi K, Schmer G, Hermodson M, Teller D, Davie EW: Inhibition of bovine Factor IX_a and Factor X_a by antithrombin-III. Biochemistry 15:368, 1976.

120. Lahiri B, Rosenberg RD, Talamo RC, Mitcheli B, Bagdasarian A, Coleman RW: Antithrombin-III: an inhibitor of human plasma kallikrein. (Abstr.) Fed Proc 33:642, 1974.

121. Lechner K, Thaler E, Niessner N, Nowotny CH, Partsch H: Antithrombin-III-Mangel und Thromboseneigung. Wien Klin Wochenschr 89:215, 1977.

122. Lechner K, Niessner H, Thaler E: Coagulation abnormalities in liver disease. Semin Thromb Hemost 4:40, 1977.

123. Leone G, Valori V, Storti S, Myers T: Inferior vena cava thrombosis in a child with familial antithrombin III deficiency. (Abstr.) Thromb Haemost 43:74, 1980.

124. Li E, Orton H, Feinman R: The interaction of thrombin and heparin. Proflavine dye binding studies. Biochemistry 13:5012, 1974.

125. Mahadoo J: Evidence for a cellular storage

pool for exogenous heparin. In Bradshaw R, Wessler S (Eds): Heparin: Structure, Cellular Functions, and Clinical Implications. Academic Press, New York, 1979, p 181.

126. Mahadoo J, Jaques L: Cellular control of heparin in blood. Med Hypotheses 5:835, 1979.

127. Mammen EF: Inhibitor abnormalities. Semin Thromb Hemost 9:42, 1983.

128. Mammen EF: Plasminogen abnormalities. Semin Thromb Hemost 9:50, 1983.

129. Mammen EF: Physiology and biochemistry of blood coagulation. In Bang Nu, Beller FK, Deutsch E, Mammen EF (Eds): Thrombosis and Bleeding Disorders: Theory and Methods. Academic Press, New York, 1971, p 1.

130. Mammen E: Oral contraceptives and blood coagulation: A critical review. Am J Obstet Gynecol 142:781, 1982.

131. Mammen EF, Thomas WR, Seegers WH: Activation of purified prothrombin to autoprothrombin II (platelet cofactor II) or autoprothrombin II-A. Thromb Diath Haemorrh 5:218, 1960.

132. Mannucci PM, Vigano S: Deficiencies of protein C, an inhibitor of blood coagulation. Lancet 2:463, 1982.

133. Mansfield AO: Alterations in fibrinolysis associated with surgery and venous thrombosis. Br J Surg 59:754, 1972.

134. Marciniak E, Farley C, DeSimone P: Familial thrombosis due to antithrombin III deficiency. Blood 43:219, 1974.

135. Marlar RA, Endres-Brooks J: Recurrent thromboembolic disease due to heterozygous protein C deficiency. (Abstr.) Thromb Haemost 50:351, 1983.

136. Marlar RA, Sills, RH, Montgomery RR: Protein C in commercial Factor IX (F IX) concentrations (CONC) and its use in the treatment of "homozygous" protein C deficiency. (Abstr.) Blood 62:303a, 1983.

137. Marsh N: Fibrinolysis in disease. In Fibrinolysis. John Wiley & Sons, New York, 1981, p 125.

138. McGehee WG, Klotz TA, Epstein DJ, Rapaport SI: Coumarin-induced necrosis in a patient with familial protein C deficiency. (Abstr.) Blood 62:304a, 1983.

139. McKay E: Immunochemical analysis of active and inactive antithrombin III. Br J Haematol 46:277, 1980.

140. Meade T: Risk associations in the thrombotic disorders. Clin Haematol 10:391, 1981.

141. Messmore HL: Natural inhibitors of the coagulation system. Semin Thromb Hemost 8:267, 1982.

142. Miller-Anderson M, Borg H, Anderson LO: Purification of antithrombin III by affinity chromatography. Thromb Res 5:439, 1974.

143. Muller-Berghaus G: Pathophysiology of generalized intravascular coagulation. Semin Thromb Hemost 3:209, 1977.

144. Murano G, Bick RL: Thrombolytic therapy. In Murano G, Bick RL (Eds): Basic Concepts of Hemostasis and Thrombosis. CRC Press, Boca Raton, FL, 1980, p 259.

145. Murano G, Williams L, Miller-Anderson M, Aronson D, King C: Some properties of antithrombin-III and its concentration in human plasma. Thromb Res 18:259, 1980.

146. Mustard J, Packham M: The role of blood and platelets in atherosclerosis and the complications of atherosclerosis. Thromb Diath Haemorrh 33:444, 1975.

147. Musumeci Y, Lanolfi R, Bizza B: Amidolytic assay of thrombin bound to α-2-macroglobulin in plasma. Haemostasis 6:98, 1977.

148. Nagagawa M, Tsuji H, Kawamura T, Okajima Y, Urano S, Okusa S, Nishizawa A, Kitani T, Watada M, Ijichi H: Familial antithrombin III deficiency and its clinical significance. Blood Vessel (Tokyo) 11:106, 1980.

149. Nagaswa H, Kim B, Steiner M, Baldini M: Inhibition of thrombin-neutralizing activity of antithrombin III by steroid hormones. Thromb haemost 47:157, 1982.

150. Nagy I, Losonczy H: The significance of the chronic anticoagulant treatment in recurrent thromboembolism caused by hereditary antithrombin III deficiency. V Congress of the International Society of Thrombosis and Haemostasis (Abstr.) 1975, p 170.

151. Naims S, Goldstein R, Proger S: Studies of coagulation and fibrinolysis of arterial and venous blood in normal subjects and patients with atherosclerosis. Circulation 27:904, 1963.

152. Nalbandian RM, Henry RL, Bick RL: Thrombotic thrombocytopenic purpura: An extended editorial. Semin Thromb Hemost 5:216, 1979.

153. Nicolaides AN, Irving D: Clinical factors and the risk of deep venous thrombosis. In Nicolaides AN (Ed): Thromboembolism: Etiology, Advances in Prevention and Management. University Park Press, Baltimore, 1975, p 193.

154. Nilsson IM: Thrombosis and treatment of thrombosis. In Nilsson IM (Ed): Hemorrhagic and Thrombotic Disease. John Wiley & Sons, New York, 1974, p 163.

155. Nilsson IM, Pandolfi M: Fibrinolytic response of the vascular wall, Thromb Diath Haemorrh 40:231, 1970.

156. Nordeman B, Nordling K, Bjork I: A differential effect of low-affinity heparin on the inhibition of thrombin and Factors X_a by antithrombin. Thromb Res 17:595, 1980.

157. O'Brien J, Etherington M, Jamieson S, Lawford P, Lincoln S, Alkjaersig N: Blood changes in atherosclerosis and long after myocardial infarction and venous thrombosis. Thromb Diath Haemorh 34:483, 1975.

158. Odegard O, Lie M, Abildgaard U: Heparin cofactor activity measured with an amidolytic method. Thromb Res 6:287, 1975.

160. Odegard O, Abildgaard U: Antithrombin-III: Critical review of assay methods: Significance of variations in health and disease. Haemostasis 7:127, 1978.

161. Penner J, Hassouna H, Hunter M, Chockley M: A clinically silent antithrombin III deficiency in an Ann Arbor family. (Abstr.) Thromb Haemost 42:186, 1979.

162. Peterson C, Kelley R, Minard B, Cawley L: Antithrombin III. Comparison of functional and immunological assays. Am J Clin Pathol 69:500, 1978.

163. Peterson R, Krull P, Finley P, Ettinger M: Changes in antithrombin-III and plasminogen induced by oral contraceptives. Am J Clin Pathol 53:468, 1970.

164. Plow EF, Edington TS: Surface markers of fibrinogen and its physiologic derivatives revealed by antibody probes. Semin Thromb Hemost 8:36, 1982.

165. Pomerantz M, Owen W: A catalytic role for heparin. Evidence of a ternary complex of heparin cofactor, thrombin, and heparin. Biochim Biophys Acta 535:66, 1978.

166. Rosenberg RD, Damus P: The purification and mechansism of action of human antithrombin-heparin cofactor. J Biol Chem 248:6490, 1973.

167. Rosenberg RD: The effect of heparin on Factor IX_a and plasmin. Thromb Diath Haemorrh 33:51, 1974.

168. Rosenberg RD: Action and interaction of antithrombin and heparin. N Engl J Med 292:146, 1975.

169. Sala N, Owen WG, Collen D: A functional assay of protein C in human plasma. Blood 63:671, 1984.

170. Sas G, Blasko G, Banhegyi D, Jako J, Palos LA: Abnormal antithrombin III (antithrombin-III "Budapest") as a cause of familial thrombophilia. Thromb Diath Haemorrh 32:105, 1974.

171. Sas G, Peto I, Banhegyi D, Blasko G, Domjan G: Heterogeneity of the "classical" antithrombin deficiency. Thromb Haemost 43:133, 1980.

172. Schipper H, Lamping R, Kahle L, ten Cate J: Antithrombin III transfusion in patients with liver cirrhosis. Thromb Haemost (Abstr.) 42:327, 1979.

173. Seegers WH, Miller KD, Andrews EB, Murphey RC: Fundamental interaction and effect of storage, other adsorbents, and blood clotting in plasma antithrombin activity. Am J physiol 169:700, 1952.

174. Seegers WH, Cole ER, Harmison CR, Monkhouse FC: Neutralization of autoprothrombin-C activity with antithrombin. Can J Biochem 42:359, 1964.

175. Seegers WH, Schroer H, Kagami M: Interactivation of purified autoprothrombin I with antithrombin. Can J Biochem 42:1425, 1964.

176. Seegers WH: Use and regulation of blood clotting mechanisms. In Seegers WH (Ed): Blood Clotting Enzymology. Academic Press, New York, 1971, p 1.

177. Seegers WH, Irwin JF, Hivegas AM: Blood coagulation: A cybernetic system modified in hemophilia. Proceedings of the IX Congress of the World Federation of Hemophilia, 1974, p 3.

178. Seegers WH, Novoa E, Henry RL, Hassouna HI: Relationship of "new" vitamin K-dependent protein C and "old" autoprothrombin II-A. Thromb Res 11:633, 1976.

179. Seligsohn U, Berger A, Abend M, Rubin L, Attias D, Zivelin A, Rapaport SI: Homozygous protein C deficiency manifested by massive venous thrombosis in the newborn. N Engl J Med 310:559, 1984.

180. Shapiro S, Anderson D: Thrombin inhibition in normal plasma. In Lundblad R, Fenton J, Mann K (Eds): Chemistry and Biology of Thrombin. Ann Arbor Science, Ann Arbor, MI 1977, p 361.

181. Sills RH, Humbert JR, Montgomery RR, Marlar R: Clinical course and therapy of an infant with severe "homozygous" protein C deficiency (Abstr.) Blood 62:310a, 1983.

182. Spaet TH, Erichson RB: The vascular wall in the pathogenesis of thrombosis. Proceedigs 2nd International Conference of Thrombosis, Basel, 1965, p 67.

183. Spero J, Lewis J, Hasiba Y: Disseminated intravascular coagulation: Findings in 346 patients. Thromb Haemost 43:28, 1980.

184. Stead N, Kaplan AP, Rosenberg RD: Inhibition of activated Factor XII by antithrombin-heparin cofactor. J Biol Chem 251:6481, 1976.

185. Stenflo J: Structure and function of Protein C. Semin Thromb Hemost 10:109, 1984.

186. Stenflow J: A new vitamin K-dependent protein: Purification from bovine plasma and preliminary characterization. J Biol Chem 251:355, 1976.

187. Stemerman MB: Vascular intimal components: Precursors of thrombosis. Prog Hemost Thromb 2:1, 1974.

188. Sveger T: Antithrombin III in adolescents. Thromb Res 15:885, 1979.

189. Teger-Nilsson A: Antithrombin in infancy and childhood. Acta Paediatr Scand 64:624, 1975.

190. Thaler E, Schmer G: A simple two-step isolation procedure for human and bovine antithrombin II/III (heparin cofactor): A comparison of two methods. Br J Haematol 31:233, 1975.

191. Thaler E, Balzar E, Kopsa H, Piggera W: Erworbener Antithrombin-III-Mangel bei Protein-

urie. Wien Klin Wochenschr 89:65, 1977.

192. Thaler E, Balzar E, Kopsa N, Piggera W: Acquired antithrombin III deficiency in patients with glomerular proteinuria. Haemostasis 7:257, 1978.

193. Thaler E, Niessner H, Kleinberger G, Gabner A: Antithrombin III replacement therapy in patients with congenital and acquired antithrombin III deficiency. (Abstr.) Thromb Haemost 42:327, 1979.

194. Thaler E, Lechner K: Antithrombin III deficiency and thromboembolism. Clin Haematol 10:369, 1981.

195. Thomas D, Merton R, Lewis W, Barrowcliffe T: Studies in man and experimental animals of a low molecular weight heparin fraction. Thromb Haemost 45:214, 1981.

196. Tomson C, Forbes C, Prentice C, Kennedy A: Changes in blood coagulation and fibrinolysis in the nephrotic syndrome. Q J Med 43:399, 1974.

197. Tullis J, Watanabe K: Platelet antithrombin deficiency: A new clinical entity. Am J Med 65:472, 1978.

198. van der Meer J, Stoepman-van Dalen E, Jansen J: Antithrombin III deficiency in a Dutch family. Am J Clin Pathol 26:532, 1973.

199. Vennerod AM, Laake K, Soleberg AK, Stormland S: Inactivation and binding of human plasma kallikrein by antithrombin III and heparin. Thromb Res 9:457, 1976.

200. Verstraete M: The place of long-term stimulation of the endogenous fibrinolytic system: Present achievements and clinical perspectives. In Davidson JF, Samama MM, Desnoyers PC (Eds): Progress in Chemical Fibrinolysis and Thrombolysis. Vol 1, Raven Press, New York, 1975, p 289.

201. Vogel G, Bottermann P, Clarmann M, Komm CH, Oberdorfer A: Antithrombin III treatment in acute liver failure. Thromb Haemost 46:373, 1981.

202. von Kaulla E, von Kaulla K: Antithrombin III and diseases. Am J Clin Pathol 48:69, 1967.

203. von Kaulla E, von Kaulla K: Deficiency of antithrombin III activity with hereditary thrombosis tendency. J Med 3:349, 1972.

204. Walker FJ: Protein S and the regulation of activated Protein C. Semin Thromb Hemost 10:131, 1984.

205. Walker F, Esmon C: The molecular mechanism of heparin action: II. Separation of functionally different heparins by affinity chromatography. Thromb Res 14:219, 1979.

206. Wessler S: Small doses of heparin and a new concept of hypercoagulability. Thromb Diath Haemorrh 33:81, 1975.

207. Wickerhauser M: A simple method for preparation of nonthrombogenic prothrombin complex. (Abstr.) Thromb Haemost 46:137, 1981.

208. Wight T: Vessel proteoglycans and thrombogenesis. Prog Hemost Thromb 5:1, 1980.

209. Williams L, Murano G: Human antithrombin III heterogeneity. Blood 57:229, 1981.

210. Wilner GD, Nossel HL, Le Roy EC: activation of Hageman factor by collagen. J Clin Invest. 47:2608, 1968.

211. Wolf M, Boyer C, Lavergne J, Larrica M: A new variant of antithrombin III. A study of three related cases. (Abstr.) Thromb Haemost 42:186, 1979.

212. Yin E, Eisenkramer L, Butler J: Heparin interaction with activated Factor X and its inhibitor. Adv Exp Med Biol 52:239, 1974.

213. Yin E: Effect of heparin on the neutralization of Factor X_a and thrombin by the plasma alpha-2-globulin inhibitor. Thromb Diath haemorrh 33:43, 1974.

214. Yue R, Gertler M, Starr T, Koutrouby R: Alterations of plasma antithrombin III levels in ischemic heart disease. Thromb Haemost 35:598, 1976.

215. Zuck T, Bergin J, Perkins R: Antithrombin III and oestrogen content of oral contraceptives. Lancet 1:831, 1973.

13
Anticoagulant Therapy

Anticoagulant therapy is in a state of evolution, with many new techniques and dosages of numerous anticoagulant and antiplatelet agents as well as new synthetic agents being subjected to multicentered double-blind prospective randomized clinical trials. At the same time, many earlier and more traditional thoughts regarding anticoagulant therapy, many centered around mystique and lack of scientifically sound information, are having to be abandoned because of recent clinical trial results and new information. Results of clinical trials may be markedly different, depending on the particular method used as an end point of the trial and depending on the particular preparation of an anticoagulant.[19] Even though the agent may be of the same generic category, different preparations may have markedly different in vivo effects. Additionally, when interpreting the results of clinical trials, the end point of the trial, whether it be clinical thrombosis, radioactive fibrinogen scanning, Doppler ultrasonography, impedance plethysmography, or thromboscintigraphy, may markedly alter the statistical end point results. In addition to the clinical examination, the modalities used for a diagnosis of thrombotic disease in clinical trials are listed in Table 13–1, including their reliability, advantages, and disadvantages.[19]

In attempting to choose an appropriate prophylactic anticoagulant or antiplatelet regimen, as well as an appropriate dose schedule, one should always keep in mind the fact that anticoagulant or antiplatelet therapy, in any form, is only prophylactic therapy, preventing further thrombus propagation, recurrent thrombosis, or development of thromboembolism. The initiation of anticoagulant or antiplatelet therapy does not ameliorate the existing disease, and it is with this very important concept in mind that anticoagulant therapy will be reviewed. For the most part, this chapter will be limited to indications and doses suggested by prospective randomized double-blind clinical trials and will also include a discussion of newer anticoagulant preparations that are becoming available for clinical trials and may become generally used in the near future.

Heparin and Heparin-like Preparations

Heparin has been in use for almost half a century and remains the most common drug for treatment of acute thrombosis and thromboembolus and for prophylaxis.[90] Despite this lengthy clinical experience, there still remains much speculation, confusion, and general misunderstanding as to the mechanisms of action of heparin.[91] In addition, ideal doses, preparations, and methods of delivery remain controversial, speculative, and in some instances largely unknown. USP heparin is a heterogeneous molecular weight preparation, with molecular weights ranging from 4000 to 40,000 daltons and the average molecular weight being approximately 15,000 to 20,000.[91,179] In addition, it should be recognized that only 30% of UPS heparin binds to antithrombin III and, thus, as will be subsequently discussed, only 30% is available to accelerate the serine protease inhibitory activity of antithrombin. The remaining 60 to 70% of USP heparin is with little or no anticoagulant activity.[91,179,180] Although the ideal doses of heparin remain unknown, it does appear that a plasma heparin level of 0.01 and 0.02 U/ml[12,21,179,193,199] is certainly adequate with respect to prevention of thrombus formation, and at this dose heparin is maximally accelerating the inhibitory activity of antithrombin III.[27,179,193,199] The most important activity of heparin is thought to be its acceleration of the inhibitory acti-

Table 13-1 Advantages and Disadvantages of Modalities for Diagnosing Deep Venous Thrombosis

Modality	Reliability	Advantage	Disadvantage
Fibrinogen ^{125}I scan	Reasonable below groin	Current thrombosis detected	Hepatitis High false-positives and false-negatives
Doppler ultrasonography	High below knee	Excellent study with experience	Affected by collaterals
Impedance plethysmography	Poor		Unreliable High false-positives and false-negatives
Ascending venography	Excellent	Definitive	Painful, rethrombosis rate is 10%
Ascending thromboscintigraphy	Excellent study	Definitive, can tell if new or old thrombus Ventilation perfusion at same time	

vity of antithrombin III against serine proteases.[21,177,193,199] However, it does appear that the mechanism of antithrombin III inhibition of thrombin (Factor IIa) versus the antithrombin inhibition activity of Factor Xa may differ with the particular preparation of heparin used;[6,12] this will be subsequently discussed.

It has been generally accepted that coagulation occurs in a cybernetic manner, with fibrin deposition and lysis occurring as a continuous process.[5,21,87,127,160] The manifestations of normal hemostasis versus increased fibrin deposition (thrombosis) or increased fibrinolysis (hemorrhage) depends on a delicate balance between the procoagulant system and associated inhibitors as well as the fibrinolytic system and its associated inhibitors.[21,75,116,127,128,159] The primary inhibitor of the procoagulant system is antithrombin III.

Antithrombins were first described in 1939 by Brinkhous and co-workers[30] and the first large survey of antithrombins was reported by Seegers and associates in 1952.[156] Earlier work considered heparin cofactor (antithrombin II) to be distinct from antithrombin III; however, it now appears that antithrombin II-heparin cofactor and antithrombin III have the same activity.[4,136] Antithrombin III has activity not only against thrombin, but also other serine proteases generated during coagulation, including Factors Xa, IXa, XIa, XIIa, plasmin, and kallikrein.[21,157,158,188] It is thought that the inhibition of Factor Xa

most closely correlates with clinical inhibition of thrombus formation, and inhibition of Factor Xa appears to be much more important than the inhibition of Factor IIa with respect to efficacy of heparin.[6,12,80,94,179] In most instances, especially with respect to antithrombin III activity against thrombin and Factor Xa this activity is markedly accelerated by the addition of heparin.

The kinetics of this heparin-antithrombin-serine protease reaction have recently been elegantly described by Yin,[199] Wessler,[193] and Kakkar[96] and are given in Table 13-2.[21]

When the hemostasis system is driven in the procoagulant direction with the attendant generation of serine proteases and eventual fibrin formation, antithrombin III consumption occurs, since antithrombin III (antithrombin) combines irreversibly with activated clotting factors,

Table 13-2 Antithrombin III and Heparin Kinetic Data*

1 U of Factor Xa can generate 50 U of thrombin
1 μg antithrombin III can inhibit 15 U of Factor Xa, in the presence of heparin at 0.01 U/mL plasma concentration
Therefore, 1 μg antithrombin III, in the presence of heparin (0.01 U/mL) potentially inhibits 750 U of thrombin
In the absence of heparin, 1 μg antithrombin III only inhibits 1 U of thrombin

* Work of Yin.[199]

and this complex is then removed from the circulation.[15] In the absence of heparin, antithrombin appears to inactivate thrombin in a progressive, irreversible manner following second order kinetics.[3] In addition, antithrombin inactivates other serine proteases, as previously discussed, although with slower reactivity in the absence of heparin than its inhibition of thrombin.[104,105,157,158,168,188] In the presence of heparin the inactivation of thrombin and Factor Xa is markedly accelerated and is almost instantaneous; however, there are differences due to the various molecular weights and other characteristics of the heparin used.[6,12,80,94] Rosenberg and Damus[151] have demonstrated that heparin interacts with antithrombin by binding to lysine residues of the antithrombin molecule, and this presumably markedly accelerates the inhibitory activity of antithrombin with respect to serine proteases. However, heparin also combines directly with thrombin and Factor Xa, and thus it is still a matter of controversy as to whether the neutralization of thrombin and Factor Xa by antithrombin is due to the interaction of heparin with antithrombin or the interaction of heparin with the particular serine protease.[81,108,189,198]

Alternatively, another proposed mechanism is that a molecule of heparin may act to bind antithrombin and thrombin or Factor Xa.[143] However, these mechanisms appear to be different with differing heparin preparations and also with respect to the antithrombin inhibition of thrombin versus the antithrombin inhibition of Factor Xa.[6,12,80,94,177] As will be discussed, differing molecular weight subspecies of heparin have markedly different activities with respect to the interaction of antithrombin III and thrombin, antithrombin III and Factor Xa, or interaction with the vasculature.[6,12,80,94,133,177,178] During the aforementioned processes heparin appears not to be consumed, and after the formation of the heparin-antithrombin-serine protease complex, heparin dissociates from the complex, thus acting as a catalyst, and then becomes available to interact with more antithrombin or serine protease.[33]

The kinetics of the heparin and serine protease interaction have been well ellucidated, providing evidence that only minute amounts of heparin, from 0.01 to 0.02 U/mL need to be present to maximally accelerate the inhibitory activity of antithrombin.[12,21,96,177,179,193,199] Endogenous heparin is rarely detected in the blood in significant amounts. However, it has been suggested that very low doses of heparin, or semisynthetic heparin analogues may release endogenous glycosaminoglycans that then activate antithrombin to inhibit serine proteases.[21,131,177,181,182] When exogenous heparin is delivered into the blood compartment, it is rapidly absorbed by the surface of endothelial cells; this endothelial-bound heparin may be far more important than heparin circulating in the bloodstream with respect to thrombus prevention in man.[89,91,120,121] In addition, it appears that the subspecies of heparin preparation used, and differing routes of delivery, may preferentially lead to more or less heparin bound to the endothelium, thus theoretically those preparations or modes of delivery that render more endothelial bound heparin and less heparin in the bloodstream may be the most efficacious for use.[89-91,120,121] In this regard it should be recognized that some of the vascular proteoglycans, other than heparin, are also able to interact with antithrombin III and enhance the rate of inhibition of thrombin and Factor Xa; this activity appears to be limited to dermatan sulfate and heparan sulfate.[78,182,194] The obvious major physiologic significance of this is implied, but not yet conclusively proved. In addition, some evidence exists that the use of ultralow-dose heparin or semisynthetic heparin analogues may accelerate endogenous vascular glycosaminoglycan-induced antithrombin-mediated inhibition of serine proteases.[97,131,181]

Most studies have revealed that the physiologic range of antithrombin in normal human blood is quite narrow and in addition decreases of antithrombin III may be of significant clinical relevance when choosing to use heparin anticoagulation.[16,21,135,177] Most patients will respond to heparin if the biologic antithrombin III level is greater than 60%; however, many will not respond if biologic antithrombin III levels are less than 40% activity.[21] In the past, increased "anticoagulant activity" of heparin has been defined by the noting of prolonged global tests of coagulation, primarily the activated partial thromboplastin time (PTT), the activated clotting time, the thrombin time, and other similar tests. However, it has been known for a long time that the prolongation of these tests does not correlate with efficacy nor do they correlate with clinical bleeding.[22,161,176] Now that the properties of different heparin preparations are becoming more clear, it is easy to explain this lack of correlation of global clotting tests and clinical efficacy of heparin. In fact, no assay yet exists to measure ideally the clinical efficacy of heparin; however, as will be discussed, the anti-Xa assay as described by Denson and Bonnar[47] using the synthetic substrate S-2222 is probably the most reasonable assay to use at the present time.[177]

Clinical Aspects

Heparin can be administered by several routes, depending on the desired effect, although it is now becoming clear that differing routes may render markedly different clinical efficacy and effects.[1] In the past the most commonly used route has been intravenous infusion; this has the advantage of an immediate onset of action as defined by global clotting tests; however, this does not correlate with efficacy and, in fact, may inversely correlate with efficacy. If heparin is going to be given intravenously, it should always be given by constant infusion because intermittent pushes are not only of unclear clinical efficacy, but are also associated with a much higher incidence of significant hemorrhagic complications.[57,66] A more popular route of heparin administration is subcutaneous injection, or so-called minidose heparin therapy. More than 18 clinical trials have now established the high degree of efficacy of subcutaneous low-dose heparin therapy for the prophylaxis of deep vein thrombosis and pulmonary embolus. These trials are summarized in Table 13–3. Four other trials

Table 13–3 Low-Dose Heparin for the Treatment and Prophylaxis of Deep Vein Thrombosis

Reference	Result
Abernethy and Harlsuck[2]	No benefit
Ballard and co-workers[9]	Benefit
Corrigan and co-workers[40]	Benefit
Covey and co-workers[41]	No benefit
Gallus and co-workers[62,63]	Benefit
Gordon-Smith and co-workers[68]	Benefit
Gruber and co-workers[71]	Benefit
International study[86]	Benefit
Kakkar and co-workers[98,99]	Benefit
Lahnborg and co-workers[106]	Benefit
Nicolaides and co-workers[132]	Benefit
Rem and co-workers[148]	Benefit
Rosenberg and co-workers[152,153]	Benefit
Scottish study[155]	Benefit
Williams[195]	Benefit

have shown that subcutaneous heparin is equally effective to intravenous heparin in treating an "active" thrombotic event,[7,15,23,139] and a new trial has revealed that ultralow-dose heparin therapy at a dose of 1 mg/kg/hour for 3 to 5 days is also highly effective.[131] This particular dosage schedule only renders a plasma heparin level of 0.007 U/mL, and it has been proposed that this ultralow-dose heparin may be causing an accelerated endogenous glycosaminoglycan interaction with antithrombin and thus inhibiting endogenous serine protease generation.[131] As will be discussed, there are clear-cut differences in plasma levels, vascular interaction, anti-IIa activity versus anti-Xa activity with differing preparations of subcutaneously delivered heparin.

In general heparin is delivered at a dosage of 20,000 to 30,000 U/24 hours by constant infusion, rendering a plasma heparin level of approximately 1 to 2 U/mL, far more than usually needed.[19] When administered subcutaneously, the usual plasma heparin level is between 0.01 and 0.1 U/mL, although this may also be more heparin than is needed.[19] Subcutaneous minidose heparin therapy is generally delivered as 2500 to 5000 U every 6 to 12 hours, depending on the clinical condition being treated. In this regard it should be recognized that heparin need not necessarily be given in the anterior abdominal wall; in fact, alternating injection sites in any subcutaneous tissue is desirable and more comfortable for the patient. Heparin administered intramuscularly is not recommended, since it may often lead to serious intramuscular hematomas. A newer route of delivery is that by intrapulmonary inhalation, which also provides very adequate plasma heparin levels and in limited trials appears to be highly efficacious with respect to prevention of thrombosis or thromboembolic disease.[24]

It has been noted that significant differences have been found between beef lung versus mucosal heparin when examined by anti-Xa assays in vivo and in vitro; however, these differences are not so pronounced when observed by global clotting tests, such as the activated PTT.[1,12,127] With both mucosal or beef lung heparin, the anti-Xa activity markedly increases with a decrease in the molecular weight; however, with beef lung heparin, the specific activity of anti-Xa is much less than that of mucosal heparin at all molecular weights. The peak heparin levels, as measured by anti-Xa assay, are 50% higher with mucosal heparin than with beef lung heparin, although with either of these preparations the PTT will be prolonged at a plasma heparin level of approximately 0.02 U/mL.[1,12,179] Thus, in general, a very low anti-Xa activity is found in most

batches of beef lung heparin and most authorities now believe that the anti-Xa activity of heparin is by far the most important activity with respect to inhibition of thrombus formation in man.[12,66,177] In this regard, the inhibition of thrombin by antithrombin-heparin is dependent on the molecular size of the heparin.[6,12,80,90,91,94,179] The inhibition of Factor Xa shows a different dependency, thereby suggesting that the heparin potentiated inhibition of Factor Xa and thrombin occur by different mechanisms.[6,12] Also, the inhibition of thrombin and Factor Xa differ in plasma versus purified systems; this has been noted by several investigators and has led to the discovery that low-density lipoprotein appears to inhibit heparin.[6,107] However, these inhibitory effects are more pronounced with respect to high molecular weight than to low molecular weight heparins.[6,107] The potentiation of anti-Xa activity is inversely proportional to the molecular weight of heparin with significant inhibitory activity increasing with decreasing molecular weight of the heparin.[6,12,80,90,91,94,179] This correlation is depicted in Figure 13–1. However, with respect to dependency on the molecular weight, thrombin-derived assay systems correlate with the PTT and other global tests of coagulation with more prolongation occurring

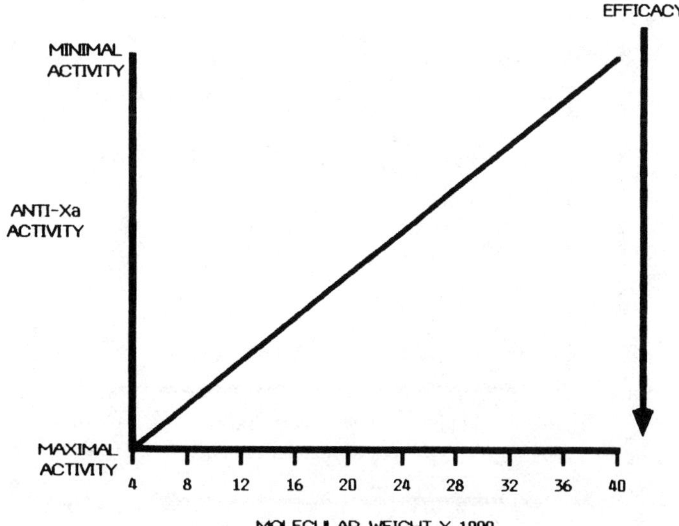

Fig. 13–1. Heparin molecular weight and anti-Xa activity.

with the higher molecular weight heparins; however, this is not thought to correlate at all with efficacy or clinical bleedability. This correlation is depicted in Figure 13–2. Thus, it is important to realize that these discrepancies may be clinically significant and relate to the mode of assay as well as the differing molecular weight distribution of heparin subspecies in various heparin fractions by trying to interpret clinical data in patients who have been delivered seemingly similar heparin preparations that, in fact, may not be similar.

It has also been recently found that an extremely low molecular weight heparin consisting of only 10 to 16 sugar units will greatly potentiate the activity of anti-Xa by antithrombin, but has no effect on the inhibition of thrombin, and therefore no prolongation of global tests of coagulation that are dependent on the inhibition of Factor IIa.[80] In addition, this extremely low molecular weight fragment has much less activity with respect to enhancing adenosine diphosphate (ADP)-induced platelet aggregation that is so commonly seen with high molecular weight heparin forms. Additionally, it has been shown that heparin when used in extremely high doses, can potentiate platelet aggregation even in the absence of ADP.[52,80,184] Platelet aggregation activity as a function of heparin molecular weight is depicted in Figure 13–3.

It is again important to realize that the anticoagulant effect of heparin is proportional to the anti-Xa inhibitory activity and not dependent on the high molecular weight portion that has significant anti-IIa activity; the anti IIa activity, however, induces significant prolongation of global tests of coagulation. Therefore, low molecular weight fractions and fragments are thought to have far more antithrombotic activity in clinical efficacy than standard heterogeneous USP heparin.

A recent study comparing four heparin preparations by the subcutaneous route has demonstrated that the highest anti-Xa activity is seen after the injection of low molecular weight sodium heparin, with a maximum effect occurring approximately 3 to 4 hours after the injection; however, with a similar preparation of sodium high molecular weight heparin, the maximum effects were seen at 1 hour.[94] Lower anti-Xa activity was seen at 1 hour with calcium heparin, which occurred at 3 to 4 hours after the injection. However, low molecular weight calcium heparin appeared equal to low molecular weight sodium heparin. Therefore this may account for why a seemingly "uniform" dose regimen

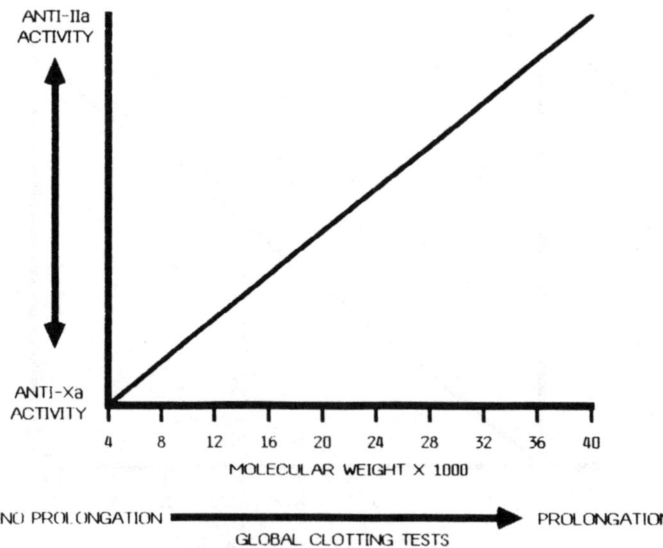

Fig. 13–2. Heparin molecular weight and global clotting tests. Anti-IIa versus anti-Xa activity.

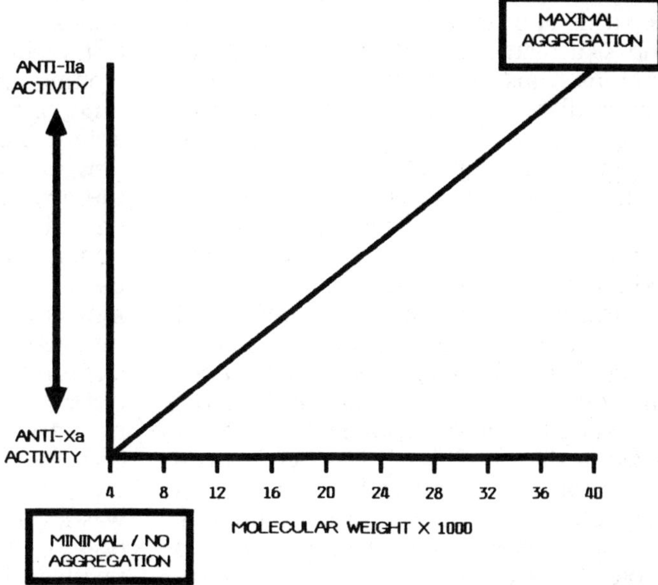

Fig. 13–3. Heparin molecular weight and platelet aggregating activity.

gives such varying degrees of clinical and laboratory discrepancies in different individual patients. Thus, the characteristics of heparin itself may have considerable effects on the plasma heparin levels after subcutaneous injection, with high levels being noted with low molecular weight heparins compared with "standard" high molecular weight heterogeneous heparins. It appears that these preparations may have significant differences in absorption from subcutaneous injection sites, with the large molecular weight species entering the circulation much more slowly.

It has also recently been noted in comparing calcium and sodium heparin salts that, when given subcutaneously, plasma heparin levels were significantly lower after the administration of a calcium heparin noted by both plasma heparin levels as well as kaolin-cephalin clotting time assays; however, no differences were noted between calcium versus sodium salt heparins when delivered intravenously.[183] When using both the Yin assay and the anti-Xa assay of Denson and Bonnar,[47] it has been noted that calcium heparin levels even though lower than sodium heparin levels were well above a minimum efficacious range (0.01 to 0.02 U/mL) by both anti-IIa and anti-Xa assay systems. It has therefore been suggested that sodium heparin may actually potentiate hemorrhage, whereas there is an extremely low incidence of any hemorrhage, including minor wound hematomas, with calcium heparin preparations.[183] This particular study, which compared calcium and sodium salts of heparin, concluded that calcium heparin is at least equal in efficacy to sodium heparin but is much less likely to produce hemorrhage.

In summary, the anti-IIa effect versus the anti-Xa effect is markedly different, depending on the molecular weight subspecies of the heparin. Anti-Xa activity increases with decreasing molecular weight of the heparin fragment or fraction, whereas the anti-IIa activity increases with increasing molecular weight of the heparin fraction. Thus, those heparins that have a higher percentage of low molecular weight components are thought to be more effective than those having a lesser percentage of low molecular weight components. An additional consideration is that mucosal heparin preparations in general appear to have much more anti-Xa activity than beef lung preparations, and an additional difference is that calcium heparins appear to be more effective in anti-Xa activity than sodium heparin preparations. Thus, among the standard heparins available today, one would want to choose calcium salt heparin of mucosal origin and a preparation containing the highest percentage of low molecular weight constituents; this would constitute the ideal heparin at present. Preliminary work has been reported on semisynthetic heparin analogues. Thus far, results reveal semisynthetic heparin analogues to be as effective as low dose heparin, and these analogues have a very strong anti-Xa activity as well as a very potent lipoprotein lipase activity.[97,181,182] It has been proposed that these semisynthetic analogues may release endogenous glycosaminoglycans and thus enhance normal physiologic protective mechanisms.[97,181,182] In addition, these semi-synthetic analogues, even though having extremely high anti-Xa activity, have minimal to absent in vitro anticoagulant activity as defined by prolongation of global tests of clotting, such as the activated PTT, thrombin time, activated clotting time, and other such tests; thus they appear to have minimal to no anti-IIa activity. Differences in differing heparin preparations are summarized in Table 13–4.

It should be noted from the aforementioned discussion that no global laboratory test, including the activated PPT, activated clotting time, whole blood recalcification time, or thrombin time, offer any predictability of efficacy or hemorrhage.[19] Spontaneous bleeding is rare with heparin therapy at any dose and in general the hazards of heparin therapy are somewhat dependent on the type of preparation used (low molecular weight versus high molecular weight, subcutaneous versus intravenous, mucosal versus beef lung) and are also related to duration of therapy, older age, sex, and surgical trauma.[117] In my experience the majority of bleeding episodes associated with heparin therapy are seen in situations in which heparin was given despite a general contraindication to anticoagulant therapy, such as peptic ulcer disease, malignant hypertension, a defect in hemostasis, the simultaneous ingestion of antiplatelet agents, or some type of invasive procedure. Occasionally, hematuria is seen in elderly females; however, this side effect is not a contraindication for continued therapy.[19,126]

An additional complication of heparin therapy in the past has been osteoporosis; however, this only generally occurs when heparin is used for a period of greater than 6 months and at a minimum dose of

Table 13–4   Characteristics of Different Heparin Preparations*

Source	
Beef lung	Porcine mucosal
Low anti-Xa activity	High anti-Xa activity
High anti-IIa activity	Low anti-IIa activity
Lower percent of low molecular weight fractions	Higher percent of low molecular weight fractions
Higher incidence hemorrhage?	Lower incidence hemorrhage?
High incidence of heparin-induced thrombocytopenia	Low incidence of heparin-induced thrombocytopenia
Lower efficacy	Higher efficacy
Salt	
Calcium	Sodium
Less hemorrhage	More hemorrhage
High anti-Xa activity	Low anti-Xa activity
Equal anti-IIa activity	Equal anti-IIa activity
Lower plasma levels (subcutaneous)	Higher plasma levels (subcutaneous)
Molecular weight	
High	Low
Low anti-Xa activity	High anti-Xa activity
High anti-IIa activity	Low anti-IIa activity
Prolonged global tests	Normal global tests
Low efficacy	High efficacy

* Ideal USP (heterogeneous molecular weight) heparin-calcium salt, mucosal origin, and highest percent of low molecular weight fractions.

10,000 U/day and this dosage regimen is rarely, if ever, used any more.[70] Heparin, unlike vitamin K antagonists, does not cross the placenta and may be used in pregnant women. About 80% of heparin is degraded by the liver and approximately 20% by the kidney. Thus, in renal or kidney failure appropriate adjustments in dosages should be made, especially if using high intravenous doses.

Heparin-induced thrombocytopenia is a major complication of heparin therapy, and heparin, in any doses, should always be accompanied by platelet counts at least every 3 days. The incidence of heparin-induced thrombocytopenia varies from less than 1% to greater than 20% depending on the study being reported.[8,14,67,72,103,144,201] Heparin-induced thrombocytopenia is much more common with beef lung heparin than with mucosal heparin, in a ratio of 4:1.[169] The usual latent period is 6 to 14 days after the initiation of heparin and a typical patient demonstrating heparin-induced thrombocytopenia is depicted in Figure 13–4. Heparin-induced thrombocytopenia occurs with intravenous or subcutaneous heparin therapy and the thrombocytopenia will usually abate 48 hours after the cessation of heparin therapy. Most instances of heparin-induced thrombocytopenia are associated with the easy demonstration of platelet associated immunoglobulin G (IgG). It was initially hoped that low molecular weight heparin fragments or fractions would be unassociated with heparin-induced thrombocytopenia; however, one recent report suggests that this may not be the case.[82] Of even greater concern is that paradoxical serious thromboembolism occurs in approximately 50% of patients with severe heparin-induced thrombocytopenia. In about 50% of individuals developing paradoxical thromboembolism a serious arterial thrombus or thromboembolus is found. In an additional 50% the patient will have an extension of an already existing thrombus, a new deep vein thrombotic event, or a pulmonary embolus. Approximately 10% of individuals developing heparin-induced thrombocytopenia and paradoxical thromboembolism will have a major cerebral vascular thrombotic event, myocardial infarction, or mesenteric vascular occlusion.

At least 18 prospective randomized

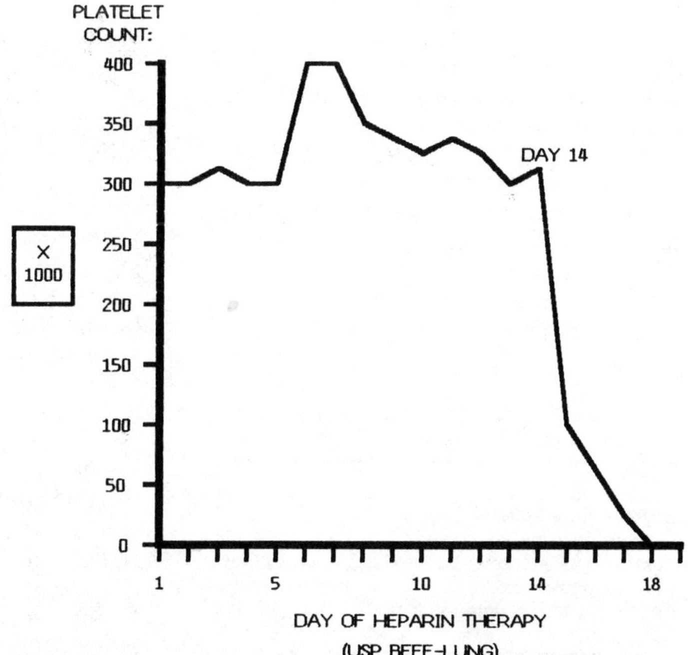

Fig. 13–4. Heparin-induced thrombocytopenia: course of a typical patient.

trials have been reported regarding the efficacy of low-dose heparin therapy; these are summarized in Table 13–3. A recent study has suggested that ultralow-dose heparin therapy may be as effective as low-dose heparin therapy, thus suggesting that perhaps the ideal dose of heparin with respect to decreasing heparin doses has not yet been established.[131] Several trials have clearly established that subcutaneous heparin is equally effective to intravenous heparin therapy in the treating of "active" thrombotic events with respect to preventing propagation of existing thrombus, recurrent thrombosis, or thromboembolism.[7,15,23,139] In addition, low-dose heparin therapy has not only been shown to be highly effective in general elective surgery, but also in surgery for malignant disease (Table 13–5). The use of low-dose heparin therapy with respect to prophylaxis in prostatic surgery and in hip surgery remains unclear, with some trials demonstrating good results and others demonstrating no differences in treated versus untreated control patients (Table 13–6). Large clinical trials evaluating the efficacy of low molecular weight heparin fragments and fractions are now underway; however, final results are not yet available. Intrapulmonary heparin is another route of delivery that is currently being explored.[24,25]

Intrapulmonary heparin was first used in 1965 when Bosner[28] subjected nine patients with chronic obstructive pulmonary disease to heparin aerosol at doses of 10,000 to 40,000 U/dose by a Bird respirator. No untoward reactions and no bleeding was noted; four of nine patients had relief of bronchospasm and two had slight increases in the whole blood clotting time. Following this Bardona and co-

Table 13–5 Low-Dose Heparin Therapy for Deep Vein Thrombosis in Malignancy

Reference	Result
Gallus and co-workers[63]	Benefit
Gordon-Smith and co-workers[68]	Benefit
Kakkar and co-workers[98]	Benefit
Rem and co-workers[148]	Marginal
Rosenberg and co-workers[152]	Benefit
Scottish study[155]	Benefit

Table 13–6 Low-Dose Heparin Therapy for Deep Vein Thrombosis in Prostatic and Orthopedic Surgery

Reference	Result
Prostatic	
Becker and co-workers[13]	No benefit
Gordon-Smith and co-workers[68]	Benefit
Kakkar and co-workers[98]	Benefit
Nicolaides and co-workers[132]	Benefit
Rem and co-workers[148]	Benefit
Rosenberg and co-workers[152]	No benefit
Williams[195]	Marginal
Orthopedic	
Dechavanne and co-workers[44]	Benefit
Evarts and Alfidi[60]	Benefit
Gallus and co-workers[62]	Benefit
Hampson and co-workers[73]	No benefit
Harris and co-workers[76]	No benefit
Hume and co-workers[84]	No benefit
Kakkar and co-workers[98]	No benefit
Morris and co-workers[124]	Benefit
Study group—Venus Thrombosis[174]	Benefit

workers subjected ten patients with asthma to heparin doses of 20,000 U by intrapulmonary aerosol, and all patients showed subjective improvement, although none revealed objective changes in spirometry. More importantly, none of these patients demonstrated a prolongation of Lee-White clotting time and no patient manifested any type of hemorrhage. In 1969 Young-Chaiyud and colleagues[200] treated 69 patients with chronic obstructive pulmonary disease with heparin aerosol given by the intrapulmonary route in a dose of 20,000 U in 1 mL of normal saline. No side effects, including hemorrhage, were noted in any patient.

Of more significance, in 1973 Molino and Bellvardo[123] delivered heparin aerosol by the intrapulmonary route to 86 patients with a variety of cardiovascular and thromboembolic disorders for prophylaxis of recurrent disease in a dosage of 100 mg (approximately 10,000 U) delivered at 12-hour intervals for a period of 5 months. Many of these patients were followed to a maximum of 5 years, and not one recurrent thrombotic or thromboembolic episode was noted, nor was any incidence of hemorrhage noted. In 1977 Thonnard-Neumann[185] delivered heparin aerosol or intravenous heparin to 60 patients with migraine or cluster headaches, and it was noted that by the intrapulmonary route, 2500 to 5000 U weekly, 86% improved and by the intravenous route 75% improved. During this period there was no change in the prothrombin time, activated PTT, and no hemorrhagic episodes were noted. In 1979 Kavanagh and Mahadoo[101] subjected human volunteers to massive doses of intrapulmonary heparin, up to 157,500 U/dose and there were no bleeding episodes, although a prolonged clotting time was noted. Mahadoo[111] delivered intrapulmonary heparin for prophylaxis of deep vein thrombosis and pulmonary emboli after major surgical procedures, and in five patients receiving intratrachial installation of heparin, rendering a plasma heparin level of 0.01 to 0.16 U/mL, two episodes of postoperative wound hematoma were noted. There were no changes in the whole blood clotting time, activated PTT, platelet count, hematocrit, or fibrinogen level. After these two wound hematomas, intrapulmonary heparin (aerosol) was used and of eight patients treated before major surgical procedures with doses of 25,000 U/kg, no wound hematomas or an other type of bleeding has been noted. In addition, at this dose no changes in the plasma heparin concentration, whole blood clotting time, antithrombin III level, or platelet count were noted.

In pharmacokinetic animal work done by Jaques and co-workers[88] it was found that doses of intrapulmonary heparin are unassociated with hemorrhage, as noted by autopsy studies. In addition, the work of these investigators utilizing electron microscopy as well as radioactive labeled heparin have revealed that heparin given by the intrapulmonary route appears to undergo immediate uptake by alveolar macrophages and capillaries and then is distributed throughout the endothelial tree, being attached to the endothelial lining, which, as previously discussed, may be the ideal place for heparin with respect to its inhibition of thrombus formation.[112,113] These same individuals have found that the greater the cellular storage pool of heparin, primarily the vascular endothelium, and the greater number of endothelial cells subjected to heparin, the more profound the clinical anticoagulant effect.[89] Mahadoo[114] and Mahadoo and

Jaques[115] have compared the pharmcokinetics and the efficacy of heparin delivered by the intravenous, intramuscular, subcutaneous, or intrapulmonary route, and these studies have provided data that now potentially accounts for the variability of clinical efficacy in man, depending on the route of administration. Specifically, the site of the heparin cellular storage pool, the vascular endothelium, appears to vary significantly with the route of administration, with evidence suggesting that endothelial-bound heparin is the major fraction involved in the prevention of thrombus formation in man and not the fraction found in plasma, and that the distribution of endothelial-bound heparin appears to be greatest by the intrapulmonary route and least by the intravenous route. This relationship is summarized in Table 13–7.

We have recently treated 18 patients who have failed traditional modes of antithrombotic therapy with intrapulmonary heparin at doses between 10,000 and 20,000 U/week for a total of 1592 patient days, or 4.3 years. Only 1 of the 18 patients had rethrombosis and this was a patient with a congenital antithrombin III deficiency. However, the use of intrapulmonary heparin even in this particular patient has markedly decreased thrombotic events, as manifested by studying her history of deep vein thrombosis and pulmonary embolus before starting intrapulmonary heparin. Our 4.3 year experience with these 18 patients have thus far demonstrated a failure rate of 1.4% per year; this recurrence rate is superior to that reported for warfarin-type therapy (3 to 38% per year) or for platelet suppressive therapy. In summary, in a limited experience, intrapulmonary heparin appears to be an

Table 13–7 Relationship of Heparin Efficacy and Dependence on Route of Administration and Endothelial Binding

Route	Endothelial Binding	Efficacy
Intravenous	Minimal	
Subcutaneous	Moderate	↓
Intrapulmonary	Maximal*	

* At present; new methods may become known in future.

extremely safe and highly effective mode of outpatient prophylaxis for deep vein thrombosis and thromboembolic disease.[24,25]

Laboratory Monitoring of Heparin Therapy

It has been demonstrated by numerous investigators that the activated PTT, thrombin time, whole blood clotting time, and other global tests of hemostasis that depend on anti-IIa activity do not correlate with plasma heparin concentration, clinical efficacy of heparin, or clinical bleeding.[19,161,176] This issue remained quite confusing for a long period of time; however, now that it has become relatively clear that the anti-IIa activity of heparin has little to do with clinical efficacy and the anti-Xa activity rendered by the low molecular weight portions is correlated with clinical efficacy; this paradox now becomes more understandable. In addition, understanding the differences between mucosal heparin versus beef lung heparin and the additional differences between calcium and sodium salts of heparin further clarify the lack of correlation between global tests of coagulation depending upon anti-IIa activity and plasma heparin levels, bleeding, or efficacy. On this note it should be appreciated that the activated PTT was developed as a screening test for hemophilia and was never intended to be used for monitoring heparin therapy.[186] Thus, the more traditional approach to adjusting a heparin dose depending on the prolongation of an activated PTT is of no clinical relevance, since it does not correlate with plasma heparin levels, bleeding, or efficacy.[19,116,176,186] The same arguments apply to other global tests of coagulation depending on anti-IIa activity, including the activated clotting time and thrombin time. If any one test were to be chosen to correlate with clinical efficacy of heparin, it should be an anti-Xa assay as described by Denson and Bonnar,[47] although this assay system is not yet generally available. However, for those using global tests of coagulation and seeing minimal to no prolongation when delivering intravenous doses of heparin or, alternatively, when seeing a patient fail heparin therapy as manifested by a thrombotic event, the obvious things that should be looked for are antithrombin III deficiency, extremely high levels of lysozyme, platelet factor 4, or extremely high levels of low-density lipoprotein; if any of these are found, an alternate mode of therapy should be considered.[6,21,54,107,179] Table 13–8 summarizes common reasons for "heparin failures."

Until anti-Xa assays become generally available, my approach to assessing heparin therapy is outlined in Figure 13–5 and is summarized as follows: when delivering subcutaneous or intrapulmonary heparin therapy, a plasma heparin level and antithrombin III level are obtained approximately 1 hour after the institution of therapy.[17] If the plasma heparin level is greater than 0.01 U/mL, it is assumed that adequate heparin is present for efficacy, and if the antithrombin III level is greater than 60%, if is assumed that adequate antithrombin III is present for anti-Xa activity. If these two criteria are met, no further laboratory monitoring is undertaken. It is again to be emphasized that this mode of monitoring may change when anti-Xa assays using the synthetic substrate S-2222 become more generally available. For those continuing to use global tests of coagulation, prolongation of the test does supply important information in that it can be assumed that if the global test of coagulation is prolonged, there are adequate levels of antithrombin III for the heparin antithrombin III interaction to occur. However, for those continuing to use global tests of coagulation, the clinicians should recognize that the results do not correlate with plasma heparin levels, clinical efficacy, or propensity to hemorrhage.

Table 13–8 Common Reasons for Heparin Failures

Hereditary or acquired Antithrombin III deficiency
Elevated levels of low-density lipoprotein
Elevated levels of lysozyme (muramidase)
Elevated levels of platelet factor 4
Elevated levels of beta-thromboglobulin

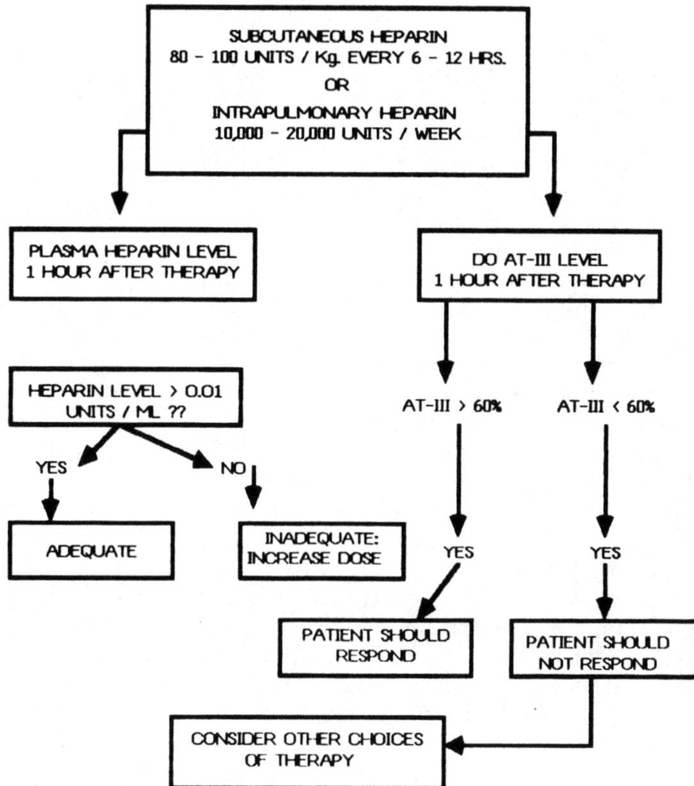

Fig. 13–5. Laboratory assessment of low-dose heparin therapy.

In summary, numerous new heparin preparations are becoming available, and it is generally recognized that differing preparations have markedly differing modes of activity. At the present time when choosing a USP heterogeneous heparin, the most effective preparations appear to be those with the highest percentage of low molecular weight material (4000 to 7000 daltons), those with a calcium salt rather than a sodium salt, and those of mucosal rather than beef lung origin. It is anticipated that within the next several years low molecular weight heparin fractions and fragments will become generally available for the treatment and prophylaxis of thrombosis and thromboembolic disease.

Oral Anticoagulants

Oral anticoagulants are of two types, the coumarins and the indanedione deriva-tives, the latter no longer being generally available and are only used in patients sensitive to the coumarin drugs.[19] Coumarin drugs are vitamin K antagonists.[46,141] All of the vitamin K antagonists interfere with the normal synthesis of the prothrombin complex factors, Factors II, VII, IX, X, and protein C; their mechanism of interference and the role of vitamin K were discussed in Chapter 1. Current evidence would suggest that the function of vitamin K is to attach calcium-binding prosthetic groups, postribosomally, onto the amino terminal regions of the prothrombin complex factors. The calcium-binding prosthetic groups have been identified as gamma-carboxyglutamic acid.[173] In the absence of vitamin K, i.e., in patients undergoing any type of coumarin-type therapy, Factors II, VII, IX, and X are synthesized but are incomplete, lacking the specific calcium-binding sites, and are thus unable to function as procoagulants because they cannot enter into enzyme substrate complex formation, as discussed in Chapter 1. However, all of these factors are present in plasma in normal immunologic concentrations, even though their biologic activity is markedly decreased, as defined by coagulation-derived assays or global tests for coagulation, such as the prothrombin time. In general, coumarins are totally absorbed from the gastrointestinal tract and are bound to plasma albumin. The onset of action of most coumarin derivatives is between 8 and 12 hours, with a maximum anticoagulant effect occurring in approximately 36 hours. Thus, in most instances the institution of coumarin derivative therapy usually requires overlap with heparin therapy. The duration of action of coumarins is approximately 72 hours.[29,147] It should be noted that Factor VII activity decreases most rapidly and best correlates with the prothrombin time determination. However, Factors IX and X depression best correlate with both the anticoagulant effect and clinical hemorrhage.[19,109] The coumarin derivatives do cross the placenta and should not be used in pregnant women. Loading doses of coumarin derivatives were used in the past, but are no longer indicated and, in fact, may potentiate hemorrhage.[48] In this regard a loading dose of coumarin simply serves to accelerate the abnormal synthesis of Factor VII but not Factors II, IX, or X.

The coumarin derivatives are associated with serious side effects, the most frequently encountered being severe hemorrhage, most commonly from the genitourinary tract. However, any vital organ is subject to serious hemorrhage, which will occur frequently in the patient with the usual contraindications to anticoagulant therapy, including malignant hypertension, the concomitant ingestion of antiplatelet agents, peptic ulcer disease, a defect in hemostasis, or recent surgery or trauma.[48,137] An extremely rare idiosyncratic reaction that can be extremely serious is that of coumarin-induced skin necrosis, which is manifested as a small vessel vasculitis that gives rise to serious skin necrosis and a violaceous rash.[129,130] Some of the patients who have demonstrated this rare and serious complication have been noted to be protein C deficient.[69] On this note, 25% of all cases involve women, who may have breast gangrene and may slough an entire breast.

The clinical and pathologic features of this rare complication have been well described.[69,129,130]

Clinical Trials and Indications

In the past coumarin derivatives have been widely used in patients with acute myocardial infarction and for prophylaxis of recurrent venous thrombosis and pulmonary embolus.[61,64,145] With respect to myocardial infarction, the only rationale for the use of coumarin in these individuals is to prevent venous thrombosis and thromboembolism while the patient is on bed rest and to prevent reinfarction. Several early studies showed significant differences between mortality, reinfarction rate, thromboembolic disease after myocardial infarction, and recurrent myocardial infarctions in patients treated with vitamin K antagonists versus those not so treated.[49] However, more recent prospective trials have failed to show any significant differences in mortality, reinfarction rate, or thromboembolic complications in these individuals.[50,145]

Many uncontrolled trials encompassing a variety of thrombotic and thromboembolic disorders, including patients considered at "high risk" for thromboembolic disease, have been conducted. Unfortunately, it is impossible to draw significant conclusions from these studies, since they have been retrospective, uncontrolled, non-randomized, and with non-uniformity of dosage regimens. Numerous randomized prospective trials, although not double-blind, have been conducted, and most of these studies have addressed a variety of disorders, including pulmonary embolization, recurrent deep vein thrombosis, and transient cerebral ischemic attacks. Results indicate a trend in decreased mortality in many high-risk patients and to a lesser degree a trend in decreased pulmonary embolization, recurrent deep vein thrombosis, and thromboembolic disease, depending on the endpoint used.[11,64,65,100,146] No significant benefit has been noted, however, in transient cerebral ischemic attacks. It is generally accepted that patients who are at high risk or who are being treated for prophylaxis of recurrent thrombotic of thromboembolic disease should be kept on coumarin-type derivitives for a period of 4 to 6 months.[19,65] However, it should also be recognized that the recurrence rate varies between 3 and 38%, depending on the series being reported, and thus in some instances the efficacy has been far inferior to that reported with low-dose heparin or antiplatelet agents.[32,56]

It can only be concluded that the efficacy of coumarin derivatives in thromboembolic disease has been highly effective in limited studies, although efficacy has been questionable in other studies. The contraindications, expense in monitoring, and the risk of serious or life-threatening hemorrhage is now causing many clinicians to rely more heavily on low-dose heparin for immediate prophylaxis and antiplatelet agents for long-term prophylaxis of patients at high risk for thrombosis or recurrent thrombotic disease.

Laboratory Monitoring

Much new information has appeared in the literature providing guidelines for monitoring of oral anticoagulant therapy. However, many laboratories are still not adopting these newer techniques. It has been demonstrated that reporting prothrombin times and percent activity has little or no meaning.[19,51,150,203] This can be readily appreciated in view of the described mechanism of action of the coumarin-type drugs and by asking the question "percent activity of what factor?" In addition, it has been shown that comparing "percent activity" has no meaning when comparing two different reagents, two different coagulation instruments, two different technologists, or two different laboratories. However, the reporting of the prothrombin time as a prothrombin index, which is obtained by dividing the control time into the patient's time, has been shown to be reasonably comparable between two different laboratories, two different technologists, two different rea-

gents, and two different coagulation instruments. Thus, most studies have advocated the use of a prothrombin index rather than percent activity.[19,51,150,203] In general, an adequate therapeutic range is defined as a prothrombin index that is 1.5 to 2.5; hemorrhage rarely occurs if the prothrombin index is less than 2.5 to 3.0.

When changing therapy from heparin to coumarin-type medications, the regimen is quite simple and well established. Some overlap is needed, since there is a delayed onset of action of coumarin drugs in heparinized patients. Exact adjustment of the prothrombin index must be empirical. The usual procedure is to start a heparinized patient on coumarin derivatives at 10 to 15 mg/day for 2 to 3 days and to cease heparin therapy when the prothrombin index is greater than 1.5 to 2.0.[19] It should be recalled that 0.75 U of heparin per mL will begin to prolong the prothrombin time. There are many drugs that interact with coumarin derivatives, many of which potentiate the activity of coumarin drugs, and others interfere with their activity. Also, coumarin drugs may enhance the action of other drugs. The most common drugs interacting with coumarin derivatives are depicted in Table 13–9, but more complete lists have been published.[164,187]

Antiplatelet Agents

Numerous antiplatelet agents have been used in both prospective as well as older retrospective clinical trials to assess efficacy in affording prophylaxis for both arterial and venous thrombotic or thromboembolic disease, including thromboembolic disease associated with prosthetic devices. Only the four most common agents will be discussed: aspirin, dipyridamole, sulfinpyrazone, and hydroxychloroquine. Interpreting data obtained in most clinical trials has been extremely difficult because in some studies only one agent was used, in other studies antiplatelet agents in combination with warfarin or heparin were used, and in others combinations of antiplatelet agents were used.[19] An additional variable complicat-

Table 13-9 Drug Interactions with Warfarin Therapy

Potentiate warfarin action	Inhibit warfarin action
Anabolic steroids	Barbiturates
Antibiotics	Corticosteroids
Chloryl hydrate	Cholystyramine
Chloramphenicol	Etchlorvynol
Clofibrate	Glutethimide
Disulfiram	Griseofulvin
Glucagon	Haloperidol
Mefenamic acid	Meprobamate
Methylphenidate	Oral contraceptives
Quinine	Rifampin
Quinidine	
Vitamin E	

Enhanced by Warfarin
Diphenylhydantoin
Chlorpropamide
Tolbutamide

ing the evaluation of these studies is the wide variety of "hypercoagulable" states studied and the end points used for the trials. This discussion addresses the results obtained in perspective randomized trials as well as my personal experience.

The antiplatelet action of aspirin is attributed to its ability to inhibit the synthesis of prostaglandins, specifically cyclo-oxygenase, thereby decreasing the production of thromboxane A_2, a compound that promotes platelet aggregability.[191] Dipyridamole is thought to inhibit cyclic adenosine monophosphate (AMP) phosphidiesterase, thus increasing cyclic AMP in the platelet, increasing phosphorylated receptor proteins that enhance calcium binding, and thus decreasing platelet aggregability and platelet adhesiveness.[122] It appears that sulfinpyrazone also inhibits prostaglandin synthesis and appears to have an action similar to that of aspirin.[191] The mechanisms of aspirin and other antiplatelet agents are given in detail, if known, in Chapter 4.

In general, a combination of two of the three antiplatelet agents is required for the most effective prophylaxis against thrombotic or thromboembolic disease, including arterial or venous events.[18,19,26,27] The most common dose for aspirin is 600 mg given twice a day, each dose with 30 mL of liquid antacid, and an ideal non-toxic plasma level is between 4 and 10 mg/dL.[38] Above 10 mg/dL patients commonly de-

velop gastric intolerance, manifested by nausea and emesis, which are the common side effects of aspirin therapy.[38] In addition, many patients complain of tinnitus at this plasma level. The usual dose of dipyridamole is 50 mg three or four times a day, and the usual dose for sulfinpyrazone is 200 mg orally three times a day. In my experience a combination of two antiplatelet agents, with differing modes of action, are required to obtain the most effective clinical response. The usual side effects of dipyridamole therapy are headaches, dizziness, nausea, flushing, and occasional syncopy. Mild gastric distress, similar to that seen with aspirin, may also be noted. Like aspirin and dipyridamole, the most common side effect of sulfinpyrazone is gastrointestinal, commonly manifested as nausea and emesis. Sulfinpyrazone, like aspirin, will aggravate or reactivate peptic ulcer disease, and this agent, like aspirin, should always be taken in conjunction with a liquid antacid. Usually a patient on antiplatelet therapy, especially when on a combination of two antiplatelet agents, will demonstrate easy and spontaneous bruising as well as mild mucosal membrane bleeding, usually manifested as gingival bleeding with toothbrushing and periodic melena.[19] These are accepted side affects of antiplatelet therapy for the prophylaxis of serious thrombic or thromboembolic disease.[19] It should be further noted that most of these agents have an antiplatelet effect for a full 7 to 10 days.[38] Thus, if a patient is ingesting these agents and is involved in trauma or requires emergency surgery, platelet concentrates may be indicated to control hemostasis.

Like other forms of anticoagulant therapy, antiplatelet therapy is in a state of flux, with numerous double-blind prospective randomized trials being conducted. The results of these trials will undoubtedly dictate more clear-cut indications for antiplatelet therapy. Alterations in platelet reactivity have been observed in patients with existing deep vein thrombosis, and many have demonstrated that venous thrombi begin with the development of a platelet (white) thrombus; this has led to the obvious suggestion that antiplatelet therapy may be indicated in venous thrombotic and thromboembolic disease.[31,79,83] The antiplatelet agent that has attracted the most attention in this regard is aspirin. The advantages of aspirin are obvious: it is extremely inexpensive and is relatively free from side effects. There have been numerous clinical trials utilizing aspirin alone or in combination for a wide variety of disorders, but there has been a lack of standardization of dosages and in many instances aspirin has been used in combination with not only another antiplatelet agent, but also with warfarin or heparin anticoagulation. Aspirin as a single agent has been subjected to double-blind prospective randomized trials for the prophylaxis of deep vein thrombosis and pulmonary embolus. There have been 13 such trials, and in nine trials a clear-cut benefit was demonstrated, one trial was questionable, and three trials revealed no benefit (Table 13–10). Aspirin in combination with dipyridamole has been utilized for the prevention of deep vein thrombosis and pulmonary embolus in general surgery, high-risk medical patients, and in orthopedic surgery in 20 trials (Table 13–11). The results were positive in 12 of these trials and without benefit in eight of them. However, the majority of trials demonstrating no benefit were limited to patients undergoing orthopedic procedures. The experience with sulfinpyrazone has been much less than that with aspirin, although Steele and co-workers[172] demonstrated a significant benefit

Table 13–10 Aspirin Trials for the Prevention of Deep Vein Thrombosis and Pulmonary Embolus

Reference	Result
Clagett and co-workers[37]	Benefit
Harris and co-workers[77]	Benefit
Hume and co-workers[85]	Marginal
Jennings and co-workers[92]	Benefit
Loew and co-workers[110]	Benefit
McKenna and co-workers[119]	No benefit
Medical Research Council[121]	Benefit
Salzman and co-workers[154]	Benefit
Shondorf and Hey[162]	No benefit
Soreff and co-workers[166]	Benefit
Stamatakis and co-workers[167]	No benefit
Weber and co-workers[190]	Benefit
Zekert and co-workers[202]	Benefit

Table 13–11 Aspirin Plus Dipyridamole Trials for the Prevention of Deep Vein Thrombosis and Pulmonary Embolus

Reference	Result
Bick[23,26]	Benefit
Clagett and co-workers[37]	Benefit
Dechavanne and co-workers[45]	No benefit
Enke and co-workers[55]	Benefit
Harris and co-workers[76,77]	Benefit
Hume and co-workers[85]	Benefit
McBride and co-workers[118]	No benefit
McKenna and co-workers[119]	Benefit
Medical Research Council[120]	No benefit
O'Brien and co-workers[134]	No benefit
Morris and Mitchell[125]	No benefit
O'Sullivan and Vellar[138]	Benefit
Parodi and co-workers[140]	Benefit
Plante and co-workers[142]	Benefit
Renney and co-workers[149]	Benefit
Shondorf and Hey[163]	No benefit
Silvergleid and co-workers[165]	No benefit
Weiss and co-workers[192]	Benefit
Wood and co-workers[196]	No benefit

when studying patients with recurrent venous thrombosis. In addition, there have been eight trials utilizing hydroxychloraquine, with five of the trials showing a benefit[34–36,74,197] and three showing no benefit.[39,85,93] Thus, although there have been some negative trials, the vast majority of trials using aspirin alone or aspirin plus dipyridamole have clearly been shown to be of benefit in decreasing the incidence of deep vein thrombosis and pulmonary embolus after elective surgery, orthopedic surgery, and in medical populations at high risk for deep vein thrombosis and pulmonary embolus.

Retrospective studies in large patient populations have revealed a decrease in the incidence of acute myocardial infarction,[29] and aspirin has clearly been shown to decrease thromboembolic disease associated with prosthetic heart valves.[43] Additional studies have shown favorable benefits of aspirin in decreasing myocardial infarction, although the results did not reach statistical significance.[53]

Dipyridamole as a single agent has been noted to decrease the rate of renal allograft rejection in patients with transplants,[102] and aspirin as a single agent has been shown to normalize platelet survival in patients with prosthetic heart valves.[175]

In this same study it was shown that sulfinpyrazone was as effective as dipyridamole, but aspirin was without effect. Sulfinpyrazone as a single agent has clearly been shown to decrease the incidence of transient cerebral ischemic attacks[59] as well as to decrease the incidence of thromboembolism in patients with rheumatic heart disease,[170] recurrent deep vein thrombosis,[58,171] and shunt thrombosis.[95] The incidence of failure in a large patient population treated with aspirin and dipyridamole demonstrated a recurrence rate comparable to most experience with warfarin-type drugs and more favorable than that reported by some investigators with warfarin-type drugs.[23] Thus, a combination of aspirin and dipyridamole for a 6-month period appears to be equally as effective as warfarin for the prevention of recurrent deep vein thrombosis and pulmonary embolus in high-risk patients.

These studies account for the majority of double-blind prospective randomized trials as well as nonrandomized trials with antiplatelet agents. It is hoped that future studies using combination therapy will allow for more clear-cut indications. However, it appears that a combination of two antiplatelet agents, each with a differing mechanism of action, appear very effective in decreasing the incidence or recurrence of deep vein thrombosis, or pulmonary embolus. In one trial just noted, many of the patients treated with aspirin and dipyridamole were at extremely high risk, because they were warfarin failures, and the vast majority of these patients did not have a recurrence on a combination of aspirin and dipyridamole.[23]

No laboratory monitoring of antiplatelet therapy is necessary; however, should one wish to document a clinical response, a template bleeding time and an aspirin tolerance test can be performed. However, a newer modality with respect to monitoring efficacy of therapy is that of platelet survival or platelet size distribution profiling, as was discussed in Chapter 4. The effects of these agents on platelet aggregation curves was also discussed in detail in Chapter 4.

Summary

The current kinetic knowledge, apparent indications, and the results of major clinical trials using anticoagulant and antiplatelet therapy have been discussed. Since many studies have been retrospective in nature, and many have been without uniform dosages and a wide variety of disorders have been studied, efficacy, at the present time, with respect to warfarin therapy, heparin versus minidose heparin therapy, and antiplatelet therapy can be expected to undergo significant changes in the future. Changes that can be anticipated are the introduction of new low molecular weight heparins, semi-synthetic heparin analogues, and new antiplatelet agents. The use of these newer agents in double-blind prospective randomized trials should provide more clear-cut indications for long-term prophylactic therapy as well as the immediate prophylaxis of high-risk patients.

References

1. Abbott WM, Warnock DF, Austen WG: The relationship of heparin source to the incidence of delayed hemorrhage. J Surg Res 22:593, 1977.
2. Abernethy EE, Hartsuck JM: Postoperative pulmonary embolism. A prospective study utilizing low-dose heparin. Am J Surg 128:739, 1974.
3. Abildgaard U: Binding of thrombin to antithrombin III. Scand J Clin Lab Invest 24:23, 1969.
4. Abildgaard U, Graven K, Godal HC: Assay of progressive antithrombin in plasma. Thromb Diath Haemorrh 34:224, 1970.
5. Alkjaersig N, Roy L, Fletcher A: Analysis of gel exclusion chromatographic data by chromatographic plate theory analysis: Application to plasma fibrinogen chromatography. Thromb Res 3:525, 1973.
6. Anderson LO, Barrowcliffe TW, Holmer E, Johnson EA, Soderstrom G: Molecular weight dependency of the heparin potentiated inhibition of thrombin and activated Factor X. Effect of heparin neutralization in plasma. Thromb Res 15:521, 1979.

7. Andersson G, Fagrell B, Holmgren K, Johnsson H, Ljungberg B, Nilsson E, Wilhelmsson S, Zetterquist S: Subcutaneous administration of heparin. A randomized comparison with intravenous administration of heparin to patients with deep vein thrombosis. Thromb Res 34:333, 1984.

8. Ansell J, Slepchuk N, Kumar R, Lopez A, Southard L, Deykin D: Heparin induced thrombocytopenia: A prospective study. Thromb Haemost 43:61, 1980.

9. Ballard RM, Bradley-Watson PJ, Johnstone FD, Kenney A, McCarthy TG, Campbell S, Weston J: Low doses of subcutaneous heparin in the prevention of deep vein thrombosis after gynecological surgery. J Obstet Gynaecol Br Commonw 80:469, 1973.

10. Bardana EJ, Edwards MJ, Pirofsky B: Heparin as treatment for bronchospasm of asthma. Ann Allergy 27:103, 1969.

11. Barker HW, Cromer HE, Hurn M, Waugh JM: The use of dicumarol in the prevention of postoperative thrombosis and embolism with special reference to dosage and safe administration. Surgery 17:207, 1945.

12. Barrowcliffe TW, Johnson EA, Eggleton CA, Thomas DP: Anticoagulant activities of lung and mucous heparins. Thromb Res 12:27, 1977.

13. Becker J, Borgstrom S, Salzman EF: Incidence of thrombosis associated with EACA administration and with combined EACA and subcutaneous heparin therapy. Acta Chir Scand 136:167, 1970.

14. Bell WR, Tomasulo PA, Alving BM, Duffy TP: Thrombocytopenia occurring during the administration of heparin; a prospective study in 52 patients. Ann Intern Med 85:155, 1976.

15. Bentley PG, Kakkar VV, Scully MF, Mac Gregor IR, Webb P, Chan P, Jones N: An objective study of alternative methods of heparin administration. Thromb Res 18:177, 1980.

16. Bick RL, Kovacs I, Fekete L: A new two-stage functional assay for antithrombin III (heparin co-factor): Clinical and laboratory evaluation. Thromb Res 8:745, 1976.

17. Bick RL, Murano G: Primary hyperfibrino-(geno)lytic syndromes. In Murano G, Bick R (Eds): Basic Concepts of Hemostasis and Thrombosis. CRC Press, Boca Raton, FL, 1980, p 181.

18. Bick RL: Treatment of bleeding and thrombosis in the patient with cancer. In Nealon T (Ed): Management of the Patient with Cancer. W.B. Saunders, Philadelphia, 1976, p 48.

19. Bick RL: Anticoagulant and antiplatelet therapy. In Murano G, Bick RL (Eds): Basic concepts of Hemostasis and Thrombosis. CRC Press, Boca Raton, FL, 1980, p 245.

20. Bick RL: Hypercoagulability and thrombosis. In Murano G, Bick RL (Eds): Basic Concepts of Hemostasis and Thrombosis. CRC Press, Boca Raton, FL, 1980, p 232.

21. Bick RL: Clinical relevance of antithrombin III. Semin Thromb Hemost 8:276, 1982.

22. Bick RL, McClain BJ: A comparison of five activated partial thromboplastin times and the activated clotting time during heparin therapy. Thromb Haemost 50:236, 1983.

23. Bick RL: Deep venous thrombosis: A clinical evaluation of 118 consecutive patients. Thromb Haemost 50:305, 1983.

24. Bick RL: The clinical use of intrapulmonary heparin. Semin Thromb Hemost. 11:213, 1985.

25. Bick RL: Intrapulmonary heparin for the long-term prevention of deep venous thrombosis and pulmonary embolism. Food and Drug Administration, Division of Cardiorenal Disease. IND # 23,746, 1985.

26. Bick RL: Disseminated intravascular coagulation. In Bick RL (Ed): Disseminated Intravascular Coagulation and Related Syndromes. CRC Press, Boca Raton, FL, 1983, p 31.

27. Bick RL, McClain BJ: Deep venous thrombosis: A laboratory evaluation of 118 consecutive patients. Thromb Haemost 50:237, 1983.

28. Bosner SW: Heparin administration as an aerosol. Vasc Dis 2:131, 1965.

29. Boston Collaborative Drug Surveillance Group: Regular aspirin intake and acute myocardial infarction. Br Med J 1:436, 1974.

30. Brinkhous KM, Smith HP, Warner ED, Seegers WH: Inhibition of blood clotting and unidentified substances which acts in conjunction with heparin to prevent the conversion of prothrombin to thrombin. Am J Physiol 125:683, 1939.

31. Bygdeman S, Eliasson R, Johnson SR: Relationship between postoperative changes in adenosine-diphosphate induced platelet adhesiveness and venous thrombosis. Lancet 1:1301, 1966.

32. Bynum LJ, Wilson JE: Low-dose heparin therapy in the long-term management of venous thromboembolism. Am J Med 67:553, 1979.

33. Carlstrom A, Lieden K, Bjork I: Decreased binding of heparin to antithrombins following the interaction between antithrombin and thrombin. Thromb Res 11:785, 1977.

34. Carter AE, Eban R, Perrett RD: Prevention of postoperative deep venous thrombosis and pulmonary embolism. Br Med J 1:312, 1971.

35. Carter AE, Eban R: Prevention of post-operative deep venous thrombosis in legs of orally

administered hydroxychloroquine sulfate. Br Med J 3:94, 1974.

36. Chrisman OD, Shook GA, Wilson TC, Short JY: Prevention of venous thromboembolism by administration of hydroxychloroquine: A preliminary report. J Bone Joint Surg 58:918, 1976.

37. Clagett GP, Brier DF, Rosoff CB, Schneider PB, Salzman EW: Effect of aspirin on postoperative platelet kinetics and venous thrombosis. Surg Forum 25:473, 1974.

38. Cohen LS: Clinical pharmacology of acetylsalicylic acid. Semin Thromb Hemost 2:146, 1976.

39. Cooke ED, Dawson MHO, Ibbotson RM, Bowcocki SA, Ainsworth ME, Pilcher MF: Failure of orally administered hydroxychloroquine sulfate to prevent venous thromboembolism following elective hip operations. J Bone Joint Surg 59:496, 1977.

40. Corrigan TP, Kakkar VV, Fossard DP: Low dose subcutaneous heparin: Optimal dose regimen. Br J Surg 61:320, 1974.

41. Covey TH, Sherman L, Baue AE: Low dose heparin in postoperative patients: A prospective coded study. Arch Surg 110:1021, 1975.

42. Craven LL: Experiences with aspirin in the nonspecific prophylaxis of coronary thrombosis. Miss Valley Med J 75:38, 1953.

43. Dale J: Prevention of arterial thromboembolism with acetylsalicylic acid in patients with prosthetic heart valves. Thromb Haemost 38:66, 1977.

44. Dechavanne M, Soudin F, Viala JJ, Kher A, Bertrix L, De Mourgues G: Prevention des thromboses veneuses. Succes de L'heparin a fortes doses lors des coxarthroses. Nouv Presse Med 3:1317, 1974.

45. Dechavanne M, Ville D, Viala JJ, Kher A, Faivre J, Pousset MB, Dejour H: Controlled trial of platelet antiaggregating agents and subcutaneous heparin in prevention of postoperative deep vein thrombosis in high risk patients. Haemostasis 4:94, 1975.

46. Denson KWE: The levels of Factors II, VII, IX, and X by antibody neutralization techniques in the plasma of patients receiving phenindione therapy. Br J Haematol 20:643, 1971.

47. Denson KWE, Bonnar J: The measurement of heparin. A method based on the potentiation of anti-Factor X_a. Thromb Diath Haemorrh 30:471, 1973.

48. Deykin D: Warfarin therapy. N Engl J Med 287:691, 1970.

49. Ebert RB: Long-term anticoagulant therapy after myocardial infarction: Final report of the veterans administration cooperative study. JAMA 207:2263, 1969.

50. Ebert RB: Anticoagulants in acute myocardial infarction: Results of a cooperative clinical trial. JAMA 225:724, 1973.

51. Editorial: Control of anticoagulants. Br Med J 1:126, 1969.

52. Eika C: On the mechanism of platelet aggregation induced by heparin, protamine, and polybrene. Scand J Haematol 9:248, 1972.

53. Elwood PC, Cochrane AL, Burr ML: A randomized controlled trial of acetylsalicylic acid in the secondary prevention of mortality from myocardial infarction. Br Med J 1:436, 1974.

54. Engelberg H: Actions of heparin relevant to the prevention of atherosclerosis. In Lundblad RL, Brown WV, Mann KS, Roberts HR (Eds): Chemistry and Biology of Heparin. Elsevier, New York, 1981, p 555.

55. Enke A, Stock CH, Dumke O: Doppelblind Studie zur postoperativen thrombiose Prophylaxe mit Dipyridamole - Acetyl Salicylsaure. Chirurg 47:670, 1976.

56. Errichetti AM, Holden A, Ansell J: Management of oral anticoagulant therapy: Experience with an anticoagulant clinic. Arch Intern Med 144:1966, 1984.

57. Estes JW, Paulin PF: Pharmacokinetics of heparin: Distribution and elimination. Thromb Diath Haemorrh 33:26, 1975.

58. Evans G, Gent M: Effect of platelet suppressive drugs on arterial venous thromboembolism. In Hirsch J, Cade JF, Gallus AS, Schonbaum E (Eds): Platelets, Drugs, and Thrombosis, Proceedings. S Karger, Basel, 1975, p 258.

59. Evans G: Effects of drugs that suppress platelet surface interaction on incidence of amarrosis fugax and transient cerebral ischemia. Surg Forum 23:239, 1972.

60. Evarts M, Alfidi J: Thromboembolism after total hip reconstruction: Failure of low doses of heparin in prevention. JAMA 225:515, 1973.

61. Gallus AS, Hirsh J: Treatment of venous thromboembolic disease. Semin Thromb Hemost 2:291, 1976.

62. Gallus AS, Hirsh J, Tuttle RJ, Trebilcock K, O'Brien SE, Carroll JJ, Minden JH, Hudecki SM: Small subcutaneous doses of heparin in prevention of venous thrombosis. N Engl J Med 288:545, 1973.

63. Gallus AS, Hirsh J, O'Brien SE, McBride JA, Tuttle RJ, Gent M: Prevention of venous thrombosis with small subcutaneous doses of heparin. JAMA :235, 1980.

64. Gallus AS, Hirsh J: Prevention of venous thromboembolism. Semin Thromb Hemost 2:232, 1976.

65. Gallus AS: Established venous thrombois and pulmonary embolism. Clin Haematol 10:583, 1981.

66. Glazier RL, Crowell EB: Randomized prospective trial of continuous vs intermittent heparin therapy. JAMA 236:1365, 1976.

67. Gollub S, Ulin AW: Heparin-induced thrombo-

cytopenia in man. J Lab Clin Med 59:430, 1962.

68. Gordon-Smith IC, LeQuesne LP, Grundy DJ, Newcombe JF: Controlled trial of two regimens of sub-cutaneous heparin in prevention of postoperative deep-vein thrombosis. Lancet 1:1133, 1972.

69. Griffin JH: Clinical studies of protein C. Semin Thromb Hemost 10:162, 1984.

70. Griffith GC, Nichols G, Asher JD: Heparin osteoporosis. JAMA 193:91, 1965.

71. Gruber UF, Fridrich R, Duckert F, Torhorst J: Prevention of postoperative thromboembolism by dextran 40, low doses of heparin, or xantinol nicotinate. Lancet 1:207, 1977.

72. Hackett T, Kelton JG, Powers P: Drug induced platelet destruction. Semin Thromb Hemost 8:138, 1982.

73. Hampson WGJ, Harris FC, Lucas HK, Roberts PH, McCall IW, Jackson PC, Powel NL, Staddon GE: Failure of low-dose heparin to prevent deep-vein thrombosis after hip replacement arthroplasty. Lancet 2:795, 1974.

74. Hanson EH, Jessing P, Lindewald H, Ostergaard P, Olesen T, Malver EI: Hydroxychloriquine sulfate in prevention of deep venous thrombosis following fracture of the hip, pelvis, or thoracolumbar spine. J Bone Joint Surg 58:1089, 1976.

75. Harpel PC, Rosenberg RD: Alpha-2-macroglobulin and antithrombin-heparin cofactor: Modulators of hemostasis and inflammatory reactions. Prog Hemost Thromb 3:145, 1976.

76. Harris WH, Salzman EW, Athanasoulis C, Waltman AC, Baum S, Sanetis RW: Comparison of warfarin, low-molecular-weight dextran, aspirin, and subcutaneous heparin prevention of venous thromboembolism following total hip replacement. J Bone Joint Surg 56:1552, 1974.

77. Harris WH, Salzman EW, Athanasoulis CA, Waltman AC, DiSanctis RW: Aspirin prophylaxis of venous thromboembolism after total hip replacement. N Engl J Med 297:1246, 1977.

78. Hatton M, Berry L, Regoeczi E: Inhibition of thrombin by antithrombin III in the presence of certain glycosaminoglycans found in the mammalian aorta. Thromb Res 13:655, 1978.

79. Hirsh J, McBride JA: Increased platelet adhesiveness in recurrent venous thrombosis and pulmonary embolism. Br Med J 2:797, 1965.

80. Holmer E, Lindahl U, Backstrom G, Thunberg L, Sandberg H, Soderstrom G, Andersson LO: Anticoagulant activities and effects on platelets of a heparin fragment with high affinity for antithrombin. Thromb Res 18:861, 1980.

81. Hook M, Bjork I, Hopwood J, Lindahl U: Anticoagulant action of heparin: Separation of high-activity and low-activity heparin species by affinity chromatography on immobilized antithrombin. FEBS Lett 66:90, 1976.

82. Horellou MH, Conard J, Lecrubier C, Samama M, Roque-D'Orbcastle O, de Fenoyl O, DiMaria G, Bernadou A: Persistent heparin induced thrombocytopenia despite therapy with low molecular weight heparin. Thromb Haemost 51:134, 1984.

83. Hume M: Platelet adhesiveness and other coagulation factors in thrombophlebitis. Surgery 59:110, 1966.

84. Hume M, Kuriakose T, Xavier ZL, Turner RH: 125-I fibrinogen and the prevention of venous thrombosis. Arch Surg 107:803, 1973.

85. Hume M, Bierhaum V, Kuriakose TX, Surprenant J: Prevention of postopertive thrombosis by aspirin. Am J Surg 133:420, 1977.

86. International Multicentre Trial. Prevention of fatal postoperative pulmonary embolism by low doses of heparin. Lancet 2:45, 1975.

87. Irwin JF, Seegers WH, Andary TJ, Fekete LF, Novoa E: Blood coagulation as a cybernetic system: Control of autoprothrombin-C (X_a) formation. Thromb Res 6:431, 1975.

88. Jaques LB, Mahadoo J, Kavanagh LW: Intrapulmonary heparin: A new procedure for anticoagulant therapy. Lancet 2:1157, 1976.

89. Jaques L, Mahadoo J: Pharmacodynamics and clinical effectiveness of heprin. Semin Thromb Hemost 4:298, 1978.

90. Jaques LB: The premises involved in the clinical use of heparin. Semin Thromb Hemost 4:275, 1978.

91. Jaques LB, McDuffie HM: The chemical and anticoagulant nature of heparin. Semin Thromb Hemost 4:277, 1978.

92. Jennings JJ, Harris WH, Sarmiento A: A clinical evaluation of aspirin prophylaxis of thromboembolic disease after total hip arthroplasty. J Bone Joint Surg 58:926, 1976.

93. Johansson E, Forsberg K, Johnsson H: Clinical and experimental evaluation of the thromboprophylactic effect of hydroxychloroquine sulfate after total hip replacement. Haemostasis 10:98, 1981.

94. Johnson EA, Kirkwood TBL, Sterling Y, Perez-Requejo JL, Ingram GIC, Bangham DR, Brozovic M: Four heparin preparations: Anti-X_a potentiating effect of heparin after subcutaneous injection. Thromb Haemost 35:586, 1976.

95. Kaegi A, Pineo FJ, Shimizu A: Arteriovenous-shunt thrombosis: Prevention by sulfinpyrazone. N Engl J Med 290:304, 1974.

96. Kakkar V: Low dose heparin in the prevention of venous thromboembolism—rationale and results. Thromb Diath Haemorrh 33:87, 1974.

97. Kakkar VV, Lawrence D, Bentley PG, de Haas HA, Ward VP, Scully MF: A comparative study of low doses of heparin and a heparin analogue in the prevention of postoperative

deep vein thrombosis. Thromb Res 13:111, 1978.

98. Kakkar VV, Spindler J, Flute PT, Corrigan T, Fossard DP, Crellin RQ: Efficacy of low-doses of heparin in prevention of deep-vein thrombosis after major surgery: A double-blind randomized trial. Lancet 2:101, 1972.

99. Kakkar VV, Field ES, Nicolaides AN, Flute PT: Low doses of heparin in prevention of deep vein thrombosis. Lancet 2:669, 1971.

100. Kakkar VV: Prevention of venous thromboembolism. Clin Haematol 10:543, 1981.

101. Kavanagh LW, Mahadoo J: Heparin by inhalation. In Bradshaw RA, Wessler S (Eds): Heparin: Structure, Cellular Functions, and Clinical Applications. Academic Press, New York, 1979, p 333.

102. Kincaide-Smith P: Modification of the vascular lesions of rejection in cadaveric renal allografts by dipyridamole and anticoagulants. Lancet 1:920, 1969.

103. King DJ, Kelton JG: Heparin-associated thrombocytopenia. Ann Intern Med 100:535, 1984.

104. Kurachi K, Schmer G, Hermodson M, Teller D, Davie EW: Inhibition of bovine Factor IX_a by antithrombin-III. Biochemistry 15:368, 1976.

105. Lahiri B, Rosenberg RD, Talamo RC, Mitcheli B, Bagdasarian A, Coleman RW: Antithrombin-III: An inhibitor of human plasma kallikrein. (Abstr.) Fed Proc 33:642, 1974.

106. Lahnborg G, Friman L, Bergstrom K, Lagergren H: Effect of low-dose heparin on incidence of postoperative pulmonary embolism detected by photoscanning. Lancet 1:329, 1974.

107. Lane DA, MacGregor IR: Low density lipoprotein: A selective inhibitor of the heparin-accelerated neutralization of Factor X_a by antithrombin III. In Lundblad RL, Brown WV, Mann KG, Roberts HR (Eds): Chemistry and Biology of Heparin. Elsevier, New York, 1981, p 301.

108. Li E, Orton H, Feinman R: The interaction of thrombin and heparin. Proflavine dye binding studies. Biochemistry. 13:5012, 1974.

109. Loeliger EA, von der Esch B, Mattern MJ, den Bracander ASH: Behaviour of Factors II, VII, IX, and X during long-term treatment with coumarin. Thromb Diath Haemorrh 9:74, 1963.

110. Loew P, Wellmer HK, Baer U, Merquet H, Rumpf P, Peterson H, Bronig G, Persch WF, Marx FJ, von Bary SM: Postoperative thromboembolic-prophylaxe mit acetylsalicylsaure. Dtsch Med Wochenschr 99:565, 1974.

111. Mahadoo J: Personal communication. March 10, 1982.

112. Mahadoo J, Hiebert LM, Wright CJ, Jaques LB: Vascular distribution of intratracheally administered heparin. Ann NY Acad Sci 370:650, 1981.

113. Mahadoo J, Hiebert LM, Jaques LB, Wright CJ: Endothelial sequestration of heparin administered by the intrapulmonary route. Artery 7:438, 1980.

114. Mahadoo J: Evidence for a cellular storage pool for exogenous heparin. In Bradshaw RA, Wessler S (Eds): Heparin: Structure, Cellular Functions, and Clinical Applications. Academic Press, New York, 1979, p 181.

115. Mahadoo J, Jaques LB: Cellular control of heparin in blood. Med Hypotheses 5:835, 1979.

116. Mammen EF: Physiology and biochemistry of blood coagulation. In Bang NU, Beller FK, Deutsch E, Mammen EF (Eds): Thrombosis and Bleeding Disorders: Theory and Methods. Academic Press, New York, 1971, p 1.

117. Mant MJ, O'Brien BD, Thong KL, Hammond GW, Birtwistle RB, Grace MG: Hemorrhagic complications of heparin therapy. Lancet 1:1133, 1977.

118. McBride JA, Turpie AGG, Kraus V, Hiltz C: Failure of aspirin and dipyridamole to influence the incidence of leg scan detected venous thrombosis after elective hip surgery. Thromb Diath Haemorrh 34:564, 1975.

119. McKenna R, Galante J, Bachman F, Wallace DL, Kaushal SP, Meredith P: Prevention of venous thromboembolism after total knee replacement by high-dose aspirin or intermittent calf and thigh compression. Br Med J 281:514, 1980.

120. Medical Research Council—Britain. Effect of aspirin on postoperative venous thrombosis. Lancet 2:441, 1972.

121. Medical Research Council. Effect of aspirin on postoperative deep venous thrombosis. Lancet 2:441, 1972.

122. Mills DCB, Smith JM: The influence on platelet aggregation of drugs that affect the accumulation of adenosine 3', 5'-cyclic monophosphate in platelets. Biochem J 121:185, 1971.

123. Molino N, Bellvardo C: Consideration on the long term use of heparin in cardiovasculopathic subjects. A new method of administration: Aerosol. Minerva Cardioangiol 22:553, 1973.

124. Morris GK, Henry APJ, Preston BJ: Prevention of deep-vein thrombosis by low-dose heparin in patients undergoing total hip replacement. Lancet 2:797, 1974.

125. Morris GK, Mitchell JPA: Preventing venous thromboembolism in elderly patients with hip fractures: Studies of low-dose heparin, dipyridamole, aspirin, and flurbiprofen. Br Med J 1:535, 1977.

126. Moser RH: Disorders produced by anticoagulants. Clin Pharmacol Ther 9:388, 1968.

127. Muller-Berghaus G: Pathophysiology of generalized intravascular coagulation. Semin

Thromb Hemost 3:209, 1977.

128. Murano G: "The Hageman Connection": Interrelationshps between complement, Kinins, and coagulation. Am J Hematol 4:409, 1978.

129. Nalbandian RM, Mader IJ, Barrett SL, Pearce JF, Rupp EC: Petechiae, ecchymoses, and necrosis of skin induced by coumarin congeners. JAMA 192:107, 1965.

130. Nalbandian RM, Beller FK, Kamp AK, Henry RL, Wolf PL: Coumarin necrosis of skin treated successfully with heparin. Obstet Gynecol 38:395, 1971.

131. Negus D, Friedgood A, Cox JJ, Peel ALG, Wells BW: Ultra-low dose intravenous heparin in the prevention of postoperative deep-vein thrombosis. Lancet 1:891, 1980.

132. Nicolaides AN, Dupont PA, Desais S, Douglas JN, Fuorides G, Lewis JD, Dodsworth H, Luck KJ, Jamieson CW: Small doses of subcutaneous sodium heparin in preventing deep venous thrombosis after major surgery. Lancet 2:890, 1972.

133. Nordeman B, Nordling K, Bjork I: A differential effect of low-affinity heparin on the inhibition of thrombin and Factor X_a by antithrombin. Thromb Res 17:595, 1980.

134. O'Brien JR. Tulevski V, Etherington M: Two in vivo studies comparing high and low aspirin dosage. Lancet 1:339, 1971.

135. Odegard O, Lie M, Abildgaard U: Heparin cofactor activity measured with an amidolytic method. Thromb Res 6:287, 1975.

137. O'Reilly RA: The pharmacodynamics of the oral anticoagulant drugs. Prog Hemost Thromb 2:175, 1974.

138. O'Sullivan EF, Vellar IDA: Assessment of the efficacy of antiplatelet drugs in the prevention of postoperative deep vein thrombosis. III Congress International Society of Thrombosis and Haemostasis, Washington, D.C., 1972, p 438.

139. Parilla H, Ansell J: Anticoagulation by constant subcutaneous heparin infusion. Thromb Haemost 47:1, 1982.

140. Parodi JG, Grandi A, Font E: El dipyridamol y el acido acetilsalicilico en la profilaxis de las thrombosis venosas postoperatorias de los membros inferiores. Dia Med 44:92, 1973.

141. Pereira M, Couri D: Studies on the site of action of dicumarol on prothrombin synthesis. Biochim Biophys Acta 237:348, 1971.

142. Plante J, Boneu B, Vaysse C, Barret A, Couzi M, Bierme R: Dipyridamole-aspirin versus low doses of heparin in the prophylaxis of deep venous thrombosis in abdominal surgery. Thromb Res 14:399, 1979.

143. Pomerantz M, Owen W: A catalytic role for heparin. Evidence of a ternary complex of heparin cofactor, thrombin, and heparin. Biochim Biophys Acta 535:66, 1978.

144. Powers PJ, Cuthbert D, Hirsh J: Thrombocytopenia found uncommonly during heparin therapy. JAMA 241:2396, 1979.

145. Prentice CRM: Myocardial infarction. Clin Haematol 10:521, 1981.

146. Pyorala T, Lampinen V: Preoperative anticoagulant treatment in gynecologic surgery. Acta Obstet Gynecol 49:215, 1970.

147. Quick AJ: Hypoprothrombinemia states. In Quick AJ (Ed): Hemorrhagic Disease and Thrombosis. Lea & Febiger, Philadelphia, 1966, p 60.

148. Rem J, Duckert F, Fridrich R, Gruber UF: Subkutane kleine Heparindozen zur Thromboseprophylaxe in der allgemeinen Chirurgic and Urologie. Schweiz Med Wochenschr 105:827, 1975.

149. Renney JTG, O'Sullivan EF, Burke PF: Prevention of postoperative deep vein thrombosis with dipyridamole and aspirin. Br Med J 2:992, 1976.

150. Report of the Working Party on Anticoagulant Therapy in Coronary Thrombosis to the Medical Research Council. Br Med J 1:335, 1969.

151. Rosenberg RD, Damus P: The purification and mechanism of action of human antithrombin-heparin cofactor. J Biol Chem 248:6490, 1973.

152. Rosenberg IL, Evans M, Pollock AV: Prophylaxis of postoperative leg vein thrombosis by low-dose subcutaneous heparin or peroparative calf muscle stimulation: A controlled clinical trial. Br Med J 1:649, 1975.

153. Rosenberg IL, Evans M, Pollock AV: Prevention of post-operative leg vein thrombosis: A comparison of low dose heparin and electrical calf muscle stimulation. Br Med J 1:153, 1974.

154. Salzman EW, Harris WH, DeSanctis RW: Reduction in venous thromboembolism by agents affecting platelet function. N Engl J Med 284:1287, 1971.

155. Scottish Study: A multi-unit controlled study: Heparin versus dextran in the prevention of deep vein thrombosis. Lancet 2:118, 1974.

156. Seegers WH, Miller KD, Andrews EB, Murphey RC: Fundamental interaction and effect of storage, other adsorbents, and blood clotting in plasma antithrombin activity. Am J Physiol 169:700, 1952.

157. Seegers WH, Cole ER, Harmison CR, Monkhouse FC: Neutralization of autoprothrombin-C activity with antithrombin. Can J Biochem 42:359, 1964.

158. Seegers WH, Schroer H, Kagami M: Interaction of purified autoprothrombin I with antithrombin. Can J Biochem 42:425, 1964.

159. Seegers WH: Use and regulation of blood clotting mechanisms. In Seegers WH (Ed): Blood Clotting Enzymology. Academic Press, New York, 1971, p 1.

160. Seegers WH, Irwin JF, Hivegas AB: Blood

coagulation: A cybernetic system modified in hemophilia. Proceedings fo the IX Congress of the World Federation of Hemophilia, 1974, p 3.

161. Shapiro GA, Huntzinger SW, Wilson JE: Variation among commercial activated partial thromboplastin time reagents in response to heparin therapy. Am. J Clin Pathol 67:477, 1977.

162. Shondorf TH, Hey D: Modified "low-dose" heparin prophylaxis to reduce thrombosis after hip joint operation. Thromb Res 12:153, 1977.

163. Shondorf TH, Hey D: Combined administration of low dose heparin and aspirin as prophylaxis of deep vein thrombosis after hip joint surgery. Haemostasis 5:250, 1976.

164. Sigel Lt, Flessa HC: Drug interactions with anticoagulants. JAMA 214:2035, 1970.

165. Silvergleid AJ, Bernstein R, Burton DS, Tanner S, Silberman JF, Schrier SL: Aspirin-persantin prophylaxis in elective hip replacement. Thromb Haemost 36:166, 1977.

166. Soreff J, Johnsson H, Diener L, Goransson L: Acetyl-salicylic acid in a trial to diminish thromboembolic complications after elective hip surgery. Acta Orthop Scand 46:246, 1975.

167. Stamatakis JP, Kakkar VV, Lawrence D, Bentley PG, Nairn D, Ward V: Failure of aspirin to prevent postoperative deep vein thrombosis in patients undergoing total hip replacement. Br Med J 1:1031, 1978.

168. Stead N, Kaplan AP, Rosenberg RD: Inhibition of activated Factor XII by antithrombin-heparin cofactor. J Biol Chem 251: 6481, 1976.

169. Stead RB, Schafer AI, Rosenberg RD, Handin RI, Josa M, Khuri SF: Heterogeneity of heparin lots associated with thrombocytopenia and thromboembolism. Am J Med 77:185, 1984.

170. Steel P, Rainwater J, Genton E: Controlled trial of sulfinpyrazone in rheumatic heart disease. Thromb Haemost 38:194, 1977.

171. Steele PP, Weily HS, Genton E: Platelet survival and adhesiveness in recurrent venous thrombosis. N Engl J Med 288:1148, 1973.

172. Steele P, Elles J, Genton E: Effects of platelet suppressant, anticoagulant, and fibrinolytic therapy in patients with recurrent venous thrombosis. Am J Med 64:441, 1978.

173. Stenflo J: Vitamin K, prothrombin, and gamma-carboxyglutamic acid. N Engl J Med 296:624, 1977.

174. Study Group—Venous Thrombosis: Small doses of subcutaneous sodium heparin in the prevention of deep vein thrombosis after elective hip operations. Br J Surg 62:348, 1975.

175. Sullivan JM, Harken DE, Gorlin R: Pharmacologic control of thromboembolic complications of cardiac-valve replacement. N Engl J Med 284:1391, 1971.

176. Teiem AN, Abildgaard R: On the value of the activated partial thromboplastin time in monitoring heparin therapy. Thromb Haemost 35:592, 1976.

177. Thaler E, Lechner K: Antithrombin III deficiency and thromboembolism. Clin Haematol 10:369, 1981.

178. Thomas D, Merton R, Lewis W, Barrowcliffe T: Studies in man and experimental animals of a low molecular weight heparin fraction. Thromb Haemost 45:214, 1981.

179. Thomas DP: Heparin. Clin Haematol 10:443, 1981.

180. Thomas DP: Heparin, low molecular weight heparin, and heparin analogues. Br J Haematol 58:385, 1984.

181. Thomas DP, Barrowcliffe TW, Merton RE, Stocks J, Dawes J, Pepper DS: In vivo release of anti-X_a clotting activity by a heparin analogue. Thromb Res 17:831, 1980.

182. Thomas DP, Merton RE, Barrowcliffe TW, Mullow B, Johnson EA: Anti-Factor X_a activity of heparan sulfate. Thromb Res 14:501, 1979.

183. Thomas DP, Sagar S, Stamatakis JD, Maffei FHA, Erdi A, Kakkar VV: Plasma heparin levels after administration of calcium and sodium salts of heparin. Thromb Res 9:241, 1976.

184. Thomas C, Forbes CD, Prentice CRM: The potentiation of platelet aggregation and adhesion by heparin in vitro and in vivo. Clin Sci Mol Med 45:485, 1973.

185. Thonnard-Neumann E: Migraine therapy with heparin: pathophysiologic basis. Headache 16:284, 1977.

186. Triplett DA, Harms CS, Koepke JA: The effect of heparin on the activated partial thromboplastin time. Am J Clin Pathol (Suppl) 70:556, 1978.

187. Udall JA: Recent advances in anticoagulant therapy. Gen Pract 11:116, 1969.

188. Vennerod AM, Laake K, Soleberg AK, Stromland S: Inactivation and binding of human plasma kallikrein by antithrombin III and heparin. Thromb Res 9:457, 1976.

189. Walker F, Esmon C: The molecular mechanism of heparin action: II. Separation of functionally different heparins by affinity chromatography. Thromb Res 14:219, 1979.

190. Weber W, Wolff U, Bromig G: Postoperative thromboembolie-prophylaxe mit colfarit. Ther Ber 43:229, 1971.

191. Weiss HJ: The pharmacology of platelet inhibition. Prog Hemost Thromb 1:199, 1972.

192. Weiss V, Jekiel M, Ritschard J, Bouvier CA: Prevention de la maladie thromboembolique post-operatoire par les antiagregants en chirurgie gynecologique. Med Hyg 35:943, 1977.

193. Wessler S: Smal doses of heparin and a new concept of hypercoagulability. Thromb Diath

Haemorrh 33:81, 1974.

194. Wight T: Vessel proteoglycans and thrombogenesis. Prog Hemost Thromb 5:1, 1980.

195. Williams HT: Prevention of psotoperative deep vein thrombosis with peri-operative subcutaneous heparin. Lancet 2:950, 1971.

196. Wood EH, Prentice CRM, McGrouther DA, Sinclair J, McNicol GP: Trial of aspirin and RA-233 in prevention of post-operative deep vein thrombosis. Thromb Diath Haemorrh 30:18, 1973.

197. Wu TK, Tsapogas MJ, Jordan FR: Prophylaxis of deep venous thrombosis by hydroxychloroquine sulfate and heparin. Surg Gynecol Obstet 145:714, 1977.

198. Yin E, Eisenkramer L, Butler J: Heparin interaction with activated Factor X and its inhibitor. Adv Exp Med Biol 52:239, 1974.

199. Yin ET: Effect of heparin on the neutralization of Factor X_a and thrombin by the plasma alpha-2-globulin inhibitor. Thromb Diath Hemorrh 33:43, 1975.

200. Young-Chaiyud P, Kettel LJ, Cugell DW: The effect of heparin aerosols on airway conductance in patients with chronic obstructive pulmonary disease. Am Rev Respir Dis 99:449, 1969.

201. Zalcberg JR, McGrath K, Daver R, Wiley JS: Heparin-induced thrombocytopenia with associated disseminated intravascular coagulation. Br J Haematol 54:655, 1983.

202. Zerkert F, Kohn P, Vormittag E, Poigenfurst J, Thien M: Thromboembolic Prophylaxe mit Acetylsalicylsaure bei Operationen wegen huftgelenknaher Fracturen. Monatsschr Unfallheilk 77:97, 1974.

203. Zucker S, Brosills E, Cooper GR: One-stage prothrombin time survey. Am J Clin Pathol 53:340, 1970.

14
Thrombolytic Therapy

In contrast to the anticoagulant drugs that are only prophylactic by impeding further growth of an existing thrombus, preventing rethrombosis, and preventing thromboembolism, the thrombolytic agents streptokinase and urokinase have the unique ability of inducing the dissolution of intravascular fibrin thrombi and the digestion of fibrinogen and other proteins, resulting in a more immediate recanalization of occluded vessels and in improved microcirculatory and macrocirculatory flow.

The most dramatic effects of pharmacologically activated fibrinolysis are usually noted when therapy is instituted early in the disease, in thrombi less than a few days old. However, recent evidence to be subsequently discussed would suggest that thrombolytic therapy may, in fact, be active in aged arterial and venous thrombi as well. Once thrombi are penetrated by fibroblasts and converted to scar tissue or have been covered by neoendothelialization, the probability of full vessel salvage is generally believed to be poor, but this is not always the case.[37] It is therefore important to establish a definitive early diagnosis, which is best achieved by visualizing intravascular thrombi by ascending venography, ascending thromboscintigraphy, or selective angiography.

Thrombolytic therapy originated with the demonstration that certain enzymes will induce the dissolution of performed fibrin clots in vitro,[14] experimentally induced intravascular thrombi in animals,[23] and superficial venous thrombi in human volunteers.[24] Of the agents tested[3] two enzymes are approved, urokinase and streptokinase, and these have received world-wide attention and have undergone numerous non-randomized as well as double-blind prospective randomized trials. This chapter summarizes the results of selected clinical trials and outlines the presently accepted therapeutic regimen for the treatment of deep vein thrombosis, massive pulmonary embolism, myocardial infarction, and arterial thrombi.[4,5,12,21,22,25,26,28,29,32,34,39–43,45,46,50] The use of thrombolytic agents in cerebral vascular disease, retinal occlusive disease, as well as the use of plasminogen in hyaline membrane disease and the subject of chemical thrombolysis using tissue plasminogen activator have received only limited attention and these studies have, in general, been associated with less encouraging results.[4,16,31]

Urokinase and Streptokinase

Urokinase is an enzyme produced by the kidney and found in the urine and is a potent activator of the fibrinolytic system. Two molecular forms of urokinase are found in current therapeutic preparations, a high molecular weight protein of 55,000 daltons and a low molecular weight protein of 34,000 daltons. The low molecular weight species is derived from the high molecular weight species by proteolysis.[3] Immunologically, the two forms are indistinguishable. Depending on the method of preparation, either one, or various proportions of each, is isolated. Kidney tissue cultures and urine are sources of urokinase, and they are extremely expensive.

Streptokinase is a bacterial enzyme synthesized by beta-hemolytic streptococci, group C. Streptokinase has a molecular weight of 47,000 daltons.[3] Streptokinase has the advantage of being far less expensive than urokinase; however, it is more commonly associated with minor allergic reactions. Table 14–1 summarizes properties of urokinase and streptokinase.[4]

Urokinase and streptokinase act on the

Table 14–1 Properties of Streptokinase and Urokinase

	Streptokinase	Urokinase
Source	Streptococci	Kidney tissue culture
Molecular weight	47,000 daltons	34,000 daltons
Half-life	10 minutes	15 minutes
Stability	Good	Good
Route	Intravenous or Intracoronary	Intravenous
Pyrogenicity	Yes	No
Antigenicity	Yes	Minimal
Dose	Uniform	Uniform
Efficacy	Equal	Equal
Retreatment	6 months	As needed
Expense	Low	High

Table 14–2 Laboratory Changes During Thrombolytic Therapy

Decreased fibrinogen
Decreased plasminogen
Decreased alpha-2-antiplasmin
Decreased clotting Factors V, VIII:C, IX, XI, XII
Prolonged activated partial thromboplastin time
Prolonged prothrombin time
Prolonged thrombin time
Elevated plasmin
Elevated fibrin(ogen) degradation products
Elevated B-beta 15–42 related peptides

endogenous fibrinolytic system by converting plasminogen to the potent nonspecific proteolytic enzyme plasmin.[30] This activation was discussed in detail in Chapter 1. Plasmin, in turn, degrades fibrin clots, and also degrades fibrinogen as well as other plasma proteins, including Factors V, VIII, IX, XI, XII, complement components, growth hormone, ACTH, and insulin.[6,8,35] Plasmin is rapidly inactivated by a variety of naturally occurring plasmin inhibitors,[2] the most important being alpha-2-antiplasmin, which acts very rapidly, and alpha-2-macroglobulin, which inhibits more slowly.[8] Since plasminogen is present in the thrombus or embolus, lysis occurs within the thrombus as well as on the surface of the thrombus.[13]

An intravenous infusion of urokinase or streptokinase is promptly followed by increased systemic fibrinolytic activity, and the effect may last for up to 12 hours after discontinuation of therapy. This activity is evident from a shortening of the euglobulin lysis time, a decrease in plasminogen levels, alpha-2-antiplasmin levels, and fibrinogen levels, and a significant increase in the amount of circulating fibrin(ogen) degradation products (FDP), and B-beta 15-42 and related peptides.[4,7] Laboratory changes with thrombolytic therapy are summarized in Table 14–2. Urinary and tissue culture urokinase have comparable fibrinolytic activities.[32] The activity of both urokinase and streptokinase is expressed in international units and is a measure of their ability to induce the lysis of a fibrin clot via the plasmin system in vitro. The half-life of both enzymes is quite short, being only 10 to 20 minutes.[4] Effective blood levels and disappearance rates of streptokinase vary with the availability of the substrate plasminogen. The efficacy of urokinase and streptokinase in the lysis of pulmonary emboli,[4,21,41,42,45] and the efficacy and lysis of deep venous thrombi[15,25,26,40,43,50] and coronary artery thrombi[5,28,29] have been established by angiography, perfusion lung scans, pulmonary arteriography, and pulmonary arterial and right heart pressure measurements, as well as ascending venography and ascending thromboscintigraphy before and after therapy.[37]

Indications

Pulmonary Embolus

Based on the results obtained in the Urokinase Pulmonary Embolism Trial (UPET)[4,21,41,42,45] and the Urokinase-Streptokinase Pulmonary Embolism Trial (USPET), sponsored by the National Heart and Lung Institute, these two thrombolytic agents are clearly indicated in adults for the lysis of acute massive pulmonary emboli or in patients with pulmonary emboli and unstable hemodynamics (Table 14–3).[37] In general, for the best thrombolytic results, treatment should be instituted as soon as possible after the onset of pulmonary embolism, but no later than 5 days after pulmonary embolus has occurred. Under these circumstances, angiographic and hemodynamic measurements demonstrate a more rapid improvement dur-

Table 14–3 Indications
for Thrombolytic Therapy

Pulmonary embolus
  Acute massive pulmonary embolus
    Defined as obstruction or significant filling defects
    involving two or more lobar pulmonary arteries, or
    the equivalent amount of emboli in smaller or other
    arteries
  Other pulmonary emboli
    Pulmonary embolus of any size associated with
    unstable hemodynamics, especially if associated
    with inability to maintain blood pressure
Deep vein thrombosis
  Extensive thrombi of any deep venous system
    (only streptokinase is approved)
  Not indicated in superficial vein thrombosis
  May be effective in both fresh (5 days old) or aged
    (up to 6 months old) venous thrombi
Acute myocardial infarction
  Indicated if symptoms are less than 6 hours old and
  ST segment elevation persists after a trial of sublin-
  gual nitroglycerin. The intracoronary route recanalizes
  about 75 to 80% of occlusions; the intravenous route
  recanalizes about 50% of occlusions
Fresh or aged arterial thrombi
  May be used intravenously (systemically) or locally

---

ing the first 24 hours of therapy than with heparin.[21,41] In addition, it has been clearly demonstrated by Sharma and co-workers[44] that the use of streptokinase and urokinase compared with heparin significantly enhanced pulmonary capillary volume and diffusion capacity at 2 weeks and 1 year later. Specifically, these investigators chose 40 patients with pulmonary embolism and evaluated the effects of heparin and of urokinase or streptokinase on pulmonary capillary volume and diffusion capacity. The capillary blood volume was found abnormally low in the heparin-treated group at both 2 weeks and at 1 year. However, pulmonary capillary blood volume and pulmonary diffusion capacity were normal at 2 weeks and 1 year in those patients who received fibrinolytic agents.[44] These results clearly indicate that fibrinolytic agents are useful in the normalization of cardiopulmonary parameters in patients with pulmonary emboli.

It has not yet been established with certainty that treatment with urokinase or streptokinase will decrease morbidity or mortality when compared with heparin therapy alone.[37] In the UPET and USPET trials urokinase was administered intravenously with a loading dose of 4400 U/kg over a period of 10 to 20 minutes followed by a continuous infusion of 4400 U/kg/hour for a period of 12 to 24 hours. Streptokinase was administered intravenously at a loading dose of 250,000 U over a period of 30 minutes followed by a continuous infusion of 100,000 U/hour for 24 hours. At the termination of thrombolytic therapy, patients received heparin for 7 to 10 days, followed by oral anticoagulants for 2 to 6 months. Clinical parameters, including pulmonary angiograms, pulmonary perfusion scans, and cardiorespiratory hemodynamics were evaluated independently by a number of panelists. To establish that the endogenous fibrinolytic system had been activated, the concentration of fibrinogen, plasminogen, and FDPs were measured in each patient (USPET) before and during infusion and at termination of therapy. As expected, the concentration of fibrinogen and plasminogen decreased, the concentration of FDPs increased, and plasminogen decreased significantly (Fig. 14–1).[4] It will be noted that a much more intense thrombolytic state is induced by streptokinase;[4] however, there is no evidence that there is any difference in efficacy between streptokinase and urokinase, and these differences appear only to be laboratory phenomena (Fig. 14–1).[37] Pulmonary angiograms, pulmonary perfusion scans, and cardiorespiratory hemodynamics showed significant improvements, (Table 14–4).[37] It was noted that there was no dramatic difference in clinical or laboratory parameters between the 12-hour and 24-hour urokinase regimen. Clinically, as mentioned, urokinase and streptokinase appear to be equally effective in pulmonary embolus.

Deep Vein Thrombosis

Several published randomized clinical trials[25,40,43,50] have established that streptokinase is effective and indicated for the lysis of acute extensive thrombi of the deep veins in adults (Table 14–5). The long-term benefits of streptokinase therapy in deep vein thrombosis as well as safety and efficacy in septic thrombophlebitis have not yet been established, although two reports[15,26] suggest some-

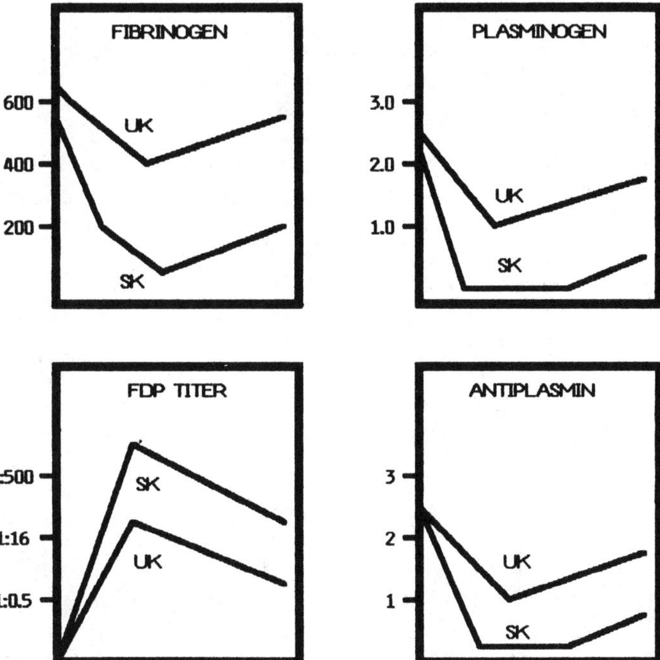

Fig. 14–1. Changes in fibrinolytic laboratory parameters during therapy with streptokinase (SK) and urokinase (UK).

Table 14–4 Efficacy of Urokinase and Streptokinase in Pulmonary Embolism

	Heparin	Strep-tokinase	Urokinase
Decrease in perfusion defect	8.3%	18.5%	16%
Decrease in pulmonary artery pressure	1.1%	5.3%	7.3%
Change in cardiac index (L/min/M²)	−0.05	+0.60	+0.045

Table 14–5 Efficacy of Streptokinase in Deep Vein Thrombosis

	Streptokinase	Heparin
Complete lysis	26%	5%
Incomplete lysis	27%	41%

what better salvage of valvular function with streptokinase and heparin than with heparin alone, indicating that the incidence of chronic venous insufficiency and the post-phlebitic syndrome are markedly decreased when thrombolytic therapy is used.[15,25] In studies on deep vein thrombosis, streptokinase was administered intravenously in a loading dose of 250,000 U over 20 to 30 minutes followed by a constant infusion of 100,000 U/hour for 72 hours. At the termination of thrombolytic therapy, patients were treated with heparin. Efficacy was documented by serial venography, which was evaluated by blinded readers.

Initially, it was thought that, as in the case of pulmonary embolism, the best results were obtained when therapy was instituted within a few days of onset of the thrombotic event. However, a recent report by Theiss and co-workers[48] has strongly indicated that old venous thrombi may also be lysed with the use of fibrinolytic therapy when applied to fresh and old thrombi of the iliac and femoral veins. Because of the widely held belief that thrombolytic therapy is capable of clearing thrombi from deep veins only when fresh thrombi are present (which may not be valid), Theiss and co-workers[48] retrospectively analyzed venographic results obtained in 85 patients with thrombosis of the iliac and femoral veins with symptoms that had been present from between

1 day and 8 weeks before thrombolytic therapy. Streptokinase, urokinase, or both drugs were successfully administered in these patients for a mean of 9 days (range, 2 to 26 days). Total or partial resolutions of the thrombotic occlusions were obtained in 94%, 82%, and 69% of patients who presented with a clot 3 days old, 7 to 14 days old, and 21 to 28 days old, respectively. With a delay of 5 to 8 weeks, the results were, however, uniformly poor, with only 1 partial recanalization seen in the seven patients. The results of this study strongly suggest that the success rate of thrombolytic therapy of iliofemoral venous thrombosis decreases only moderately during the first 2 weeks after the appearance of symptoms; patients who come to therapy with a delay of up to 2 weeks should therefore be considered for thrombolytic therapy as if they had presented with a "fresh" deep venous thrombotic event.[48] With a delay of more than 2 weeks, but no more than 4 weeks, the chances of success are clearly reduced so that thrombolytic therapy should be reserved for particularly young or severely affected patients at this stage of the disease.[48] If there has been a delay of greater than 4 weeks, a favorable outcome occurs so rarely that thrombolytic therapy, if attempted at all, is only justified in the most desperate cases, such as bilateral iliac thrombosis or thrombosis of the inferior vena cava.[48] These investigators also conclude that for aged iliofemoral venous thrombi, fibrinolytic therapy should usually be extended beyond the customary 3 days and should be continued until either complete recanalization has been proved by ascending venography or until a significantly prolonged fibrinolytic attempt (10 to 14 days) has guaranteed that all that is possible has been achieved in a given patient. They also found in this study that the poorest category of patients may often require the successive use of streptokinase and urokinase in those instances where urokinase had not been used initially.[48]

Arterial thrombi have also been successfully treated with thrombolytic therapy. Slanie and co-workers[46] reported on local thrombolysis in arterial occlusive disease. They studied a series of 38 patients in whom intra-arterial catheters were used to infuse streptokinase or urokinase just proximal to an acute thromboembolic occlusion in 20 limbs or to perfuse streptokinase directly into the obstructing thrombus material in 23 extremities with subacute or chronic occlusions by advancing the catheter stepwise until the distal open segment of the artery was reached. The dose of streptokinase used in this study varied between 50,000 and 400,000 U and was administered over 1 to 4 hours. Patency was achieved in 16 of 20 acute occlusions and 16 of 23 chronically occluded vessels within this time. A systemic thrombolytic state of 12 to 24 hours duration was observed when the total dose of streptokinase exceeded 80,000 U. In nine patients thrombolysis was immediately followed by angioplasty. This study strongly suggests that the advantage of this technique is rapid, effective, low cost, and highly successful thrombolysis even in chronic femoral or popliteal arterial occlusions, and local thrombolytic therapy should be applied to patients in who systemic thrombolysis would be considered contraindicated due to old age or other reasons.[46]

Further evidence for the efficacy of streptokinase in chronic arterial disease comes from work of Martin[34] who reported on 475 arterial occlusions treated with streptokinase given over a period of 3 days. The occlusions were divided into 257 isolated femoral artery thrombi, 177 iliac artery thrombi, and 41 aortic obstructions. The dose used was a continuous streptokinase regimen at 100,000 U/hour. In subdividing the group of femoral occlusions there were 225 chronic occlusions and 32 occlusions that were nonchronic, including reocclusions after transluminal catheter placement, and vascular surgery or thrombotic events after angiography. The success rate was quite remarkable. In patients undergoing thrombolytic treatment during the first 2 weeks after femoral occlusion a clearance rate was established in 75%. Femoral artery occlusions of 2 to 6 weeks revealed a 57% recanalization rate with streptokinase and in patients having a 6-week to 3-month old femoral artery thrombus there was a 38% recanalization and clearance rate.[34] However, it was noted that femoral artery occlusions older than 6 months did not respond to thrombolytic therapy.[34] Recanalization was documented by angiography before and after successfully conducted streptokinase therapy.

Myocardial Infarction

A newer indication for thrombolytic therapy is that of acute myocardial infarction, which has become widely accepted, very popular, and appears to be extremely effective. Excellent reviews regarding thrombolytic therapy for acute myocardial infarction have recently been published.[5,20,28,29] For many years, it was thought that acute myocardial infarction was secondary to coronary artery spasm and not thrombi. However, DeWood and colleagues[17] finally determined that the prevalence of total coronary artery occlusion during the early hours of myocardial infarction was associated with a high rate of coronary artery thrombus. Specifically, 90% of 517 patients with a documented acute myocardial infarction undergoing angiography and left ventriculography within 24 hours after the onset of symptoms demonstrated intracoronary thrombi. However, the incidence of intracoronary thrombi fell to 54% if the patients were studied within 12 to 24 hours after the onset of symptoms, suggesting that spontaneous thrombolysis can occur in some patients with acute myocardial infarction.

Thus, the concept of intracoronary thrombolysis using streptokinase was developed with the major purpose being to salvage myocardium by immediately recanalizing the coronary vasculature and thus preserving left ventricular function.[28,29] In general, patients selected for intracoronary thrombolysis are those who have a history of onset of chest pain of less than 6 hours' duration, and demonstrate typical ST segment elevations that persist after sublingual nitroglycerin.[28,29] Patients excluded from coronary artery thrombolysis are those with contraindications to thrombolytic therapy, such as recent surgery, cardiopulmonary resusitation, or recent cerebral vascular accident.[28,29,37] Some investigators also exclude patients with cardiogenic shock, although some studies have suggested that thrombolytic therapy with streptokinase can lead to dramatic reversal of cardiogenic shock.[38,29] Various dosages are used for intracoronary streptokinase, the most common being initiated with a bolus of 10,000 to 30,000 U followed by a continuous infusion of 2000 to 4000 U/minute with the infusion being continued until recanalization of the vessel is documented or until a maximal dose of 500,000 U has been administered.[5,28,29] The response to thrombolysis is monitored angiographically every 15 minutes during infusion of streptokinase, although the sudden relief of chest pain, the new onset of arrhythmias, or the rapid resolution of ST segment elevations are clinical markers of potential recanalization.[28,29] In general, the average time from the onset of intracoronary streptokinase to recanalization is approximately 30 minutes, and the average dose of streptokinase required is approximately 65,000 U.[28,29] If successful recanalization occurs, there is a rapid early rise in creatine kinase MB activity, with peak levels generally being reached 8 to 15 hours after the onset of symptoms with successful recanalization of coronary arteries.[28,29] After streptokinase therapy, heparin is initiated, since the patient is rendered hypercoagulable because the patient may have a defective fibrinolytic system after thrombolytic activation.[37]

Numerous trial results have been reported in the literature. The European Cooperative Study Group with streptokinase treatment in acute myocardial infarction has reported that streptokinase administered to medium risk myocardial infarction patients admitted to a coronary care unit within 12 hours after the onset of typical symptomatology significantly reduces mortality at 6 months.[20] In addition, Markis and co-workers[33] studied nine patients with acute myocardial infarction, and approximately 4 hours after the onset of chest pain each patient was treated with intracoronary streptokinase. Occluded coronary arteries were opened within 20 minutes, and the effect of thrombolysis on myocardial salvage was assessed by thallium-201 scans. At 2 weeks and at 3 months, the patients were restudied, and it was found that in the majority of patients the immediate recanalization of thrombosed coronary arteries significantly salvaged jeopardized myocardium.[33] Khaja and co-workers[27] and Anderson and co-workers[1] in two separate randomized trials studied intracoronary thrombolytic therapy in acute myocardial infarction in 40 and 50 patients, respectively. In the first study the average time to initiation of therapy was 5.4 hours, and reperfusion was established in 60% of streptokinase-treated patients and only 10% of placebo patients.[27] Antiplatelet therapy was initiated on the day after intervention. Left ventricular function, angiographic ejection fraction, and regional wall motion measured before and immediately after intervention as well as radionuclear ejection fraction measured at the time of treatment, at 12 days, and at 5 months demonstrated no significant differences between control and placebo groups.[27] In the second group, however, the average time to reinitiation of therapy was 4 hours. Reperfusion was established in 81% of streptokinase-treated patients and both patient groups were treated with subcutaneous heparin and antiplatelet agents following this. The ejection fraction and wall motion studies, enzyme changes, and electrocardiographic changes were significantly improved much more rapidly than in the streptokinase group.[1]

Timmis and co-workers[49] prospectively evaluated 116 consecutive patients undergoing thrombolysis for coronary artery thrombus. Hemorrhage was minor and was documented in about 25% of patients and was not related to a preexisting bleeding diathesis or to the streptokinase dose. As expected, a net reduction in fibrinogen concentration and elevation of FDPs were noted in all patients and also did not correlate with bleeding. These investigators suggest that sequential fibrinogen profiles may be erroneous in that FDP interference with the quantitation of fibrinogen and the bleeding noted is a consequence of the powerful anticoagulant effect of FDPs, specifically the interference with fibrin monomer polymerization and platelet dysfunction, as well as possibly the concomitant administration of heparin at the conclusion of catheterization.[49]

In properly selected patients, however, hemorrhagic complications are generally confined to hematoma formations at arterial puncture sites and localized oozing at venous puncture sites.[37] In addition, reperfusion-associated arrhythmias may occur in as many as 80% of patients treated with intracoronary streptokinase, with the most common arrhythmias being accelerated idioventricular rhythm. This occurs in more than 50% of patients who demonstrate successful recanalization and frequent premature ventricular contractions.[28,29] However, ventricular tachycardia and ventricular fibrillation are extremely rare.

Although there has been a long-standing and very good experience with intracoronary streptokinase, more and more clinicians are now treating patients with intravenous streptokinase.[28,29] Intracoronary streptokinase, in general, causes recanalization of coronary arteries in approximately 75% of patients when infused directly into the thrombosed coronary artery and when infused with the first 6 hours of the onset of chest pain and evidence of infarction.[28,29] On the other hand, systemic intravenous streptokinase infusion only results in recanalization in approximately 50% of patients with acute myocardial infarction.[28,29] However, intravenous streptokinase can be carried out much more rapidly than intracoronary streptokinase because the former can be initiated immediately and the intracoronary route requires more team effort, mobilization of equipment and of catheterization laboratory personnel, and cardiopulmonary bypass standby.

Stampfer and co-workers[47] reported on the effect of intravenous streptokinase in acute myocardial infarction and summarized mortality data obtained in eight randomized trials in which streptokinase was infused intravenously for period of up to 72 hours after the onset of symptoms of myocardial infarction. Although the tabulated results of all of these trials appear favorable, it is imperative to keep in mind that the summary encompasses selected trials performed within a 10-year period ending in 1979, thus bridging the introduction of the coronary care unit, the use of antiarrhythmic drugs and other ancillary therapy, and the introduction of early ambulatory programs. This renders the process of "pooling" the data from these eight randomized trials difficult to interpret.[38]

Complications of Therapy

Bleeding

Activation of the fibrinolytic system by thrombolytic therapy, urokinase or streptokinase, results in a seriously compromised hemostatic system.[37] This is attributed to a generalized intravascular proteolytic process induced by systemically circulating plasmin. As a consequence, hemorrhage in varying degrees occasionally occurs. In initial reports from the USPET and UPET trials, severe spontaneous bleeding, including cerebral, retroperitoneal, and gastrointestinal, was documented in slightly less than 5% of the patients treated.[37] In addition, several fatalities due to cerebral hemorrhage have occurred. Less severe spontaneous bleeding, such as superficial hematomas, hematuria, and hemoptysis have also been observed during therapy at approximately twice the frequency as that occurring during heparin therapy alone.[37] In several instances, spontaneous bleeding has been traced to concomitant anticoagulant treatment, which is contraindicated during thrombolysis.[37] Oozing blood from sites of percutaneous trauma is frequent; hence, all invasive procedures, especially arterial punctures and intramuscular injections, must be avoided and intravenous punctures kept to a minimum before and during treatment with streptokinase and urokinase.[37] Although the initial UPET and USPET trial reports noted numerous hemorrhagic complications of therapy, at a more recent NIH Consensus Panel Meeting it was noted that the hemorrhagic complications in community hospital settings were much less than those noted during the early trials.[18,19,36]

Allergic Reactions

Reactions representing possible anaphylaxis have been observed in approximately 3% of patients treated with streptokinase for venous thrombosis or pulmonary embolism. These ranged in severity from minor breathing difficulty to bronchospasm, periorbital swelling, or angioneurotic edema. Other mild or allergic reactions, urticaria, itching, flushing, nausea, headache, or musculoskeletal pain have been observed in approximately 12% of patients, and these mild or allergic reactions are not correlated with the dose of streptokinase. Transient elevation or lowering of systolic blood pressure of greater than 25 mm Hg has been observed in less than 2% of patients. Relatively mild allergic reactions, including bronchospasm and skin rash, have been reported, although rarely with urokinase. With the purer preparations of streptokinase now available, allergic reactions appear much less than those just cited.

Fever

Streptokinase is nonpyrogenic in standard animal tests; however, 30% of patients treated with streptokinase have shown increases in body temperature of 1.5 F or more, and the incidence of a temperature of greater than 104 F has been reported to be about 3.5%. Febrile reactions with urokinase occur in approximately 3% of patients. Like the allergic reactions, the purer and newer preparations of streptokinase appear to be associated with far fewer incidences of febrile episodes. Table 14–6 lists absolute contraindications for fibrinolytic therapy, Table 14–7 lists warnings for the use of thrombolytic therapy in patients who may be at high risk, Table 14–8 lists adverse reactions to streptokinase and urokinase, Table 14–9 summarizes the types of bleeding and appropriate management for bleeding in patients undergoing thrombolytic therapy, and Table 14–10 summarizes the allergic reactions and appropriate management associated with thrombolytic therapy.

Laboratory Monitoring

Both streptokinase and urokinase are given by fixed dose regimen and no lab-

Table 14–6 Contraindications to Thrombolytic Therapy

Active internal bleeding
Hemorrhagic diathesis
Recent (within 2 months) cerebrovascular accident, intracranial or intraspinal surgery
Intracranial neoplasm

Table 14–7 Warnings for the Use of Thrombolytic Therapy (Increased Hemorrhagic Risk)

Recent (10 days) surgery, delivery, biopsy, or puncture of noncompressible artery
Recent (10 days) gastrointestinal bleeding
Recent trauma or cardiopulmonary resuscitation
Severe hypertension
Left heart thrombus (mitral stenosis or atrial fibrillation)
Subacute bacterial endocarditis
Pregnancy
Cerebrovascular disease
Diabetic hemorrhagic retinopathy
Past severe allergy to streptokinase
Septic thrombophlebitis
Occluded arteriovenous cannula with infection
Any other condition in which bleeding constitutes a potential hazard

Table 14–8 Adverse Reactions to Thrombolytic Agents

Streptokinase	Urokinase
Bleeding	Bleeding
Allergic reactions	Mild allergic reactions
Fever	Fever rarely
Local Phlebitis	

Table 14–9 Hemorrhagic Syndromes with Streptokinase and Urokinase

Type of Bleeding	Management
Severe	Discontinue therapy
Cerebral	immediately
Retroperitoneal	Volume expanders
Gastrointestinal	Avoid plasma
Moderate	Packed red cells
Hemoptysis	Aminocaproic acid
Hematuria	
Mild	
Superficial hematoma	
Oozing from intravenous or intra-arterial punctures	

Table 14–10 Allergic Reactions with Streptokinase and Urokinase

Reaction*	Management
Minor dyspnea (SK)	Mild reactions
Bronchospasm (SK and UK)	Continue therapy and administer anti-histamine and corti-costeroids
Periorbital edema (SK)	
Angioneurotic edema (SK)	
Urticaria (SK and UK)	
2.5%	
12%	Severe reactions
Pruritus (SK and UK)	Discontinue therapy
Flushing (SK)	Intravenous corti-costeroids
Nausea (SK)	
Headache (SK)	Antihistamines
Myalgias (SK)	Epinephrine

* SK: streptokinase; UK: urokinase.

oratory test is noted to correlate with either bleeding or efficacy,[4,37] thus it needs to be strongly emphasized that the doses are not changed based on laboratory monitoring. Any changes made are associated with clinical bleeding.[9,37] Both agents are given by a fixed dose regimen, with streptokinase being infused intravenously as a 250,000 U loading dose over 30 minutes followed by 100,000 U/hour for 24 to 72 hours. Intracoronary streptokinase, used for acute myocardial infarction, is generally given as a 10,000 to 20,000 U loading dose followed by 2000 to 4000 U/minute for 60 minutes. The intracoronary route is usually not associated with a significant systemic thrombolytic state, such as that noted with intravenous urokinase or streptokinase. Urokinase likewise is administered on a fixed dose regimen and the dose is not changed based on any laboratory parameters. The usual intravenous dose is 4400 U/kg/hour for 12 to 24 hours. Many physicians and laboratory personnel remain unclear and confused as to appropriate laboratory monitoring procedures that should be performed to monitor the use of these agents, especially when used systemically. It is again important to realize that the dose of these agents is not changed, regardless of changes in laboratory parameters.[9] Thus, no dose adjustment at all is made based upon laboratory tests or alterations of laboratory tests; the only dose adjustment ever made is the immediate cessation of streptokinase or urokinase should significant clinical bleeding occur.[9,37] The recommended monitoring procedures are dictated by previously noting that no laboratory tests or combination of tests in hemostasis correlate at all with the efficacy of streptokinase and urokinase nor has any laboratory test been shown to correlate with predisposition to hemorrhage while receiving these agents.[4,9,37] Thus, it is possible to keep laboratory testing at a minimum while still providing useful information for the clinician. The recommended monitoring test is therefore the thrombin time.[9,37]

Before subjecting a patient to systemic thrombolytic therapy, a careful baseline clinical hemostasis history, prothrombin time, activated partial thromboplastin time, hemoglobin, hematocrit, and platelet count must be obtained.[9] Most patients deemed candidates for thrombolytic therapy have been placed on heparin before consideration of thrombolytic therapy. Thus, a thrombin time should be done before commencing thrombolytic therapy, and this should not be started until heparin has been stopped and the thrombin time has returned to less than two times normal. During thrombolysis the thrombin time will be prolonged; however, no regimented frequency of performing the thrombin time during therapy has yet been devised or recommended, and it is only noted that the thrombin time will usually be prolonged during therapy.[9] It is reasonable to obtain a thrombin time approximately 4 hours after starting therapy to document a systemic thrombolytic effect; however, prolongation of the thrombin time does not correlate with clinical bleeding or efficacy.[4,9,37] It is important to repeat a thrombin time after cessation of thrombolytic therapy and before reinstituting heparin therapy. Heparin should not be reinstituted until thrombolytic therapy is discontinued and the thrombin time has returned to less than two times prolonged. After this is noted, heparin can be safely reinstituted. The reinstitution of some type of anticoagulant therapy is extremely important, since patients are considered to be hypercoagulable after thrombolytic therapy because they have usually

almost totally depleted the fibrinolytic system.[37]

In summary, during systemic use of urokinase and streptokinase the laboratory monitoring test that is recommended and necessary is the thrombin time. This is obtained after cessation of heparin and before commencing thrombolytic therapy, and thrombolytic therapy is withheld until the thrombin time has returned to less than two times prolonged. There is no advantage to performing multiple thrombin times during thrombolytic therapy because they do not correlate with efficacy or bleeding, although a single determination approximately 4 hours after starting therapy is reasonable. After cessation of thrombolytic therapy, a repeat thrombin time should be performed and heparin not reinstituted until the thrombin time has returned to less than 2 times prolonged. One exception to this general monitoring procedure is for a patient who has undergone systemic thrombolytic therapy and then becomes a candidate for an invasive procedure, usually transluminal angioplasty or a cardiopulmonary bypass procedure. In this instance the patient who has previously undergone systemic thrombolytic therapy should also have a fibrinogen level performed and the fibrinogen level should be greater than 100 mg/dL before proceeding with an invasive procedure or angioplasty.[9] In this instance it is extremely important to choose carefully a fibrinogen determination system that is reliable and not influenced by the presence of FDPs, which may give false evaluations of fibrinogen levels in a post-thrombolytic therapy patient.[10,11]

Summary

Data reported in the studies described indicate that both urokinase and streptokinase are capable of inducing a systemic thrombolytic state in man, and their use is definitely superior to heparin alone in accelerating the rate of clot dissolution and vessel recanalization. These agents can be safely employed in humans, provided therapy is supervised by a physician highly competent in the management of thrombohemorrhagic phenomena.

It is important to note that although no differences in mortality have been detected between pulmonary embolism patients on thrombolytic agents and on heparin, it is apparent that particularly patients with massive pulmonary emboli receive considerable benefit from the rate of return of cardiopulmonary hemodynamics toward normal, including diffusion capacity and capillary blood volume, at least up to 1 year. In addition, thrombolytic therapy has been shown to be highly successful for new and aged venous thrombi and evidence would suggest that the use of thrombolytic therapy in individuals with deep vein thrombosis will significantly reduce the incidence of postphlebitic syndrome and chronic venous insufficiency. It is also clear that aged or fresh arterial thrombi are capable of being lysed up to those being present for 6 months. It is amply clear that the use of intracoronary and intravenous streptokinase is highly successful in salvaging myocardium and left ventricular function. In general, patients not responding to conventional anticoagulants are, in most instances, excellent candidates for thrombolytic therapy, which is a much safer alternative than embolectomy.

References

1. Anderson JL, Marshall, HW, Bray BE, Lutz JR, Frederick PR, Yanowitz FG, Datz FL, Klausner SC, Hagan AO: A randomized trial of intracoronary streptokinase in the treatment of acute myocardial infarction. N Engl J Med 308:1312, 1983.
2. Aoki N, Moroi M, Matsuda M, Tachiya K: The behavior of α-2-plasmin inhibitor in fibrinolytic states. J Clin Invest 60:361, 1977.
3. Bang NU: Physiology and biochemistry of fibrinolysis. In Bang NU, Beller FK, Deutsh E, Mammen EF (Eds): Thrombosis and Bleeding Disorders. Academic Press, New York, 1971, p 292.
4. Bell WR: Thrombolytic therapy: A comparison between urokinase and streptokinase. Semin Thromb Hemost 2:1, 1975.
5. Bell WR, Meek AG: Guidelines for the use of thrombolytic agents. N Engl J Med 301:1266, 1979.
6. Bick RL: Syndromes associated with hyperfibrino(geno)lysis. In Bick RL (Ed): Disseminated Intravascular Coagulation and Related Syndromes. CRC Press, Boca Raton, FL, 1983, p 105.
7. Bick RL: Clinical implications of molecular markers in hemostasis and thrombosis. Semin Thromb Hemost 10:290, 1984.
8. Bick RL: Basic mechanisms of hemostasis pertaining to DIC. In Bick RL (Ed): Disseminated Intravascular Coagulation and Related Syndromes. CRC Press, Boca Raton, FL, 1983, p 1.
9. Bick RL: Laboratory monitoring of thrombolytic therapy. Summary report of the American Society of Clinical Pathologists. ASCP Press, Chicago, 1984.
10. Bick RL, McClain BJ: A comparison of Dade and DuPont fibrinogen assays in patients with DIC, thromboembolic disease, and during thrombolytic therapy. Am J Clin Pathol 82:372, 1984.
11. Bick RL, Wheeler A, Camposano N: A comparative study of the DuPont antithrombin and fibrinogen assay systems. Am J Clin Pathol 83:541, 1985.
12. Brogden RN, Splight TM, Avery GS: Streptokinase: A review of its clinical pharmacology, mechanisms of action and therapeutic uses. Drugs 5:357, 1973.
13. Chesterman CN, Allington MJ, Sharp A: Relationship of plasminogen activator to fibrin. Nature [N Biol] 238:15, 1972.
14. Christensen LR: Streptococcal fibrinolysis: A proteolytic reaction due to a serum enzyme activated by streptococcal fibrinolysin. J Gen Physiol 28:363, 1945.
15. Common HH, Seaman AJ, Rosch J, Porter JM, Dotter CT: Deep vein thrombosis treated with streptokinase or heparin. Angiology 27:645, 1976.
16. Davidson JF, Samama MM, Desnoyers PC: Progress in Chemical Fibrinolysis and Thrombolysis, vol 1. Raven Press, New York, 1975.
17. DeWood MA, Spores J, Notske MD: Prevalence of total coronary occlusion during early hours of transmural myocardial infarction. N Engl J Med 303:897, 1980.
18. Editorial: Thrombolytic therapy in thrombosis. A National Institute of Health Consensus Development Conference Ann. Intern Med 93:141, 1980.
19. Editorial: Are we using fibrinolytic agents often enough? Ann Intern Med 93:136, 1980.
20. European Cooperative Study Group for Streptokinase Treatment in Acute Myocardial Infarction. N Engl J Med 301:797, 1979.
21. Fratantoni JC, Ness P, Simon TL: Thrombolytic therapy: current status. N Engl J Med 293:1073, 1975.
22. Hirsh J: Dosage regimens for streptokinase

treatment: Evaluation of a standard dosage schedule. Australas Ann Med 19 (Suppl):12, 1970.

23. Johnson AJ, Tillett W: The lysis in rabbits of intravascular blood clots by the streptococcal fibrinolytic system (streptokinase). J Exp Med 95:449, 1952.

24. Johnson AJ, McCarty W: Some aspects of the mechanism of thrombolysis. Thromb Diath Haemorrh 5:391, 1961.

25. Kakkar VV, Flanc C, Howe CT, O'Shea M, Flute PT: Treatment of deep vein thrombosis. A trial of heparin, streptokinase and Arvin. Br Med J 1:806, 1969.

26. Kakkar VV: Results of streptokinase therapy in deep venous thrombosis. Postgrad Med J (Suppl) 49:60, 1973.

27. Khaja F, Walton JA, Brymer JF, Lo E, Osterberger L, O'Neill WW, Colfer HT, Weiss R, Lee T, Kurian T, Goldberg AD, Pitt B, Goldstein S: Intracoronary fibrinolytic therapy in acute myocardial infarction. N Engl J Med 308:1305, 1983.

28. Laffel GL, Braunwald E: Thrombolytic therapy: A new strategy for the treatment of acute myocardial infarction: Part I. N Engl J Med 311:710, 1984.

29. Laffel GL, Braunwald E: Thrombolytic therapy: A new strategy for the treatment of acute myocardial infarction: Part II. N Engl J Med 311:770, 1984.

30. Mammen EF: Thrombolytic therapy. Semin Thromb Hemost 2:1, 1975.

31. Mammen EF: Venous thromboembolism Semin Thromb Hemost 2:203, New York, 1976.

32. Marder VJ, Donahoe JF, Bell WR, Branley JJ, Kwaan HC, Sasahara AA, Barlow GH: Comparison of in vivo biochemical effects of human urokinase prepared from urinary and tissue cultures sources. (Abstr.) Thromb Hemost 38:195, 1977.

33. Markis JE, Malagold M, Parker JA, Silverman KJ, Barry WH, Als AV, Paulin S, Grossman W, Braunwald E: Myocardial salvage after intracoronary thrombolysis with streptokinase in acute myocardial infarction. N Engl J Med 305:777, 1981.

34. Martin M: Systemic streptokinase treatment of arterial occlusions—clinical results. In Streptokinase in Chronic Arterial Disease. CRC Press, Boca Raton, FL, 1982, p 59.

35. McNicol GP: The fibrinolytic system. Postgrad Med J (Supp.) 49:10, 1973.

36. Medical News: Comments on NIH thrombolytic therapy consensus panel. Greater use of fibrinolytic agents urged. JAMA 243:2275, 1980.

37. Murano G, Bick RL: Thrombolytic therapy. In Murano G, Bick RL (Eds): Basic Concepts of Hemostasis and Thrombosis. CRC Press, Boca Raton, FL, 1980, p 259.

38. Murano G: Editorial Comment. Semin Thromb Hemost 9:137, 1983.

39. Paoletti R, Sherry S: Thrombosis and Urokinase. Academic Press, New York, 1977.

40. Robertson BR, Nilsson IM, Nylander G: Thrombolytic effect of streptokinase as evaluated by phlebography of deep venous thrombi of the leg. Acta Chir Scand 134:203, 1968.

41. Sasahara AA, Hyers TM, Cole CM: The urokinase pulmonary embolism trial. Circulation. (Suppl II) 47:1, 1973.

42. Sasahara AA, Bell WR, Simon TL, Stengle JM, Sherry S: The phase II urokinase-streptokinase pulmonary embolism trial. Thromb Diath Haemorrh 3:464, 1975.

43. Seaman AJ, Common HH, Rosch J, Dotter CT, Proter JM, Lindell TD, Lawler WL, Schlueter WJ: Deep vein thrombosis treated with streptokinase or heparin: A randomized study. Angiology 27:549, 1976.

44. Sharma GVRK, Burleson VA, Sasahara AA: Effect of thrombolytic therapy on pulmonary-capillary blood volume in patients with pulmonary embolism. N Engl J Med 303:842, 1980.

45. Sherry S: Streptokinase, urokinase: Do they really work? Mod Med 44:72 (Nov 1), 1976.

46. Slanie J, Ezenhofer V, Karnik R: Local thrombolysis in arterial occlusive disease. Angiology 35:231, 1984.

47. Stampfer MJ, Goldhaber SZ, Yosuf S, Peto R, Hennekens CH: Effect of intravenous streptokinase on acute myocardial infarction. N Engl J Med 307:1180, 1982.

48. Theiss W, Wirtzfeld A, Fink U, Maubach P: The success rate of fibrinolytic therapy in fresh and old thrombosis of the iliac and femoral veins. Angiology 34:61, 1983.

49. Timmis GC, Gangadhran V, Ramos RG, Hauser AM, Westyeer DC, Stewart J, Goodfliesh R, Gordon S: Hemorrhage and the products of fibrinogen digestion after intracoronary administration of streptokinase. Circulation 69:1146, 1984.

50. Tsapogas JM, Peabody RA, Wu KT, Karmody AM, Devaraj KT, Eckert C: Controlled study of thrombolytic therapy in deep vein thrombosis. Surgery 74:973, 1973.

Index